Nutrition-Infection
Interactions and Impacts on
HUMAN
HEALTH

Nutrition-Infection Interactions and Impacts on
HUMAN HEALTH

Edited by
MOHAN PAMMI
JESUS G. VALLEJO
STEVEN A. ABRAMS

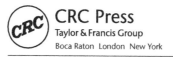

CRC Press
Taylor & Francis Group
Boca Raton London New York

CRC Press is an imprint of the
Taylor & Francis Group, an **informa** business

CRC Press
Taylor & Francis Group
6000 Broken Sound Parkway NW, Suite 300
Boca Raton, FL 33487-2742

First issued in paperback 2016

Version Date: 20140612

ISBN 13: 978-1-138-03376-4 (pbk)
ISBN 13: 978-1-4665-8049-7 (hbk)

Library of Congress Cataloging-in-Publication Data

Nutrition-infection interactions and impacts on human health / editors, Mohan Pammi, Jesus G. Vallejo, Steven A. Abrams.
   p. ; cm.
   Includes bibliographical references and index.
   ISBN 978-1-4665-8049-7
   I. Pammi, Mohan, editor. II. Vallejo, Jesus G., editor. III. Abrams, S. A. (Steven A.) editor.
   [DNLM: 1. Nutritional Physiological Phenomena--immunology. 2. Food. 3. Immunity. 4. Infection. 5. Nutrition Disorders. QU 145]

RM216
613.2--dc23   2014022374

Visit the Taylor & Francis Web site at
http://www.taylorandfrancis.com

and the CRC Press Web site at
http://www.crcpress.com

Contents

Preface ix
Editors xi
Contributors xiii

Chapter 1   Role of Nutrition in Human Health and Disease 1

                 David C. Hilmers and Steven A. Abrams

Chapter 2   Interaction of Nutrition and Immunity 17

                 Ebenezer Satyaraj and John E. Morley

Chapter 3   Micronutrient Deficiency and Immunity 39

                 Sarah E. Cusick and Chandy C. John

Chapter 4   Infection–Nutrition Interaction: Perspectives from the
                 Developing World in Transition 59

                 Noel W. Solomons and Anne-Marie Chomat

Chapter 5   Role of Oxidative Stress and Inflammation in Nutrition–
                 Infection Interactions and the Potential Therapeutic Strategy
                 Using Antioxidants and Modulating Inflammation 81

                 Elena Puertollano and Maria A. Puertollano

Chapter 6   Nutrient–Drug Interactions 107

                 Kathleen M. Gura

Chapter 7   HIV and Micronutrient Supplementation 153

                 Elaine A. Yu, Julia L. Finkelstein, and Saurabh Mehta

Chapter 8   Tuberculosis and Human Nutrition 179

                 Kee Thai Yeo and Anna Mandalakas

Chapter 9   Impact of Malaria and Parasitic Infections on Human Nutrition 221

                 Athis Rajh Arunachalam, Vedanta S. Dariya, and Celia Holland

Chapter 10 Gut Microbiome in the Nutrition–Infection Interaction: A Focus
on Malnourished Children 247

Dorottya Nagy-Szakal, Richard Kellermayer, and Sanjiv Harpavat

Chapter 11 Enteric Syndromes Leading to Malnutrition and Infections............257

Vi Lier Goh and Praveen S. Goday

Chapter 12 Relationship of Probiotics, Prebiotics, Synbiotics to Infections,
Immunity, and Nutrition...287

Diomel de la Cruz and Josef Neu

Chapter 13 Immunonutrients and Evidence for Their Use in Hospitalized
Adults Receiving Artificial Nutrition...309

Philip C. Calder

Chapter 14 Impact of Infection–Nutrient Interactions in Infants, Children,
and Adolescents..333

Renán A. Orellana and Jorge A. Coss-Bu

Chapter 15 Aging and Effects of Nutrient–Infection Interactions.....................357

Sung Nim Han

Chapter 16 Future Strategies and Research Directions in Nutrition–
Infection Interactions That Will Enhance Human Health 377

Mohan Pammi, Jesus G. Vallejo, and Steven A. Abrams

Index..391

Preface

Our intention is to summarize the current state-of-the-art evidence on nutrition–infection interactions and its impact on health and disease, including state-of-the-art clinical and basic science research.

Nutrition and infection are often at cross-roads interacting with each other, influencing human health in a way that has implications for both the developed and developing world. Infectious morbidity is huge in the malnourished, both in the deficient and excess nutritional states. Infections, both systemic and gastrointestinal, significantly affect enteral nutrition and absorption. A book that describes nutrition–infection interactions is not only extremely useful but also essential for health-care staff, nutritionists, and epidemiologists. We strongly believe that such a book will not only improve care of patients in health-care facilities but also the health of the vulnerable population.

The book's first chapter explores the role of nutrition in health and disease, especially the effects of malnutrition, both undernutrition and overnutrition. We then describe the relation between malnutrition and immunity followed by a chapter exploring micronutrient deficiency and immunity. The concept of nutrition–infection interaction pertaining to the developing world in transition is introduced. The final common pathway for many human diseases may be unbalanced inflammation and oxidant injury. A chapter discussing the role of oxidant stress and therapy with antioxidants explores the inflammation concept. An interesting link in nutrition–infection interactions is how nutrients and drugs interact, both anti-infective drugs and others. Nutrient–drug interactions are extensively reviewed in Chapter 6. We devote the next few chapters to nutrient–infection interactions in specific infections. We discuss the interactions in human immunodeficiency virus, tuberculosis, malaria, and parasitic infections, with special emphasis on nutritional interventions. The role of the gastrointestinal tract and its influence on nutrition, focusing on the human gastrointestinal microbiota and enteric syndromes, are presented next. The human gastrointestinal microbiome is essential in the maturation of immune responses and prevention of pathogen colonization, both of which influence infectious risk. The pattern of gastrointestinal microbiota is altered by the dietary intake and conversely alters dietary components, which in turn affect nutrient absorption and immune responses. Modifying indigenous microbiota for health benefits is discussed in the chapter on probiotics and prebiotics. Current research lays emphasis on immunonutrients that can enhance immunity and prevent infections, and a chapter that discusses immunonutrients has been included. We also discuss infection–nutrition interactions in special age groups: children, adolescents, and the elderly. We close the book with a review on nutritional and anti-infective strategies emerging from the horizon and identify future research directions.

The chapters are penned by outstanding, internationally reputable authors who have published significantly in their field. We have kept in mind the broad audience to this book and hence tailored to enhance the book's applicability to both the developed and the developing world. We sincerely hope that we have conveyed our perspective on nutrition–infection interactions to everyone's benefit.

Mohan Pammi
Jesus G. Vallejo
Steven A. Abrams

Editors

Mohan Pammi, MD, PhD, MBBS, MRCPCH, is an assistant professor in the Section of Neonatology, Department of Pediatrics at Texas Children's Hospital and Baylor College of Medicine, Houston, Texas, United States. He has significant interest in nutrition–infection interactions and immunonutrients such as lactoferrin and probiotics. He has published basic science and translational science articles on lactoferrin. His research laboratory is focused on *Staphylococcus* and *Candida* infections and in novel strategies in preventing and treating these infections. He has extensive experience in conducting systematic reviews for the Cochrane Collaboration and is interested in dissemination of evidence-based medicine.

Jesus Vallejo, MD, is a professor in the Section of Pediatric Infectious Diseases, Department of Pediatrics at Baylor College of Medicine and Texas Children's Hospital, Houston, United States. He is a nationally renowned infectious disease specialist, and the focus of his research is on the role of innate immunity in infections, specifically viral myocarditis.

Steven A. Abrams, MD, is a professor at the US Department of Agriculture/ Agricultural Research Service Children's Nutrition Research Center and Section of Neonatology, Department of Pediatrics at Texas Children's Hospital, Baylor College of Medicine, Houston, Texas, United States. He is an internationally known neonatologist and nutrition expert, and collaborates with other researchers in Latin America, the Middle East, and India. Dr. Abrams has authored numerous publications and is a member of the Committee on Nutrition of the American Academy of Pediatrics and has served on multiple Institute of Medicine committees.

Contributors

Steven A. Abrams
Department of Pediatrics
Baylor College of Medicine
Houston, Texas

Athis Rajh Arunachalam
Department of Pediatrics
Baylor College of Medicine
Houston, Texas

Philip C. Calder
Faculty of Medicine
University of Southampton
Southampton General Hospital
Southampton, United Kingdom

Anne-Marie Chomat
Center for Studies of Sensory
  Impairment, Aging and Metabolism
  (CeSSIAM)
Guatemala City, Guatemala

Jorge A. Coss-Bu
Department of Pediatrics–Critical Care
Baylor College of Medicine
Houston, Texas

Sarah E. Cusick
Division of Global Pediatrics
University of Minnesota
Minneapolis, Minnesota

Vedanta S. Dariya
Department of Pediatrics
Baylor College of Medicine
Houston, Texas

Diomel de la Cruz
Department of Pediatrics
University of Florida-Shands Hospital
  for Children
Gainesville, Florida

Julia L. Finkelstein
Division of Nutritional Sciences
Cornell University
Ithaca, New York

Praveen S. Goday
Department of Pediatric
  Gastroenterology and Nutrition
Medical College of Wisconsin
Milwaukee, Wisconsin

Vi Lier Goh
Department of Pediatric
  Gastroenterology and Nutrition
Boston University
Boston, Massachusetts

Kathleen M. Gura
Clinical Pharmacist GI/Nutrition Team
  Leader, Surgical Programs
Boston Children's Hospital
Boston, Massachusetts

Sung Nim Han
Department of Food and Nutrition
College of Human Ecology
Seoul National University
Seoul, Korea

Sanjiv Harpavat
Department of Pediatrics–
  Gastroenterology
Baylor College of Medicine
Houston, Texas

David C. Hilmers
Department of Pediatrics
Baylor College of Medicine
Houston, Texas

Celia Holland
Department of Zoology
School of Natural Sciences
Trinity College
Dublin, Ireland

Chandy C. John
Division of Global Pediatrics
University of Minnesota
Minneapolis, Minnesota

Richard Kellermeyer
Department of
    Pediatrics–Gastroenterology
Baylor College of Medicine
Houston, Texas

Anna Mandalakas
Department of Pediatric Medicine,
    Retrovirology and Global Health
Baylor International Pediatric AIDS
    Initiative
and
Childhood TB Initiative
Global Tuberculosis and
    Mycobacteriology Program
Baylor College of Medicine
Texas Children's Hospital
Houston, Texas

Saurabh Mehta
Division of Nutritional Sciences
Cornell University
Ithaca, New York

John E. Morley
Department of Internal Medicine
Saint Louis University School of
    Medicine
St. Louis, Missouri

Dorottya Nagy-Szakal
Department of Pediatrics–
    Gastroenterology
Baylor College of Medicine
Houston, Texas

Josef Neu
Department of Pediatrics
University of Florida-Shands Hospital
    for Children
Gainesville, Florida

Renán Orellana
Department of Pediatrics–Critical Care
Baylor College of Medicine
Houston, Texas

Mohan Pammi
Department of Pediatric
    Medicine—Neonatology
Baylor College of Medicine
Houston, Texas

Elena Puertollano
Department of Food and Nutritional
    Sciences
The University of Reading
Reading, United Kingdom

Maria A. Puertollano
Department of Health Sciences
Faculty of Experimental Sciences
University of Jaén
Jaén, Spain

Ebenezer Satyaraj
Nutritional Immunology
NRC-St. Louis, Petcare Basic Research
St. Louis, Missouri

Noel W. Solomons
Center for Studies of Sensory
    Impairment, Aging and Metabolism
    (CeSSIAM)
Guatemala City, Guatemala

Jesus G. Vallejo
Department of Pediatrics–Infectious
    Disease
Baylor College of Medicine
Houston, Texas

Kee Thai Yeo
Rainbow Babies and Children's
    Hospital
Cleveland, Ohio

Elaine A. Yu
Division of Nutritional Sciences
Cornell University
Ithaca, New York

1 Role of Nutrition in Human Health and Disease

David C. Hilmers and Steven A. Abrams

CONTENTS

Introduction...1
Definitions of Malnutrition 2
Fetal Health...3
Early Infancy...4
Nutrition in Ages 1–5, the Critical Years 4
    New Concepts Relating Infectious Diseases to Severe Malnutrition,
    Use of Antibiotics 6
    Malaria and Iron Supplementation...7
School-Age Children 7
    Hidden Hunger...8
Adolescence 8
Pregnancy..9
Adults.. 11
Geriatrics... 11
References.. 13

INTRODUCTION

Adequate nutrition is the key to health through all stages of life. It is the fuel that powers each of the cellular mechanisms that allow us to exist in a functional state of good health. Imbalances, surfeits, or deficiencies in macronutrients (protein, carbohydrates, fats) or micronutrients (iron, zinc, vitamins, etc.) can lead to pathologic derangements and death. This is true through all stages of life, whether as an embryo or as an aging adult. Malnutrition often begins *in utero* and its effects can persist through a lifetime, causing chronic disease, suboptimal quality of life, and enormous costs to society. Malnutrition in women of childbearing age can result in intrauterine growth retardation (IUGR) and low-birth-weight infants. This cycle can persist through generations without appropriate intervention.

One of the Millennium Development Goals is to reduce by 50% the proportion of individuals who are affected by malnutrition and hunger from the prevalence seen in 1990.[1] While there has been some success in children <5 years of age with a reduction in the prevalence of underweight children in developing countries from 29% in 1990 to 18% in 2010, the improvements have not been uniform throughout all regions. Because of population increases, the number of children who are malnourished has scarcely changed. The world's population is projected to reach 9 billion in 2050, and the means by which to continue these improvements in global nutritional status without irreparable ecologic harm remains problematic.[2]

This chapter will serve as an introduction to later sections of the book, and while it does not intend to encompass the entire spectrum of the effects of nutrition on health, it will focus on key nutritional issues related to the major phases of the life cycle and inform the reader about selected recent advances and controversies.

DEFINITIONS OF MALNUTRITION

Malnutrition generally describes the imbalance between the supply of nutrients that are delivered and the demand for nutrients to supply all the functions required for growth, development, and maintenance.[3] As this is particularly important in

TABLE 1.1
Definitions of Malnutrition

Classification	Definition	Grading	
Gomez	Weight below % median weight for age (WFA)	Mild (grade 1)	75%–90% WFA
		Moderate (grade 2)	60%–74% WFA
		Severe (grade 3)	<60% WFA
Waterlow	z-Scores (SD) below median weight for height (WFH)	Mild	80%–90% WFH
		Moderate	70%–80% WFH
		Severe	<70% WFH
WHO (wasting)	z-Scores (SD) below median WFH	Moderate	$-3\% \le z\text{-Score} < -2$
		Severe	$z\text{-Score} < -3$
WHO (stunting)	z-Scores (SD) below median height for age (HFA)	Moderate	$-3\% \le z\text{-Score} < -2$
		Severe	$z\text{-Score} < -3$
Adult classification	BMI (weight/height^2)	Obese	>30.0
		Overweight	25–30
		Normal	20–25
		Marginal	18.5–20
		Mild	17–18.5
		Moderate	16–17
		Severe	<16
Mean upper arm circumference	Mid upper arm circumference in inches	Normal	Males >23
			Females >22
		Malnourished	Males <23
			Females <22

Source: Adapted from http://www.medicalcriteria.com/site/index.php?option=com_content&view=article&id=275%3Amalnutrition&catid=66%3Anutrition&Itemid=80&lang=en. Accessed May 15, 2013.

the stages of development through which an individual passes, a number of classifications have been made to categorize and define the grades of malnutrition (see Table 1.1). The Gomez classification is a weight-based system using a percentage of the median weight for age to grade the degree of malnutrition (mild, moderate, severe). This is called "underweight." The Waterlow classification uses weight-for-height z-scores (standard deviation) below the median for age, again based on a percentage. Low percentages on this scale are also called "wasting." The World Health Organization (WHO) uses the same criteria for wasting but bases their definition of moderate and severe wasting on the z-score. Stunting is measured by the height-for-age z-score and under the WHO classification is "severe" when <-3 and moderate when between -2 and -3. There are other means of evaluating malnutrition, such as mean upper arm circumference (MUAC) and body mass index (BMI), which is weight divided by the height squared. The latter definition is being increasingly used in children, particularly in monitoring trends in obesity, but has been traditionally most commonly applied to adults.[4–7]

Classically, "mild" malnutrition has been defined as between -1 and -2 standard deviations ("z-score") below the median measurement. "Moderate" malnutrition is defined as between -2 and -3 z-score and "severe" malnutrition as below -3 z-score. These terms will be used throughout this book when used to describe the epidemiology and severity of malnutrition.

FETAL HEALTH

IUGR refers to the lack of proper increase in weight and length of the fetus *in utero*. In developing countries, the most common cause is malnutrition, leading to either stunting or underweight in the mother or lack of appropriate weight gain during pregnancy. Infectious diseases such as diarrhea, respiratory illnesses, malaria (particularly with placental involvement), and human immunodeficiency virus/acquired immunodeficiency syndrome (HIV/AIDS) are important causes of IUGR. Iron deficiency during pregnancy certainly plays a large role as well, whether due to menorrhagia, parasitosis, or inadequate intake of bioavailable iron. In industrialized countries, smoking is one of the most important causes of IUGR along with inadequate weight gain during pregnancy and low maternal weight. Tobacco use is also an emerging problem in mothers in developing countries in recent years.

Although much attention has been placed on macronutrient delivery, there is increasing concern about the role of inadequate fetal micronutrient status and short- and long-term consequences of this deficiency. In particular, there is concern about bone health and immunological health related to poor newborn status of calcium and vitamin D. Neonatal hypocalcemia, rickets, and long-term health risks may be associated with poor calcium and vitamin D status in the neonatal period related to poor fetal health and delivery of IUGR infants. Controversy exists over the specific role of poor vitamin D status at birth on short- and long-term health; however, some studies link this to conditions including pulmonary and allergic disease, as well as long-term bone health. Much more research is needed to understand these relations and the possibility of a further link to other conditions, including diabetes or infectious diseases.[8–10]

EARLY INFANCY

It is universally accepted that prenatal nutrition and early childhood nutrition are key to long-term health and development. An essential element in enhancing health is supporting breast-feeding throughout at least the first year of life and further encouraging the introduction of age-appropriate solid foods. There are few contraindications to breast-feeding, and these are extensively discussed in the literature. However, it is not these contraindications that are responsible for most infants not receiving breast milk during the first year of life. Rather, it is the complex social structure of families and societies and ready availability of breast milk alternatives that lead to most failure to start or to early cessation of breast-feeding. The global introduction of the Baby Friendly Hospital Initiative has been critical throughout both developed and emerging market countries in supporting and enhancing breast-feeding. This initiative is an effort by the United Nations Children Fund and WHO to ensure that hospital maternities become centers of breast-feeding support. A maternity facility can be designated "baby-friendly" when it does not accept free or low-cost samples of breast milk substitutes, feeding bottles, or nipples, and has implemented specific steps to support successful breast-feeding.[11] However, this mostly affects the introduction of breast-feeding, not the early weaning that is common. A compelling volume of data demonstrate the importance of breast-feeding in lower-income locations in decreasing the severity, including deaths, from diarrhea and other infectious conditions.[12–14]

A second key issue is the introduction and timing of the introduction of solid foods. The WHO and many other international groups recommend exclusive breast-feeding for the first 6 months of life. Some controversy exists about whether slightly earlier introduction, especially of iron-fortified foods, should be considered not sooner than 4 months of age. Recent studies support the early use of meat products when culturally appropriate to provide heme iron to infants in the second 6 months of life. In many cultures, the use of inappropriate weaning foods, such as coffee, may be harmful to nutrition and development.[15]

When infant formula is provided, it is important to ensure that it is provided as safely as possible. Risks of contamination, especially with powder forms of formula, in early life exist, particularly in developing countries where a safe supply of water cannot be ensured. Other risks include the possibility of errors, intentional or accidental, in diluting formula. Although advocacy for breast-feeding is crucial, the common use of infant formulas should not be ignored, and health advocacy for safely preparing and providing infant formulas is important.

NUTRITION IN AGES 1–5, THE CRITICAL YEARS

It is well documented that undernutrition in the first years of life can have profound effects on productivity; development of chronic diseases such as diabetes, coronary/cerebral vascular disease, hypertension, and dyslipidemias; and quality of life in later years. In nations with high rates of undernutrition, particularly in women of childbearing age and in children, this can result in substantial economic and societal costs, including decreases in gross domestic product and increased health-care expenditures for chronic diseases. Studies show that suboptimal growth due to poor nutrition *in utero* and in the first 2 years of life can cause irreparable problems with academic performance, economic status, and short stature, and that poor women with undernutrition as children are more likely to bear offspring with low birth weight. Therefore, it can be concluded that national health policies that address the issue of childhood and maternal undernutrition are extremely cost-effective.[16]

The critical period for growth is in the first 2 years of life when growth faltering can result in stunting and underweight. It is during this time that poor nutrition, including lack of protein, caloric intake, and micronutrients such as iron, zinc, vitamin A, and iodine, can have a profound effect on future growth and the ability to recover from infections such as diarrhea and pneumonia.[17]

Rates of stunting and underweight in children remain high in developing countries, with improvements seen in some countries, notably China. In South and Central America and the Caribbean, rates of stunting are nearly four times higher than the rates of underweight. On the other hand, in other developing countries worldwide, stunting is only one to two times as common and the rates tend to change in parallel with one another as do rates of improvement. Lack of progress is often a result of natural phenomena (droughts, natural disasters), man-made events (war and large-scale refugee displacement), and disease (HIV/AIDS). Progress seems to occur where there are improving socioeconomic conditions, the absence of warfare, and stable governments that invest wisely in the health of their people through expansion of health-care systems and nutritional programs.[18]

Low-birth-weight rates are falling in the developing world, although slowly. Rates are low and stable in developing countries in the Western Hemisphere. The rates are highest in South Asia with a drop over the past 20 years from 34% to 27%. Overall, the incidence of low birth weight in Asia is now 18%. Improvement in maternal nutrition is likely to be among the most beneficial interventions to reduce the prevalence of low birth weight, as there appears to be a correlation between improvements in prepregnancy maternal weights and lower rates of low birth weight. Ameliorating rates of iron deficiency could have similar benefits. Thus, prioritizing nutrition in this age group can benefit not only the current but also future generations.[18]

Anemia continues to be a major cause of morbidity and mortality, and the most common cause in both the developed and developing world is iron deficiency. In nonpregnant women, the rates of anemia continue to hover around 45% in Africa and Asia, and are even higher in pregnant females. In children, prevalences of >60% have been seen in some regions of Africa. The cost of anemia in terms of time lost from work, reduced productivity, and poor cognitive development is enormous. There is a close relation between anemia and infectious diseases, including malaria, tuberculosis, HIV, and parasitosis. Despite improvements in controlling these infectious diseases and the implementation of programs to supplement iron, fortify foods, and diversify diets, there has been little change seen in the rates of iron deficiency and anemia. This must be one of the highest-priority challenges in nutrition for policy-making bodies.[18]

Recent statistics show that despite supplementation campaigns and programs to combine vitamin A with immunizations, vitamin A deficiency continues to be highly prevalent in developing countries in children and in women of childbearing age. In Southern Asia and Central and West Africa, >40% of children are deficient. This is a leading cause of blindness in those affected and also can cause reduced resistance to infectious diseases, particularly measles. A series of studies have shown that vitamin A supplementation programs that are often combined with immunization campaigns in children between the ages of 6 months and 5 years can decrease all-cause mortality by about 23%–24%. The mechanism by which such dramatic results are achieved is not clear. Yet, at a cost of pennies per dose, this represents one of the most cost-effective programs to reduce childhood morbidity and mortality and is implemented in about 70 countries worldwide. There have been mixed results in the use of this strategy in children <6 months of age, and there is no sufficient data to recommend vitamin A supplementation in infants in this group.[19,20]

Progress is being made to reduce the rates of iodine deficiency. Iodine deficiency can lead to hypothyroidism, which, if left untreated, can result in permanent intellectual deficit and growth retardation. It has been shown that in areas where iodination of salt is increasing, the rates of goiter are decreasing. In countries where iodination is widely used, the rates of goiter have decreased from 12.0% to 10.5%.[2]

In addition to malnutrition caused by inadequate intake and absorption of micronutrients, it can also be caused by derangements in body function caused by limited intake of macronutrients. The latter has also been classically named "protein–energy malnutrition" (PEM). Within this broad category, there is edematous PEM or "kwashiorkor," nonedematous or "marasmus," and a condition with features of both or "mixed." Marasmus is associated with low caloric intake and the resulting consequences of prolonged inadequate energy consumption. There has been a great deal of investigation into the origin and pathophysiology of kwashiorkor; however, as yet, there is no single mechanism that explains all of its features. It seems to be more common in wet climates and often occurs after illnesses and natural disasters.

There has been increasing use of ready-to-use foods with long shelf lives in the treatment and prevention of malnutrition. They can be used at home and do not require water, which reduces the risk of bacterial contamination. The first products to be produced were ready-to-use therapeutic foods (RUTF) with very dense caloric content, intended for use in cases of severe malnutrition. A number of studies have shown their efficacy in the treatment of this condition.[21–23] Recently, lower-energy dense products called ready-to-use supplemental foods have been designed to treat or prevent moderate malnutrition. These foods usually contain peanuts or other high-fat-containing, locally grown products as the main substrate, as well as a slurry of micronutrients, milk powders, and other ingredients.[24,25]

New Concepts Relating Infectious Diseases to Severe Malnutrition, Use of Antibiotics

The use of lipid-based formulas for treating childhood malnutrition has allowed many children with uncomplicated acute severe malnutrition (height-for-weight z-score of <−3.0) to receive therapy as outpatients. The RUTFs have improved outcomes and have freed inpatient beds to care for more severe cases requiring hospitalization. However, despite these incremental improvements, 10%–15% of children still do not recover. There has been discussion about whether the routine use of antibiotics in treatment of all cases of uncomplicated acute severe malnutrition is warranted or not, even in those not displaying systemic signs of infection or with good appetites. To address this question, a randomized trial was performed in Malawi in which 2767 children were assigned to either placebo or one of two antibiotics (cefdinir or amoxicillin), both of which cost less than $10 for the course of treatment. Both the risks of treatment failure and mortality were lower in the two groups receiving antibiotics than in those receiving placebo. The mortality rates were 35.6% lower in the amoxicillin group and 44.3% lower in the cefdinir cohort. The authors felt that these antibiotics are probably effective in lowering infections caused by translocation of bacteria across compromised intestinal mucosal barriers in malnourished children.[26]

MALARIA AND IRON SUPPLEMENTATION

There continues to be controversy over the use of iron supplementation in children and pregnant women in malaria endemic areas. While chronic iron deficiency can have severe developmental, physical, and cognitive consequences, it may also decrease the susceptibility to infections such as malaria. However, it is also known that anemia is the cause of increased morbidity and mortality during acute episodes of malaria and placental malarial infections can have an impact on the birth weight and survival of fetuses. A cross-sectional study in central Sudan looked at the relation between anemia and placental malaria. It showed that there was a strong protective effect (odds ratio 0.2, confidence interval [CI] 0.1–0.6) against placental malaria by the presence of anemia.[27]

A prospective study with 727 preschool children in Malawi showed a lower incidence of malaria parasitemia and clinical malaria in children with iron deficiency at baseline during a year of follow-up (hazard ratio [HR] 0.55 [CI 0.41–0.74] and HR 0.49 [CI 0.33–0.73], respectively). The authors conclude that iron deficiency is protective against malaria in young children and that general use of iron supplementation must be implemented with caution and with careful preventive measures against malaria.[28]

A Cochrane systematic review from June 2011 using 71 trials in >45,000 children completed up to that time came to the conclusion that iron alone or with antimalarial treatment does not increase the risk of malarial episodes or mortality when usual malaria surveillance and treatment is provided. This was similar in groups with anemia or with normal hemoglobin. They noted that iron treatment for anemia resulted in a higher risk for clinical cases of malaria only in trials in areas where malaria surveillance and treatment was not routinely performed. Furthermore, it was noted that iron supplementation during acute attacks did not result in treatment failure. They conclude that iron supplementation alone or with antimalarial treatment does not increase the risk of cases of malaria when malaria surveillance and treatment are performed.[29]

SCHOOL-AGE CHILDREN

From age 5 to 9 years, children usually experience slow but steady growth before the spurt that occurs during adolescence. Evidence seems to indicate that catch-up growth is unlikely for those who were stunted at 2 years of age and even less likely if they consume nutritionally deficient diets, are exposed to infectious diseases, or experience lack of sanitation and clean water. Anemia continues to be highly prevalent during this period, and chronic iron deficiency often affects their school performance and growth.

Programs that have shown success in improving academic achievement include school feeding programs. Other initiatives that have been tested in this population for use in schools include diet diversification, micronutrient-fortified beverages, dual fortification of salt with iodine and iron, staple food fortification, and school-based supplementation programs.[30–32]

HIDDEN HUNGER

The term "hidden hunger" has been used recently to refer to micronutrient deficiencies caused by the use of energy-dense, nutritionally poor foods. This is often seen in developing countries where affordable, nutritious foods are unavailable either for reasons of poor distribution systems or high cost. However, this phenomenon is being seen in developed countries where children and adolescents consume large amounts of high-calorie soft drinks or juices and fast foods. This situation can develop during periods of economic downturns or in the presence of so-called food deserts, primarily in inner cities, where fast-food outlets and convenience stores abound with a corresponding paucity of supermarkets and poor access to fresh produce. Neighborhood violence and increasing time spent indoors watching television or using electronic gadgets can lead to sedentary lifestyles and lack of exposure to sunlight leading to vitamin D deficiency. Either overt micronutrient deficiencies, which are more likely found in developing countries, or more subtle deficiencies, common in industrialized regions, can have significant neurocognitive and growth consequences. Supplementation can overcome specific deficiency states; however, ensuring a reliable supply and distribution of tablets can be problematic in remote areas and in developing countries. Other means of improving micronutrient intake are discussed elsewhere in this chapter. In developed nations, some authors have expressed concern about oversupplementation, particularly in children whose parents already are feeding their offspring an adequate diet. Studies have shown that minority children, who are at highest risk for developing micronutrient deficiencies from hidden hunger, are the least likely to be taking supplements. National Health and Nutrition Examination Survey (NHANES) data from 2003 to 2006 showed that even with the use of supplements, more than one-third of US children 2–18 years old did not have adequate calcium and vitamin D intake.[33–35]

ADOLESCENCE

During adolescence and puberty, individuals experience some of the most profound physiological and behavioral changes in their lives. There are many physiologic, hormonal, growth, and lifestyle changes that occur during adolescence that make optimal nutritional status during this period critical to adult well-being and productivity. This is a period of rapid growth with nearly 50% of adult weight obtained during puberty and 20% of final adult height. There are significant changes in body shape and composition with marked changes in proportions of fat, muscle, body water, and bone density in both sexes. Growth hormone, gonadal releasing factors, and hormones play a crucial role in the formation of these changes leading from childhood to adulthood. As a result, proper nutrition is critical.[36]

Undernutrition appears to delay the onset of menarche. Better-nourished females appear to have an earlier and more rapid growth spurt; however, undernourished females tend to start their spurt later, which subsequently lasts longer. These patterns appear to be equivalent in terms of effects on final adult height. However, the undernourished female is more likely to become pregnant while still in her growth phase. This results in smaller birth weights due to competition between the fetus for nutrients necessary for growth of both the mother and child.[37]

An example of the nutritional problems associated with adolescence, anorexia nervosa, is not due to lack of access to adequate food intake but to poor inappropriate body image and fear of gaining weight. More frequently diagnosed in developed countries, it has one of the highest mortality rates of any mental illness. While it can occur in any age group and in any socioeconomic class, it appears to be most common in 9–12-year-old females, often of middle or upper class strata, although it can persist throughout life. It is felt that the pressures of adolescence, the desire for perfection, and changing norms of beauty prominently displayed in the media may play key roles in its pathogenesis. Recent studies show that although ghrelin levels, a hormone inducing appetite, are normal or elevated in patients with anorexia nervosa, intravenous infusion of ghrelin can have a small, but positive, effect on caloric intake. Several other novel strategies for improving outcomes include zinc supplementation, Marinol (a synthetic form of the active ingredient in marijuana), and n-3 fatty acids.[38–40]

Another alarming trend is the increased rates of obesity in adolescents, mostly in developed countries but now increasingly prevalent in developing nations. Data from the 2009–2010 NHANES showed that 18.4% of US adolescents are obese, using the criteria for obesity of ≥95%ile of the age- and sex-specific growth charts.[41]

The burden of disease worldwide secondary to obesity continues to increase. Estimates using trend data indicate that the number of obese individuals now has passed 2 billion. Certain fat patterns, particularly truncal obesity, are thought to have greater implications for chronic disease. These patterns are more prevalent in populations in Latin America, Southern Asia, the Middle East, and parts of Africa. Owing to the enormous expense involved in the implementation of strategies to prevent and treat the complications of obesity, many countries cannot afford to address the explosion of diabetes, hypertension, and hyperlipidemia (metabolic syndrome) that will inevitably result.[42]

PREGNANCY

Iron supplementation with or without folic acid has long been shown to improve iron stores and to prevent anemia in pregnant women. Low hemoglobin levels are known to affect birth weight and fetal outcomes. Researchers examined the Cochrane Pregnancy and Childbirth Group's Trials Register and ongoing trials and looked at the outcomes with oral supplements, which either contained iron or did not, during pregnancy. The risk of low-birth-weight infants (<2500 g), maternal anemia, and iron deficiency were lower in the iron-supplemented women. Mean birth weights and hemoglobin levels were significantly greater, and there was no evidence of an increase of risk of placental malaria in malaria-endemic areas. Side effects were marginally higher in the iron-supplemented groups, and there was increased risk of hemoglobin concentrations >130 g/L during pregnancy. The researchers concluded that iron supplementation is effective in preventing the adverse consequences of iron deficiency but side effects and the higher risk of greater than desired hemoglobin levels indicate a need to examine dosing requirements more closely.[43]

It is known that multiple vitamin and mineral deficiencies can coexist in pregnant women because of increased demands by the fetus. It would seem logical that multiple-micronutrient supplementation would be at least as effective as iron or an iron–folate combination alone. Twenty-three trials involving >75,000 women were examined in a recent Cochrane Database review. The researchers found that there was a statistically significant decrease in the number of low-birth-weight and small-for-gestational-age newborns in the multiple-micronutrient supplementation group as compared with the iron–folate groups. However, there was no difference in other outcomes such as preterm birth, miscarriage, and maternal or neonatal mortality. There were insufficient data to examine other important outcomes such as neural tube defects, neurodevelopmental outcomes, side effects, and relative costs. The authors conclude that there seems to be a beneficial impact on the important parameters of low birth weight and small for gestational age, but more studies are needed to assess the proper dosages and regional differences in maternal and birth outcomes.[44]

Folic acid supplementation during pregnancy and in women of childbearing age has been encouraged to reduce the risk of neural tube defects and appears to have contributed to an decrease in the incidence of this devastating condition.[45] A recent Cochrane systematic review looked at 31 trials involving 17,771 women. The researchers concluded that there was no impact on the risk of preterm birth, stillbirths or neonatal deaths, predelivery anemia, and hemoglobin or folate levels. However, there was an improvement in mean birth weight and the incidence of megaloblastic anemia.[46]

Another recent Cochrane review examined outcomes in pregnant women taking either daily iron + folate or intermittent (one to three times weekly) supplements. The motivation for this review was that while supplementation is important during pregnancy in iron-deficient women, noncompliance, side effects such as nausea or constipation, and a tenuous supply chain can make daily supplementation problematic in low-resource areas with high rates of anemia. The authors conclude that the quality of the evidence is limited, but intermittent regimens appear to give similar maternal and infant outcomes but have fewer side effects.[47]

Other researchers have examined the evidence for vitamin D supplementation during pregnancy. The trials seem to indicate that pregnant women taking supplements have higher levels of vitamin D at term, as measured by levels of 25-hydroxyvitamin D. There appeared to be a marginally significant improvement in the risk of low-birth-weight babies; however, the authors suggest that more rigorous trials are needed to determine the effect of vitamin D supplementation on birth outcomes and maternal/child safety.[48]

ADULTS

The most productive years of persons in any population are during adulthood, roughly at age 18–65 years. Malnutrition, either in the form of overnutrition or undernutrition, can have significant social and economic impacts on a nation. BMI (weight/height^2) is an imperfect measure but has been traditionally used to determine relative levels of overweight or underweight. Underweight can be mild (BMI 17.0–18.49), moderate (BMI 16.0–16.99), or severe (<16.0). Likewise, overweight can be mild (BMI 25.0–29.99), moderate (BMI 30.0–39.99), or severe (BMI >40.0). Evidence shows that there is a U-shaped curve for mortality/morbidity, with the lowest levels for normal and mildly obese adults and increasing rates above a BMI of 30.0 and below 18.5. Productivity also generally decreases with either underweight or overweight as work capacity declines. A dramatic shift has been seen recently, with areas predominately showing undernutrition previously now have higher rates of overweight than underweight. This includes some parts of North Africa, the Middle East, and Latin America. Part of this shift has come from the greater availability of high-calorie foods with low nutritional value and the sedentary lifestyles that have become the norm in a highly interconnected world.[49]

Increasingly, underweight has been associated with chronic conditions such as malabsorption (Crohn's disease, ulcerative colitis), infectious diseases such as HIV/AIDS and tuberculosis, and cancer. A person with diseases such as these enters a vicious cycle wherein anorexia causes decreased intake, and the increased metabolic demands caused by the disease process further reduce dwindling body reserves and the ability of the immune system to fight the effects of the disease. Obesity has caused an epidemic of diabetes, hyperlipidemia, and hypertension, the so-called metabolic syndrome. When left unchecked, these conditions can lead to congestive heart failure, coronary and cerebrovascular disease, blindness, chronic renal failure, diabetic ulcers, and a host of related conditions. By far, the major causes of end-stage renal disease (ESRD) in the United States are hypertension and diabetes, and the cost of ESRD reached \$42.5 billion in 2009 and continues to climb as more individuals qualify for dialysis each year.[50]

GERIATRICS

Malnutrition is increasingly being recognized as a cause of morbidity among the elderly. In industrialized countries, the average age of populations has increased as life expectancy increases. It is expected that the percentage of adults >65 years old in Japan will reach 25% by 2020. Body weight and muscle mass appear to decrease after age 60, with a typical loss of weight of >5%. Whereas in younger adults, mortality appears to increase with BMI <18.5, this relation appears to start at a BMI of 22–23 in the elderly.[51]

In a recent prospective cohort study in France, malnutrition was found to be the strongest predictor of short-term mortality in the elderly visiting the emergency department. Cross-sectional studies have shown that PEM in the elderly is highly predictive of mortality, whether the individual is institutionalized or living in the community. In addition, the risk of hip fracture resulting from falls also increases with worsening hypovitaminosis D, as this condition negatively affects bone health. Lower levels of 25-hydroxyvitamin D in the elderly are often the result of decreased outdoor activity and decreased sunlight exposure. Studies have shown that fall rates themselves increase as vitamin D levels decline in the elderly. There is a wide range of observational data that support the critical role of vitamin D in the elderly; however, the mechanism and exact role remains controversial. It has been suggested that vitamin D is implicated in higher rates of coronary artery disease, cancer, myopathy, muscle strength, functional limitation, global cognitive decline, and disability.[51–56]

There are a number of factors that can lead to malnutrition in the elderly, even in developed countries. These include loss of loved ones and support networks and physical debility, resulting in the inability to obtain nutritious foods. The elderly can "outlive" their retirement funds, leaving them with a limited budget to maintain a healthy diet. Depression, dementia, and even mild cognitive impairment often make it difficult to make wise food choices. Loss of loved ones may lead to anorexia. Debility resulting from chronic conditions such as cardiovascular or cerebrovascular, endocrine, renal, or neoplastic diseases may cause impairments in physical condition or increased nutrient requirements. Long lists of prescribed medications for chronic medical conditions may depress appetite or interfere with gastrointestinal tract absorption. Fear of falling or fractures may limit their willingness to exercise or to leave home, further isolating the elderly and preventing them from obtaining vital exercise and sunlight, with resulting weakened bones and depressed appetite. Decreased sensory input from taste, smell, or sight is a natural part of aging and may lead to decreased appetite. Loss of teeth or ill-fitting dentures may cause dysphagia and further depress dietary intake. Malnutrition, as in other age groups, can affect the elderly by decreasing immune response and increasing susceptibility to infections.[57]

The practice of enteral "comfort" feedings for patients with advanced dementia or receiving palliative care has been controversial. On the one hand, family members and caregivers are loath to see their loved ones or patients "starving to death." On the other hand, evidence demonstrating a benefit in quality of life, nutritional status, or mortality is lacking, and the expenditure of health-care resources to place and maintain a percutaneous gastrostomy tube or other enteral feeding device is high. A Cochrane review of studies examining this topic has concluded that there is no evidence to support such a practice although there are a very large number of patients receiving this intervention. As policy makers examine means by which to bring health-care costs under control, practices such as this at the end of life will likely undergo increased scrutiny.[58,59]

The Mini Nutritional Assessment is a widely used, validated means of evaluation for nutritional deficits in the elderly. In a retrospective pooled analysis of multinational studies describing the prevalence of malnutrition in the elderly from 12 countries, across five continents but primarily in Europe, 46.2% of subjects were at risk of malnutrition and 22.8% were classified as overtly malnourished. A study in Switzerland found that about 1% of healthy elderly living in the community were malnourished, but the rates were 4% in outpatients receiving home care, 5% with Alzheimer's living at home, 20% in hospitalized elderly, and 37% in institutionalized elderly. These studies demonstrate that even in developed countries, malnutrition is a serious problem in the elderly and contributes both to degradation in the quality of life and life expectancy. The risk for malnutrition in developing countries is even higher given the more tenuous social support systems in place.[60–62]

REFERENCES

1. Millennium Development Goals reports. Available at http://www.un.org/millenniumgoals/reports.shtml. Accessed June 5, 2013.
2. World Health Statistics. Available at http://www.who.int/gho/publications/world_health_statistics/2012/en/. Accessed June 6, 2013.
3. World Hunger and Poverty Facts and Statistics. Available at http://www.worldhunger.org/articles/Learn/world%20hunger%20facts%202002.htm.
4. Gomez F, Galvan RR, Cravioto J, Frenk S. Malnutrition in infancy and childhood, with special reference to kwashiorkor. *Adv Pediatr.* 1955;7:131–69.
5. Waterlow JC. Classification and definition of protein–calorie malnutrition. *Br Med J.* 1972;3(5826):566–9.
6. Waterlow JC, Buzina R, Keller W, Lane JM, Nichaman MZ, Tanner JM. The presentation and use of height and weight data for comparing the nutritional status of groups of children under the age of 10 years. *Bull World Health Organ.* 1977;55(4):489–98.
7. Grover Z, Ee LC. Protein energy malnutrition. *Pediatr Clin North Am.* 2009;56(5): 1055–68.
8. Jones AP, Palmer D, Zhang G, Prescott SL. Cord blood 25-hydroxyvitamin D3 and allergic disease during infancy. *Pediatrics.* 2012;130:e1128.
9. Morales E, Romieu I, Guerra S, Ballester F, Rebagliato M, Vioque J, Tardón A et al. INMA Project. Maternal vitamin D status in pregnancy and risk of lower respiratory tract infections, wheezing, and asthma in offspring. *Epidemiology.* 2012;23:64–71.
10. Camargo CA Jr, Ingham T, Wickens K, Thadhani R, Silvers KM, Epton MJ, Town GI, Pattemore PK, Espinola JA, Crane J; New Zealand Asthma and Allergy Cohort Study Group. Cord-blood 25-hydroxyvitamin D levels and risk of respiratory infection, wheezing and asthma. *Pediatrics.* 2012;127:e180.
11. Baby-Friendly Hospital Initiative (BFHI). Available at http://www.unicef.org/programme/breastfeeding/baby.htm. Accessed June 5, 2013.
12. Merten S, Dratva J, Ackermann-Liebrich U. Do baby-friendly hospitals influence breastfeeding duration on a national level? *Pediatrics.* 2005;116:e702–8.
13. Huffman SL, Combest C. Role of breast-feeding in the prevention and treatment of diarrhoea. *J Diarrhoeal Dis Res.* 1990;8(3):68–81.
14. Section on Breastfeeding. Breastfeeding and the use of human milk. *Pediatrics.* 2012;129:e827.
15. World Health Organization (WHO). Maternal, newborn, child and adolescent health. Available at http://www.who.int/maternal_child_adolescent/documents/infant_feeding/en/. Accessed June 5, 2013.
16. Victora CG, Adair L, Fall C, Hallal PC, Martorell R, Richter L, Sachdev HS; Maternal and Child Undernutrition Study Group. Maternal and child undernutrition: Consequences for adult health and human capital. *Lancet.* 2008;371(9609):340–57. doi: 10.1016/S0140-6736(07)61692-4. Review. Erratum in: *Lancet.* 2008;371(9609):302. PubMed PMID: 18206223.
17. United Nations Administrative Committee on Coordination/Sub-Committee on Nutrition (ACC/SCN). Fourth Report on The World Nutrition Situation. 2000. Available at http://www.ifpri.org/sites/default/files/pubs/pubs/books/4thrpt/4threport.pdf.

18. United Nations System Standing Committee on Nutrition (UNSCN). Sixth Report on the World Nutrition Situation. 2010. Available at http://www.unscn.org/files/Publications/RWNS6/html/.

19. Imdad A, Herzer K, Mayo-Wilson E, Yakoob MY, Bhutta ZA. Vitamin A supplementation for preventing morbidity and mortality in children from 6 months to 5 years of age. *Cochrane Database Syst Rev*. 2010;(12):CD008524. doi: 10.1002/14651858. CD008524.pub2. Review. PubMed PMID: 21154399.

20. The World Bank. Vitamin A supplementation coverage rate (% of children ages 6–59 months). Available at http://data.worldbank.org/indicator/SN.ITK.VITA.ZS. Accessed June 3, 2013.

21. Sunguya BF, Poudel KC, Mlunde LB, Otsuka K, Yasuoka J, Urassa DP, Mkopi NP, Jimba M. Ready to Use Therapeutic Foods (RUTF) improves undernutrition among ART-treated, HIV-positive children in Dar es Salaam, Tanzania. *Nutr J*. 2012;11:60. doi: 10.1186/1475-2891-11-60. PubMed PMID: 22931107; PubMed Central PMCID: PMC3478224.

22. Singh AS, Kang G, Ramachandran A, Sarkar R, Peter P, Bose A. Locally made ready to use therapeutic food for treatment of malnutrition a randomized controlled trial. *Indian Pediatr*. 2010;47(8):679–86. PubMed PMID: 20972285.

23. Nackers F, Broillet F, Oumarou D, Djibo A, Gaboulaud V, Guerin PJ, Rusch B, Grais RF, Captier V. Effectiveness of ready-to-use therapeutic food compared to a corn/soy-blend-based pre-mix for the treatment of childhood moderate acute malnutrition in Niger. *J Trop Pediatr*. 2010;56(6):407–13. doi: 10.1093/tropej/fmq019. Epub March 23, 2010. PubMed PMID: 20332221.

24. Santini A, Novellino E, Armini V, Ritieni A. State of the art of ready-to-use therapeutic food: A tool for nutraceuticals addition to foodstuff. *Food Chem*. 2013;140(4):843–9. doi: 0.1016/j.foodchem.2012.10.098. Epub November 12, 2012. PubMed PMID:23692774.

25. Dewey KG, Arimond M. Lipid-based nutrient supplements: How can they combat child malnutrition? *PLoS Med*. 2012;9(9):e1001314. doi: 10.1371/journal.pmed.1001314.

26. Trehan I, Goldbach HS, LaGrone LN, Meuli GJ, Wang RJ, Maleta KM, Manary MJ. Antibiotics as part of the management of severe acute malnutrition. *N Engl J Med*. 2013;368(5):425–35. doi: 10.1056/NEJMoa1202851. PubMed PMID: 23363496.

27. Adam I, Ehassan EM, Mohmmed AA, Salih MM, Elbashir MI. Decreased susceptibility to placental malaria in anaemic women in an area with unstable malaria transmission in central Sudan. *Pathog Glob Health*. 2012;106(2):118–21. doi: 10.1179/2047773212Y.0000000011. PubMed PMID: 22943548.

28. Jonker FA, Calis JC, van Hensbroek MB, Phiri K, Geskus RB, Brabin BJ, Leenstra T. Iron status predicts malaria risk in Malawian preschool children. *PLoS One*. 2012;7(8):e42670. doi: 10.1371/journal.pone.0042670. Epub August 16, 2012. PubMed PMID: 22916146; PubMed Central PMCID: PMC3420896.

29. Okebe JU, Yahav D, Shbita R, Paul M. Oral iron supplements for children in malaria-endemic areas. *Cochrane Database Syst Rev*. 2011;(10):CD006589. doi: 10.1002/14651858.CD006589.pub3. Review. PubMed PMID: 21975754.

30. Abrams SA, Mushi A, Hilmers DC, Griffin IJ, Davila P, Allen L. A multinutrient-fortified beverage enhances the nutritional status of children in Botswana. *J Nutr*. 2003;133(6):1834–40. PubMed PMID: 12771326.

31. Anderson M, Thankachan P, Muthayya S, Goud RB, Kurpad AV, Hurrell RF, Zimmerman MB. Dual fortification of salt with iodine and iron: A randomized, double-blind, controlled trial of micronized ferric pyrophosphate and encapsulated ferrous fumarate in southern India. *Am J Clin Nutr*. 2008;88(5):1378–87. PubMed PMID: 18996875.

32. Miller J, Marek T. *Class Action: Improving School Performance in the Developing World through Better Health and Nutrition*. Washington, DC: World Bank, 1996.

33. Burchi F, Fanzo J, Frison E. The role of food and nutrition system approaches in tackling hidden hunger. *Int J Environ Res Public Health.* 2011;8:358–73.
34. Cole CR. Preventing hidden hunger in children using micronutrient supplementation. *J Pediatr.* 2012;161(5):777–8. doi: 10.1016/j.jpeds.2012.06.053. Epub August 4, 2012. PubMed PMID: 22867986.
35. Bailey RL, Fulgoni VL 3rd, Keast DR, Lentino CV, Dwyer JT. Do dietary supplements improve micronutrient sufficiency in children and adolescents? *J Pediatr.* 2012;161(5):837–42. doi: 0.1016/j.jpeds.2012.05.009. Epub June 18, 2012. PubMed PMID: 22717218; PubMed Central PMCID: PMC3477257.
36. Kulin HE, Bwibo N, Mutie D, Santner S. The effect of chronic childhood malnutrition on pubertal growth and development. *Am J Clin Nutr.* 1982;36:527–36.
37. Gopalan C. Motherhood in early adolescence, in *Combating Undernutrition.* Special Publication Series 3. New Delhi: NFI, 304–305, 1987.
38. Ayton AK, Azaz A, Horrobin DF. Rapid improvement of severe anorexia nervosa during treatment with ethyl-eicosapentaenoate and micronutrients. *Eur Psychiatry.* 2004;19(5):317–9. doi: 10.1016/j.eurpsy.2004.06.002.PMID 15276668.
39. Birmingham CL, Su J, Hlynsky JA, Goldner EM, Gao M. The mortality rate from anorexia nervosa. *Int J Eat Disord.* 2005;38(2):143–6. doi: 10.1002/eat.20164. PMID 16134111.
40. Hotta M, Ohwada R, Akamizu T, Shibasaki T, Takano K, Kangawa K. Ghrelin increases hunger and food intake in patients with restricting-type anorexia nervosa: A pilot study. *Endocr J.* 2009;56(9):1119–28. doi: 10.1507/endocrj.K09E-168. PMID 19755753.
41. Ogden CL, Carroll MD, Kit BK, Flegal KM. Centers for Disease Control and Prevention, Atlanta, GA. Available at http://www.cdc.gov/nchs/data/databriefs/db82.pdf. Accessed June 3, 2013.
42. Popkin BM, Adair LS, Ng SW. Global nutrition transition and the pandemic of obesity in developing countries. *Nutr Rev.* 2012;70(1):3–21. doi: 10.1111/j.1753-4887.2011.00456.x. Review. PubMed PMID: 22221213; PubMed Central. PMCID: PMC3257829.
43. Peña-Rosas JP, De-Regil LM, Dowswell T, Viteri FE. Daily oral iron supplementation during pregnancy. *Cochrane Database Syst Rev.* 2012;12:CD004736. doi: 10.1002/14651858.CD004736.pub4. Review. PubMed PMID:23235616.
44. Haider BA, Bhutta ZA. Multiple-micronutrient supplementation for women during pregnancy. *Cochrane Database Syst Rev.* 2012;11:CD004905. doi: 10.1002/14651858.CD004905.pub3. Review. PubMed PMID: 23152228.
45. Rosenthal J, Casas J, Taren D, Alverson CJ, Flores A, Frias J. Neural tube defects in Latin America and the impact of fortification: A literature review. *Public Health Nutr.* 2013:1–14. Epub ahead of print. PubMed PMID: 23464652.
46. Lassi ZS, Salam RA, Haider BA, Bhutta ZA. Folic acid supplementation during pregnancy for maternal health and pregnancy outcomes. *Cochrane Database Syst Rev.* 2013;3:CD006896. doi: 10.1002/14651858.CD006896.pub2. PubMed PMID:23543547.
47. Peña-Rosas JP, De-Regil LM, Dowswell T, Viteri FE. Intermittent oral iron supplementation during pregnancy. *Cochrane Database Syst Rev.* 2012;7:CD009997. doi: 10.1002/14651858.CD009997. Review. PubMed PMID: 22786531.
48. De-Regil LM, Palacios C, Ansary A, Kulier R, Peña-Rosas JP. Vitamin D supplementation for women during pregnancy. *Cochrane Database Syst Rev.* 2012;2:CD008873. doi: 0.1002/14651858.CD008873.pub2. Review. PubMed PMID: 22336854.
49. Pan WH, Yeh WT, Chen HJ, Chuang SY, Chang HY, Chen L, Wahlqvist ML. The U-shaped relationship between BMI and all-cause mortality contrasts with a progressive increase in medical expenditure: A prospective cohort study. *Asia Pac J Clin Nutr.* 2012;21(4):577–87. PubMed PMID: 23017316.
50. U.S. Department of Health and Human Services. Kidney Disease Statistics for the United States. Available at http://kidney.niddk.nih.gov/kudiseases/pubs/kustats/. Accessed June 6, 2013.

51. Sinclair A, ed. *Diabetes in Old Age*. Wiley, Hoboken, NJ. 2009; 211–2, section 15.2.2. ISBN: 978-0-470-06562-4.

52. Gentile S, Lacroix O, Durand AC, Cretel E, Alazia M, Sambuc R, Bonin-Guillaume S. Malnutrition: A highly predictive risk factor of short-term mortality in elderly presenting to the emergency department. *J Nutr Health Aging*. 2013;17(4):290–4. doi: 10.1007/s12603-012-0398-0. PubMed PMID: 23538647.

53. Suzuki T, Kwon J, Kim H, Shimada H, Yoshida Y, Iwasa H, Yoshida H. Low serum 25-hydroxyvitamin D levels associated with falls among Japanese community-dwelling elderly. *J Bone Miner Res*. 2008;23(8):1309–17. doi: 10.1359/jbmr.080328. PubMed PMID: 18410227.

54. Flicker L, Mead K, MacInnis RJ, Nowson C, Scherer S, Stein MS, Thomasx J, Hopper JL, Wark JD. Serum vitamin D and falls in older women in residential care in Australia. *J Am Geriatr Soc*. 2003;51(11):1533–8. PubMed PMID: 14687381.

55. Annweiler C, Schott AM, Rolland Y, Blain H, Herrmann FR, Beauchet O. Dietary intake of vitamin D and cognition in older women: A large population-based study. *Neurology*. 2010;75(20):1810–6. doi: 10.1212/WNL.0b013e3181fd6352. PubMed PMID: 21079183.

56. Wilkins CH, Birge SJ, Sheline YI, Morris JC. Vitamin D deficiency is associated with worse cognitive performance and lower bone density in older African Americans. *J Natl Med Assoc*. 2009;101(4):349–54. PubMed PMID: 19397226; PubMed Central PMCID: PMC2801439.0.

57. Birt M. Another Tsunami Warning: Caring for Japan's Elderly. Available at http://www.nbr.org/research/activity.aspx?id=131. Accessed April 21, 2013.

58. Malmgren A, Hede GW, Karlström B, Cederholm T, Lundquist P, Wirén M, Faxén-Irving G. Indications for percutaneous endoscopic gastrostomy and survival in old adults. *Food Nutr Res*. 2011;55. doi: 10.3402/fnr.v55i0.6037. Epub July 20, 2011. PubMed PMID: 21799666; PubMed Central PMCID: PMC3144742.

59. Sampson EL, Candy B, Jones L. Enteral tube feeding for older people with advanced dementia. *Cochrane Database Syst Rev*. 2009;(2):CD007209. doi: 10.1002/14651858.CD007209.pub2. Review. PubMed PMID: 19370678.

60. Calvo I, Olivar J, Martínez E, Rico A, Díaz J, Gimena M. MNA® Mini Nutritional Assessment as a nutritional screening tool for hospitalized older adults; rationales and feasibility. *Nutr Hosp*. 2012;27(5):1619–25. doi: 10.3305/nh.2012.27.5.5888. PubMed PMID: 23478714.

61. Guigoz Y, Lauque S, Vellas BJ. Identifying the elderly at risk for malnutrition. The Mini Nutritional Assessment. *Clin Geriatr Med*. 2002;18(4):737–57. Review. PubMed PMID: 12608501.

62. Kaiser MJ, Bauer JM, Rämsch C, Uter W, Guigoz Y, Cederholm T, Thomas DR et al. Mini Nutritional Assessment International Group. Frequency of malnutrition in older adults: A multinational perspective using the mini nutritional assessment. *J Am Geriatr Soc*. 2010;58(9):1734–8. doi: 10.1111/j.1532-5415.2010.03016.x. PubMed PMID:20863332.

2 Interaction of Nutrition and Immunity

Ebenezer Satyaraj and John E. Morley

CONTENTS

Introduction... 17
   Cells and Processes Involved in Nutrition and the Immune System
   Have Coevolved 18
Diet and Immunity: History and Renewed Focus 20
   Why Is It Important to Ensure Immune Health? 20
   What Impacts Immune Health? 21
      Malnutrition/Overnutrition 21
      Metabolic Disease: Diabetes Mellitus 21
   Effect of Age on the Immune System 23
      Immune Response in Neonates 23
      Immune Response Changes with Aging 24
      Stress 24
   How Can Nutrition Influence the Immune System? 25
      Gut Is the Largest "Immune Organ" 25
      Gut-Associated Lymphoid Tissue (GALT) Plays an Important Role in
      the Development of the Immune System 26
      Efficient Antigen Presentation Is Fundamental for Efficient
      Immune Response 26
      Nutrition Interacts with the Immune System at Multiple Levels 27
References 31

INTRODUCTION

The fundamental role of the immune system is to preserve the integrity of the organism. While fulfilling its role, the immune system is influenced by several factors, both internal and external, including genetics, age, reproductive phase, health and disease, nutrition, environment, and resident microbiota—both symbiotic and pathogenic. Of all the factors that shape the immune response and influence its response, only nutrition provides both the building blocks and the energy that are essential for its function. Interestingly, until recently, the role of nutrition was understood to be precisely that, to provide sustenance for the immune system. As current thinking evolves, nutrition is increasingly being recognized as a powerful driving force that shapes key physiological and pathological responses and underwrites evolutionary biology. The immune system is also significantly influenced by nutrition, as we shall review in this chapter.

CELLS AND PROCESSES INVOLVED IN NUTRITION AND THE IMMUNE SYSTEM HAVE COEVOLVED

Both nutritional awareness (nutrient metabolism) and pathogen sensing (immunity) are essential for survival—the former sustains and the latter preserves life. It is no surprise that nutrient metabolism and immunity have codeveloped organ systems and signaling pathways during evolution [1]. We see many examples of this in nature. In the common fruit fly, *Drosophila melanogaster*, both immune and metabolic responses are controlled by the same organ, namely the "fat body" [2]. While higher organisms have evolved different organ systems for immune and metabolic response, the evolutionary relation is still retained, for example, (a) the close proximity of immune cells such as macrophages and Kupffer cells in tissues actively involved in nutrient metabolism, such as adipose and liver tissue [1], (b) the observation that remodeling of adipose tissue often accompanies certain inflammatory diseases, such as the development of panniculitis during inflammatory bowel disease [3], and (c) the inflammatory stress brought on by obesity [4].

Importantly, this evolutionary relation is hardwired at the molecular level in cells involved in metabolic and immune processes, and this has significant biological consequences. Both adipocytes and macrophages secrete cytokines in response to bacterial products such as lipopolysaccharide (LPS) [5]. Preadipocytes can differentiate into macrophages, and transcriptional profiling reveals that they are genetically related [6,7]. Mutations in genes of the insulin signaling pathway have significant effects on immune response, as shown in some elegant studies done in the *Drosophila* model. Chico, an adaptor protein—a *Drosophila* homolog of vertebrate insulin receptor substrates—when altered by mutation, affects the resistance of flies to bacterial pathogens. Libert et al. [8] have shown that flies homozygous for mutant *chico* showed greater resistance to bacterial pathogens as compared with the wild-type or heterozygous flies. Also using the *Drosophila* model, Becker et al. [9] have shown that antimicrobial peptides can be activated in response to nuclear forkhead transcription factor (FOXO) activity. FOXO is key transcription factor that adapts metabolism to nutrient conditions and is one of the most evolutionarily ancient downstream effectors of the insulin signaling pathway [10,11]. *In vivo* experiments have shown that FOXO binds to regulatory regions of the AMP promoter (i.e., drosomysin) [10]. FOXO interacts with target of rapamycin (TOR) and AMP-activated protein kinase, which are key molecules that integrate information on cellular nutritional status by sensing both qualitative and quantitative changes in nutrients, particularly branched-chain amino acids and glucose [11]. In a recent review, MacIver et al. [12] describe how T lymphocytes regulate their metabolic process predominantly by using an ATP-generating process as quiescent T cells. However, upon activation, T cells switch to higher metabolic flux through growth-promoting pathways by using metabolic intermediates into biosynthetic pathways needed for proliferation. This switch to match cellular metabolic demands is orchestrated by several transcription regulators through the Glut1/mammalian TOR (mTOR) pathways. These studies show that the interaction between nutrition and immune function is mediated by nutrient signaling pathways that not only involve the monitoring of energy status but also perhaps involve specific nutrients and metabolites.

Given this close relation, it is not a surprise that nutrient deficiency or excess can negatively influence immune status and susceptibility to infection, and compromise overall health. Protein–energy undernutrition has been shown to lead to numerous negative effects on the immune system (Table 2.1). Protein–energy undernutrition increases the risk for a variety of infections such as urinary tract infections, pneumonia, abscesses, and meningitis [13], as well as a variety of fungal and other atypical infections [14]. The classic example is a young child with marasmus who develops an infection resulting in cytokine release, inflammation, and capillary leak with third spacing of albumin. Low serum albumin causes edema, and the child now has kwashiorkor with an even higher chance of infection if the child does not receive adequate protein and calorie replacement [15].

On the other end of the spectrum, overnutrition can also adversely affect the immune system. For instance, adipose tissue in obesity has been shown to produce higher levels of proinflammatory cytokines such as tumor necrosis factor (TNF)-α [16], resulting in low-grade inflammation leading to impaired immune response, metabolic syndrome, and associated diseases such as insulin resistance, type 2 diabetes, and atherosclerosis [17]. The good news is that this relation can also be used to proactively enhance immune health.

TABLE 2.1
Examples of the Effects of Protein–Energy Undernutrition on the Immune System

	Effect
Thymus	Atrophy
Delayed hypersensitivity	Decreased
Helper induced T cells (CD4$^+$)	Decreased
Cytotoxic suppressor T cells (CD8$^+$)	Mild decrease
CD4$^+$/CD8$^+$	Decreased
Mitogen lymphocyte proliferation	Decreased
Circulating immune complexes	Decreased
Response to immunization	Decreased
Neutrophil function	Decreased
Cytokines	
IL-3	Increased
IL-4	Increased
IL-6	Increased
IL-2	Decreased
IFN-α	Decreased
TGF	Decreased
GM-CSF	Decreased

DIET AND IMMUNITY: HISTORY AND RENEWED FOCUS

The understanding of the impact of diet on the immune system is not new; references are seen in the writings of ancient Egyptians and Indians. Hippocrates, the father of Western medicine, is believed to have recommended his students to evaluate diet in order to understand human disease. However, the earliest scientific evidence implicating the role of nutrition in immune function was from observations made by J.F. Menkel in 1810, describing thymic atrophy in malnourished patients in England [18]. These observations, among others, gave birth to nutritional immunology, which continued to evolve as a scientific discipline with the study of nutritional deficiencies caused by malnutrition sometimes referred to as nutritionally acquired immune deficiency syndrome [18]. Since its early beginnings in the 1800s, and with new evolving concepts in the vitamin era of the early 1900s, the emphasis in nutritional immunology was on the impact of nutrient deficiencies on the immune system. While malnutrition still remains a global problem, many of the detrimental effects of malnutrition can be addressed by correcting the specific underlying nutritional problem. With the advances made in agriculture, in the developed world, the current challenge, however, is related to an aging population, stress, and dietary overindulgence. Unlike immune deficiency caused by malnutrition, age-related immune deficiencies (life stage) and immune deficiency due to stress or dietary overindulgence need a more comprehensive strategy. Such immune deficiencies cannot be simply addressed by correcting nutritional problems and are therefore more difficult to evaluate, understand, and manage. Hence, the paradigm shift in today's research emphasis in nutritional immunology, is shifting from malnutrition to addressing impaired immune status because of age, stress, and diet.

WHY IS IT IMPORTANT TO ENSURE IMMUNE HEALTH?

The benefits of good immune health go beyond protection from infections. Immune health or the lack thereof, has profound metabolic consequences and new research indicates that it can affect several body systems, including cognition and brain aging [19]. In addition, the immune system plays an important role in recognizing and attacking cancer cells and an abnormal immune system can lead to autoimmunity [20]. At a fundamental level, a healthy immune system affords protection by preventing infectious agents from entering the host and establishing an active infection. This is the critical "barrier" function, otherwise called as the "first line of defense" role of the immune system. When the immune system is compromised, this barrier weakens and pathogens invade, causing disease. This triggers an active immune response to neutralize and eliminate the infectious agent, involving physiological changes including fever, inflammation, and cellular responses such as generation of T cells and antibodies that can specifically target the pathogen. While such a full-blown immune response is critical for survival, it nevertheless comes with a price; it is a metabolically costly endeavor, using precious resources. To put this in perspective, a 1°C increase in body temperature (fever associated with active infection) involves an energy expenditure equal to a 70-kg person walking 45 km $(9.4 \times 10^6$ J) [21]. This implies that repeated immune activation to combat infection can be a significant drain on metabolic resources and will unfavorably compete with energy-demanding functions such as reproduction, lactation, and growth because, evolutionarily, "protection" is assigned a higher priority. Repeated immune activation has other secondary consequences, the so-called collateral damage such as increased oxidative stress, which is especially harmful in the elderly. A healthy immune system capable of preventing infections thus has profound positive metabolic implications. Recent research done in rodents and persons with age-related dementia suggests that poor immune health can negatively influence cognition and brain aging [19]. The SAMP8 mouse, an animal model of Alzheimer's disease, has increased cytokines and free radical production leading to oxidative damage [22]. These effects can be reversed with α-lipoic acid [23], and there are some data suggesting that α-lipoic acid may improve memory in humans with Alzheimer's disease [24]. Clearly, a healthy immune system has implications that go well beyond disease prevention.

WHAT IMPACTS IMMUNE HEALTH?

Malnutrition/Overnutrition

As already alluded to, protein–energy undernutrition is associated with a variety of immune defects and infections. Patients with a variety of cytokine-associated illnesses develop cachexia—a condition associated with anorexia, loss of fat and muscle, anemia, low albumin, and a variety of immune system abnormalities [25].

Similarly, overnutrition can lead to a number of deficits in the immune system [26]. Besides the inflammatory response produced by excess adipocytes, leptin is a proinflammatory hormone produced in excess in obesity [27]. While the anti-inflammatory hormone adiponectin has reduced levels in obese persons, leptin increases lymphopoiesis, resulting in T-cell proliferation and an increase in thymocyte survival [28]. Nonesterified fatty acids activate Toll-like receptors, leading to an inflammatory response. This low-grade inflammatory response places obese persons at an increased risk for nosocomial and viral infections, tuberculosis, *Helicobacter pylori*, and a worse outcome, as shown in the 2009 influenza A pandemic [29,30].

The increase in viral infections is most probably due to the decrease in the immune sentinel dendritic cells [31]. These cells are regulated by Toll-like receptors, and upregulation of these receptors leads to fewer CD83 dendritic cell markers. These are cells that play an important role in CD83 T-cell priming to respond to viral infections. Obesity impairs response to hepatitis vaccination, which is reversed after gastric bypass with weight loss [29]. The major alterations in obesity, in response to a foreign antigen, are an increase in short-lived effector cells, decreased memory precursors and antigen-specific memory T cells, resulting in a decline in activation-induced cell death over time [32,33]. The effects of obesity on the immune system are summarized in Table 2.2. Epidemiologically, obesity has been linked to a variety of cancers, including breast, endometrium, colon, gastric, and pancreatic cancers, as well as leukemia [34,35]. The mechanism by which obesity is postulated to cause cancers is by the PI3K/Akt/mTOR pathway (Figure 2.1) [36].

Metabolic Disease: Diabetes Mellitus

Diabetes mellitus often decreases tissue zinc [37]. This is due to both a decreased absorption of zinc and an increased loss of zinc in the urine [38,39]. Zinc deficiency is associated with a decrease in T-cell numbers and a decreased phytomitogen

TABLE 2.2
Alterations in the Immune System in Obesity

- Decreased dendritic cells → decreased CD^{8-} T cells
- Increased short-lived effector cells and decreased memory precursors and antigen-specific memory T cells → ↓induced cell death
- Increased leptin → ↑macrophage activation → ↑TNF-α, IL-6, IL-12, IL-10, IL-1β macrophage, inflammatory protein-1
- Increased leptin→ ↑T-cell proliferation → ↑IL-2 → CD8 T-cell proliferation → ↑IFN-δ
- Increased leptin → ↑NK function
- Increased leptin → ↑intracellular adhesion molecule
- Decreased adiponectin → ↓nitric oxide and other reactive oxygen species
- Increased Toll-like receptors → ↓CD83 dendritic cells
- Impaired response to hepatitis B and tetanus vaccine
- Increased resistin → ↑ICAM-1, UCAM-1, E-selectin, and NK cell function
- Decreased visfaten → ↑TNF-α, IL-6, IL-8
- Visceral fat → ↓regulating T cells → ↓B1 antibody–producing cells → ↓IgA and IgM → ↓antibodies to influenza

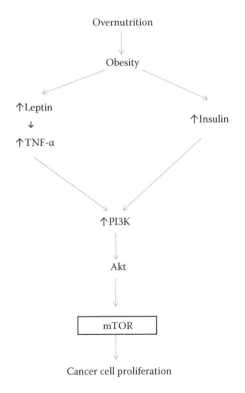

FIGURE 2.1   Putative mechanism by which overnutrition causes cancer.

response by T cells [40]. Natural killer (NK) cell activity is decreased in the presence of zinc deficiency [41,42]. Zinc is necessary for the dendritic cell response to Toll-like receptor 4 [43]. Zinc deficiency reduces the T-helper type 1 (Th1) cytokine response, whereas it does not activate the Th2 cytokine response [41].

In the absence of disease, age and stress are other important factors influencing the immune status. The immune response of a neonate and or an older animal may be less adequate than an adult, making them more susceptible to infection [44]. Aging is also characterized by low-level chronic inflammation that contributes to the declining ability of the immune system to respond and regulate immune response [45]. Stress, in particular chronic stress, has been shown to have a significant negative impact on the immune system irrespective of the age of the subject [46].

EFFECT OF AGE ON THE IMMUNE SYSTEM

Immune Response in Neonates

Neonatal immune responses tend to be not as strong as in an adult animal [47]. While neonates are capable of responding to an immune challenge, their immune responses tend to exhibit a Th2 bias [44]. A Th1 immune response is characterized by proinflammatory cytokines such as interferon (IFN)-γ, interleukin (IL)-6, and TNF-α, and hence is more effective in preventing infectious diseases. In contrast, Th2-biased immune response is predominated by anti-inflammatory cytokines such as IL-10, IL-4, and transforming growth factor (TGF)-β and is not as effective in dealing with microbial infections, making neonates more susceptible to infections. Neonatal deficiency of innate cellular immunity includes a decreased production of IFNs, IL-12/IL-23, IL-18, and other proinflammatory cytokines, and an impaired type-1 response of macrophages to IFN-γ, LPS (the primary constituent of the outer membrane of gram-negative bacteria), as well as to multiple Toll-like receptor ligands [48].

There are several cellular and molecular reasons for this Th2 bias: (a) As compared with adult cells, neonatal antigen-presenting cells (APCs) are less efficient in antigen presentation because of their reduced capacity to express the crucial costimulatory molecules CD86 and CD40 and upregulate MHC class II molecules [49]. MHC class II molecules and costimulatory molecules are required to present antigens to CD4$^+$ T cells to initiate an immune response. (b) The feto-placental environment tends to be immunosuppressive and Th2 biased owing to locally acting cytokines and hormones, and these influence neonatal immune responses [44]. (c) Neonatal B cells, which also function as APCs, have altered signaling due to lowered MHC class II molecules as well as lowered accessory signaling molecules. Lack of upregulation of CD40 (accessory signaling molecules) and CD40L (receptor for CD40) tends to dampen B-cell response as well as their ability to class switch immunoglobulin production contributing to the Th2 bias. (d) Neonatal Th1 cells undergo apoptosis because of the unique receptors they express. In a recent study, Lee et al. have shown that although a primary immune response from neonatal T cells includes a significant Th1 component, the Th1 cells generated have unique characteristics. They tend to have high levels of IL-13Rα1, which heterodimerizes with IL-4Rα. As the immune response progresses, due to the lack of appropriate dendritic cells (DCs), the immune response is dominated by IL-4, which binds the IL-13Rα1–IL-4Rα

complex expressed on the Th1 cells and induces apoptosis, eliminating the Th1 cells and resulting in a Th2 bias. As the neonate ages, a significant number of appropriate DCs start accumulating especially in the spleen. These DCs produce IL-12, and this IL-12 triggers the downregulation IL-13Rα1 on the Th1 cells, rescuing them from IL-4-induced apoptosis. This study underlines the need for cytokines such as IL-12 to initiate a Th1-biased immune response [50].

Immune Response Changes with Aging

Aging brings changes to both the humoral and cellular immune responses. These include defects in the hematopoietic bone marrow and defects in lymphocyte migration, maturation, and function. Aging also involves involution of the thymus, which contributes to loss of immune function with increasing age [51].

With age, the immune system loses plasticity, resulting in lowered response. Immune plasticity is the ability of the immune system to remodel itself to respond appropriately to danger signals that include pathogens, tissue damage, and oxidative stress, and to a quiescent state once the danger has passed. One of the reasons for this declining immune plasticity is the chronic metabolic stress associated with aging [52]. This results in reduced immune response and a lower cellular capacity in DNA repair, leading to a condition described as "immunosenescence," which increases the risk of age-related diseases, i.e., cancer and infection [53,54]. Declining immune plasticity leads the cells of the immune system to undergo cell death or necrosis triggered by oxidative stress [55].

Stress

Stress, both physical and mental, has a significant negative impact on the immune system, irrespective of age. Both major and minor stressful events have been shown to have a profound influence on immune responses in both animal and human studies. One of the hallmarks of chronic stress is the general increase in levels of oxidative stress, and oxidative stress gradually erodes immune plasticity. Research in this area has spawned a new discipline called "psychoneuroimmunology"—the study of the interaction between the psychological process and the nervous and immune systems [56]. Using vaccine responses as an indicator of immune status [57–62], researchers have demonstrated that among medical students taking exams, the level of stress lowered response to vaccine (virus-specific antibody and T-cell responses to hepatitis B vaccine were lower), while the degree of social support increased vaccine response. Another good example of chronic stress is the stress associated with caregiving for a spouse with Alzheimer's disease, which was associated with a poorer response [59] to an influenza virus vaccine when compared with well-matched control subjects [59]. Vaccine responses demonstrate clinically relevant alterations in an immunological response to challenge under well-controlled conditions and therefore can be used as a surrogate for responses to an infectious challenge. Individuals who respond poorly to vaccines tend to have greater susceptibility to the pathogens when compared with those with better vaccine responses. Burns et al., among others, have shown that adults who show poorer responses to vaccines also experience higher rates of clinical illness, as well as longer-lasting infectious episodes [63,64].

Cohen et al. showed that human volunteers who were inoculated with five different strains of respiratory viruses showed a dose-dependent relation between stress and clinical symptoms observed after infection [65]. Therefore, from these vaccine studies, it is clear that stress puts individuals at greater risk for more severe illnesses.

At the molecular level, stress delays inflammation by reducing efficiency of CD62L-mediated immune surveillance by phagocytes [66]. Stress decreases IFN-γ secretion by lymphocytes and may decrease antigen presentation efficiency by downregulating MHC class II molecule expression on APCs, and delay or impair immune responses to vaccination.

Hormones play an important role in the effect of stress on the immune system. Stress sets into motion physiological changes that help the organism cope with the stressor (fight or flight response). However, chronic stress results in sustained activation of stress responses, which include activation of the hypothalamic–pituitary–adrenal axis and the sympathetic–adrenal–medullary axis, resulting in the production of glucocorticoid (GC) hormones and catecholamine. GC receptors are expressed by a variety of immune cells and bind cortisol, interfering with nuclear factor-κB function, which in turn regulates the activity of cytokine-producing immune cells. Sustained release of stress hormones negatively influences the immune system. Several models have been proposed to explain the mechanism of action of stress hormones on the immune cells [67]. GC affects the expression of cytokines, costimulatory molecules, and adhesion molecules, which influences immune cell migration, differentiation, proliferation, and effector function [68–70]. Adrenergic receptors bind epinephrine and norepinephrine and activate the cAMP response element binding protein, inducing the transcription of a variety of immune response genes, including genes for cytokines. Elevated levels of catecholamines produced during stress can modify immune response genes [71]. Stress is another key factor that can negatively influence the immune status of an animal irrespective of its age.

Malnutrition (both undernutrition and overnutrition), metabolic disease, age, and stress clearly can undermine the immune status in the absence of other immune system-associated diseases. Immunodeficiency, irrespective of etiology, can severely undermine health, triggering debilitating diseases such as infections, malignancies, and autoimmune diseases. Hence, there is a critical need to evaluate immune status and address deviations that, if managed effectively, can significantly enhance the quality of life.

How Can Nutrition Influence the Immune System?

Gut Is the Largest "Immune Organ"

Besides being the gateway for nutrient intake, the gut is the largest immune organ, containing >65% of all the immune cells in the body and >90% of all immunoglobulin-producing cells [72,73]. In an adult human, the intestine contains 3-fold greater Ig-producing cells (about 7×10^{10}) as compared with the bone marrow (2.5×10^{10}) [74]. It is estimated that approximately 3 g of secretory IgA is secreted daily into the lumen of an adult human [75]. Thus, a significant part of the immune system interacts with what we eat.

Gut-Associated Lymphoid Tissue (GALT) Plays an Important Role in the Development of the Immune System

Research conducted with germ-free animals has documented that stimuli from environmental antigens, especially the gut microbiota, are essential for the development of a healthy immune system [76]. Germ-free animals tend to have a very underdeveloped immune system, clearly underscoring the role played by symbiotic microbiota and associated environmental antigens. The GALT therefore offers a unique opportunity for immunomodulation through the diet. The GALT is unique in its ability to be exposed to a diverse array of antigens from food (roughly 10–15 kg of food per year per human), and from the >1000 species of commensal microorganisms (10^{12} mL per milliliter of colon content, making them the most numerous cells in the body), and yet remains quiescent until it encounters a threat, such as a pathogen. This is initiated by molecules called PAMPs expressed by microbial pathogens. PAMPs, which stands for pathogen-associated molecular patterns, are highly conserved motifs present in these microorganisms. PAMPs include LPS from the gram-negative cell wall, peptidoglycan, lipotechoic acids from the gram-positive cell wall, the sugar mannose (common in microbial glycolipids and glycoproteins but rare in mammals), bacterial DNA, N-formyl methionine found in bacterial proteins, double-stranded RNA from viruses, and glucans from fungal cell walls. Most dietary immune-modulating strategies involve targeting PAMP receptors of the GALT by using appropriate ingredients.

Efficient Antigen Presentation Is Fundamental for Efficient Immune Response

Efficient antigen presentation to T lymphocytes, by APCs such as macrophages, is a prerequisite for an effective immune response. APCs set the tone of the immune response through the costimulatory molecules they express and the cytokines they secrete. APC function is central to the altered immune response that is characteristic of the neonatal immune system, immune response of an aging immune system, and immune response during stress. In all three cases, due to the lack of immune-potentiating cytokines such as IL-1 and IL-12, APCs responding to an immune challenge are not able to upregulate MHC class II molecules and costimulatory molecules such as CD86. Lack of these cytokine signals also modifies the immune response, reducing its efficiency and giving it a Th2 bias. The resulting immune response therefore tends to be not as efficient. The approach to address this deficiency hinges on providing the required signaling to the APCs [77]. Receptors on immune cells present in the gut serve this function and are the primary targets of strategies for immunomodulation through diet. These receptors have evolved to respond to molecules in microbial pathogens collectively called PAMPs (described in the paragraph above). Examples include yeast β-glucans [78], yeast mannans [79], and nucleic acids [80]. Probiotics interact with the immune system by virtue of their PAMP molecules such as LPS [81]. These molecules, also referred to as immune response modifiers (IRMs), primarily initiate a local proinflammatory cytokine secretion that activates local APCs to upregulate MHC class II and costimulatory molecules, enabling them to present antigens efficiently to T lymphocytes. IRMs provided through diet enhance APC efficiency. APCs in the gut continually process and present antigens to T lymphocytes in the GALT, while the GALT is quiescent to the myriad antigenic stimuli it receives through diet (when it encounters a pathogen, it is able to initiate a more efficient immune response). The enhanced immune activity induced by dietary IRMs in the GALT (mucosal immune system) spreads to the entire immune system, by the trafficking of activated lymphocytes, cytokines, and the significant overlap with the nonmucosal immune system [82].

Nutrition Interacts with the Immune System at Multiple Levels

Nutrition and the immune system interact at multiple levels and, for simplicity, can be considered in a framework of four stages. Stages I and II are passive because they involve providing the immune system with essential nutrients. Stages III and IV focus on modifying the immune response by using agents such as IRMs that primarily target the PAMP receptors in the gut and involve more active approaches in enhancing immune status.

Stage I: Complete Nutrition

At the primary level, the focus revolves around dietary energy, protein, vitamins (vitamins A, C, and E) and minerals such as Zn, Mg, and Fe [83]. Minerals such as Ca^+ and Mg^+ drive signaling mechanisms in the immune system and are therefore also important for enhanced immune response. Providing basic nutrition is the very least that we can do for the immune system.

Stage II: Optimizing Macronutrients and Micronutrients

The second stage involves optimizing key nutrients that are critical for immune cells. The immune system has a need for certain nutrients, and providing greater amounts of these key nutrients will optimize immune function. A temporary deficiency of a key nutrient can negatively affect the immune system. For example, during strenuous exercise, muscle cells preferentially use glutamine as their energy source and, as a result, there is a reduction of glutamine levels in circulation. Glutamine is also the preferred energy source for immune cells, and because of low levels of glutamine in circulation after a strenuous exercise, immune cells cannot function efficiently if challenged, making these athletes vulnerable to infections immediately after vigorous bouts of exercise [84].

The key ingredients needed for a healthy immune system would include optimal levels and high quality of proteins in diet. At a molecular level, proteins make up the structural components and mediate key processes of the immune system. Receptors, cytokines, immunoglobulins, complement components, bactericidal proteins, etc., are all proteins. A source of high-quality protein in diets is therefore important for a healthy immune system. Vitamins (vitamins A, C, and E) and minerals such as Zn, Mg, and Fe are also critical for the normal functioning of the immune system.

Addressing oxidative stress and subsequent damage to cellular DNA is another example of this strategy. Aging and other environmental stressors tend to increase the levels of oxidative damage to cellular DNA, including immune cells. Cells have the ability to repair damage in response to injury or stress. However, beyond a point, the damage can be irreparable and result in cell death by apoptosis. Oxidative DNA damage due to free radicals produced during cellular metabolism is one of the primary causes of cell death [85]. Increased apoptosis can break immune tolerance to self-antigens, resulting in autoimmunity [86]. Immunosenesence is characterized by a decreased response to mitogens and decreased cytokine production, and changes in signal transduction have been associated with aging (reviewed in ref. 83). Various strategies can help address senescence, tissue damage, and apoptosis associated with aging, including the following:

1. **Caloric restriction (CR):** Apart from increasing the life span [87], data from laboratory animals have demonstrated that CR reduces immunosenescence [88]. Recent data from a CR study conducted in Labrador retriever dogs clearly show that CR can help retard immunosenescence [89]. There are two caveats to CR: first, CR only works in animals that are younger than middle age and, second, primate studies have failed to show convincing evidence for CR in older animals [90].

2. **Antioxidants:** Increased levels of antioxidants such as vitamin C [91], vitamin E [83], and carotenoids (β-carotene, α-carotene, lycopene, astaxanthin, etc.) can prevent damage mediated by free radicals. There are a number of reports documenting the benefits of carotenoids in dogs, particularly in older animals [92–94]. However, the effect of antioxidants in humans is less clear; a large meta-analysis suggested that antioxidant vitamins in healthy persons may increase mortality [95].

3. **Prebiotics:** Prebiotics that help maintain normal gut organisms also fall into this category. Intestinal microbiota play an important role in keeping the immune system primed to prevent colonization by pathogenic microbes (Figure 2.2). However, under certain conditions, such as antibiotic therapy, gastrointestinal infections, stress, or old age, the normal biota in the gastrointestinal tract is perturbed, leading to either a change in the bacteria due to overgrowth of harmful bacteria (e.g., *Clostridium difficile*). Prebiotics such as inulin help maintain a healthy commensal population in the gut under stress [96]. Probiotics have been shown to decrease the production of mRNA for TNF-α and IL-6, as well as to reduce sCD14, a marker of activated macrophages, in older persons receiving oligosaccharides [97]. Probiotics have been shown to prevent antibiotic-induced diarrhea in humans [97].

The first two stages are passive approaches in "immunonutrition." These are passive because they focus on providing dietary energy, protein, vitamins, minerals, and antioxidants, and manage caloric intake to help the immune system function optimally. Stages III and IV are considerably different and involve a more proactive approach at managing the immune system to obtain the desired outcome.

Stage III: Active Modulation of the Immune System

In stage III, the emphasis is on active interaction with the immune system to modulate its function toward a desired goal. Examples would include the following:

1. Reversing the Th2 bias and restoring Th1 response by enabling efficient antigen presentation: A Th1 (proinflammatory) response is important for protection against microbial infections. The Th1 component of the immune system is

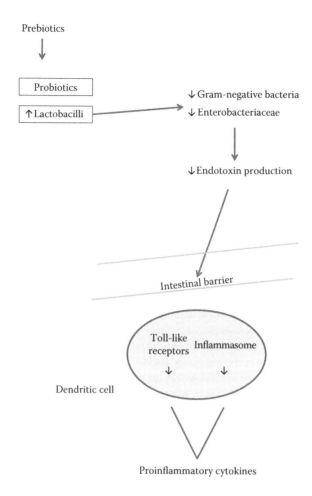

FIGURE 2.2 Mechanisms by which prebiotics and probiotics decrease inflammation.

boosted by stimulating the immune system with probiotic bacteria or PAMP-expressing moieties (e.g., yeast β-glucans). Probiotics (*Enterococcus faecium*, *Lactobacilli* sp., *Bifidobacteria* sp., etc.) in the diet have been shown to enhance immune status in humans [98] and several other species [99]. Milk bioactives from bovine colostrum have been shown to have immune-enhancing effects in both human and murine studies, making bovine colostrum an interesting immunomodulating ingredient. Colostrum contains immunoglobulins, cytokines, lactoferrin, and lactoperoxidase, each of which can influence the immune system [100]. Mice fed milk bioactives produced significantly higher serum and intestinal antibodies to several antigens (influenza virus, diphtheria and tetanus toxin, poliomyelitis vaccine, ovalbumin, and cholera toxin subunit) [101]. In another study, mice fed milk bioactives had enhanced resistance to pneumococcal infection [102,103]. In a recently published study, Satyaraj et al. [104] have shown that dogs fed a diet supplemented with bovine colostrum had significantly enhanced immune function. In an *in vitro* study conducted with human monocytes, Biswas et al. [105] report that coculture with bovine colostrum without antigenic stimulus induced a dose-dependent production of IL-12 by CD 14$^+$ monocytes but did not induce IFN-γ production. Interestingly, in the same study, bovine colostrum differentially affected stimuli-induced IFN-γ production: it enhanced IFN-γ in response to weak antigenic stimulation and inhibited IFN-γ in response to strong antigenic stimulation. As discussed earlier, IL-12 and IFN-γ are cytokines involved in the Th1 polarization required for a successful immune response toward intracellular pathogens such as bacteria and viruses. In a clinical study conducted in highly trained cyclists, supplementation with low-dose bovine colostral protein concentrate favorably modulated immune parameters during normal training and after an acute period of intense exercise, which contributed to lowering of the incidence of upper respiratory illness [106]. In a study conducted with adult dogs, we evaluated the immune-enhancing effect of bovine colostrum. Our results demonstrated that adding bovine colostrum significantly enhanced their immune status, as measured by their response to canine distemper vaccine as well as the increased level of GALT activity measured by IgA production. Colostrum-supplemented diets also enhanced immune status in cats, as evidenced by increased rabies vaccine response and increased GALT activity also measured by IgA production [107]. Stimulating the immune cells in the gut likely leads to a cascade of immune cell activation that results in the secretion of cytokines that reach the rest of the immune cells through the circulation, resulting in the overall activation of the immune system and an increase in the production of IgA in the gut.

2. Managing inflammation better will prevent further damage: Chronic inflammation is central to the pathophysiology of a number of diseases, including cardiovascular diseases and neurological diseases (Alzheimer's, impaired cognition) [108]. Physiologically, the effects of inflammation are mediated by prostaglandins and leukotrienes, all end products of the arachidonic acid metabolism. A diet rich in docosahexaenoic acid and omega-3 fatty acids can control the damaging effects of inflammation because of the reduction in the levels of active prostaglandins and leukotrienes, and can be an effective strategy in addressing the effects of chronic inflammation. Reduced inflammation not only improves the quality of life by preventing a number of cardiovascular and neurological diseases but also helps prevent autoimmunity by reducing the exposure of the immune system to self-antigens.

Stage IV: "Personalized Nutrition"—Predictive, Preventive, and Personalized Nutrition

Interaction between diet, environment, and genome ultimately defines health status and can be critical in influencing chronic disease [109–112]. During the last few decades, the science of pharmacogenomics, which deals with the genetic basis underlying disease susceptibility and variable drug response in individuals, has brought about a paradigm shift in the pharmaceutical industry by moving it from a "one drug fits all" toward personalized therapy. This process has been greatly accelerated by advances in the "omics" fields: single nucleotide polymorphism analysis, transcriptomics (cDNA analysis), proteomics, and metabolomics. A good example of genetic variability affecting disease is breast cancer therapy with the drug trastuzumab (Herceptin®, a humanized monoclonal antibody against the HER2 receptor developed by Genentech Inc.) linked to HER2 overexpression. Individuals expressing low levels of the HER2 receptor respond poorly to Herceptin [113,114]. Another example is the influence of genetic variability on cytochrome P450 monooxygenase system enzymes (P450 family of enzymes are important for the metabolism of most drugs) and drug toxicity in individual patients [115].

The concept of "personalized medicine" is now being explored in nutrition. Although "personalized nutrition" is still in its infancy, it is practiced in principle as in the dietary management of diabetes or maintaining a healthy lipid profile to manage risk of cardiovascular disease. For a practical personalized diet strategy, there are two basic requirements: a clear understanding of the pathogenesis and the availability of cost effective and reliable biomarkers to either identify susceptibility or diagnose disease. Biomarkers are an objectively measured characteristic that indicates normal biological processes, pathological processes, or pharmacological responses to a therapeutic intervention. The ultimate goal here is to modify the physiology through a "personalized" dietary regimen and reduce the risk of disease, thereby enhancing the quality of life.

Induction of a local Th2 bias in persons with inflammatory bowel disease by using dietary means is an example of a targeted approach to immunomodulation. Probiotic microbes have been characterized on the basis of the cytokine responses they induce. Certain bacteria induce secretion of anti-inflammatory cytokines such as IL-10, TGF-β, and IL-13 [116]. These probiotic agents provides the opportunity to explore probiotic-fortified diets that will help patients with inflammatory bowel diseases. Similarly, TGF-β-rich ingredients, such as colostrum and whey proteins, are being increasingly used to effectively address localized inflammatory conditions in the gut, especially with diets for inflammatory bowel diseases.

In summary, as research advances our understanding of complex physiological networks in health and disease, the role played by the immune system and its interaction with diet takes a whole new meaning. As our understanding of the relation between nutrition and the immune system matures, a variety of diet-based approaches to address immune needs will become available, both for us and our pets. The food we eat can clearly deliver several other benefits beyond basic nutrition, and this is the promise of immunonutrition. Current evidence supports well-balanced nutrient-enriched food to be more effective in improving health than highly processed individual nutrients.

REFERENCES

1. Hotamisligil GS. Inflammation and metabolic disorders. *Nature*. 2006 Dec 14;444:860–7.
2. Hoffmann JA, Reichhart JM. *Drosophila* innate immunity: An evolutionary perspective. *Nat Immunol*. 2002 Feb;3:121–6.
3. Karagiannides I, Pothoulakis C. Obesity, innate immunity and gut inflammation. *Curr Opin Gastroenterol*. 2007 Nov;23:661–6.
4. Fain JN. Release of inflammatory mediators by human adipose tissue is enhanced in obesity and primarily by the nonfat cells: A review. *Mediators Inflamm*. 2010;2010:513948.

5. Akira S, Hemmi H. Recognition of pathogen-associated molecular patterns by TLR family. *Immunol Lett.* 2003 Jan 22;85:85–95.
6. Charriere G, Cousin B, Arnaud E, Andre M, Bacou F, Penicaud L, Casteilla L. Preadipocyte conversion to macrophage. Evidence of plasticity. *J Biol Chem.* 2003 Mar 14;278:9850–5.
7. Khazen W, M'bika JP, Tomkiewicz C, Benelli C, Chany C, Achour A, Forest C. Expression of macrophage-selective markers in human and rodent adipocytes. *FEBS Lett.* 2005 Oct 24;579:5631–4.
8. Libert S, Chao Y, Zwiener J, Pletcher SD. Realized immune response is enhanced in long-lived puc and chico mutants but is unaffected by dietary restriction. *Mol Immunol.* 2008 Feb;45:810–7.
9. Becker T, Loch G, Beyer M, Zinke I, Aschenbrenner AC, Carrera P, Inhester T, Schultze JL, Hoch M. FOXO-dependent regulation of innate immune homeostasis. *Nature.* 2010 Jan 21;463:369–73.
10. Hay N. Interplay between FOXO, TOR, and Akt. *Biochim Biophys Acta.* 2011 Nov;1813:1965–70.
11. Kapahi P, Chen D, Rogers AN, Katewa SD, Li PW, Thomas EL, Kockel L. With TOR, less is more: A key role for the conserved nutrient-sensing TOR pathway in aging. *Cell Metab.* 2010 Jun 9;11:453–65.
12. MacIver NJ, Michalek RD, Rathmell JC. Metabolic regulation of T lymphocytes. *Annu Rev Immunol.* 2013;31:259–83.
13. Morley JE. Undernutrition in older adults. *Fam Pract.* 2012;29 Suppl 1:i89–93.
14. Kaiser FE, Morley JE. Idiopathic CD4[+] T lymphopenia in older persons. *J Am Geriatr Soc.* 1994 Dec;42:1291–4.
15. Grover Z, Ee LC. Protein energy malnutrition. *Pediatr Clin North Am.* 2009 Oct;56:1055–68.
16. Leoni MC, Pizzo D, Marchi A. Adipocytokines: Potential biomarkers for childhood obesity and anorexia nervosa. *Minerva Pediatr.* 2010 Apr;62:171–8.
17. Hotamisligil GS, Shargill NS, Spiegelman BM. Adipose expression of tumor necrosis factor-alpha: Direct role in obesity-linked insulin resistance. *Science.* 1993 Jan 1;259:87–91.
18. Beisel WR. History of nutritional immunology: Introduction and overview. *J Nutr.* 1992 Mar;122:591–6.
19. Kipnis J, Derecki NC, Yang C, Scrable H. Immunity and cognition: What do age-related dementia, HIV-dementia and 'chemo-brain' have in common? *Trends Immunol.* 2008 Oct;29:455–63.
20. Fernandes G, West A, Good RA. Nutrition, immunity, and cancer—A review. Part III: Effect of diet on the diseases of aging. *Clin Bull.* 1979;9:91–106.
21. Romanyukha AA, Rudnev SG, Sidorov IA. Energy cost of infection burden: An approach to understanding the dynamics of host–pathogen interactions. *J Theor Biol.* 2006 Jul 7;241:1–13.
22. Morley JE, Armbrecht HJ, Farr SA, Kumar VB. The senescence accelerated mouse (SAMP8) as a model for oxidative stress and Alzheimer's disease. *Biochim Biophys Acta.* 2012 May;1822:650–6.
23. Farr SA, Price TO, Banks WA, Ercal N, Morley JE. Effect of alpha-lipoic acid on memory, oxidation, and lifespan in SAMP8 mice. *J Alzheimers Dis.* 2012;32:447–55.
24. Hager K, Kenklies M, McAfoose J, Engel J, Munch G. Alpha-lipoic acid as a new treatment option for Alzheimer's disease—A 48 months follow-up analysis. *J Neural Transm Suppl.* 2007;72:189–93.
25. Evans WJ, Morley JE, Argilés J, Bales C, Baracos V, Guttridge D, Jatoi A et al. Cachexia: A new definition. *Clin Nutr.* 2008 Dec;27:793–9.
26. de Heredia FP, Gomez-Martinez S, Marcos A. Obesity, inflammation and the immune system. *Proc Nutr Soc.* 2012 May;71:332–8.

27. Craft MK, Reed MJ. Immunologic changes in obesity. *Crit Care Clin.* 2010 Oct;26:629–31.

28. Procaccini C, Carbone F, Galgani M, La Rocca C, De Rosa, V, Cassano S, Matarese G. Obesity and susceptibility to autoimmune diseases. *Expert Rev Clin Immunol.* 2011 May;7:287–94.

29. Milner JJ, Beck MA. The impact of obesity on the immune response to infection. *Proc Nutr Soc.* 2012 May;71:298–306.

30. Karlsson EA, Beck MA. The burden of obesity on infectious disease. *Exp Biol Med (Maywood).* 2010 Dec;235:1412–24.

31. O'Shea D, Corrigan M, Dunne MR, Jackson R, Woods C, Gaoatswe G, Moynagh PN, O'Connell J, Hogan AE. Changes in human dendritic cell number and function in severe obesity may contribute to increased susceptibility to viral infection. *Int J Obes (Lond).* 2013 Feb 26;37(11):1510–3.

32. Federico A, D'Aiuto E, Borriello F, Barra G, Gravina AG, Romano M, De Palma R. Fat: A matter of disturbance for the immune system. *World J Gastroenterol.* 2010 Oct 14;16:4762–72.

33. Kaminski DA, Randall TD. Adaptive immunity and adipose tissue biology. *Trends Immunol.* 2010 Oct;31:384–90.

34. Hursting SD, Dunlap SM. Obesity, metabolic dysregulation, and cancer: A growing concern and an inflammatory (and microenvironmental) issue. *Ann N Y Acad Sci.* 2012 Oct;1271:82–7.

35. Vucenik I, Stains JP. Obesity and cancer risk: Evidence, mechanisms, and recommendations. *Ann N Y Acad Sci.* 2012 Oct;1271:37–43.

36. Yehuda-Shnaidman E, Schwartz B. Mechanisms linking obesity, inflammation and altered metabolism to colon carcinogenesis. *Obes Rev.* 2012 Dec;13:1083–95.

37. Levine AS, McClain CJ, Handwerger BS, Brown DM, Morley JE. Tissue zinc status of genetically diabetic and streptozotocin-induced diabetic mice. *Am J Clin Nutr.* 1983 Mar;37:382–6.

38. Kinlaw WB, Levine AS, Morley JE, Silvis SE, McClain CJ. Abnormal zinc metabolism in type II diabetes mellitus. *Am J Med.* 1983 Aug;75:273–7.

39. Niewoehner CB, Allen JI, Boosalis M, Levine AS, Morley JE. Role of zinc supplementation in type II diabetes mellitus. *Am J Med.* 1986 Jul;81:63–8.

40. Chasapis CT, Loutsidou AC, Spiliopoulou CA, Stefanidou ME. Zinc and human health: An update. *Arch Toxicol.* 2012 Apr;86:521–34.

41. Honscheid A, Rink L, Haase H. T-lymphocytes: A target for stimulatory and inhibitory effects of zinc ions. *Endocr Metab Immune Disord Drug Targets.* 2009 Jun;9: 132–44.

42. Bao B, Prasad AS, Beck FW, Godmere M. Zinc modulates mRNA levels of cytokines. *Am J Physiol Endocrinol Metab.* 2003 Nov;285:E1095–102.

43. Kitamura H, Morikawa H, Kamon H, Iguchi M, Hojyo S, Fukada T, Yamashita S, Kaisho T, Akira S, Murakami M, Hirano T. Toll-like receptor-mediated regulation of zinc homeostasis influences dendritic cell function. *Nat Immunol.* 2006 Sep;7:971–7.

44. Morein B, Abusugra I, Blomqvist G. Immunity in neonates. *Vet Immunol Immunopathol.* 2002 Sep 10;87:207–13.

45. Ungvari Z, Buffenstein R, Austad SN, Podlutsky A, Kaley G, Csiszar A. Oxidative stress in vascular senescence: Lessons from successfully aging species. *Front Biosci.* 2008;13:5056–70.

46. Tausk F, Elenkov I, Moynihan J. Psychoneuroimmunology. *Dermatol Ther.* 2008 Jan;21:22–31.

47. Toman M, Faldyna M, Knotigova P, Pokorova D, Sinkora J. Postnatal development of leukocyte subset composition and activity in dogs. *Vet Immunol Immunopathol.* 2002 Sep 10;87:321–6.

48. Marodi L. Neonatal innate immunity to infectious agents. *Infect Immun.* 2006 Apr;74:1999–2006.
49. Marshall-Clarke S, Reen D, Tasker L, Hassan J. Neonatal immunity: How well has it grown up? *Immunol Today.* 2000 Jan;21:35–41.
50. Lee HH, Hoeman CM, Hardaway JC, Guloglu FB, Ellis JS, Jain R, Divekar R, Tartar DM, Haymaker CL, Zaghouani H. Delayed maturation of an IL-12-producing dendritic cell subset explains the early Th2 bias in neonatal immunity. *J Exp Med.* 2008 Sep 29;205:2269–80.
51. Gruver AL, Hudson LL, Sempowski GD. Immunosenescence of ageing. *J Pathol.* 2007 Jan;211:144–56.
52. Mocchegiani E, Santarelli L, Costarelli L, Cipriano C, Muti E, Giacconi R, Malavolta M. Plasticity of neuroendocrine-thymus interactions during ontogeny and ageing: Role of zinc and arginine. *Ageing Res Rev.* 2006 Aug;5:281–309.
53. Pawelec G, Solana R. Immunosenescence. *Immunol Today.* 1997 Nov;18:514–6.
54. Makinodan T. Patterns of age-related immunologic changes. *Nutr Rev.* 1995 Apr;53: S27–31.
55. Mocchegiani E, Giacconi R, Cipriano C, Muzzioli M, Gasparini N, Moresi R, Stecconi R, Suzuki H, Cavalieri E, Mariani E. MtmRNA gene expression, via IL-6 and glucocorticoids, as potential genetic marker of immunosenescence: Lessons from very old mice and humans. *Exp Gerontol.* 2002 Jan;37:349–57.
56. Kav Vedhara MIMRI. *Human Psychoneuroimmunology.* Oxford University Press, USA, 2005.
57. Kiecolt-Glaser JK, McGuire L, Robles TF, Glaser R. Emotions, morbidity, and mortality: New perspectives from psychoneuroimmunology. *Annu Rev Psychol.* 2002;53: 83–107.
58. Kiecolt-Glaser JK, Cacioppo JT, Malarkey WB, Glaser R. Acute psychological stressors and short-term immune changes: What, why, for whom, and to what extent? *Psychosom Med.* 1992 Nov;54:680–5.
59. Kiecolt-Glaser JK, Glaser R, Gravenstein S, Malarkey WB, Sheridan J. Chronic stress alters the immune response to influenza virus vaccine in older adults. *Proc Natl Acad Sci U S A.* 1996 Apr 2;93:3043–7.
60. Morag M, Morag A, Reichenberg A, Lerer B, Yirmiya R. Psychological variables as predictors of rubella antibody titers and fatigue—A prospective, double blind study. *J Psychiatr Res.* 1999 Sep;33:389–95.
61. Vedhara K, Cox NK, Wilcock GK, Perks P, Hunt M, Anderson S, Lightman SL, Shanks NM. Chronic stress in elderly carers of dementia patients and antibody response to influenza vaccination. *Lancet.* 1999 Feb 20;353:627–31.
62. Jabaaij L, van HJ, Vingerhoets JJ, Oostveen FG, Duivenvoorden HJ, Ballieux RE. Modulation of immune response to rDNA hepatitis B vaccination by psychological stress. *J Psychosom Res.* 1996 Aug;41:129–37.
63. Burns EA, Lum LG, Seigneuret MC, Giddings BR, Goodwin JS. Decreased specific antibody synthesis in old adults: Decreased potency of antigen-specific B cells with aging. *Mech Ageing Dev.* 1990 Apr 30;53:229–41.
64. Patriarca PA. A randomized controlled trial of influenza vaccine in the elderly. Scientific scrutiny and ethical responsibility. *JAMA.* 1994 Dec 7;272:1700–1.
65. Cohen S, Tyrrell DA, Smith AP. Psychological stress and susceptibility to the common cold. *N Engl J Med.* 1991 Aug 29;325:606–12.
66. Kehrli ME, Burton JL, Nonnecke BJ, Lee EK. Effects of stress on leukocyte trafficking and immune responses: Implications for vaccination. *Adv Vet Med.* 1999;41: 61–81.
67. Padgett DA, Glaser R. How stress influences the immune response. *Trends Immunol.* 2003 Aug;24:444–8.

68. Mirani M, Elenkov I, Volpi S, Hiroi N, Chrousos GP, Kino T. HIV-1 protein Vpr suppresses IL-12 production from human monocytes by enhancing glucocorticoid action: Potential implications of Vpr coactivator activity for the innate and cellular immunity deficits observed in HIV-1 infection. *J Immunol.* 2002 Dec 1;169:6361–8.

69. Ashwell JD, Vacchio MS, Galon J. Do glucocorticoids participate in thymocyte development? *Immunol Today.* 2000 Dec;21:644–6.

70. Russo-Marie F. Macrophages and the glucocorticoids. *J Neuroimmunol.* 1992 Oct;40:281–6.

71. Shaywitz AJ, Greenberg ME. CREB: A stimulus-induced transcription factor activated by a diverse array of extracellular signals. *Annu Rev Biochem.* 1999;68:821–61.

72. Bengmark S. Immunonutrition—Concluding remarks. *Nutrition.* 1999 Jan;15:57–61.

73. Brandtzaeg P, Halstensen TS, Kett K, Krajci P, Kvale D, Rognum TO, Scott H, Sollid LM. Immunobiology and immunopathology of human gut mucosa: Humoral immunity and intraepithelial lymphocytes. *Gastroenterology.* 1989 Dec;97:1562–84.

74. Brandtzaeg P, Johansen FE. Mucosal B cells: Phenotypic characteristics, transcriptional regulation, and homing properties. *Immunol Rev.* 2005 Aug;206:32–63.

75. Conley ME, Brown P, Bartelt MS. IgG subclass potential of surface IgM-negative and surface IgM-positive human peripheral blood B cells. *Clin Immunol Immunopathol.* 1987 May;43:211–22.

76. Cebra JJ. Influences of microbiota on intestinal immune system development. *Am J Clin Nutr.* 1999 May;69:1046S–51S.

77. Murtaugh MP, Foss DL. Inflammatory cytokines and antigen presenting cell activation. *Vet Immunol Immunopathol.* 2002 Sep 10;87:109–21.

78. van Nevel CJ, Decuypere JA, Dierick N, Molly K. The influence of *Lentinus edodes* (Shiitake mushroom) preparations on bacteriological and morphological aspects of the small intestine in piglets. *Arch Tierernahr.* 2003 Dec;57:399–412.

79. Pietrella D, Mazzolla R, Lupo P, Pitzurra L, Gomez MJ, Cherniak R, Vecchiarelli A. Mannoprotein from *Cryptococcus neoformans* promotes T-helper type 1 anticandidal responses in mice. *Infect Immun.* 2002 Dec;70:6621–7.

80. Holen E, Bjorge OA, Jonsson R. Dietary nucleotides and human immune cells. II. Modulation of PBMC growth and cytokine secretion. *Nutrition.* 2006 Jan;22:90–6.

81. Saavedra JM. Use of probiotics in pediatrics: Rationale, mechanisms of action, and practical aspects. *Nutr Clin Pract.* 2007 Jun;22:351–65.

82. Hannant D. Mucosal immunology: Overview and potential in the veterinary species. *Vet Immunol Immunopathol.* 2002 Sep 10;87:265–7.

83. Hughes DA, Darlington LG, Bendich A (eds.). *Diet and Human Immune Function.* Humana Press, Totowa, NJ, 2004.

84. Gleeson M, Pyne DB, McDonald WA, Bowe SJ, Clancy RL, Fricker PA. *In-vivo* cell mediated immunity in elite swimmers in response to training. *J Sci Med Sport.* 2004 Mar;7:38–46.

85. Cooke MS, Evans MD, Dizdaroglu M, Lunec J. Oxidative DNA damage: Mechanisms, mutation, and disease. *FASEB J.* 2003 Jul;17:1195–214.

86. Cline AM, Radic MZ. Apoptosis, subcellular particles, and autoimmunity. *Clin Immunol.* 2004 Aug;112:175–82.

87. Barger JL, Walford RL, Weindruch R. The retardation of aging by caloric restriction: Its significance in the transgenic era. *Exp Gerontol.* 2003 Nov;38:1343–51.

88. Pahlavani MA. Influence of caloric restriction on aging immune system. *J Nutr Health Aging.* 2004;8:38–47.

89. Greeley EH, Kealy RD, Ballam JM, Lawler DF, Segre M. The influence of age on the canine immune system. *Vet Immunol Immunopathol.* 1996 Dec;55:1–10.

90. Morley JE, Chahla E, Alkaade S. Antiaging, longevity and calorie restriction. *Curr Opin Clin Nutr Metab Care.* 2010 Jan;13:40–5.

91. Anderson R, Smit MJ, Joone GK, Van Staden AM. Vitamin C and cellular immune functions. Protection against hypochlorous acid-mediated inactivation of glyceraldehyde-3-phosphate dehydrogenase and ATP generation in human leukocytes as a possible mechanism of ascorbate-mediated immunostimulation. *Ann N Y Acad Sci.* 1990;587:34–48.

92. Massimino S, Kearns RJ, Loos KM, Burr J, Park JS, Chew B, Adams S, Hayek MG. Effects of age and dietary beta-carotene on immunological variables in dogs. *J Vet Intern Med.* 2003 Nov;17:835–42.

93. Kim HW, Chew BP, Wong TS, Park JS, Weng BB, Byrne KM, Hayek MG, Reinhart GA. Dietary lutein stimulates immune response in the canine. *Vet Immunol Immunopathol.* 2000 May 23;74:315–27.

94. Kim HW, Chew BP, Wong TS, Park JS, Weng BB, Byrne KM, Hayek MG, Reinhart GA. Modulation of humoral and cell-mediated immune responses by dietary lutein in cats. Vet Immunol Immunopathol. 2000 Mar 15;73:331–41

95. Bjelakovic G, Nikolova D, Gluud LL, Simonetti RG, Gluud C. Antioxidant supplements for prevention of mortality in healthy participants and patients with various diseases. *Cochrane Database Syst Rev.* 2012;3:CD007176.

96. Flickinger EA, Fahey GC, Jr. Pet food and feed applications of inulin, oligofructose and other oligosaccharides. *Br J Nutr.* 2002 May;87 Suppl 2:S297–300.

97. Schiffrin EJ, Thomas DR, Kumar VB, Brown C, Hager C, Van't Hof MA, Morley JE, Guigoz Y. Systemic inflammatory markers in older persons: The effect of oral nutritional supplementation with prebiotics. *J Nutr Health Aging.* 2007 Nov;11:475–9.

98. Gill HS, Guarner F. Probiotics and human health: A clinical perspective. *Postgrad Med J.* 2004 Sep;80:516–26.

99. Benyacoub J, Czarnecki-Maulden GL, Cavadini C, Sauthier T, Anderson RE, Schiffrin EJ, von der WT. Supplementation of food with *Enterococcus faecium* (SF68) stimulates immune functions in young dogs. *J Nutr.* 2003 Apr;133:1158–62.

100. Artym J, Zimecki M, Paprocka M, Kruzel ML. Orally administered lactoferrin restores humoral immune response in immunocompromised mice. *Immunol Lett.* 2003 Oct 9;89:9–15.

101. Low PP, Rutherfurd KJ, Gill HS, Cross ML. Effect of dietary whey protein concentrate on primary and secondary antibody responses in immunized BALB/c mice. *Int Immunopharmacol.* 2003 Mar;3:393–401.

102. Bounous G, Gervais F, Amer V, Batist G, Gold P. The influence of dietary whey protein on tissue glutathione and the diseases of aging. *Clin Invest Med.* 1989 Dec;12:343–9.

103. Bounous G, Batist G, Gold P. Immunoenhancing property of dietary whey protein in mice: Role of glutathione. *Clin Invest Med.* 1989 Jun;12:154–61.

104. Satyaraj E, Reynolds A, Pelker R, Labuda J, Zhang P, Sun P. Supplementation of diets with bovine colostrum influences immune function in dogs. *Br J Nutr.* 2013 Dec;110(12):2216–21.

105. Biswas P, Vecchi A, Mantegani P, Mantelli B, Fortis C, Lazzarin A. Immunomodulatory effects of bovine colostrum in human peripheral blood mononuclear cells. *New Microbiol.* 2007 Oct;30:447–54.

106. Shing CM, Peake J, Suzuki K, Okutsu M, Pereira R, Stevenson L, Jenkins DG, Coombes JS. Effects of bovine colostrum supplementation on immune variables in highly trained cyclists. *J Appl Physiol.* 2007 Mar;102:1113–22.

107. Gore AM, Satyaraj E, Labuda J, Pelker R, Sun P. Supplementation of diets with bovine colostrum influences immune and gut function in kittens, personal communication.

108. Casserly IP, Topol EJ. Convergence of atherosclerosis and Alzheimer's disease: Cholesterol, inflammation, and misfolded proteins. *Discov Med.* 2004 Jun;4:149–56.

109. Ames BN, Gold LS. The causes and prevention of cancer: The role of environment. *Biotherapy.* 1998;11:205–20.

110. Ames BN. DNA damage from micronutrient deficiencies is likely to be a major cause of cancer. *Mutat Res.* 2001 Apr 18;475:7–20.
111. Kaput J, Swartz D, Paisley E, Mangian H, Daniel WL, Visek WJ. Diet–disease interactions at the molecular level: An experimental paradigm. *J Nutr.* 1994 Aug;124:1296S–305S.
112. Milner JA. Molecular targets for bioactive food components. *J Nutr.* 2004 Sep;134:2492S–8S.
113. Goldenberg MM. Trastuzumab, a recombinant DNA-derived humanized monoclonal antibody, a novel agent for the treatment of metastatic breast cancer. *Clin Ther.* 1999 Feb;21:309–18.
114. Baselga J, Norton L, Albanell J, Kim YM, Mendelsohn J. Recombinant humanized anti-HER2 antibody (Herceptin) enhances the antitumor activity of paclitaxel and doxorubicin against HER2/neu overexpressing human breast cancer xenografts. *Cancer Res.* 1998 Jul 1;58:2825–31.
115. Touw DJ. Clinical implications of genetic polymorphisms and drug interactions mediated by cytochrome P-450 enzymes. *Drug Metabol Drug Interact.* 1997;14:55–82.
116. Ma D, Forsythe P, Bienenstock J. Live *Lactobacillus rhamnosus* [corrected] is essential for the inhibitory effect on tumor necrosis factor alpha-induced interleukin-8 expression. *Infect Immun.* 2004 Sep;72:5308–14.

3 Micronutrient Deficiency and Immunity

Sarah E. Cusick and Chandy C. John

CONTENTS

Iron 40
    Iron Deficiency and Immunity 40
    Importance of Iron Homeostasis in Immunity 41
    Summary 43
Vitamin A 43
    Vitamin A Function 44
    Mucosal Immunity 44
    Vitamin A and Cellular Immunity 45
    Vitamin A and Humoral Immunity 46
    Summary 46
Zinc 47
    Key *In Vivo* and *In Vitro* Models of Zinc Deficiency 47
    Zinc and IL-2 Expression in HuT-78 Cells 48
    Zinc and B-Lymphocyte Development and Function 48
    Zinc and Infectious Disease 49
    Zinc and Sickle Cell Disease 49
    Summary 49
Vitamin D 50
    Vitamin D and Macrophage Function 50
    Vitamin D and Dendritic Cells 51
    Vitamin D and Cellular Immunity 51
    Vitamin D and Humoral Immunity 52
    Summary 52
References 52

More than two billion people worldwide are deficient in at least one micronutrient [1,2]. Micronutrient deficiencies are sometimes referred to as hidden hunger because they are often not clinically apparent until severe; however, they can have significant health consequences even at subclinical levels [3]. Deficiency of iron, vitamin A, and zinc together account for >10% of deaths among children younger than 5 years, as well as approximately 10% of the disability-adjusted life years, that is, years of life lost because of ill health, early death, or disability among children in this age group

39

[4]. These figures, however, do not take into full account the interaction between micronutrient deficiency and infection [5].

While micronutrient deficiencies each have specific or unique consequences, such as the established relation between iron deficiency in infancy and neurobehavioral impairment, the contribution of vitamin A deficiency to childhood blindness, and the necessity of zinc for optimal linear growth, each of these micronutrients, as well as others, additionally plays an integral role in immunity. Micronutrient deficiencies rarely occur in isolation, making the specific immune consequence of a single nutrient deficiency difficult to parse out, particularly *in vivo*. Results from *in vitro* and animal models, confirmed by improved immunological outcomes with supplementation in human populations, however, have established associations between specific micronutrients and immunologic functions.

This chapter will focus on four micronutrients for which deficiency is common in children, particularly in low-income countries: iron, vitamin A, zinc, and vitamin D. A number of other micronutrients, such as selenium, vitamin C, and vitamin E, also play an important role in immunity; however, deficiency of these micronutrients is uncommon, so they will not be covered in this chapter.

IRON

Iron deficiency is the most common micronutrient deficiency worldwide, affecting >2 billion people [2]. Of all micronutrients, the relation between iron and immunity is perhaps the most complex. A cofactor for ribonucleotide reductase, the enzyme that initiates DNA synthesis, iron is essential for cell replication and thus sustainment of an effective immune response [6,7]. However, iron is also the prize of an intense battle between the host and the invading pathogen. A carefully orchestrated sequence of steps that collectively restrict iron not only from the pathogen but also from the host is the hallmark of a potent immune response to infection, making correction of iron deficiency with supplemental iron, particularly in areas of high frequency of infection, a difficult and potentially dangerous undertaking. The complex interrelatedness between iron and infection is underscored by the fact that it is the only micronutrient whose body status is regulated by a protein, hepcidin, that also is a mediator of the immune response [8].

IRON DEFICIENCY AND IMMUNITY

While little evidence exists to support systematic deficits in humoral immunity in iron-deficient individuals, specific impairments in cell-mediated immunity have been widely reported and reviewed [6,7,9]. Several investigators have reported decreased numbers of T cells and thymic atrophy in iron deficiency, with the reduction proportional to the severity of iron deficiency in both pregnant women and children [6,9–11]. Many [12,13], but not all [14], report an impaired T-lymphocyte proliferative response to a variety of antigens in iron-deficient individuals, perhaps explaining the repeated finding that iron-deficient patients are also more likely than their iron-sufficient counterparts to have an impaired cutaneous delayed hypersensitivity to *Candida*, mumps, diphtheria, tuberculin, trichophyton, and streptokinase–streptodornase [7,9,12,13,15]. This impairment in T-lymphocyte proliferation and resulting delayed cutaneous sensitivity appears to be reversible with iron treatment [7,15].

The reported deficits in cell-mediated immunity with iron deficiency are likely attributable to the essential role of iron in several enzymes affecting immunity, including not only ribonucleotide reductase, which initiates DNA synthesis, but also several additional peroxide-generating and nitric oxide (NO)–generating enzymes critical for immune cell function [6].

Iron also plays a role in the production of cytokines by T cells. Lower levels of specific cytokines, including interleukin (IL)-6 [14,16], IL-2 [17,18], and IL-4 [19], have been reported in iron-deficient individuals. Ekiz et al. [14] hypothesized that lower levels of IL-6 may explain impaired natural killer activity reported in both iron-deficient humans and animals [20–22]. However, lower cytokine levels in iron deficiency may not normalize after iron repletion [17], suggesting that iron deficiency alone may not be the cause of the lower cytokine levels and/or that prior changes induced by iron deficiency cannot be reversed by later iron supplementation.

Finally, as reviewed by Dallman [7], there is strong evidence suggesting that iron deficiency impairs the bactericidal activity of neutrophils and macrophages [12,14], likely as a result of lower levels of the iron-containing enzyme myeloperoxidase, which produces reactive oxygen intermediates that kill intracellular pathogens [6,22]. Ekiz et al. [14] similarly found that the oxidative burst activity and phagocytic activity of monocytes was significantly reduced in children versus those without iron deficiency.

IMPORTANCE OF IRON HOMEOSTASIS IN IMMUNITY

Iron deficiency undoubtedly impairs multiple aspects of the host immune response; however, careful maintenance of body iron homeostasis, including protecting host iron from invading pathogens, is also a critical component of a healthy immune system. Nearly all bacteria require iron for their own survival, and >500 iron-binding bacterial siderophores that tightly bind and capture host iron have been identified [8]. The large portion of the genome of many pathogenic bacteria that is dedicated to iron acquisition pathways highlights the critical nature of host iron for bacterial survival. Human hosts, in turn, have intricate mechanisms for keeping iron away from pathogens at both the systemic and cellular levels, a phenomenon coined "nutritional immunity" [23]. Disturbance of the delicate iron balance between host and pathogen, whether by iron supplementation, other nutritional deficiency, or infection, has the potential to prolong the course of infection or increase its severity.

Systemic and cellular iron statuses interact to achieve overall body iron homeostasis and optimal immune protection [24–26]. On a systemic level, the hepatic antimicrobial protein hepcidin is the principal orchestrator of body iron homeostasis, linking the sites of iron absorption, iron storage, and erythropoiesis [8,27]. High serum iron levels upregulate hepcidin secretion by the liver and downregulate gut iron absorption. Low serum iron in turn downregulates hepcidin production and increases intestinal absorption [28,29]. Hepcidin also binds directly to the protein ferroportin, the only known exporter of iron that is located primarily on macrophages and enterocytes, causing its destabilization and degradation and trapping iron within the reticuloendothelial or intestinal cell [30], where it is predominantly stored as ferritin.

In addition to dietary cues, hepcidin production is also strongly induced by inflammatory cytokines, particularly IL-6, through the STAT3/BMP6 pathway [8,28]. Recent work has revealed that the proinflammatory cytokines tumor necrosis factor α (TNF-α), TGF-β, and IL-22 also stimulate hepcidin production and that hepcidin upregulation, along with reduced transferrin saturation, represents a component of the acute-phase response to *Candida albicans* and influenza A virus *in vivo* [28]. Agonists of Toll-like receptor 4 (TLR4) in macrophages can also stimulate local production of hepcidin, which functions in an autocrine manner to further downregulate ferroportin and withhold iron [31,32]. These findings collectively suggest that hepcidin plays a role in the innate immune response in addition to being a key mediator of body iron homeostasis [28].

The collective effect of increased hepcidin and consequent downregulated expression of ferroportin is withdrawal of iron from extracellular pathogens. Much of the iron withheld as part of the inflammatory response is trapped as ferritin in cells of the mononuclear phagocyte system, primarily macrophages [24–26,33,34]. Macrophages have multiple means of acquiring iron, including primarily phagocytosis of senescent erythrocytes, but also uptake of transferrin-bound iron through membrane-bound transferrin receptors and acquisition of molecular iron by the divalent metal transporter-1 [25,26,34]. Upregulation of these iron acquisition pathways by proinflammatory cytokines is concomitant with hepcidin-induced iron trapping, leading to profound hypoferremia (i.e., low serum iron) and hyperferritinemia (i.e., high ferritin) [35]. In cases of chronically high hepcidin levels and trapped iron, an anemia, often called the anemia of chronic disease, develops. This anemia can occur regardless of dietary iron status and is not refractory to supplemental iron [36].

Several mechanisms that are part of the inflammatory response further withhold iron from pathogens. Lactoferrin, a protein that binds ferric iron, is produced by neutrophils during inflammation and is considered to be an iron scavenger at sites of infection and mucosal surfaces [36]. Lipocalin-2 is an acute-phase response protein produced by neutrophils and macrophages in response to bacterial stimulation of TLRs. Lipocalin-2 captures iron-rich bacterial siderophores, protecting against sepsis and limiting iron-mediated oxidative stress [36–38]. Nramp1 is a recently identified protein that pumps iron across the phagolysosomal membrane in macrophages, effectively removing the metal from the phagosomal space [36,39].

The proinflammatory cytokine–induced withdrawal of iron from extracellular compartments, however, is not without cost. Iron loading of macrophages can promote the growth and virulence of phagocytosed intracellular pathogens, including bacteria such as *Salmonella*, *Escherichia coli*, *Chlamydia*, and *Mycobacterium tuberculosis*; viruses, including HIV; and protozoans, including malaria [24–26,34]. These pathogens have access to the labile iron pool, the metabolically active fraction of cytosolic iron that is available for metabolic purposes [34], and many have evolved iron-capturing mechanisms that evade host defenses. Although lipocalin-2 can hinder iron acquisition by intracellular pathogens, as evidenced by lipocalin-2 knockout mice having increased mortality after exposure to Enterobacteriaceae [40,41], both

Salmonella and *M. tuberculosis* can biochemically modify the protein, sterically prohibiting the binding of lipocalin-2 to siderophores [33,34,42]. Both bacteria, along with *Chlamydia pneumonia* and *Francisella tularensis*, can also acquire ionic iron by upregulating Dmt1 mRNA [34]. Mycobacteria colocalize with transferrin-bound iron in macrophage endosomes and thus are able to take advantage of host iron while avoiding activation of bactericidal mechanisms [34].

While proinflammatory cytokines affect iron homeostasis, iron can also have a profound effect on the inflammatory response. In addition to intracellular pathogens benefiting directly from retained iron, the iron loading of macrophages is also associated with reduced production of TNF-α and IL-6 and impairment of macrophage ability to kill intracellular pathogens through interferon (IFN)-γ-induced expression of NO [24,34,43]. Iron blocks the transcription of inducible or type 2 NO synthase 2 (iNOS or NOS2), the key enzyme of NO production. Recent work by Nairz et al. [43] revealed that NO upregulates ferroportin expression in mouse and human cells and that NOS2 knockout macrophages exhibit increased iron storage and reduced iron egress on account of reduced ferroportin expression. Iron accumulation after infection of NOS2 knockout macrophages with *Salmonella typhimurium* resulted in reduced production of proinflammatory cytokines, including TNF-α, IL-12, and IFN-γ, and reduced pathogen control. The authors proposed that the NOS2–ferroportin axis is an important determinant of iron homeostasis and immune function of macrophage, and serves as a counterbalance to the hepcidin-induced degradation of ferroportin and resulting iron storage during infection.

SUMMARY

In summary, iron and iron homeostasis influence host immune response and immunity to specific pathogens in multiple ways. Iron deficiency does not appear to play a major role in humoral immunity; however, it has important effects on cellular immunity, including a reduction in total number of T cells, reduced lymphocyte proliferation, and decreased production of IL-2, IL-4, and IL-6. In addition, the interplay of factors in iron homeostasis, including iron sequestration and withholding by hepcidin and other proteins including lipocalin-2 and lactoferrin, is critical in regulation of infection; however, the resulting excess iron in macrophages may benefit intracellular pathogens. The balance of adequate iron for optimal host immune response, storage of iron, and avoidance of excess iron availability to pathogens is therefore key to effective control of infection, and the difficulty of achieving this complex balance makes iron supplementation in areas endemic for infections, particularly intracellular pathogens such as malaria, *Salmonella*, and *M. tuberculosis*, a complicated endeavor.

VITAMIN A

Vitamin A deficiency is the second most common nutritional deficiency worldwide, affecting approximately 200 million children younger than 5 years [44]. In addition to being the world's leading cause of preventable blindness, vitamin A deficiency is strongly associated with increased morbidity and mortality in young children, likely as a result of the vitamin's vital role in immune function. The immune-potentiating properties of vitamin A have been recognized since the early 20th century when Edward Mellanby and Harry Green first called the micronutrient an "anti-infective agent" [45]. Scrimshaw et al. [46] similarly noted in 1968 that "no nutritional deficiency is more consistently synergistic with infectious disease than that of vitamin A." Clinically, numerous studies have definitively established the beneficial effects of vitamin A administration to children age 6 months to 5 years, including reductions in all-cause mortality, diarrhea-related and possibly measles-related mortality, diarrhea and measles incidence, and vision problems [47,48]. The mechanisms by which protection from infection and infection-related mortality occurs are still not fully understood; however, a growing body of work has established the necessity of sufficient vitamin A to support several aspects of both innate and acquired immunity, including maintenance of mucosal barriers, activation and differentiation of T cells, modulation of gut immune homeostasis, protection against prolonged inflammation through modulation of the T helper 1 (Th1)/Th2 balance, and expansion of B-cell subsets.

Vitamin A Function

The widespread immune-modulating effects of vitamin A are mediated primarily by its acid derivatives, namely all-*trans*-retinoic acid and 9-*cis*-retinoic acid [49,50], which bind two families of nuclear receptors, the retinoic acid receptors (RARs) and the retinoid X receptors (RXRs). RARs and RXRs form homodimers or heterodimers and bind to retinoic acid response elements (RAREs) located in the regulatory regions of multiple genes, including approximately 100 genes that RAR and RXR are known to regulate directly and >500 genes regulated by the involvement of RAR/RXR with other transcription factors.

Mucosal Immunity

Vitamin A deficiency impairs mucosal immunity in the eye and in the respiratory, gastrointestinal, and genitourinary tracts [50]. Adequate vitamin A is required for epithelial cell maintenance and may regulate both keratinization and mucin production at the transcriptional level. During deficiency, the ciliated columnar epithelial cells of the respiratory tract are replaced by stratified, keratinized epithelium [50,51]. Protective secretions of these cells, including mucin, secretory IgA, and lactoferrin, are also limited. Vitamin A deficiency similarly leads to loss of microvilli, goblet cells, and mucin in the small intestine [50,52]. These vitamin A deficiency–induced epithelial cell changes diminish crucial barrier protection to pathogens and likely explain the repeated finding of increased respiratory infection and diarrhea in vitamin A–deficient children. Similar keratinizing changes have also been reported in the bladder, ureter, kidney, and uterus of vitamin A–deficient individuals, perhaps predisposing vitamin A–deficient children to a greater frequency of urinary tract infections [50,53].

Supplementation with vitamin A has been shown to improve mucosal function in some of these areas. As reviewed by Villamor and Fawzi [54], vitamin A supplementation consistently improves markers of intestinal integrity in young children, particularly when the children are severely malnourished or experiencing severe infection. The benefits of supplementation on respiratory infection are less evident, likely due to the multifactorial etiology of respiratory infections.

VITAMIN A AND CELLULAR IMMUNITY

Retinoic acid is required in the bone marrow for terminal differentiation of myeloid cells, including neutrophils, macrophages, and dendritic cells (DCs) and is essential for their function [55,56]. Vitamin A deficiency in animals impairs neutrophil function, including chemotaxis, adhesion, phagocytosis, and ability to generate reactive oxidant molecules, although the overall number of neutrophils appears unaffected [50,57]. Macrophage function is similarly impaired. *In vivo* treatment with all-*trans*-retinol significantly enhanced the phagocytic activity and production of reactive oxygen species in Kupffer cells of rats, while peripheral blood monocytes from vitamin A–treated rats also had increased respiratory burst activity [58,59]. Vitamin A also affects macrophage cytokine production, upregulating the production of TGF-β, IL6, and IL-1 in human monocytes [50,54]. In contrast, vitamin A supplementation of deficient children lowers concentrations of the proinflammatory cytokines TNF-α and IL-6 after exposure to specific pathogens [50,54]. These findings likely reflect the multiple pathways through which vitamin A may affect *in vivo* cytokine production, including through preferential differentiation of naïve precursor CD4$^+$ T cells into Th2 cells, perhaps by activation of specific transcription factors, discussed below [60].

Retinoic acid also has profound effects on the maturation of DCs, not only by affecting the strength and quality of antigen-specific T- and B-cell responses, but also by playing a specific key role in gut immune homeostasis [60,61]. A series of studies by Iwata et al. [62,63] revealed that expression of two molecules integral for the migration of gut-homing T cells, cell-surface chemokine receptor (CCR9), and $\alpha_4\beta_7$ integrin was dependent on retinoic acid and was significantly reduced in vitamin A–deficient mice. Work by the same group and others showed that specific subsets of DCs are themselves able to generate retinoic acid from retinol and that retinoic acid increased the expression of CCR9 and $\alpha_4\beta_7$ and increased T-cell chemotactic activity [61]. These retinoic acid–generating, gut-associated DCs, located in Peyer's patches and mesenteric lymph nodes of the intestine, play a critical role in gut immune function through the homing of T cells, generation of regulatory T cells (Tregs), and modulation of the Th1/Th2/Th17 balance [55,56,60]. During retinoic acid deficiency, an unusual subset of DCs develop that have an enhanced ability to induce Th17 cells but a decreased ability to produce Tregs, worsening tissue inflammation [55,64,65].

Vitamin A deficiency in children has been shown to reduce T-cell counts, particularly CD4$^+$ naïve T cells [54,66,67] and can also alter the function and differentiation of T cells in response to antigens, specifically enhancing differentiation of CD4$^+$ naïve T cells into Th1 cells while limiting the production of Th2 cells [55,60,68]. Vitamin A deficiency promotes differentiation into Th1 cells, while vitamin A supplementation promotes differentiation into Th2 cells. Vitamin A may act on T-cell differentiation directly, through specific transcription factors [60], or indirectly, through modulation of DCs or increased production of counterbalancing Tregs. Vitamin A supplementation has been associated with reduced incidence of intestinal parasitic infection, including *Giardia* and *Ascaris* [54]. This protection may be due to upregulation of the Th2 response, which is critical in immune protection from intestinal parasites.

As reviewed by Ross [60], a third major subset of T helper cells, Th17 have also recently been identified. These cells, which play a major role in the inflammatory response, are activated in the presence of TGF-β and IL-6. Th17 cells promote inflammation, particularly at mucosal barriers, and like Th1 cells, Th17 cells can cause excessive activation and tissue damage if left unchecked. Vitamin A has been shown to reduce Th17 cell commitment, perhaps through upregulation of counterbalancing Tregs. In the presence of TGF-β but low IL-6, Treg differentiation is favored [60]. The balance between Th17 and Foxp3+ Tregs under the influence of retinoic acid has emerged as a critical player in the maintenance of normal mucosal immunity, particularly in the intestine [55,60,61].

Vitamin A and Humoral Immunity

In addition to the induction of Tregs in the gut, vitamin A is also required for B cell–mediated IgA antibody responses. Vitamin A deficiency is associated with defective IgA production and defective transport of IgA across the epithelial cell barrier in mucosal tissues [55,69]. Retinoic acid directly affects antibody class switching of B cells and can also act through DC and T cells to promote antibody production [55]. Vitamin A may also protect against infectious disease by enhancing antibody responses to T-cell-dependent and type II T-cell-independent antigens. However, studies of antibodies to measles and tetanus vaccines in children receiving concurrent vitamin A have shown variable results. Some studies show no difference in measles antibody seroconversion and/or levels [70–72]; however, others show an increase in seroconversion or levels [73]. Similarly, some trials suggest also that antibody titers against tetanus toxoid are higher in children if vitamin A is administered before vaccination [54], particularly if the child is vitamin A deficient; however, others document no difference in antibodies to tetanus in those given vitamin A concurrently with immunization [74]. The most compelling evidence of vitamin A's effects on long-term antibody levels comes from a follow-up study that showed that children given concurrent vitamin A at the time of measles vaccination at 9 months of age were more likely to have protective measles antibody titers at age 6–8 years than those who had not received vitamin A [75]. However, vitamin A also appears to have complex interactions with age, sex, and vaccine antigen, and may negatively or beneficially affect immune responses and adverse effects to vaccines, depending on vaccine given, sex, and age at time of vaccine administration [76].

Summary

Vitamin A is essential for optimal immune function, playing a critical role in the maintenance of barrier immunity, modulation of gut immune homeostasis, protection against excess inflammation through modulation of the Th1/Th2/Th17 balance, and expansion of B-cell subsets. This wide range of roles in immunity likely explains the repeated findings of benefit of vitamin A supplementation in reducing all-cause child mortality, diarrhea incidence and persistence, and the severity of certain infectious diseases, including measles. More research is needed to establish a clear benefit between vitamin A and malaria and also the benefit or possible harm of administering vitamin A concurrently with childhood vaccinations.

ZINC

Zinc is present in all human body tissues and fluids and is the second most abundant trace mineral after iron [77]. Zinc is required for the function of >100 enzymes and plays a critical role in protein, carbohydrate, and lipid metabolism and DNA synthesis [78]. While the importance of zinc in plant and animal health has been known since the 1930s, its essentiality for human health was not recognized until the 1960s, when, during studies in the Middle East, Prasad et al. [79–81] identified a group of zinc-deficient dwarfs who did not survive past 25 years of age. Their death was due to infection; however, the exact cause was unclear. Since that time, studies by Prasad and other groups have collectively demonstrated several specific and essential functions of zinc in immune function. Clinical studies reinforce their findings, with zinc supplementation significantly and consistently reducing the incidence of pneumonia and diarrhea [82–87], the first and second leading causes of death, respectively, of children younger than 5 years worldwide [88]. Zinc also has established benefit in strengthening immunity in patients with sickle cell disease (SCD) or malaria as well as in the elderly [79,89]. Finally, zinc sufficiency in the prenatal period helps ensure continued immune competence throughout the first years of life [80].

KEY *IN VIVO* AND *IN VITRO* MODELS OF ZINC DEFICIENCY

Two series of studies by Prasad et al., one involving an *in vivo* human model of zinc deficiency and one using HuT-78 cells, a human Th0 malignant lymphoblastoid cell line, have established the foundation of current knowledge of the effects of zinc deficiency on immunity [79–81,90]. In the human model, male volunteers 20–45 years of age underwent baseline, zinc-depletion, and zinc-repletion phases that induced a specific zinc deficiency and permitted the investigators to assess both the effect of deficiency on immune function as well as the effect of zinc repletion on any observed consequence [91,92].

A primary finding was that the activity of thymulin, the thymus-specific hormone that promotes T-lymphocyte maturation, cytotoxicity, and IL-2 production, was significantly impaired even with mild zinc deficiency [93]. Zinc repletion corrected this deficit. Concentrations of the Th1 cytokines IL-2, IFN-γ, and TNF-α were also significantly lower in the zinc-depletion phase, but were restored by zinc repletion. Concentrations of the Th2 cytokines IL-4, IL-6, and IL-10 were unaffected [91]. This latter finding suggested an imbalance of Th1 and Th2 in zinc-deficient individuals, a finding that has been replicated by others [94]. Natural killer cell lytic activity was also reduced by zinc deficiency, likely due to diminished production of IL-2 [79]. Finally, zinc deficiency reduced, and zinc repletion corrected, the CD4+ to CD8+ ratio, suggesting that zinc may be required for regeneration of new CD4+ T lymphocytes. The percentage of CD8+CD73+ T lymphocytes, cytotoxic T-lymphocyte precursors, was also decreased [79,91].

Others have similarly reported decreased concentrations and depressed function of T lymphocytes in zinc-deficient mice and humans. As reviewed by Shankar and Prasad [80], several authors have reported suppressed delayed hypersensitivity responses and reduced cytotoxic activity during zinc deficiency. Zinc also appears to modify lymphocyte surface molecules that govern cell-to-cell interaction, including the enhancement of the transcription and translation of ICAM-1 on the surface of lymphoid cells.

Finally, zinc is an antioxidant and may protect lymphocytes from oxidative damage during immune activation [95]. Zinc upregulates metallothionein production in lymphocytes that also has antioxidant activity [80,96]. Daily zinc supplementation (45 mg) of healthy volunteers for 8 weeks in one study resulted in decreased plasma levels of lipid peroxidation products and DNA adducts. These markers did not change significantly in volunteers who received placebo [97].

Zinc and IL-2 Expression in HuT-78 Cells

In vitro findings in HuT-78 cells by Prasad [90] provided mechanistic explanation to the observed *in vivo* deficits in cell-mediated immunity. Using HuT78, a human malignant T-lymphoblastoid cell line, investigators found that the gene expression of IL-2 was 50% lower in zinc-deficient cells stimulated with phytohemagglutinin/phorbol myristate acetate than in zinc-sufficient cells [98]. They additionally found decreased gene expression of receptors IL2-α and IL2-β, and demonstrated that this decrease was at least in part attributable to decreased activation of NF-Kβ in zinc-deficient cells. NF-Kβ is a zinc finger protein in the promoter region of IL-2 and IL-2Rα. IL-2 mediates the activation of T lymphocytes by triggering peripheral T lymphocytes to enter the S phase of the cell cycle and divide; thus, these findings of reduced IL-2 and IL-2 receptor expression in zinc-deficient cells likely explain the lymphopenia reported in zinc-deficient individuals [79].

Zinc and B-Lymphocyte Development and Function

Zinc deficiency in mice is associated with a significant reduction of B-lymphocyte development in bone marrow, resulting in fewer B lymphocytes in the spleen. Pre-B and immature B lymphocytes appear to be most affected, with a much smaller effect on mature B lymphocytes observed [80]. Zinc deficiency also impairs B-lymphocyte antibody responses. T-cell-dependent antibody responses appear to be more inhibited than T-cell-independent responses, although zinc-deficient mice exhibited a reduced antibody recall response to both T-dependent and T-independent antigens for which they had previously been immunized [80].

ZINC AND INFECTIOUS DISEASE

Diarrhea is the second leading cause of death among children younger than 5 years in the developing world [88]. Placebo-controlled trials conducted in a variety of geographic regions have demonstrated that zinc supplementation has a consistent and strong effect on the reduction of diarrhea prevalence and incidence [82–86]. The beneficial effect appears to extend beyond the period of supplementation [99,100]. A 1998 meta-analysis of nine randomized, controlled trials of zinc supplementation in low-income countries in Latin America, Africa, southeast Asia, and the western Pacific found that zinc supplementation was associated with an overall 18% reduction in the incidence of diarrhea and a 25% reduction in the prevalence of diarrhea [82]. An updated 2010 review of 10 studies found that zinc supplementation reduced the proportion of diarrheal episodes that lasted >7 days, risk of hospitalization, and all-cause mortality, and reduced diarrhea-specific mortality by 23% [101].

Zinc supplementation also has an established effect of reducing the incidence of acute lower respiratory infections, including pneumonia, the leading cause of death in children younger than 5 years [88]. A pooled analysis of trials of zinc supplementation in India, Jamaica, Peru, and Vietnam found that zinc-supplemented children had an overall 41% reduction in the incidence of pneumonia compared with non-supplemented children [78,82]. Some trials have shown a benefit of zinc supplementation on malaria morbidity [102,103]; however, recent large trials [104,105] failed to show a benefit and a meta-analysis concluded that there is insufficient evidence that zinc supplementation reduces malaria incidence [106]. A recent study of combined vitamin A and zinc supplementation showed a reduction in malaria incidence in the group receiving supplementation, suggesting that combined therapy with vitamin A and zinc may reduce malaria morbidity than either therapy alone [107].

ZINC AND SICKLE CELL DISEASE

In patients with SCD, frequent hemolysis in the context of diminished zinc reabsorption due to renal tubular damage increases the daily requirement for zinc. This requirement is frequently not met, leaving many SCD patients zinc deficient. SCD patients have diminished immunity, marked by depressed peripheral T-lymphocyte numbers, a reduced $CD4^+/CD8^+$ lymphocyte ratio, loss of delayed hypersensitivity, lower natural killer cell activity, and lower production of IL-2 [108]. Zinc supplementation has been shown to restore these indices to near-normal values, and in a placebo-controlled trial, zinc decreased the incidence of *Staphylococcus aureus* pneumonia, *S. pneumoniae* tonsillitis, and *E. coli* urinary tract infections in SCD patients [109].

SUMMARY

Zinc is essential for thymulin activity, IL-2 production, and T-lymphocyte proliferation. It also maintains the balance between Th1 and Th2 cells and B-lymphocyte antibody responses. Zinc supplementation in children reduces the incidence and severity of diarrhea and acute lower respiratory infections, the two leading causes of mortality in children younger than 5 years worldwide. An ameliorative effect of zinc on malaria morbidity is less clear; however, administration of zinc with vitamin A or other micronutrients may strengthen the beneficial relation reported by some.

VITAMIN D

The discovery that vitamin D has significant beneficial effects on human health besides its well-known classic effects on calcium homeostasis and bone health has been relatively recent [110–112]. Important immune-modulating effects, particularly with respect to infectious and autoimmune disease, but also in cancer and cardiovascular disease, are among these "nonclassic effects" of vitamin D. Total circulating vitamin D, referred to as 25(OH)D, is the sum of vitamin D photosynthesized in the skin in response to UVB rays from the sun along with dietary vitamin D consumed in food and supplements [111,113]. The 25(OH)D threshold to defined deficiency was originally set at <20 ng/mL (<50 nmol/L), a level that would be protective against rachitic disease. However, the finding that the inverse relation with vitamin D and parathyroid hormone exists until 25(OH)D is between 30 and 40 ng/mL has led many experts to accept a 25(OH)D level of 21–29 ng/mL as representative of vitamin D "insufficient" [111,114]. Using this cutoff of <30 ng/mL, it is estimated that 1 billion people worldwide are vitamin D insufficient, causing vitamin D deficiency to be referred to as a worldwide pandemic [111,114,115]. As described in the next section, vitamin D insufficiency not only increases the risk of skeletal disease but also potentially disrupts immune homeostasis.

VITAMIN D AND MACROPHAGE FUNCTION

The first link between vitamin D and immunity came with reports in the early 1980s of the ability of vitamin D to stimulate differentiation of precursor macrophages into more mature phagocytic macrophages [116–118]. The findings that macrophages of different maturational stages exhibited different levels of both 1α-hydroxylase, the enzyme that catalyzes the conversion of 25(OH)D into the active form of vitamin D, 1,25-dihydroxyvitamin D3 $(1,25(OH)_2D_3)$, and also the vitamin D receptor (VDR) [116,117], supported these findings, as did the finding that IFN-γ stimulated the synthesis of $1,25(OH)_2D_3$ [119].

Work by Liu et al. in 2006 [120] provided a mechanistic explanation for the reported role of vitamin D as a powerful macrophage stimulator. Using DNA array analysis, Liu et al. found that activation of TLR2/1 in human macrophages upregulated the expression of both VDR and the gene for 1α-hydroxylase, leading to induction of cathelicidin, an antimicrobial protein, and subsequent enhanced intracellular killing of M. tuberculosis [120]. Prior studies had revealed that the 1,25(OH)2D–VDR complex directly stimulated transcriptions of the gene for cathelicidin, LL-37, through a VDRE within the LL-37 gene promoter [110,121]. The investigators additionally demonstrated that the vitamin D status of the individual affected the size of the cathelicidin response, showing that the sera of African Americans, a group known to have lower serum 25(OH)D, was less efficient than that of sera from Caucasian donors in supporting cathelicidin mRNA induction [120]. A subsequent study by Adams et al. [122] confirmed these findings, demonstrating that *in vivo* supplementation with vitamin D increased the levels of TLR2/1-induced LL-37. This work established localized synthesis of $1,25(OH)_2D_3$ as a key link between TLR activation and antibacterial responses in innate immunity [120].

As reviewed by Hewison [110], subsequent work has revealed that antibacterial activity of vitamin D metabolites is not restricted to macrophages, but also occurs in bronchial epithelial cells, myeloid cell lines, decidual and trophoblastic cells of the placenta, and keratinocytes. Cathelicidin is also not the only antibacterial protein whose production is known to be upregulated by $1,25(OH)_2D$ [110]. Work by Wang et al. [123] revealed that *DEFB4*, the gene for antibacterial protein β-defensin, is similarly stimulated by $1,25(OH)_2D_3$, although apparently in conjunction with NF-κB [110].

VITAMIN D AND DENDRITIC CELLS

The activity of vitamin D and its metabolites in modulation of the immune response is also evident in DCs, the principal antigen-presenting cells of the innate immune system and a link between the innate and adaptive immune systems. Brennan et al. [124] first reported that DCs express VDR in 1987. Studies by Adorini and Kumar [reviewed in 110,116] demonstrated that $1,25(OH)_2D_3$ and its synthetic analogs inhibited DC differentiation and maturation and limited their antigen-presenting capacity, particularly among myeloid DCs. This decreased DC maturation was concomitant with increased expression of Tregs [125]. Vitamin D thus promotes a tolerogenic and immunosuppressive phenotype.

This tolerogenic phenotype is further supported by DC expression of 1α-hydroxylase and VDR. As reviewed by Hewison [110,116], 1α-hydroxylase activity increases as DCs mature; however, mature DCs express lower levels of VDR than immature DCs. This structure promotes a tolerogenic phenotype in that locally produced $1,25(OH)_2D_3$ permits an initial T-cell response while preventing overstimulation of T cells.

VITAMIN D AND CELLULAR IMMUNITY

While the initial link between vitamin D and improved immunity against *M. tuberculosis* was in the innate immune system and upregulated antibacterial activity of macrophages through TLR1/2 stimulation, more recent work has highlighted the complementary and strengthening role of vitamin D in the adaptive immune system. T cells express VDR, and several investigators have demonstrated that cytokines from different T-cell subsets have different effects on innate immune responses to vitamin D. For example, Fabri et al. [126] showed that IFN-γ, a Th1 cytokine, enhances TLR1/2 activation and consequent production of cathelicidin and β-defensin, while IL-4, a Th2 cytokine, attenuates the TLR1/2 response. Lemire et al. [127] demonstrated that vitamin D promotes a T-cell shift from Th1 to Th2 *in vitro*, but subsequent experiments in mice failed to confirm these findings and suggest that the effect of vitamin D on T-cell subsets *in vivo* is more complex [110]. The predominant evidence, however, suggests that vitamin D deficiency promotes a Th1-dominant environment, while sufficiency promotes a Th2-dominant environment. Thus, vitamin D deficiency promotes a Th1-dominant environment, while Th1 cytokines, perhaps in feedback response, enhance TLR1/2 activation and the production of cathelicidin and β-defensin.

Although the mechanism has not been fully identified, vitamin D also plays a key role in the regulation of Th17 cytokines. In animal models of the gastrointestinal inflammatory disease colitis, treatment with $1,25(OH)_2D_3$, the active form of vitamin D, reduced the expression of Th17 [110,116]. Finally, vitamin D promotes the action of suppressor cells, or Tregs, both through the direct stimulatory action of $1,25(OH)_2D_3$ on VDR on regulatory IL-10-producing CD4+/CD25+ Treg T cells and also by the promotion of immature DCs and enhanced tolerogenic Treg activity. This action may explain the beneficial role of vitamin D in autoimmune disease [110,116].

VITAMIN D AND HUMORAL IMMUNITY

Like T cells, B cells also express VDR, and recent work by Chen et al. [128] clearly demonstrated that 1,25(OH)2D3 can directly affect B-cell homeostasis. In patients with systemic lupus erythematosus, 1,25(OH)2D3 inhibited the proliferation of activated B cells and induced their apoptosis, while initial cell division was unaffected. Development of plasma cells and post-switch memory B cells was also impaired. Chen et al. also found that B cells from patients with lupus expressed mRNA for 1α-hydroxylases and 24-hydroxylase in addition to VDR. Their results, clearly demonstrating the immune modulating effects on B cells, underscore the potential beneficial role vitamin D therapy may play in the treatment of B-cell-mediated autoimmune disorders.

SUMMARY

Recognition of the role of vitamin D in immunity is relatively recent but rapidly increasing. Vitamin D stimulates the maturation of macrophages and is the apparent link between TLR activation and subsequent killing of intracellular pathogens such as *M. tuberculosis* through the production of antibacterial proteins, including cathelicidin. Through modulation of DC maturation and stimulation, vitamin D and its metabolites permit an initial T-cell response, but prevent overstimulation, causing many to describe vitamin D as promoting a tolerogenic phenotype. Vitamin D stimulation of Tregs and maintenance of Th1/Th2/Th17 balance further supports this description and likely explains the beneficial role of vitamin D in autoimmune disease.

REFERENCES

1. Ramakrishnan, U., Prevalence of micronutrient malnutrition worldwide. *Nutr Rev*, 2002. **60**(5 Pt 2): S46–52.
2. Stoltzfus, R., Defining iron-deficiency anemia in public health terms: A time for reflection. *J Nutr*, 2001. **131**(2S–2): 565S–7S.
3. Muthayya, S. et al., The global hidden hunger indices and maps: An advocacy tool for action. *PLoS One*, 2013. **8**(6): e67860.

4. Black, R.E. et al., Maternal and child undernutrition: Global and regional exposures and health consequences. *Lancet*, 2008. **371**(9608): 243–60.

5. Habicht, J.P., Malnutrition kills directly, not indirectly. *Lancet*, 2008. **371**(9626): 1749–50; author reply 1750.

6. Beard, J.L., Iron biology in immune function, muscle metabolism and neuronal functioning. *J Nutr*, 2001. **131**(2S–2): 568S–79S; discussion 580S.

7. Dallman, P.R., Iron deficiency and the immune response. *Am J Clin Nutr*, 1987. **46**(2): 329–34.

8. Drakesmith, H. and A.M. Prentice, Hepcidin and the iron–infection axis. *Science*, 2012. **338**(6108): 768–72.

9. Oppenheimer, S.J., Iron and its relation to immunity and infectious disease. *J Nutr*, 2001. **131**(2S–2): 616S–33S; discussion 633S–5S.

10. Hershko, C., Iron, infection and immune function. *Proc Nutr Soc*, 1993. **52**(1): 165–74.

11. Kuvibidila, S. et al., Influence of iron-deficiency anemia on selected thymus functions in mice: Thymulin biological activity, T-cell subsets, and thymocyte proliferation. *Am J Clin Nutr*, 1990. **51**(2): 228–32.

12. Chandra, R.K. and A.K. Saraya, Impaired immunocompetence associated with iron deficiency. *J Pediatr*, 1975. **86**(6): 899–902.

13. Joynson, D.H. et al., Defect of cell-mediated immunity in patients with iron-deficiency anaemia. *Lancet*, 1972. **2**(7786): 1058–9.

14. Ekiz, C. et al., The effect of iron deficiency anemia on the function of the immune system. *Hematol J*, 2005. **5**(7): 579–83.

15. Macdougall, L.G. et al., The immune response in iron-deficient children: Impaired cellular defense mechanisms with altered humoral components. *J Pediatr*, 1975. **86**(6): 833–43.

16. Feng, X.B., X.Q. Yang, and J. Shen, Influence of iron deficiency on serum IgG subclass and pneumococcal polysaccharides specific IgG subclass antibodies. *Chin Med J (Engl)*, 1994. **107**(11): 813–6.

17. Thibault, H. et al., The immune response in iron-deficient young children: Effect of iron supplementation on cell-mediated immunity. *Eur J Pediatr*, 1993. **152**(2): 120–4.

18. Sipahi, T. et al., Serum interleukin-2 and interleukin-6 levels in iron deficiency anemia. *Pediatr Hematol Oncol*, 1998. **15**(1): 69–73.

19. Kuvibidila, S.R. et al., Iron deficiency reduces serum and in vitro secretion of interleukin-4 in mice independent of altered spleen cell proliferation. *Nutr Res*, 2012. **32**(2): 107–15.

20. Dhur, A., P. Galan, and S. Hercberg, Iron status, immune capacity and resistance to infections. *Comp Biochem Physiol A Comp Physiol*, 1989. **94**(1): 11–9.

21. Hallquist, N.A. et al., Maternal-iron-deficiency effects on peritoneal macrophage and peritoneal natural-killer-cell cytotoxicity in rat pups. *Am J Clin Nutr*, 1992. **55**(3): 741–6.

22. Spear, A.T. and A.R. Sherman, Iron deficiency alters DMBA-induced tumor burden and natural killer cell cytotoxicity in rats. *J Nutr*, 1992. **122**(1): 46–55.

23. Weinberg, E.D., Modulation of intramacrophage iron metabolism during microbial cell invasion. *Microbes Infect*, 2000. **2**(1): 85–9.

24. Collins, H.L., Withholding iron as a cellular defence mechanism—Friend or foe? *Eur J Immunol*, 2008. **38**(7): 1803–6.

25. Recalcati, S., M. Locati, and G. Cairo, Systemic and cellular consequences of macrophage control of iron metabolism. *Semin Immunol*, 2012. **24**(6): 393–8.

26. Weiss, G., Iron and immunity: A double-edged sword. *Eur J Clin Invest*, 2002. **32 Suppl 1**: 70–8.

27. Ganz, T., Hepcidin and iron regulation, 10 years later. *Blood*, 2011. **117**(17): 4425–33.

28. Armitage, A.E. et al., Hepcidin regulation by innate immune and infectious stimuli. *Blood*, 2011. **118**(15): 4129–39.
29. Nemeth, E. and T. Ganz, The role of hepcidin in iron metabolism. *Acta Haematol*, 2009. **122**(2–3): 78–86.
30. Nemeth, E. et al., Hepcidin regulates cellular iron efflux by binding to ferroportin and inducing its internalization. *Science*, 2004. **306**(5704): 2090–3.
31. Peyssonnaux, C. et al., TLR4-dependent hepcidin expression by myeloid cells in response to bacterial pathogens. *Blood*, 2006. **107**(9): 3727–32.
32. Theurl, I. et al., Autocrine formation of hepcidin induces iron retention in human monocytes. *Blood*, 2008. **111**(4): 2392–9.
33. Cherayil, B.J., S. Ellenbogen, and N.N. Shanmugam, Iron and intestinal immunity. *Curr Opin Gastroenterology*, 2011. **27**(6): 523–8.
34. Nairz, M. et al., The struggle for iron—A metal at the host-pathogen interface. *Cell Microbiol*, 2010. **12**(12): 1691–702.
35. Scharte, M. and M.P. Fink, Red blood cell physiology in critical illness. *Crit Care Med*, 2003. **31**(12 Suppl): S651–7.
36. Wessling-Resnick, M., Iron homeostasis and the inflammatory response. *Annu Rev Nutr*, 2010. **30**: 105–22.
37. Correnti, C. and R.K. Strong, Mammalian siderophores, siderophore-binding lipocalins, and the labile iron pool. *J Biol Chem*, 2012. **287**(17): 13524–31.
38. Srinivasan, G. et al., Lipocalin 2 deficiency dysregulates iron homeostasis and exacerbates endotoxin-induced sepsis. *J Immunol*, 2012. **189**(4): 1911–9.
39. Canonne-Hergaux, F. et al., The Nramp1 protein and its role in resistance to infection and macrophage function. *Proc Assoc Am Physicians*, 1999. **111**(4): 283–9.
40. Berger, T. et al., Lipocalin 2-deficient mice exhibit increased sensitivity to *Escherichia coli* infection but not to ischemia–reperfusion injury. *Proc Natl Acad Sci U S A*, 2006. **103**(6): 1834–9.
41. Flo, T.H. et al., Lipocalin 2 mediates an innate immune response to bacterial infection by sequestrating iron. *Nature*, 2004. **432**(7019): 917–21.
42. Raffatellu, M. et al., Lipocalin-2 resistance confers an advantage to *Salmonella enterica* serotype Typhimurium for growth and survival in the inflamed intestine. *Cell Host Microbe*, 2009. **5**(5): 476–86.
43. Nairz, M. et al., Nitric oxide-mediated regulation of ferroportin-1 controls macrophage iron homeostasis and immune function in *Salmonella* infection. *J Exp Med*, 2013. **210**(5): 855–73.
44. World Health Organization, Global prevalence of vitamin A deficiency in populations at risk 1995–2005. *WHO Global Database on Vitamin A Deficiency*, 2009. Geneva: World Health Organization.
45. Green, H.N. and E. Mellanby, Vitamin A as an anti-infective agent. *Br Med J*, 1928. **2**(3537): 691–6.
46. Scrimshaw, N.S., C.E. Taylor, and J.E. Gordon, Interactions of nutrition and infection. *World Health Organization Monograph Series*, 1968. Geneva: World Health Organization, 329 pp.
47. Mayo-Wilson, E. et al., Vitamin A supplements for preventing mortality, illness, and blindness in children aged under 5: Systematic review and meta-analysis. *BMJ*, 2011. **343**: d5094.
48. Sudfeld, C.R., A.M. Navar, and N.A. Halsey, Effectiveness of measles vaccination and vitamin A treatment. *Int J Epidemiol*, 2010. **39 Suppl 1**: i48–55.
49. Chambon, P., A decade of molecular biology of retinoic acid receptors. *FASEB J*, 1996. **10**(9): 940–54.
50. Semba, R.D., The role of vitamin A and related retinoids in immune function. *Nutr Rev*, 1998. **56**(1 Pt 2): S38–48.

51. McDowell, E.M., K.P. Keenan, and M. Huang, Effects of vitamin A-deprivation on hamster tracheal epithelium. A quantitative morphologic study. *Virchows Arch B Cell Pathol Incl Mol Pathol*, 1984. **45**(2): 197–219.

52. Rojanapo, W., A.J. Lamb, and J.A. Olson, The prevalence, metabolism and migration of goblet cells in rat intestine following the induction of rapid, synchronous vitamin A deficiency. *J Nutr*, 1980. **110**(1): 178–88.

53. Brown, K.H., A. Gaffar, and S.M. Alamgir, Xerophthalmia, protein–calorie malnutrition, and infections in children. *J Pediatr*, 1979. **95**(4): 651–6.

54. Villamor, E. and W.W. Fawzi, Effects of vitamin a supplementation on immune responses and correlation with clinical outcomes. *Clin Microbiol Rev*, 2005. **18**(3): 446–64.

55. Kim, C.H., Retinoic acid, immunity, and inflammation. *Vitam Horm*, 2011. **86**: 83–101.

56. Manicassamy, S. and B. Pulendran, Retinoic acid–dependent regulation of immune responses by dendritic cells and macrophages. *Semin Immunol*, 2009. **21**(1): 22–7.

57. Twining, S.S. et al., Vitamin A deficiency alters rat neutrophil function. *J Nutr*, 1997. **127**(4): 558–65.

58. Erickson, K.L., E.A. Medina, and N.E. Hubbard, Micronutrients and innate immunity. *J Infect Dis*, 2000. **182 Suppl 1**: S5–10.

59. Hoglen, N.C. et al., Modulation of Kupffer cell and peripheral blood monocyte activity by in vivo treatment of rats with all-*trans*-retinol. *Liver*, 1997. **17**(3): 157–65.

60. Ross, A.C., Vitamin A and retinoic acid in T cell-related immunity. *Am J Clin Nutr*, 2012. **96**(5): 1166S–72S.

61. Cassani, B. et al., Vitamin A and immune regulation: Role of retinoic acid in gut-associated dendritic cell education, immune protection and tolerance. *Mol Aspects Med*, 2012. **33**(1): 63–76.

62. Iwata, M., Retinoic acid production by intestinal dendritic cells and its role in T-cell trafficking. *Semin Immunol*, 2009. **21**(1): 8–13.

63. Iwata, M. et al., Retinoic acid imprints gut-homing specificity on T cells. *Immunity*, 2004. **21**(4): 527–38.

64. Kang, S.G. et al., High and low vitamin A therapies induce distinct FoxP3+ T-cell subsets and effectively control intestinal inflammation. *Gastroenterology*, 2009. **137**(4): 1391–402.e1–6.

65. Saurer, L., K.C. McCullough, and A. Summerfield, In vitro induction of mucosa-type dendritic cells by all-trans retinoic acid. *J Immunol*, 2007. **179**(6): 3504–14.

66. Semba, R.D. et al., Abnormal T-cell subset proportions in vitamin-A-deficient children. *Lancet*, 1993. **341**(8836): 5–8.

67. Stephensen, C.B., Vitamin A, infection, and immune function. *Annu Rev Nutr*, 2001. **21**: 167–92.

68. Carman, J.A., S.M. Smith, and C.E. Hayes, Characterization of a helper T lymphocyte defect in vitamin A-deficient mice. *J Immunol*, 1989. **142**(2): 388–93.

69. Mora, J.R. and U.H. von Andrian, Role of retinoic acid in the imprinting of gut-homing IgA-secreting cells. *Semin Immunol*, 2009. **21**(1): 28–35.

70. Bahl, R. et al., Vitamin A administered with measles vaccine to nine-month-old infants does not reduce vaccine immunogenicity. *J Nutr*, 1999. **129**(8): 1569–73.

71. Cherian, T. et al., Effect of vitamin A supplementation on the immune response to measles vaccination. *Vaccine*, 2003. **21**(19–20): 2418–20.

72. Semba, R.D. et al., Effect of vitamin A supplementation on measles vaccination in nine-month-old infants. *Public Health*, 1997. **111**(4): 245–7.

73. Benn, C.S. et al., Randomised trial of effect of vitamin A supplementation on antibody response to measles vaccine in Guinea-Bissau, west Africa. *Lancet*, 1997. **350**(9071): 101–5.

74. Newton, S. et al., Vitamin a supplementation does not affect infants' immune responses to polio and tetanus vaccines. *J Nutr*, 2005. **135**(11): 2669–73.

75. Benn, C.S. et al., Effect of vitamin A supplementation on measles-specific antibody levels in Guinea-Bissau. *Lancet*, 2002. **359**(9314): 1313–4.
76. Benn, C.S., Combining vitamin A and vaccines: Convenience or conflict? *Dan Med J*, 2012. **59**(1): B4378.
77. World Health Organization and Food and Agriculture Organization of the United Nations. *Vitamin and Mineral Requirements in Human Nutrition*, 2nd ed., 2004. Geneva, Rome: World Health Organization, FAO, xix, 341 pp.
78. Brown, K.H. et al., International Zinc Nutrition Consultative Group (IZiNCG) technical document #1. Assessment of the risk of zinc deficiency in populations and options for its control. *Food Nutr Bull*, 2004. **25**(1 Suppl 2): S99–203.
79. Prasad, A.S., Effects of zinc deficiency on Th1 and Th2 cytokine shifts. *J Infect Dis*, 2000. **182**(Suppl 1): S62–8.
80. Shankar, A.H. and A.S. Prasad, Zinc and immune function: The biological basis of altered resistance to infection. *Am J Clin Nutr*, 1998. **68**(2 Suppl): 447S–63S.
81. Prasad, A.S., Zinc and immunity. *Mol Cell Biochem*, 1998. **188**(1–2): 63–9.
82. Bhutta, Z.A. et al., Prevention of diarrhea and pneumonia by zinc supplementation in children in developing countries: Pooled analysis of randomized controlled trials. Zinc Investigators' Collaborative Group. *J Pediatr*, 1999. **135**(6): 689–97.
83. Ruel, M.T. et al., Impact of zinc supplementation on morbidity from diarrhea and respiratory infections among rural Guatemalan children. *Pediatrics*, 1997. **99**(6): 808–13.
84. Sazawal, S. et al., Zinc supplementation in young children with acute diarrhea in India. *N Engl J Med*, 1995. **333**(13): 839–44.
85. Sazawal, S. et al., Zinc supplementation reduces the incidence of persistent diarrhea and dysentery among low socioeconomic children in India. *J Nutr*, 1996. **126**(2): 443–50.
86. Sazawal, S. et al., Efficacy of zinc supplementation in reducing the incidence and prevalence of acute diarrhea—A community-based, double-blind, controlled trial. *Am J Clin Nutr*, 1997. **66**(2): 413–8.
87. Sazawal, S. et al., Zinc supplementation reduces the incidence of acute lower respiratory infections in infants and preschool children: A double-blind, controlled trial. *Pediatrics*, 1998. **102**(1 Pt 1): 1–5.
88. Bryce, J. et al., WHO estimates of the causes of death in children. *Lancet*, 2005. **365**(9465): 1147–52.
89. Ballester, O.F. and A.S. Prasad, Anergy, zinc deficiency, and decreased nucleoside phosphorylase activity in patients with sickle cell anemia. *Ann Intern Med*, 1983. **98**(2): 180–2.
90. Prasad, A.S., Zinc: Mechanisms of host defense. *J Nutr*, 2007. **137**(5): 1345–9.
91. Beck, F.W. et al., Changes in cytokine production and T cell subpopulations in experimentally induced zinc-deficient humans. *Am J Physiol*, 1997. **272**(6 Pt 1): E1002–7.
92. Rabbani, P.I. et al., Dietary model for production of experimental zinc deficiency in man. *Am J Clin Nutr*, 1987. **45**(6): 1514–25.
93. Prasad, A.S. et al., Serum thymulin in human zinc deficiency. *J Clin Invest*, 1988. **82**(4): 1202–10.
94. Wieringa, F.T. et al., Reduced production of immunoregulatory cytokines in vitamin A- and zinc-deficient Indonesian infants. *Eur J Clin Nutr*, 2004. **58**(11): 1498–504.
95. Bray, T.M. and W.J. Bettger, The physiological role of zinc as an antioxidant. *Free Radic Biol Med*, 1990. **8**(3): 281–91.
96. Cousins, R.J., Absorption, transport, and hepatic metabolism of copper and zinc: Special reference to metallothionein and ceruloplasmin. *Physiol Rev*, 1985. **65**(2): 238–309.
97. Prasad, A.S. et al., Antioxidant effect of zinc in humans. *Free Radic Biol Med*, 2004. **37**(8): 1182–90.
98. Prasad, A.S. et al., Zinc enhances the expression of interleukin-2 and interleukin-2 receptors in HUT-78 cells by way of NF-kappaB activation. *J Lab Clin Med*, 2002. **140**(4): 272–89.

99. Behrens, R.H., A.M. Tomkins, and S.K. Roy, Zinc supplementation during diarrhoea, a fortification against malnutrition? *Lancet*, 1990. **336**(8712): 442–3.

100. Lira, P.I., A. Ashworth, and S.S. Morris, Effect of zinc supplementation on the morbidity, immune function, and growth of low-birth-weight, full-term infants in northeast Brazil. *Am J Clin Nutr*, 1998. **68**(2 Suppl): 418S–24S.

101. Walker, C.L. and R.E. Black, Zinc for the treatment of diarrhoea: Effect on diarrhoea morbidity, mortality and incidence of future episodes. *Int J Epidemiol*, 2010. **39**(Suppl 1): i63–9.

102. Bates, C.J. et al., A trial of zinc supplementation in young rural Gambian children. *Br J Nutr*, 1993. **69**(1): 243–55.

103. Shankar, A.H. et al., The influence of zinc supplementation on morbidity due to *Plasmodium falciparum*: A randomized trial in preschool children in Papua New Guinea. *Am J Trop Med Hyg*, 2000. **62**(6): 663–9.

104. Muller, O. et al., Effect of zinc supplementation on malaria and other causes of morbidity in west African children: Randomised double blind placebo controlled trial. *BMJ*, 2001. **322**(7302): 1567.

105. Veenemans, J. et al., Effect of supplementation with zinc and other micronutrients on malaria in Tanzanian children: A randomised trial. *PLoS Med*, 2011. **8**(11): e1001125.

106. Haider, B.A. and Z.A. Bhutta, The effect of therapeutic zinc supplementation among young children with selected infections: A review of the evidence. *Food Nutr Bull*, 2009. **30**(1 Suppl): S41–59.

107. Zeba, A.N. et al., Major reduction of malaria morbidity with combined vitamin A and zinc supplementation in young children in Burkina Faso: A randomized double blind trial. *Nutr J*, 2008. **7**: 7.

108. Prasad, A.S. et al., Immunological effects of zinc deficiency in sickle cell anemia (SCA). *Prog Clin Biol Res*, 1989. **319**: 629–47; discussion 648–9.

109. Prasad, A.S. et al., Effect of zinc supplementation on incidence of infections and hospital admissions in sickle cell disease (SCD). *Am J Hematol*, 1999. **61**(3): 194–202.

110. Hewison, M., Vitamin D and immune function: An overview. *Proc Nutr Soc*, 2012. **71**(1): 50–61.

111. Holick, M.F., Vitamin D deficiency. *N Engl J Med*, 2007. **357**(3): 266–81.

112. Van Belle, T.L., C. Gysemans, and C. Mathieu, Vitamin D in autoimmune, infectious and allergic diseases: A vital player? *Best Pract Res Clin Endocrinol Metab*, 2011. **25**(4): 617–32.

113. Gibson, R.S., *Principles of Nutritional Assessment*, 2nd ed. 2005. New York: Oxford University Press, xx, 908 pp.

114. Dawson-Hughes, B. et al., Estimates of optimal vitamin D status. *Osteoporos Int*, 2005. **16**(7): 713–6.

115. Holick, M.F. and T.C. Chen, Vitamin D deficiency: A worldwide problem with health consequences. *Am J Clin Nutr*, 2008. **87**(4): 1080S–6S.

116. Hewison, M., Vitamin D and the immune system: New perspectives on an old theme. *Endocrinol Metab Clin North Am*, 2010. **39**(2): 365–79, table of contents.

117. Koeffler, H.P. et al., Gamma-interferon stimulates production of 1,25-dihydroxyvitamin D3 by normal human macrophages. *Biochem Biophys Res Commun*, 1985. **127**(2): 596–603.

118. Tanaka, H. et al., 1 Alpha,25-dihydroxyvitamin D3 induces differentiation of human promyelocytic leukemia cells (HL-60) into monocyte-macrophages, but not into granulocytes. *Biochem Biophys Res Commun*, 1983. **117**(1): 86–92.

119. Kreutz, M. et al., 1,25-Dihydroxyvitamin D3 production and vitamin D3 receptor expression are developmentally regulated during differentiation of human monocytes into macrophages. *Blood*, 1993. **82**(4): 1300–7.

120. Liu, P.T. et al., Toll-like receptor triggering of a vitamin D–mediated human antimicrobial response. *Science*, 2006. **311**(5768): 1770–3.

121. Gombart, A.F., N. Borregaard, and H.P. Koeffler, Human cathelicidin antimicrobial peptide (CAMP) gene is a direct target of the vitamin D receptor and is strongly up-regulated in myeloid cells by 1,25-dihydroxyvitamin D3. *FASEB J*, 2005. **19**(9): 1067–77.
122. Adams, J.S. et al., Vitamin D–directed rheostatic regulation of monocyte antibacterial responses. *J Immunol*, 2009. **182**(7): 4289–95.
123. Wang, T.T. et al., Cutting edge: 1,25-Dihydroxyvitamin D3 is a direct inducer of antimicrobial peptide gene expression. *J Immunol*, 2004. **173**(5): 2909–12.
124. Brennan, A. et al., Dendritic cells from human tissues expr ess receptors for the immunoregulatory vitamin D3 metabolite, dihydroxycholecalciferol. *Immunology*, 1987. **61**(4): 457–61.
125. Gregori, S. et al., Regulatory T cells induced by 1 alpha,25-dihydroxyvitamin D3 and mycophenolate mofetil treatment mediate transplantation tolerance. *J Immunol*, 2001. **167**(4): 1945–53.
126. Fabri, M. et al., Vitamin D is required for IFN-gamma-mediated antimicrobial activity of human macrophages. *Sci Transl Med*, 2011. **3**(104): 104ra102.
127. Lemire, J.M. et al., Immunosuppressive actions of 1,25-dihydroxyvitamin D3: Preferential inhibition of Th1 functions. *J Nutr*, 1995. **125**(6 Suppl): 1704S–8S.
128. Chen, S. et al., Modulatory effects of 1,25-dihydroxyvitamin D3 on human B cell differentiation. *J Immunol*, 2007. **179**(3): 1634–47.

4 Infection–Nutrition Interaction

Perspectives from the Developing World in Transition

Noel W. Solomons and Anne-Marie Chomat

CONTENTS

Introduction of Basic Concepts and Frameworks 60
Nature of Coadaptation in Evolution 60
Social Power and Physical Well-Being 61
Classic Narrative of the Interaction of Malnutrition and Infection 62
Malnutrition in All of Its Forms and Emerging Infectious Diseases..................62
Infection and Nutrition: The Undernutrition Paradigms..64
Infection and Enhanced Risk of Undernutrition 64
Undernutrition and Aggravation of Infectious Consequences 66
Undernutrition and Diminished Infectious Consequences................................68
Infection and Nutrition: The Overnutrition Paradigms...70
Infection, Improved Nutrition, and Enhanced Risk of Overnutrition 70
Increased Adiposity, and Overweight/Obesity and Immune Function...............71
Increased Adiposity and Overweight/Obesity..73
Iron Supplementation and Increased Reserves 73
Conclusions and Future Perspectives..74
References..75

Half a century of explosive population growth, scientific expansion in immunology and molecular biology, changing population demography, and evolving infections and nutritional epidemiology places the interaction of nutrition and infection into a myriad of new and relevant contexts.

Solomons [1]

59

INTRODUCTION OF BASIC CONCEPTS AND FRAMEWORKS

NATURE OF COADAPTATION IN EVOLUTION

It is a fundamental underpinning of evolutionary biology that the survival of the species, rather than any individual within the species, is the highest-order imperative. That one species is dependent on numerous others is also axiomatic. In the case of plants, this could be the insects that pollinate, the other plants that offer shade or support, and all of those dead organisms whose decay in the soil or water fertilizes and nourishes. In the case of animals, it is not only all of the organisms of both kingdoms that supply food but also organisms that play a role in anatomy or metabolism, from the bacteria that devour desquamated skin cells to the normal intestinal flora. In this context, greater diversity of species in an ecosystem enhances the chances of the mutual survival of all [2,3]. The nature of evolution, the course it has taken, and the mechanism of inheritance of traits are essential to understanding the interaction of infection and the host, notably for our consideration here, the human host.

Interspecies—and sometimes even intraspecies—relations can be described across a gamut of types from symbiotic and commensal to parasitic and ultimately pathogenic. This also describes a spectrum of decreasing harmony and increasing tension and stress. Infectious experience has been instrumental in human evolution. For instance, in an ecosystem in which humans were entrenched with a given microbial adversary, the function of the tribe would be enhanced where the productivity of adults is not hampered by sequelae of severe past infections. Those with a constitutional resistance to such an organism would logically have greater reproductive fitness by virtue of arriving to adulthood alive (survivors) and unscathed (not disabled). This is the manner by which a selection would operate on the human side in order to aid future generations to better cope with the agent and thrive in this forced coexistence. At the same time, since survival of all births would expand the tribal group to overpopulation of their hunting tract, the nonsurvival in the face of this and other pathogens represents the pruning mechanism for population stability.

Humans are, and have always been, part of an ecosystem made up of innumerable other organisms. Microbes likely played a determining role in the evolution of *Homo sapiens* and of human civilization, while the health of individuals and of populations is highly dependent on the maintained balance between humans and the organisms they harbor. The long history of hominid–parasite coevolution has played a selective role in the biological evolution of humans, and of the human ecosystem. On an individual level, populations of microbes inhabit the skin and mucosa, forming part of the normal human physiology; if microbe numbers grow beyond their typical ranges or populate atypical areas of the body, disease can occur.

The adult intestine contains approximately 100 trillion microbes—a number 10 times greater than the number of cells in the human body. The gut microbiota is established at birth and is modulated by a number of environmental factors both during infancy and later in life. The gut microbiota has coevolved with the host and exhibits metabolic features that are vital to human health, such as vitamin synthesis and xenobiotic metabolism [4,5]. The metabolic activity performed by these bacteria is equal to that of a virtual organ. Indeed, research suggests that the relation between gut flora and humans is a mutualistic, symbiotic relation, as microbes perform a host of useful functions such as fermenting unused energy substrates, training and maintaining the immune system, preventing growth of harmful organisms, producing vitamins for the host (such as biotin and vitamin K), and producing hormones to direct the host to store fats [4–6].

These evolutionary–biological points and principles are essential to understanding the intricacies of the biological relations of our theme. In no way, however, in this post-Hippocratic age, are we advocating any enduring respect for any fitness competition in contemporary societies. To the contrary, clinical and public health ethics oblige extending equivalent access to quality therapeutic and preventative health care to all individuals.

Social Power and Physical Well-Being

Access to food is one of the first and most fundamental of all human rights. Where food is lacking, it becomes impossible to live with dignity, and the rights to a healthy life and peaceful coexistence are undermined. Food insecurity at the household level has become an increasing public problem with increasing wealth inequality [7] and intermittent inflation of staple food prices [8].

The concept of malnutrition stretches to encompass excess as well as deficiency. Worldwide, 925 million people, or 14% of the world's population, are undernourished [9]. Overall, women and children account for the highest proportion of the chronically hungry. Meanwhile, obesity has become a worldwide epidemic. Rates of obesity are increasing worldwide, not only in adults but also in children. In 2008, >1.4 billion adults were overweight; of these, more than 200 million men and 300 million women were obese. In addition, >40 million children under the age of 5 years were overweight in 2010 [10]. Poverty is also seen as a strong risk factor for excessive weight because quality foods are beyond the means of the poor.

Malnutrition has become a significant impediment to development in rich and poor countries alike. At the individual level, both hunger and obesity can reduce a person's physical fitness, increase susceptibility to illness, and shorten life span. In addition, children deprived of adequate nutrients during development can develop permanently reduced mental capacity. At the national level, poor eating hampers educational performance, curtails economic productivity, increases the burden of health care, and reduces general well-being.

Confronting this epidemic of poor eating will have widespread benefits; however, policy responses have been wildly off the mark in addressing the problem. Efforts to eliminate hunger often focus on technological quick fixes aimed at boosting crop yields and producing more food rather than addressing the socioeconomic causes of hunger, such as meager incomes, inequitable distribution of land, and the disenfranchisement of women. Efforts to reduce overeating single out affected individuals—through fad diets, diet drugs, or the like—while failing to promote prevention and education about healthy alternatives in a food environment full of heavily marketed, nutritionally suspect, "supersized" junk food. The result: half of humanity, in both rich and poor nations, is malnourished today, despite recent decades of global food surpluses [11].

CLASSIC NARRATIVE OF THE INTERACTION OF MALNUTRITION AND INFECTION

The classic formulation of the interaction of nutrition and infection comes from the work of Nevin Scrimshaw in his masters dissertation work at the Harvard School of Public Health, published first as a review article [12] and then as a World Health Organization monograph [13], both with the title of "Interaction of Nutrition and Infection." The essence of the Scrimshaw–Taylor–Gordon thesis is that impaired nutrition and infections interact in a dynamic manner with interactions, which are generally either greater than the simple sum of the respective components (synergism) or less than the additive combination (antagonism). The four quadrants of these interactions are described schematically in Box 4.1.

BOX 4.1   SCHEMATIC RELATIONS OF SYNERGISTIC AND ANTAGONISTIC INTERACTIONS OF MALNUTRITION AND INFECTION

Synergistic interactions	Undernutrition aggravates infection	Infection aggravates undernutrition
Antagonistic interactions	Undernutrition produces resistance to infection	Infection produces resistance to undernutrition

---

That one of the arcane terms for tuberculosis is "consumption" is revealing of a cultural appreciation of the negative imposition of infection on nutritional status. The pathogen specificity and the immune mechanisms have emerged as interesting, as discussed below. Perhaps equally entrenched is the concept that frail persons were more likely to succumb to infections. It turns out that this is nuanced in terms of characteristics of infection such as initial susceptibility, duration, and severity. Challenging to logic on first instance is how having fewer nutrients could be protective against infection; however, ample evidence for this phenomenon, and its mechanisms, are emerging. Even the strange interaction in the lower right-hand quadrant, of infection enhancing nutrient status, has gained substantiation over the decades.

MALNUTRITION IN ALL OF ITS FORMS AND EMERGING INFECTIOUS DISEASES

Although Scrimshaw and colleagues [12,13] contemplated nutrient excess in their treatise as part of logical symmetry, they failed to develop the corresponding matrix for overnutrition. This is not difficult to rationalize given the concentration of nutritional science and public health in the post-war and decolonization period on the situations in low-income countries of Africa, Asia, and Latin America. Protein–energy malnutrition (PEM), manifested by poor linear growth, underweight, or both, was the dominant concern from the end of World War II through the 1970s [14,15]. Micronutrient deficiencies (hidden hunger) emerged and surpassed PEM in interest and awareness in the 1980s, specifically with concerns for vitamin A, iron, and iron deficiencies [16]. These concerns fit nicely into the "undernutrition" paradigm of the matrix in Box 4.1. It was not until the worldwide pandemic of overweight and obesity, first recognized in developed countries in the late 1990s [17], came into prominence that an even more comprehensive and complex dimension to the infection–malnutrition interaction became evident. In the new millennium, the public health imperative to understand malnutrition in all of its forms, i.e., both overnutrition and undernutrition, has become an imperative [18].

The burden of overweight was first recognized in affluent nations, and among the affluent elite of developing societies [19]. On the epidemiological front, however, the concept of transitions, specifically "epidemiological transition" [20] and "nutrition transition" [21], would emerge in a sequential manner to complicate the panorama. Classic concepts of these two transitions are outlined in Box 4.2. With respect to the nutritional status of populations, problems of deficit and deficiency persisted as public health problems in low-income settings, keeping the paradigm of Box 4.1 relevant. However, the poor of the world were also becoming overweight and obese within the broader framework of malnutrition, presenting the more challenging panorama for evaluation and response.

BOX 4.2

EPIDEMIOLOGICAL TRANSITION

Conceptually, the theory of epidemiologic transition focuses on the complex change in patterns of health and disease *and* on the interactions between these patterns and their demographic, economic and sociologic determinants and consequences.

Source: A.R. Omran, *Milbank Memorial Fund Quarterly* 49, 509, 1971.

NUTRITION TRANSITION

Several major changes seem to be emerging, leading to a marked shift in the structure of diet and the distribution of body composition in many regions of the world: a rapid reduction in fertility and aging of the population, rapid urbanization, the epidemiologic transition, and economic changes affecting populations in different and uneven ways. These changes vary significantly over time. In general, we find that problems of under- and overnutrition often coexist, reflecting the trend in which an increasing proportion of people consume the types of diets associated with a number of chronic diseases.

Source: B.M. Popkin, *Nutrition Review*, 52, 285, 1994.

Through the first half of the 20th century, undernutrition and infection were the main drivers of morbidity and mortality in Africa, Asia, and Latin America, and life expectancies were low. On these continents, few lived deeply enough into middle and late adulthood to worry about noncommunicable, degenerative diseases. This panorama began to change, however, with the epidemiological transition. In part because of immunizations, antimicrobial medications, and sanitary measures to control infections, introduced after World War II, infections became more survivable and overall survival to later adulthood advanced rapidly. Today, only in Africa is infectious death more common than that from noncommunicable diseases. One can conclude that the infection part of the interaction is receding from historical dimensions, while what remains confronts its traditional counterpart in undernutrition and a new partner in overnutrition and nutrient excess, all in the subtropical and tropical and socioeconomically deprived continents.

As infection per se becomes a less important sector of the mortality panorama, the epidemiology of lethal infections is undergoing constant change. Small pox, measles, pneumonia, meningitis, poliomyelitis, diphtheria, pertussis, typhoid, yellow fever, leprosy, tuberculosis, schistosomiasis, cholera, and malaria represent a litany of classic lethal transmissible diseases for which either immunizations, antimicrobial therapy, or both emerged and became generalized during the 20th century. All have demonstrable interactions with malnutrition. It is, however, the domains of the "emerging" infectious diseases and to some extent "reemerging" infections, notably tuberculosis and malaria from the previous list, which are escaping from the traditional control measures through drug resistance [22,23], that confront the imbalances in nutritional status, and to some extent play out on a stage that includes developed and developing countries alike.

INFECTION AND NUTRITION: THE UNDERNUTRITION PARADIGMS

The classic narrative, based on the formulation of Scrimshaw et al. [12,13], has two paradigms related to undernutrition. This includes the experience of infections as promoting nutrient deficiency, on the one hand, and undernutrition, related to deficiency of macronutrients or micronutrients, to predisposing to more infections or more serious consequences of infections, on the other hand.

INFECTION AND ENHANCED RISK OF UNDERNUTRITION

Infections of all varieties, i.e., viral, bacterial, chlamydial, fungal, protozoal, helminthic, and ectoparasitic infections, can impair the nutritional status of energy and the range of macronutrients and micronutrients, as documented in the classic Scrimshaw et al. monograph [13]. Obviously, not all pathogens affect the same organisms, nor do infectious processes equally affect all nutrients. The interactions have been exhaustively catalogued since 1968, and it is not the intention here to reproduce the entire litany. More important is to explore the biological fundamentals. Nutritional deficiencies derive from lack of intake, maldigestion and malabsorption, excessive wasting, poor utilization, and increased requirements [24], and all of these can act alone or in combination in the prodrome, active period, and convalescence of infections. For example, intestinal infections reduce appetite, impair uptake systems, and enhance fecal excretion [25]. Fever produces energy consumption and wasting of nutrients into the urine [26].

As mentioned, the term "consumption" for tuberculosis dates back centuries. It is also a classic observation that the edematous form of PEM, kwashiorkor, was often induced in children with marginal diets by an episode of acute infection, such as measles [14]. This relation took on a modern context since the 1980s in the advent of the pandemic of acquired immunodeficiency syndrome (AIDS). One of the original terms for what would be known as AIDS was "slim disease" [27] because of the emaciated status of the patients in late-stage human immunodeficiency virus (HIV) infection. Concerning the pathogenesis in this context, it ranges from decreased intake due to margination, loss of appetite, and oral candidiasis, to intestinal infections such as intractable *Cryptosporidium* diarrhea to the cachectic effects of proinflammatory cytokines [28].

Febrile illnesses, with the activation of the acute-phase response, can even lead to excessive renal loss of nutrients that do not usually pass in the urine, such as vitamin A [29]. Moreover, in young children, even without superimposed HIV, intestinal cryptosporidiosis can produce undernutrition [30]. This latter finding, finally, is similar to observations in some, but not all, settings for intestinal colonization with the protozoal organism, *Giardia intestinalis* [31].

Respiratory and gastrointestinal infections are the most common childhood infectious illnesses worldwide. Beginning in the 1970s and consistently shown to the present has been the pervasiveness of infectious diarrhea as a factor in growth retardation [32]. As nutritional impairment is a risk factor for diarrhea, it required prospective studies to disentangle the two-way interaction. The adverse nutritional effects can readily be explained by impaired absorption and transintestinal wasting of nutrients [33].

Certain parasites that inhabit the lumen of the intestine have a high requirement for iron for their growth and reproduction. Among these are *Entamoeba histolytica* in the protozoan family, and hookworm (*Ancylostoma duodenale, Necator americanus*) and whipworm (*Trichuris trichiura*) among the nematodes. These organisms obtain their iron by ingesting red blood cells of the host and provoke additional bleeding to gain access to the mucosal blood vessels. With infections of short-term or low intensity, the host can upregulate iron absorption to compensate for the parasite-related losses. Another nematode that can cause iron loss through bleeding is the schistosome. The intestinal variety, *Schistosoma mansoni*, can produce a colonic polyposis by invading mucosal blood vessels and produce bloody diarrhea; the bladder variety, *Schistosoma haematobium*, inhabits the vasculature of the lower urinary tract, leading to blood loss in urine.

Similarly, it perhaps can be generalized that human and animal filarial parasites (thread worms), which burrow into internal tissues causing diseases from onchocerciasis (river blindness) to infections with worm of the *Wuchereria* and *Brugia* genera (elephantiasis), have a high vitamin A requirement for their production of the infective microfilaria [34]. Presumably as a consequence, hypovitaminosis A is more common in filarial patients.

In terms of program and policy implications, Dewey and Mayers [35] have raised the question of "What is less clear is whether infection reduces the effectiveness of nutrition interventions or, vice versa, whether malnutrition lessens the impact of infection control strategies." With regard to the former, they conclude that nutrition interventions are less effective in the context of recurrent childhood infections. Eradicating the background infection may not be indispensable for obtaining a desirable nutritional impact.

UNDERNUTRITION AND AGGRAVATION OF INFECTIOUS CONSEQUENCES

Nutritional deficiency states enhance the risk of adverse consequences of infections. Again, from the classic treatise [13], having adequate status was thought to convey resistance to infectious disease (primarily in laboratory animals), in accordance with the Scrimshaw synthesis. Although examples of the interaction were documented with almost every nutritional deficiency, some were much more prominent as associated with infectious risk. The mechanism is presumed to be an impairment of function or regulation of the innate and/or acquired immune systems in the host defense [1,36–38]. This can range from a nutrient-related dermatosis that weakens the barrier protection to a metabolic disruption that suppresses thymus-dependent lymphocytes.

In a classic set of observations in rural Bangladeshi villages, Black et al. [39] demonstrated that the duration and intensity—but not incidence—of diarrhea was exacerbated in children with low weight for height. Subsequently, however, many instances of nutrient deficiencies predisposing individuals to greater incidences of infections have been documented. Death is the most serious outcome of any illness. A decade ago, Caulfied et al. [40] produced a model based on the interaction of low weight for age and four common childhood infections: diarrhea, pneumonia, malaria, and measles. They concluded that "A significant proportion of deaths in young children worldwide is attributable to low weight-for-age, and efforts to reduce malnutrition should be a policy priority" [40]. This has more recently been refined in an analysis of all-cause mortality in relation to the predictive strength of either stunting or wasting or underweight and their interplay in combinations [41].

Following undernutrition defined by anthropometric indices, vitamin A deficiency has received the greatest attention concerning childhood infections. Vitamin A was known as the "anti-infective" vitamin early in the history of the discovery of vitamins [42,43]. In a large epidemiological surveillance study in the north of the island of Sumatra in Indonesia, published in 1983 [44], initial evidence showed that preschool children with marginal vitamin A status (mild xerophthalmia) had a four times greater mortality rate during 18 months than their unaffected peers. Three years later, the results of a randomized field intervention involving 26,000 preschoolers receiving 6-monthly dosing with 200,000 IU of vitamin A during a 12-month period were published [45]. The high-dose supplementation induced a 34% greater reduction in mortality from childhood infections. Seven years later, a total of seven experiences had become available for collective analysis from Africa and Asia. Five were conducted with high-dose supplements, one with weekly low-dose supplements, and one with fortification of monosodium glutamate (MSG) condiment. The weighted average of decreased mortality risk was 22% [46]. On the basis of this experience, periodic high-dose supplementation to this age group became an international recommendation for countries suspected of having vitamin A deficiency as a measure to promote child survival.

Several lessons and insights can be derived. Not all individuals in these trials were themselves vitamin A deficient. Moreover, the periodic high-dose administration of vitamin A improves liver stores only transiently. The antimortality effects with periodic supplementation interventions could be a pharmacological effect of the high pulse dose of vitamin A. Of note was the fact that the greatest relative reductions of mortality in the seven trials were in the weekly supplementation [47] and the MSG fortification [48], the two measures likely to produce sustainable increments in liver vitamin reserves. The mechanism of life sparing with vitamin A interventions is unknown; however, it would seem that it reduces the lethality of infections. Rahmathullah et al. [49] observed no difference in the incidence of infections across their treatment groups despite a 54% reduction in mortality in the group receiving the low-dose weekly supplement.

Zinc status and infection has undergone similar scrutiny to that of vitamin A [50]. The deficiency of zinc has been suspected to be widespread across low-income countries. A major limitation for this trace element is the lack of a good clinical biomarker of zinc status, either at the population or individual level. Nevertheless, zinc supplementation trials of various doses, to various age groups, and in various geographic areas have tried to explore the interaction of nutrition and infection.

As reviewed by Penny [51], adjunctive therapy with oral zinc supplementation during acute diarrhea, in conjunction with use of oral rehydration solution, is universally recommended, independent of patients' zinc status. This measure is estimated to reduce mortality from this infection by 23% in children 12–59 months. Penny concluded from a compilation of studies that "daily zinc supplements for all children >12 months of age in zinc deficient populations are estimated to reduce diarrhea incidence by 11%–23%. The greatest impact is in reducing multiple episodes of diarrhea." Zinc is also efficacious in reducing dysentery and persistent diarrhea. Finally, she estimated from her review that prophylactic supplementation of zinc could reduce pneumonia rates by up to 19% [51].

A specific focus on zinc status and infectious risk has emerged in relation to the elderly and their tendency to develop pneumonia [52]. Barnett and colleagues [52] reviewed evidence showing that low zinc status is commonly reported in the elderly, impairs immune function, decreases resistance to pathogens, and is associated with increased incidence and duration of pneumonia; it also augments the use and duration of antibiotic treatment, and increases the overall mortality risk in the elderly. As yet, no randomized controlled trials are available to confirm the causality. Similarly, by virtue of its role in cellular immunity, Cuevas and Koyanagi [50] proposed that zinc has a potential role in tropical intracellular infections such as lepromatous leprosy and leishmaniasis.

It is unlikely that infections will have a major impact on vitamin D status, even with decreased appetite or impaired absorption, as the major factor in vitamin D acquisition is exposure to sunlight in tropical countries. However, it has only recently been appreciated that tropical latitude is no guarantee of full vitamin D repletion.

A review of vitamin D status in Latin America and the Caribbean showed surprisingly consistent rates of insufficient and deficient circulating levels of the biomarker 25-hydroxyvitamin D [53]. These epidemiological insights highlighted its relevance in developing countries. Vitamin D plays an immunomodulating role in cells of the immune system [54,55]. The role of the vitamin in tuberculosis control is interesting as patients in sanatoriums were treated with solariums in the era before antituberculosis drugs, and the stimulation of vitamin D synthesis is probably at the basis of whatever beneficial effects were documented. Its active metabolite, 1,25-dihydoxyvitamin D, has long been known to enhance the immune response to mycobacteria *in vitro* [56]. Results of a randomized trial of vitamin D–fortified milk versus nonfortified milk in schoolchildren during the winter in Mongolia produced a 50% reduction in acute respiratory infection symptoms [57]. It remains to be determined if reversing the unexpectedly widespread deficiency in vitamin D will modulate host susceptibility to infection in the developing world.

An unusual and potentially menacing interaction between nutritional status and infection has been explored by Beck and collaborators [58,59] using a murine model of coxsackievirus infection. It focuses on the transformation of nonvirulent organisms to virulent pathogens with their passage through a micronutrient-deficient host. The coxsackievirus produces a benign and self-limited infection in well-nourished mice; however, selenium deficiency converts it into a lethal infection. The virus isolated from the deficient animals becomes virulent and causes a fatal infection when inoculated into selenium-replete mice. It was postulated that the oxidant milieu in the unprotected tissues in selenium-deficient mice favors mutation of the virus into the more virulent organism. Any human analogy of such a situation could lead to devastating pandemics in communities in which micronutrient deficiencies are rampant.

Recent medical hypothesis suggests that simple fasting and short-term withholding of macronutrients may favor the advance of hepatitis C virus (HCV) in individuals infected by this organism. Shlomai and Shaul [60] have created a "metabolovirus model" based on the observations on the influence of liver kinase metabolism and hepatic immune responses to the invading virus. In synthesis, they state, "Thus, our hypothesis sets the stage for viral manipulation by controlling food intake, and opens additional avenues towards food or nutritional therapy as an effective anti-HBV weapon."

Therefore, we might address the alternative formulation of the Dewey and Mayers [35] query, that is, "whether malnutrition lessens the impact of infection control strategies." Here they attest to confluent evidence that improving nutritional status can reduce the severity of diarrheal infection. Hence, programs aimed at supporting growth and diminishing micronutrient deficiencies can, in some instances, be considered as infection-control strategies.

UNDERNUTRITION AND DIMINISHED INFECTIOUS CONSEQUENCES

Both hosts and pathogens require many of the same nutrients and compete for these nutrients for the growth of the host and the proliferation and virulence of the pathogen. This sets the stage for a competitive nutrition–infection interaction known as "nutritional immunity," a term coined by E.D. Weinberg in 1975 [61,62]. His observations were based on the requirements of microbial pathogens and parasites for iron. He synthesizes the theory as follows: "Hosts attempt to withhold growth-essential iron from invading bacteria, fungi, and protozoa. Clinical conditions in which hosts are stressed by excess quantities of iron in specific fluids, tissues, or cells result in enhanced susceptibility to infection" [77]. Certain bacteria have binding receptors (siderophores) with high affinity to capture and hold iron. Humans and other higher organisms have their physiological mechanisms to regulate and control internal exposure to iron. Drakesmith and Prentice [63] comment: "Iron lies at the center of a battle for nutritional resource between higher organisms and their microbial pathogens." The iron status of the human host affects the pathogenicity of numerous infections including malaria, HIV-1, and tuberculosis. As another example, experimental studies show that amoebas are much less virulent in both animals and humans with restricted iron reserves. Denic and Agarwal [64] suggest that the phenomenon of nutritional immunity represents an adaptation in evolution to humans living in closer proximity, with consequent risk of epidemics. The lower bioavailability of iron in plant-based diets from agricultural crops resulted in hosts with a lesser offering of iron for the pathogens of the plagues of antiquity.

Another substantial example of nutritional immunity can be found in investigations on murine *Plasmodiun* infections, mimicking human malaria [65,66]. For this invasive protozoal organism to propagate from host to host, it must proliferate in circulating red blood cells. To the extent that the blood corpuscle resists the initial invasion, it serves as a base of operation for reproduction. If the cell membrane were to collapse on contact with the *Plasmodium*, the cell is shut down as a "nursery." The deprivation of vitamin E would act to make cell membranes exquisitely sensitive to oxidative destruction. With two species of mouse *Plasmodium*, vitamin E depletion produced protection against infectious mortality after inoculation as compared with the vitamin E–replete control. That this effect operates through direct oxidative debilitation of the red cell was indicated by the fact that mutant mice unable to mobilize cellular or humoral immune resistance to the protozoa were equally protected against mortality [66]. The authors recur to traditional Chinese medicine with the speculation that "Nutritional manipulation of host oxidative stress status may be a useful adjunct therapy in patients undergoing treatment with pro-oxidant antimalarials such as drugs of the qinghaosu family" [65].

An interesting interaction of this nature has been demonstrated in experimental models of the aforementioned threadworm parasites (filaria); whereas the presence of adult worms drains the vitamin A nutrition of the host, preexisting hypovitaminosis A limits the fertility of the female worms, as reflected by the reduced total body loads of the microfilaria [34].

Finally, evidence is only beginning to emerge, but the notions of nutritional immunity with iron deficiency have focused workers on other trace elements whose concentrations fluctuate with infection and inflammation and which may be essential to human pathogens. Specifically, LeGrand and Alcock [67] postulate an evolved mechanism called "immune brinksmanship" related to the acute-phase response. The stress generated is harmful not only for the host but also for the pathogen. The stimulation of zinc-sequestering proteins (metallothioneins), mediated by cytokines, has the effect of reducing the concentration of cellular and circulating zinc, limiting the supply to pathogens that might be zinc dependent for their proliferation. Kehl-Fe and Skaar [68] ratify the notion of zinc withholding and pathogen resistance, and add evidence that manganese can also be involved in an analogous role.

INFECTION AND NUTRITION: THE OVERNUTRITION PARADIGMS

The classic narrative [12,13] correspondingly has two paradigms related to nutrient excess and overnutrition. This includes, logically, the experience of infections as promoting better nutrition, although this has practical contradictions. It also embraces the proposition that overnutrition makes one more prone to infections or more serious consequences of infections.

INFECTION, IMPROVED NUTRITION, AND ENHANCED RISK OF OVERNUTRITION

This is the quadrant of the Scrimshaw treatise that has virtually defied exemplification. Considering the malabsorptive and catabolic concomitants of infections described above, it is not surprising. Bacteria of the normal colonic microflora elaborate essential nutrients, notably folic acid and vitamin K. Upper intestinal bacterial overgrowth might be considered a quasi-infectious state, as it has proliferation of otherwise commensal organisms resident in an abnormal anatomical site and causing pathological harm [69,70]. Enhanced folic acid status is a documented consequence of bacterial overgrowth in the upper small intestine [71].

Obesity is a form of energy storage overnutrition. It may be related to microorganisms either in a strictly noninfectious, commensal relation as part of the normal large intestinal flora, or in more classic (invasive organism) relations. The most intriguing is the former context, in which the floral pattern of the commensal resident intestinal microbial flora (microbiome) assorts with a lean or an obese phenotype. Forced feeding of excess energy loads altered the bacterial community in both types; however, the lean group had greater fecal energy loss. Upon completion of energy loading, the microbiota returned to their original—and distinct—phenotype-specific patterns [72]. Taking the emerging microbiome research into context, there is reason to suspect that the intestinal flora has a direct functional role in regulating the metabolic responses governing energy balance in the human host [73].

The less solid but potentially more powerful microbiological relation comes from the exploration of obesity as an infectious disease. In a pioneering conceptual piece, Dhurandhar [74] introduced the term "infectobesity." He illustrated laboratory experiments in which a series of viruses (canine distemper virus, scrapie agent, Borna disease virus, Rous-associated virus 7, and several human adenoviruses—SMAM-1 avian adenovirus, and human adenoviruses Ad36 and Ad37) have been shown to produce obesity in rodent models. He concludes in his classic review: "Although the exact mechanism of pathogen-induced obesity is unclear, infection attributable to certain organisms should be included in the long list of potential etiological factors for obesity" [74]. While the relative contribution of these pathogens to human obesity is unknown, these data give a new perspective to the pathogenesis of obesity and imply an infectious origin, at least in some human beings.

INCREASED ADIPOSITY, AND OVERWEIGHT/OBESITY AND IMMUNE FUNCTION

Although the effects of obesity on the development of metabolic and cardiovascular problems are well studied, much less is known about its impact on immune function and infectious disease. As we will review below, data suggest that some infections are more common in obese people than those of normal weight. While this increase in susceptibility has been documented for a handful of infections, a significant number remain unexplored. In addition, while several possible mechanisms for increased susceptibility to infection have been suggested, the exact systemic impact of obesity on infection susceptibility has not been fully investigated [75].

In the hospital setting, obese patients are more likely to develop secondary infections and complications such as sepsis, pneumonia, bacteremia, and wound and catheter-related infections—which have been associated with increased length of stay and increased risk of death. Obese patients in the intensive care unit (ICU) setting are reported to have higher mortality than normal-weight patients, possibly owing to a higher risk of these complications [76]. In addition, obesity has been found to be independently associated with *Staphylococcus aureus* nasal carriage, which is a risk factor for surgical-site infections.

Overweight and obesity have also been associated with an increased risk of periodontitis [77]. However, data are insufficient to determine whether obesity is a risk factor for periodontal disease or whether periodontitis might increase the risk of weight gain [77]. Interestingly, one cohort study has shown that in nondiabetics, the severity of periodontal disease is associated with the development of glucose intolerance [78].

Obesity can profoundly alter lung mechanics, diminish exercise capacity, and augment airway resistance, resulting in an increased work of breathing and impaired gas exchange. Obesity is closely associated with obstructive sleep apnea, a syndrome often accompanied by an increased risk for aspiration as well as chronic inflammation of the lower and upper respiratory tracts [76]. Hospitalized obese patients have been shown to be at an increased risk for pulmonary aspiration and community-related respiratory tract infections [79,80]. Increased body mass index (BMI) and weight gain have also been found to be associated with increased risk for community-acquired pneumonia in women and with increased susceptibility to acute respiratory infections in overweight children [81–83].

Overweight also has an adverse effect on chronic hepatitis C virus (HCV) liver disease, with diminished response to antiviral therapy and more rapid progression [84–87]. Specifically, obesity has been shown to increase the risk of hepatic steatosis and fibrosis in nondiabetic patients with chronic HCV infection. Experimental and clinical evidence also suggest that HCV infection may contribute to the development of insulin resistance and diabetes [77].

Obesity may increase the risk for *Helicobacter pylori* colonization and infection [88]. Obese patients are also at an increased risk for biliary disease and its infectious complications. Several studies indicate an association between obesity and severe pancreatitis as well as its local complications—pancreatic pseudocysts, abscess, and necrosis [89,90]. The severity of acute pancreatitis in obese patients and in patients with central fat distribution seems to be related to the amplification of the systemic inflammatory reaction that occurs owing to the secretion of adipokines from adipose tissues [91].

Recent studies have consistently shown that obesity increases the risk of urinary tract infections (UTIs). In addition, obese individuals are more likely to develop pyelonephritis than the nonobese [92]. Obesity has also been shown to be a risk factor for UTI in pregnant women and during the postpartum period [93]. Obesity has also been shown to be a risk factor for UTI in men with diabetes, after traumatic injury, and in the ICU. There are no data on the effect of obesity on the outcome of UTI [77].

Obesity causes changes in skin barrier function, the lymph system, collagen structure and function, and wound healing. Evidence suggests that the vascular supply is impaired in obese persons and that obesity affects both macrocirculation and microcirculation [94]. Being overweight and obese has been associated with a wide range of skin diseases, and with an increased risk of cellulitis, erysipelas, and recurrent soft-tissue infections compared to nonobese persons [77]. Fungal foot infections (tinea pedis and toenail onychomycosis) have been found to be more common in obese than nonobese patients [76].

Obesity has recently been found to constitute an independent risk factor for increased severity of infection and death from the 2009 H1N1 pandemic influenza strain [95]. Obesity has also been shown to be a risk factor for mortality in patients with H1N1 infection–related community-acquired bacterial pneumonia [96–98]. Data on the impact of obesity on the outcome of influenza virus infections other than H1N1 are rare, although data suggest that severely obese patients are at increased risk for respiratory hospitalization during influenza seasons [99].

Evidence is accumulating that obese individuals may respond differently to vaccination and various drugs such as antibiotics, further affecting the outcome of infections. Despite the growing prevalence of obesity worldwide, little is known about the impact of obesity on the response to vaccination. However, a number of studies have shown an association between obesity and poor antibody response to hepatitis B vaccines [75]. It has also been reported that antibody response to standard tetanus immunization is lower in overweight than in controls with lower BMIs [100]. Obesity has also been associated with impaired immune response to influenza vaccination in humans [101]. A decrease in pre-B and immature B cells may be responsible for the impact of obesity on reducing the antibody response vaccination. Despite limited data, it appears that vaccine responses in obese individuals may be very different from vaccine responses in lean individuals. This suggests that obese adults/children may not be receiving the full benefits of our current immunization protocols [75].

There are also no well-established guidelines about the management of infections in obese patients, including specific recommendations about dose adjustment of therapy with antimicrobial agents. Obese patients show increased volume distribution and clearance for vancomycin, which best correlates with total body weight; vancomycin serum concentrations should be obtained to ensure that the administered doses are adequate. The volume distribution of aminoglycosides is also increased in obese compared with normal-weight patients. Thus, dosages of vancomycin and aminoglycosides may require an adjustment in obese patients, based on the estimated fraction of the excess body weight. There are limited data about the pharmacokinetics of other classes of antimicrobial agents in obese individuals [76].

Increased Adiposity and Overweight/Obesity

Obesity is defined as a state of excess adiposity, and its cause, although multifactorial, is primarily prolonged positive energy balance. Several comorbidities are associated with obesity, especially immune dysfunction. Alterations in inflammation and the immune cell function in the obese play a significant role in nearly all pathophysiological effects of obesity. However, few studies have addressed how this may affect host defense. Despite strong epidemiological evidence in humans and mice that a state of excess adiposity greatly increases susceptibility to infections, much remains to be learned about obesity-related immune impairment [102].

An intact and functioning immune response is critical for protection against infectious disease. Nutrition and immunocompetence are intimately linked, and states of imbalanced nutrition such as obesity can easily deregulate immune function. While no specific mechanism has been defined to decrease immune response to infectious disease in the obese host, several obesity-associated changes could affect the immune response [76]. In obese individuals, the overall number of circulating lymphocytes appears to be altered, with decreased numbers of CD8$^+$ T cells and increased or decreased numbers of CD4$^+$ T cells [75]. Alterations in T-cell subsets appear to be linked to an increase in proinflammatory cytokines, such as tumor necrosis factor-α (TNF-α), and deregulated expression of other cytokines. Reduced macrophage dendritic cell function and natural killer cell impairment have also been observed in obese individuals [75]. Finally, obesity has also been associated with a low-grade inflammatory state, which has been implicated in the development of several disease states such as type 2 diabetes mellitus and atherosclerosis, possibly due to the ability of adipocytes and immune cells within adipose tissue to secrete inflammatory mediators such as TNF-α and interleukin-6 [103]. Moreover, the capacity of lymphocytes to respond to antigen and mitogen stimulation appears to be reduced [101]. Several studies have assessed immune function in obese individuals after weight loss or dietary restriction. The majority showed increased immune responsiveness and improvement [75].

Iron Supplementation and Increased Reserves

With iron, the overexposure to mineral is the converse of the situation of the aforementioned nutritional immunity [61,62], centered on deprivation of iron and the virulence of assorted pathogens. Oral iron supplementation is the recommended measure for both preventing and treating iron deficiency and iron deficiency anemia. We have a recent, graphic narrative experience of apparent implication of the antagonistic relation of iron and infection from an oral iron supplementation trial, randomized and controlled among young children on the Zanzibari island of Pemba in Tanzania [104]; this is an area of holo-endemic transmission of *Falciparum* malaria, and nonimmune infants and toddlers experience the brunt of the potentially fatal complications. Among the most eye-opening findings were that children in the treatment arms receiving 12.5 mg of elemental iron (with or without zinc) were much more susceptible to adverse outcomes (hospitalization or death) than were those receiving only zinc or no supplements. Within this superficial assortment, it was found that those who were iron replete and not anemic in the iron-exposed groups were most vulnerable to adverse consequences, as compared with anemic and iron-deficient recipients, who had a nutritional need for the nutrient. The malaria organism, *Plasmodium*, attacks red blood cells for their prodigious requirements for iron. A panel convened by the World Health Organization in Lyon, France, in 1987 called for a moratorium on routine oral iron supplementation in regions of high malaria transmission.

Tuberculosis and HIV infections are additional widespread human infections in which iron status and iron exposure may have an important role. It was speculated as early as 1973 [105] that iron may promote tuberculosis, and the epidemiology of African iron overload shows an increased susceptibility to tuberculous infection [106]. It has long been known through *in vitro* experiments that iron promotes the growth of *Mycobacterium tuberculosis* [107]; however, studies show that it also downregulates the immune response within infected macrophage cells [108]. Finally, as obligatorily intracellular and iron-dependent organisms, retrovirus virulence has been postulated to be influenced by host iron status. In a randomized clinical trial of iron supplementation in Africa, however, twice-weekly supplementation with 60 mg of oral iron failed to influence the viral load of HIV patients [109].

CONCLUSIONS AND FUTURE PERSPECTIVES

Globalization and modernization are bound to continue apace, probably accelerating in their advance into the new millennium. They will alter exposures for the human population in terms of the variety, preparation, and processing of foods and their nutritional content, and in the virulence and transmission mechanisms for established and emerging human pathogens. One hopes that time consolidates the distribution of wealth and social assurance; however, population expansion and political instability could produce the opposite progression.

Climate change is a reality, with poorly predictable consequences for climatic manifestations, and even more uncertain interactions with food production and commerce and transmission of communicable diseases. Loss of wilderness habitat may reduce the interaction of humans with classic soil parasites, whereas expanding irrigation systems may intensify the contact with others.

Malarial resistance to all forms of control seems to be advancing, and organisms, notably the tuberculosis bacillus and varieties of staphylococci, among others, are developing multiple resistances to antibiotics. These reexpose humans to the infectious danger from organisms that once were under reasonable control in the antibiotic era. An increasing proportion of the population will be the elderly, a situation that is associated with declining immunological regulation and patency and with challenges to obtaining a balanced and adequate diet.

An expected constant within all of the anticipated disruptions and reorderings in the material environment and social organizations will be the operation of the interaction of nutrition and infection, albeit with new dietary styles and emergent human pathogens. Biological and medical sciences also face a brave new world of technological innovation, especially within the domain of molecular genetics and biotechnology. These tools of unprecedented potential to understand issues of parasitic virulence, human host defense immunity, and functional nutritional status will be at the disposition of the clinical, public health, and research communities. Where nutritional status assessment is challenging and the interaction with infection is based on nutrient supplementation, the plausibility of a pharmaceutical effect—rather than a nutritional deficiency consequence—needs to be kept in focus. To the extent, however, that awareness of the paradigms and principles of the interaction of malnutrition and infection are remembered and considered in therapeutic and public health decisions and in investigations to resolve new challenges, they should constitute guidance for the appropriate and maximally beneficial application of 21st century technical capacity.

REFERENCES

1. N.W. Solomons, "Malnutrition, immunity and infection," in *Diet, Immunity and Inflammation*, eds. Calder P.L., Yaqoob P. (Cambridge, UK: Woodhouse Publishing, Ltd), Chapter 27, September 2013: 686–717.
2. J.D. Bever, T.G. Platt and E.R. Morton, "Microbial population and community dynamics on plant roots and their feedbacks on plant communities," *Annual Review of Microbiology* 66 (2012): 265–283.
3. T. Johns and P.B. Eyzaguirre, "Linking biodiversity, diet and health in policy and practice," *Proceedings of the Nutrition Society* 65 (2006): 182–189.
4. F. Guarner and J.R. Malagelada, "Gut flora in health and disease," *Lancet* 361 (2003): 512–519.
5. C.L. Sears, "A dynamic partnership: Celebrating our gut flora," *Anaerobe* 11(5) (2005): 247–251.
6. A.M. O'Hara and F. Shanahan, "The gut flora as a forgotten organ," *European Molecular Biology Organization* 7 (2006): 688–693.
7. P.K. Pathak and A. Singh, "Trends in malnutrition among children in India: Growing inequalities across different economic groups," *Social Science and Medicine* 73 (2011): 576–585.
8. The World Bank, "Poverty reduction and Equity Group," *Food Price Watch* 13 (2013), accessed July 29, 2013, http://siteresources.worldbank.org/EXTPOVERTY/Resources/336991-1311966520397/Food-Price-Watch-March-2013.pdf.
9. The Food and Agriculture Organization, "World hunger and poverty facts and statistics 2010," *Global Issue*, accessed July 29, 2013, http://www.worldhunger.org/articles/Learn/world%20hunger%20facts%202002.htm.
10. The World Health Organization, "Obesity: Preventing and managing the global epidemic, Report of the WHO consultation," *World Health Organization Technical Report Series* 894 (2000): 1–253.
11. The WorldWatch Institute, "Innovations that nourish the planet," *State of the World 2011*, accessed July 29, 2013, http://blogs.worldwatch.org/nourishingtheplanet/wp-content/uploads/2011/03/SOW-2011-Ch-1-Final.pdf.
12. N.S. Scrimshaw, C.E. Taylor and J.E. Gordon, "Interactions of nutrition and infection," *American Journal of Medical Science* 237 (1959): 367–403.
13. N.S. Scrimshaw, C.E. Taylor and J.E. Gordon, "The interaction of nutrition and infection," *WHO Monograph Series* 57 (1968).
14. N.S. Scrimshaw and M. Behar, "Protein malnutrition in young children," *Science* 133 (1961): 2039–2047.
15. J.C. Waterlow, "Childhood malnutrition—The global problem," *Procedures of the Nutrition Society* 38 (1979): 1–9.

16. G.F. Maberly et al., "Programs against micronutrient malnutrition: Ending hidden hunger," *Annual Review of Public Health* 15 (1994): 277–301.
17. P.T. James et al., "The worldwide obesity epidemic," *Obesity Research* 9(S4) (2001): 228S–233S.
18. R. Uauy and N.W. Solomons, "Diet, nutrition, and the life-course approach to cancer prevention," *Journal of Nutrition* 135(S12) (2005): 2934S–2945S.
19. C.A. Monteiro et al., "Shifting obesity trends in Brazil," *European Journal of Clinical Nutrition* 54 (2000): 342–346.
20. A.R. Omran, "The epidemiologic transition: A theory of the epidemiology of population change," *Milbank Memorial Fund Quarterly* 49 (1971): 509–538.
21. B.M. Popkin, "The nutrition transition in low-income countries: An emerging crisis," *Nutrition Review* 52 (1994): 285–298.
22. K.C. Chang et al., "WHO group 5 drugs and difficult multidrug-resistant tuberculosis: A systematic review with cohort analysis and meta-analysis," *Antimicrobial Agents and Chemotherapy* 57 (2013): 4097–4104.
23. A. Nzila, Z. Ma and K. Chibale, "Drug repositioning in the treatment of malaria and TB," *Future Medicinal Chemotherapy* 3 (2011): 1413–1426.
24. V. Herbert, "The five possible causes of all nutrient deficiency: Illustrated by deficiencies of vitamin B12," *American Journal of Clinical Nutrition* 26 (1973): 77–86.
25. N.W. Solomons, "Pathways to the impairment of human nutritional status by gastrointestinal pathogens," *Parasitology* 107 (1993): S19–S35.
26. G.T. Keusch and M.J. Farthing, "Nutrition and infection," *Annual Review of Nutrition* 6 (1986): 131–154.
27. D. Serwadda et al., "Slim disease: A new disease in Uganda and its association with HTLV-III infection," *Lancet* 2 (1985): 849–852.
28. G.T. Keusch and M.J. Farthing, "Nutritional aspects of AIDS," *Annual Review of Nutrition* 10 (1990): 475–501.
29. A.K. Mitra et al., "Urinary retinol excretion and kidney function in children with shigellosis," *American Journal of Clinical Nutrition* 68 (1998): 1095–1103.
30. K. Mølbak et al., "*Cryptosporidium* infection in infancy as a cause of malnutrition: A community study from Guinea-Bissau, West Africa," *American Journal of Clinical Nutrition* 65 (1997): 149–152.
31. T.L. Duffy et al., "Prevalence of giardiasis in children attending semi-urban daycare centers in Guatemala and comparison of 3 *Giardia* detection tests," *Journal of Health and Population Nutrition* 31 (2013): 290–293.
32. W. Checkley et al., "Multi-country analysis of the effects of diarrhoea on childhood stunting," *International Journal of Epidemiology* 37 (2008): 816–830.
33. R.L. Guerrant et al., "The impoverished gut—A triple burden of diarrhoea, stunting and chronic disease," *National Review of Gastroenterology and Hepatology* 10 (2013): 220–229.
34. D.M. Storey, "Filariasis: Nutritional interactions in human and animal hosts," *Parasitology* 107 (S1) (1993): S147–S158.
35. K.G. Dewey and D.R. Mayers, "Early child growth: How do nutrition and infection interact?" *Maternal and Child Nutrition* 7 (S3) (2011): S129–S142.
36. S. Hughes and P. Kelly, "Interactions of malnutrition and immune impairment, with specific reference to immunity against parasites," *Parasite Immunology* 28 (2006): 577–588.
37. N.W. Solomons, "Malnutrition and infection: An update," *British Journal of Nutrition* 98 (2007): S5–S10.
38. S. Maggini et al., "Selected vitamins and trace elements support immune function by strengthening epithelial barriers and cellular and humoral immune responses," *British Journal of Nutrition* 98 (S1) (2007): S29–S35.

39. R.E. Black, K.H. Brown and S. Becker, "Malnutrition is a determining factor in diarrheal duration, but not incidence, among young children in a longitudinal study in rural Bangladesh," *American Journal of Clinical Nutrition* 39 (1984): 87–94.
40. L.E. Caulfield et al., "Undernutrition as an underlying cause of child deaths associated with diarrhea, pneumonia, malaria, and measles," *American Journal of Clinical Nutrition* 80 (2004): 193–198.
41. C.M. McDonald et al., "The effect of multiple anthropometric deficits on child mortality: Meta-analysis of individual data in 10 prospective studies from developing countries," *American Journal of Clinical Nutrition* 97 (2013): 896–901.
42. B.A. Underwood, "Was the 'anti-infective' vitamin misnamed?" *Nutrition Review* 52 (1994): 140–143.
43. A.C. Ross and C.B. Stephensen, "Vitamin A and retinoids in antiviral responses" *Federation for American Societies for Experimental Biology Journal* 10 (1996): 979–985.
44. A. Sommer et al., "Increased mortality in children with mild vitamin A deficiency," *Lancet* 2 (1983): 585–588.
45. A. Sommer et al., "Impact of vitamin A supplementation on childhood mortality. A randomised controlled community trial," *Lancet* 1 (1986): 1169–1173.
46. G.H. Beaton et al., "Effectiveness of vitamin A supplementation in the control of young child morbidity and mortality in developing countries," Geneva, *Administrative Committee on Coordination/Subcomission on Nutrition* (United Nations), 1993.
47. Muhilal et al., "Vitamin A-fortified monosodium glutamate and health, growth, and survival of children: A controlled field trial," *American Journal of Clinical Nutrition* 48 (1988): 1271–1276.
48. L. Rahmathullah et al., "Reduced mortality among children in southern India receiving a small weekly dose of vitamin A," *New England Journal of Medicine* 323 (1990): 929–935.
49. L. Rahmathullah et al., "Diarrhoea, respiratory infections, and growth are not affected by a weekly low-dose vitamin A supplement: A masked, controlled field trial in children in southern India," *American Journal of Clinical Nutrition* 54 (1991): 568–577.
50. L.E. Cuevas and A. Koyanagi, "Zinc and infection: A review," *Annals of Tropical Paediatrics* 25 (2005): 149–160.
51. M.E. Penny, "Zinc supplementation in public health," *Annals of Nutrition and Metabolism* 62 (S1) (2013): S31–S42.
52. J.B. Barnett, D.H. Hamer and S.N. Meydani, "Low zinc status: A new risk factor for pneumonia in the elderly?" *Nutrition Review* 68 (2010): 30–37.
53. A. Brito et al., "Less than adequate vitamin D status and intake in Latin America and the Caribbean: A problem of unknown magnitude," *Food and Nutrition Bulletin* 34 (2013): 52–64.
54. V. Lagishetty, N.Q. Liu and M. Hewison, "Vitamin D metabolism and innate immunity," *Molecular and Cellular Endocrinology* 347 (2011): 97–105.
55. R.W. Chesney, "Vitamin D and the Magic Mountain: The anti-infectious role of the vitamin," *Journal of Pediatrics* 156 (2010): 698–703.
56. A.R. Martineau, "Old wine in new bottles: Vitamin D in the treatment and prevention of tuberculosis," *Procedures of the Nutrition Society* 71 (2012): 84–89.
57. C.A. Jr. Camargo et al., "Randomized trial of vitamin D supplementation and risk of acute respiratory infection in Mongolia," *Pediatrics* 130 (2012): e561–e567.
58. M.A. Beck, "Selenium and host defence towards viruses," *Procedures of the Nutrition Society* 58 (1999): 707–711.
59. M.A. Beck and C.C. Matthews, "Micronutrients and host resistance to viral infection," *Procedures of the Nutrition Society* 59 (2000): 581–585.
60. A. Shlomai and Y. Shaul, "The 'metabolovirus' model of hepatitis B virus suggests nutritional therapy as an effective anti-viral weapon," *Medical Hypotheses* 78 (2008): 53–57.

61. E.D. Weinberg, "Nutritional immunity: Host's attempt to withhold iron from microbial invaders," *Journal of the American Medical Association* 231 (1975): 39–41.
62. E.D. Weinberg, "Infection and iron metabolism," *American Journal of Clinical Nutrition* 30 (1977): 1485–1490.
63. H. Drakesmith and A.M. Prentice, "Hepcidin and the iron–infection axis," *Science* 338 (2012): 768–772.
64. S. Denic and M.M. Agarwal, "Nutritional iron deficiency: An evolutionary perspective," *Nutrition* 23 (2007): 603–614.
65. D.W. Taylor et al., "Vitamin E-deficient diets enriched with fish oil suppress lethal *Plasmodium yoelii* infections in athymic and scid/bg mice," *Infection and Immunology* 65 (1997): 197–202.
66. O.A. Levander et al., "Protection against murine cerebral malaria by dietary-induced oxidative stress," *Journal of Parasitology* 81 (1995): 99–103.
67. E.K. LeGrand and J. Alcock, "Turning up the heat: Immune brinksmanship in the acute-phase response," *The Quarterly Review of Biology* 87 (2012): 3–18.
68. T.E. Kehl-Fe and E.P. Skaar, "Nutritional immunity beyond iron: A role for manganese and zinc," *Current Opinion in Chemical Biology* 14 (2010): 218–224.
69. M. Gracey, "Intestinal absorption in the contaminated small-bowel syndrome," *Gut* 12 (1971): 403–410.
70. P.W. Broido, S.L. Gorbach and L.M. Nyhus, "Microflora of the gastrointestinal tract and the surgical malabsorption syndromes," *Surgical Gynecology and Obstetrics* 135 (1972): 449–460.
71. R.M. Batt and J.O. Morgan, "Role of serum folate and vitamin B12 concentrations in the differentiation of small intestinal abnormalities in the dog," *Research in Veterinary Science* 32 (1982): 17–22.
72. R. Jumpertz et al., "Energy-balance studies reveal associations between gut microbes, caloric load, and nutrient absorption in humans," *American Journal of Clinical Nutrition* 94(1) (2011): 58–65.
73. S.F. Clarke et al., "The gut microbiota and its relationship to diet and obesity: New insights," *Gut Microbes* 3 (2012): 186–202.
74. N.V. Dhurandhar, "Infectobesity: Obesity of infectious origin," *Journal of Nutrition* 131 (2001): 2794S–2797S.
75. E.A. Karlsson and M.A. Beck, "The burden of obesity on infectious disease," *Experimental Biology and Medicine* 235 (2010): 1412–1424.
76. M.E. Falagas and M. Kompoti, "Obesity and infection," *Lancet Infectious Diseases* 6 (2006): 438–446.
77. R. Huttunen and J. Syrjänen, "Obesity and the risk and outcome of infection," *International Journal of Obesity* 37 (2013): 333–340.
78. T. Saito et al., "The severity of periodontal disease is associated with the development of glucose intolerance in non-diabetics: The Hisayama study," *Journal of Dental Research* 83 (2004): 485–490.
79. S.M. Koenig, "Pulmonary complications of obesity," *American Journal of Medical Science* 321 (2001): 249–279.
80. A. Jubber, "Respiratory complications of obesity," *International Journal of Clinical Practice* 58 (2004): 573–580.
81. E.B. Rimm et al., "Prospective study of cigarette smoking, alcohol use, and the risk of diabetes in men," *British Medical Journal* 310 (1995): 555–559.
82. I. Baik et al., "A prospective study of age and lifestyle factors in relation to community-acquired pneumonia in US men and women," *Archives in Internal Medicine* 160 (2000): 3082–3088.

83. W. Jedrychowski et al., "Predisposition to acute respiratory infections among overweight preadolescent children: An epidemiologic study in Poland," *Public Health* 112 (1998): 189–195.
84. O. Lo Iacono et al., "The impact of insulin resistance, serum adipocytokines and visceral obesity on steatosis and fibrosis in patients with chronic hepatitis C," *Alimentary Pharmacology and Therapeutics* 25 (2007): 1181–1191.
85. A. Delgado-Borrego et al., "Influence of body mass index on outcome of pediatric chronic hepatitis C virus infection," *Journal of Pediatric Gastroenterology and Nutrition* 51 (2010): 191–197.
86. V. Ortiz et al., "Contribution of obesity to hepatitis C-related fibrosis progression," *American Journal of Gastroenterology* 97 (2002): 2408–2414.
87. L. Massard et al., "Natural history and predictors of disease severity in chronic hepatitis C," *Journal of Hepatology* 44 (S1) (2006): S19–S24.
88. E. Arslan, H. Atilgan and I. Yavasoglu, "The prevalence of *Helicobacter pylori* in obese subjects," *European Journal of Internal Medicine* 20 (2009): 695–697.
89. J. Martinez et al., "Is obesity a risk factor in acute pancreatitis? A meta-analysis," *Pancreatology* 4 (2004): 42–48.
90. J. Martinez et al., "Obesity is a definitive risk factor of severity and mortality in acute pancreatitis: An updated meta-analysis," *Pancreatology* 6 (2006): 206–209.
91. L. Sempere et al., "Obesity and fat distribution imply a greater systemic inflammatory response and a worse prognosis in acute pancreatitis," *Pancreatology* 8 (2008): 257–264.
92. M.J. Semins et al., "The impact of obesity on urinary tract infection risk," *Urology* 79 (2012): 266–269.
93. T.S. Usha Kiran et al., "Outcome of pregnancy in a woman with an increased body mass index," *BJOG: An International Journal of Obstetrics and Gynecology* 112 (2005): 768–772.
94. G. Yosipovitch, A. DeVore and A. Dawn, "Obesity and the skin: Skin physiology and skin manifestations of obesity," *Journal of the American Academy of Dermatology* 56 (2007): 917–920.
95. O.W. Morgan et al., "Morbid obesity as a risk factor for hospitalization and death due to 2009 pandemic influenza A (H1N1) disease," *Public Library of Science One* 5 (2010): e9694.
96. R. Riquelme et al., "Predicting mortality in hospitalized patients with 2009 H1N1 influenza pneumonia," *The International Journal of Tuberculosis and Lung Disease* 15 (2011): 542–566.
97. L. Fezeu et al., "Obesity is associated with higher risk of intensive care unit admission and death in influenza A (H1N1) patients: A systematic review and meta-analysis," *Obesity Review* 12 (2011): 653–659.
98. M.D. Van Kerkhove et al., "Risk factors for severe outcomes following 2009 influenza A (H1N1) infection: A global pooled analysis," *Public Library of Science Medicine* 8 (2011): e1001053.
99. J.C. Kwong, M.A. Campitelli and L.C. Rosella, "Obesity and respiratory hospitalizations during influenza seasons in Ontario, Canada: A cohort study," *Clinical Infectious Disease* 53 (2011): 413–421.
100. A. Eliakim et al., "Reduced tetanus antibody titers in overweight children," *Autoimmunity* 39 (2006): 137–141.
101. P.A. Sheridan et al., "Obesity is associated with impaired immune response to influenza vaccination in humans," *International Journal of Obesity* 36(8) (2011): 1072–1077.
102. J.J. Milner and M.A. Beck, "The impact of obesity on the immune response to infection," *Procedures of the Nutrition Society* 71 (2012): 298–306.

103. C. Power, S.K. Miller and P.T. Alpert, "Promising new causal explanations for obesity and obesity-related diseases," *Biological Research for Nursing* 8 (2007): 223–233.
104. S. Sazawal et al., "Effects of routine prophylactic supplementation with iron and folic acid on admission to hospital and mortality in preschool children in a high malaria transmission setting: Community-based, randomised, placebo-controlled trial," *Lancet* 367 (2006): 133–143.
105. I. Kochan, "The role of iron in bacterial infections, with special consideration of host-tubercle bacillus interaction," *Current Topics in Microbiology and Immunology* 60 (1973): 1–30.
106. I. Kasvosve et al., "African iron overload," *Acta Clinica Belgica* 55 (2000): 88–93.
107. T.M. Hoette et al., "Immune interference in *Mycobacterium tuberculosis* intracellular iron acquisition through siderocalin recognition of carboxymycobactins," *ACS Chemical Biology* 6 (2011): 1327–1331.
108. J. Serafín-López et al., "The effect of iron on the expression of cytokines in macrophages infected with *Mycobacterium tuberculosis*," *Scandinavian Journal of Immunology* 60 (2004): 329–337.
109. A. Olsen et al., "Low-dose iron supplementation does not increase HIV-1 load," *Journal of Acquired Immune Deficiency Syndrome* 36 (2004): 637–638.

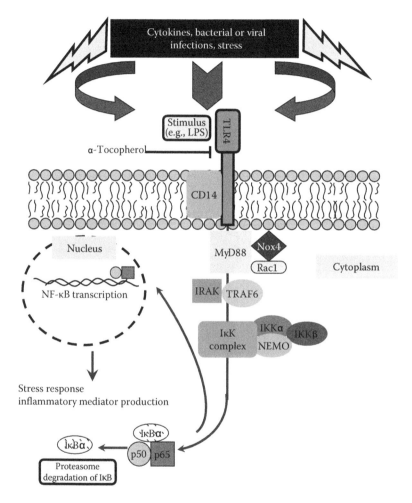

FIGURE 5.2 Oxidative stress signaling pathway and gene expression in sepsis. IκK, IκB kinase complex; IRAK, interleukin-1 receptor-associated kinase; LPS, lipopolysaccharide; MyD88, myeloid differentiation protein 88; NEMO, NF-κB essential modifier; NF-κB, nuclear factor-κB; Nox4, NADPH oxidase; TLR4, Toll-like receptor 4; TRAF6, tumor necrosis factor receptor-associated factor 6. (From Puertollano, M.A. et al., *Curr Top Med Chem.*, 11, 1752, 2011.)

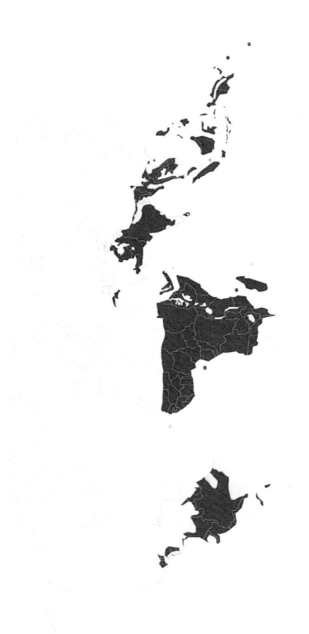

Malaria, countries or areas at risk of transmission, 2010

■ Countries or areas where malaria transmissions occurs
□ Countries or areas with limited risk of malaria transmission

FIGURE 9.2 Areas of high incidence of malaria. Note: This map is intended as a visual aid only and not as a definitive source of information about malaria endemicity. (From Global Malaria Programme: Information for travellers, 2011. Available at http://www.who.int/malaria/travellers/en/.)

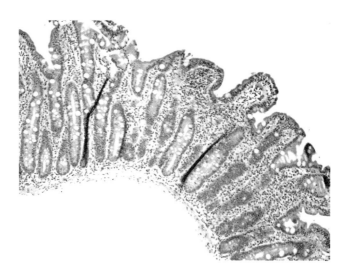

FIGURE 11.1 Histological findings of celiac disease with increased density of intraepithelial lymphocytes, villous atrophy, and crypt hyperplasia. (Picture courtesy of Dr. Michael O'Brien, MD MPH, Boston Medical Center.)

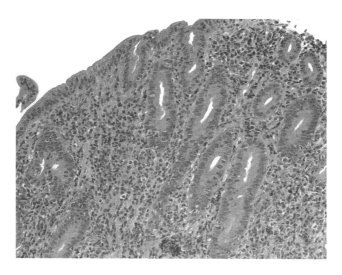

FIGURE 11.2 Histological findings in AIE with villous atrophy, mucosal mononuclear cell infiltration, and decreased number of goblet cells. (Picture courtesy of Dr. Michael O'Brien, MD MPH, Boston Medical Center.)

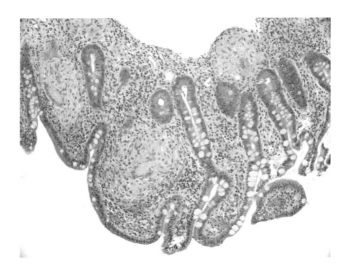

FIGURE 11.3 Granuloma seen in the terminal ileum in a patient with Crohn's disease. (Picture courtesy of Dr. Michael O'Brien, MD MPH, Boston Medical Center.)

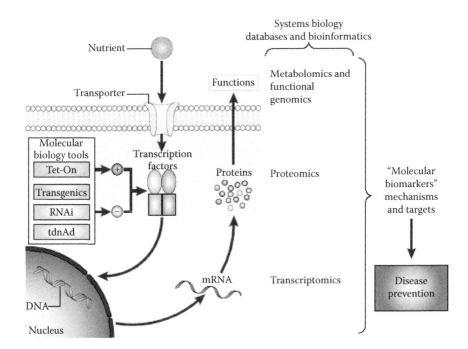

FIGURE 16.1 Nutrigenomics and systems biology in nutrition: "smart" combination of molecular nutrition and nutrigenomics. Molecular biology tools related to transcriptomics, proteomics, metabolomics, and functional genomics will determine the effects of nutrients, "nutrient signatures." These signatures will enhance the discovery of nutritional biomarkers that relate to personalized or general strategies for disease prevention and assessment of disease risk. These biomarkers will allow early dietary intervention to reverse the onset of diet-related diseases and to regain homeostasis. (Reprinted by permission from McMillan Publishers Ltd., *Nat Rev Genet*, Muller, M. and S. Kersten, Nutrigenomics: Goals and strategies, 4, 4, 315–22, copyright 2003.)

5 Role of Oxidative Stress and Inflammation in Nutrition–Infection Interactions and the Potential Therapeutic Strategy Using Antioxidants and Modulating Inflammation

Elena Puertollano and Maria A. Puertollano

CONTENTS

Introduction 82
Oxidative Stress: Protective Role of Antioxidants 84
Dietary Antioxidants and Host Natural Resistance to Infection 87
    Vitamins and Host Resistance to Infection 89
        Vitamin C 89
        Vitamin E 89
        β-Carotene 92
    Trace Elements and Host Resistance to Infection 92
        Selenium 93
        Iron 96
        Zinc 96
        Copper 97
Other Natural Antioxidants Contained in Foods: A Brief Description 97
References 100

INTRODUCTION

The immune system of vertebrate organisms may be described as a highly effective and complex network of cells and factors, perfectly orchestrated and coordinated, that protects the host from infectious and pathogenic microorganisms. It recognizes and destroys foreign agents through two primary defense mechanisms: innate immunity and acquired immunity. The innate immune system (nonspecific immune response) is present at birth and includes physiologic barriers (skin, mucous membranes, body temperature, low pH, and special chemical mediators such as complement and interferon [IFN]), specialized cells (natural killer [NK] cells, and phagocytes including neutrophils, monocytes, and macrophages, which can engulf, kill, and digest whole microorganisms), and inflammatory mediators. On the other hand, the acquired immune system (specific immune response) is acquired later in life (immunization or exposition to pathogens) and includes special cells called B lymphocytes and T lymphocytes that are capable of secreting a large variety of specialized chemicals (antibodies and cytokines) to regulate the immune response (Figure 5.1).

The innate arm of immunity prevents the entry of foreign microorganisms into the body, playing a crucial role in the early control of infectious agents, as well as in the initiation and subsequent course of the acquired immunity. Therefore, innate response constitutes the first line (early phase) of defense against pathogens. It is obvious that innate immunity represents an important mechanism that rapidly destroys and eliminates microorganisms. In fact, innate immunity is the most efficient mechanism to eliminate intracellular growth microorganisms. Innate resistance does not distinguish among microorganisms and does not change in intensity upon reexposure. On the other hand, acquired immunity requires the identification of molecules from an invading agent. The recognition of antigens is carried out by B lymphocytes and T lymphocytes, which constitute the main arm of acquired immunity and produce antibodies (B cells) or recognize the antigens on the surface of cells (B or T cells). T lymphocytes can be divided into two fundamental groups: (i) T-helper 1 (Th1) lymphocytes, which are regulated by interleukin-12 (IL-12) and IFN-γ, produce proinflammatory cytokines (such as IL-2 or IFN-γ), and activate macrophages, NK cells, and cytotoxic T lymphocytes; (ii) Th2 lymphocytes, which are regulated by IL-4, and are specialized in the production of cytokines with an anti-inflammatory activity such as IL-4, IL-5, IL-10, and IL-13. Hence, infection with intracellular pathogens will induce the differentiation along the Th1 pathway, whereas infection with extracellular pathogens will promote the differentiation along the Th2 pathway. Once the body has identified the antigen, the immune system response to a second exposition is faster and more effective the next time that antigen is recognized. Thus, the infectious agent is eliminated and immunological memory remains (Figure 5.1).

The innate immune system is capable of recognizing a limited group of conserved components of bacteria, parasites, fungi, or viruses, known as pathogen-associated molecular patterns (PAMPs), which have therefore been called pattern recognition receptors (PRRs). Host cells express various PRRs that detect diverse PAMPs, varying from lipids, lipopolysaccharides, lipoproteins, proteins, and nucleic acids. As a consequence, identification of these PAMPs by PRRs promotes the activation of intracellular signaling pathways that conclude in the release of proinflammatory

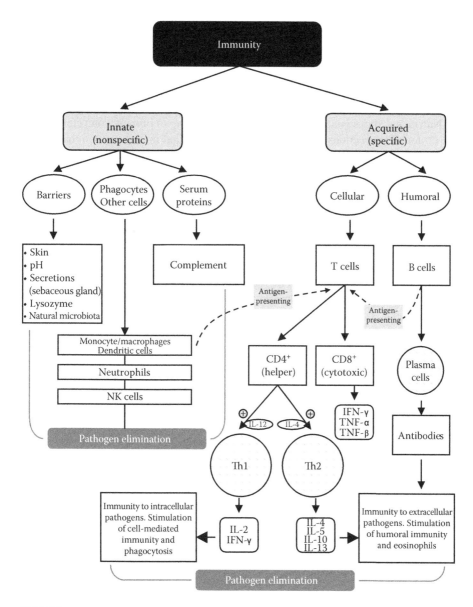

FIGURE 5.1 Schematic representation of both innate and acquired immune response. IFN-γ, interferon-γ; IL, interleukin; NK, natural killer. (From Puertollano, M.A. et al., *Curr Top Med Chem.*, 11, 1752, 2011.)

cytokines, chemokines, or IFNs, thus preparing the organism to the presence of infection (Wolowczuk et al., 2008). PRRs comprise the members of the Toll-like receptor (TLR) family, the nucleotide-binding oligomerization domain receptors (NOD-like receptors, NLRs), and the retinoic acid–inducible gene-like helicases (RIG-like helicases, RLHs) (Yoneyama et al., 2005). Both TLRs and NLRs have shown a critical role in host protection against microbial infections and in homeostasis of commensal microbiota (Takeda et al., 2003).

However, many of the protective functions of immune cells depend on cell membrane fluidity. It is clear that lipid peroxidation decreases membrane fluidity, which adversely affects immune responses. Therefore, the relevance of antioxidants is particularly critical for the functionality of the immune system.

Nutritional status is an important factor contributing to immunocompetence, and the profound interactions among nutrition, infection, and immune system have been widely recognized (Scrimshaw and SanGiovanni, 1997; Klasing and Leshchinsky, 2000). Nowadays, it is clearly established that nutritional deficiency is related to an inadequate function of immune response, especially cell-mediated immunity, phagocyte activity, cytokine production, or antibody synthesis. In addition to protein–energy malnutrition, deficiencies of trace elements, vitamins, and essential fatty acids are responsible for an impairment of immunity (Chandra, 1999). It is obvious that an inadequate immune functionality increases the risk and incidence of infections, leading to augmentation in morbidity and mortality rates. Moreover, infections exacerbate micronutrient deficiencies by reducing nutrient intake, increasing losses, and interfering with utilization by altering the activity of metabolic pathways (reviewed in Wintergerst et al., 2007). In the past years, numerous investigations have focused on the role of nutrition and particularly on the contribution of dietary antioxidants to an optimum and adequate functioning of the immune system. Since antioxidants constitute our first line of defense against free radical damage and are crucial for maintaining optimum health, the need for antioxidants becomes even more critical with increased exposure to free radicals, which promote harmful activities associated with injury to cells and the body, causing damage to cell membranes, enzymes, and DNA.

The immune system is especially sensitive to oxidative stress. Cells that constitute the immune system depend on cell–cell communication, through membrane-bound receptors, to carry out an adequate transmission of signals. Cell membranes are rich in phospholipids, which, if peroxidized, can lead to a loss of membrane integrity or to an alteration of membrane fluidity (Baker and Meydani, 1994), and as a result both cell functions and intracellular signaling are intensely impaired. It has been demonstrated that exposure to potential prooxidants can involve a reduction in cell membrane receptor expression in those cells that are not suitably protected by antioxidants (Gruner et al., 1986). For these reasons, it is obvious that adequate amounts of neutralizing antioxidants not only are required to protect cells against oxidative stress but also to prevent damage of the immune cells, reducing morbidity and mortality. By contrast, insufficient intake and status of dietary antioxidants may lead to a profound suppression of immune functions, which increases the risk of sepsis and predisposition to infections.

OXIDATIVE STRESS: PROTECTIVE ROLE OF ANTIOXIDANTS

Oxidative stress can be defined as an imbalance between tissue oxidants and antioxidants. As oxidant agents, free radicals are composed of atoms or molecules highly reactive due to the unpaired electrons in the outer orbital. To this broad group belongs reactive oxygen species (ROS), such as superoxide anion $\left(O_2^{\bullet-}\right)$, hydroxyl radical ($^{\bullet}OH$), and hydrogen peroxide (H_2O_2), as well as reactive nitrogen species (RNS), which include nitric oxide (NO) and peroxynitrite ($ONOO^-$). ROS or free radicals in organisms are continually generated within cells as a consequence of a normal aerobic metabolism and as an immune system strategy to eliminate invading agents. For example, $O_2^{\cdot-}$ plays an essential role in the intracellular killing of microorganisms by activated phagocytes. Nevertheless, all the major classes of biomolecules are vulnerable to free radical damage. As a result, free radicals cause strand breaks in DNA, which potentially can lead to subsequent misrepair and tumor cell generation. In addition, the continuous generation may also cause oxidative damage to lipids or proteins, and consequently their accumulation may lead to the oxidative destruction of cells. Thereby, long-chain lipids (especially polyunsaturated fatty acids, which contain double bonds) are more susceptible to free radical attack leading to lipid oxidative destruction of fatty acids called lipid peroxidation, a key consequence of oxidative stress (De Pablo and Alvarez de Cienfuegos, 2000). ROS react with the double bond of polyunsaturated lipids, producing unstable lipid peroxides that may cause cell death (Mishra, 2007). Therefore, oxidative stress may be described as a circumstance in which ROS or free radicals exert important toxic effects on cells.

ROS are mainly produced by leukocytes and by the respiratory mitochondrial chain. They are essential for cell signaling and for bacterial defense (Valko et al., 2007). The physiological protection systems to neutralize free radicals are constituted by (i) endogenous antioxidants, which may be both nonenzymatic and enzymatic and by (ii) exogenous antioxidants (Table 5.1). All these molecules are defined as substances that inhibit or delay oxidation when present in adequate amounts, and they constitute the antioxidant defenses due mainly to their capability to transform ROS into stable and undamaging compounds or by scavenging both ROS and RNS with a redox-based mechanism (Valko et al., 2007).

Oxygen radicals are identified as mediators of various chronic disorders such as diabetes, cancer, rheumatoid arthritis, brain dysfunctions, and immune alterations. Accordingly, cells that constitute the immune system are particularly sensitive

TABLE 5.1
Endogenous and Exogenous Antioxidants

Endogenous		Exogenous
Enzymatic	**Nonenzymatic**	**Exogenous**
Superoxide dismutases	Glutathione	Vitamin A
Glutathione peroxidases	Uric acid	Vitamin E (α and γ tocopherols)
Catalase	Bilirubin	Vitamin C
	Thiols	Carotenoids (β-carotene, lycopene)
	Albumin	Flavonoids and other related polyphenols
		Metallothionein
		Coenzyme Q10

Source: Puertollano, M.A. et al., 2013. Natural antioxidants and resistance to infection. In: *Bioactive Food as Dietary Interventions for Arthritis and Related Inflammatory Diseases*, Watson, R.R. and Preedy, V.R., Eds. San Diego: Academic Press, 157–174.

to oxidative stress because cell membranes are mainly composed of fatty acids. In addition, many immune cells produce ROS as part of the body's defense against infection; however, the production of ROS by phagocytic immune cells can damage the cells themselves if they are not sufficiently protected by antioxidants. Levels of ROS are balanced by the neutralizing activity of antioxidant molecules and enzymes, thereby preventing intense damage to the host. Hence, it is very easy to assume that cells of the immune system require more concentrations of antioxidants than other types of cells to neutralize the excess of ROS accumulation. Obviously, the oxidant/antioxidant balance is a crucial determinant that contributes to improve immune

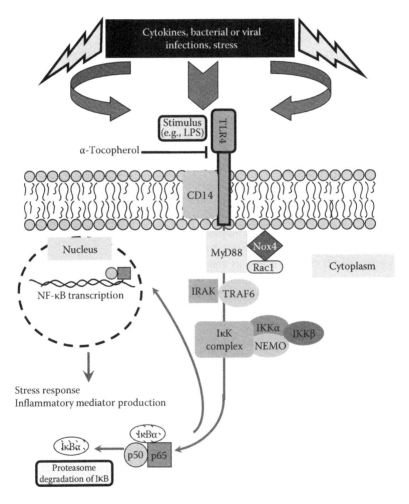

FIGURE 5.2 **(See color insert.)** Oxidative stress signaling pathway and gene expression in sepsis. IκK, IκB kinase complex; IRAK, interleukin-1 receptor-associated kinase; LPS, lipopolysaccharide; MyD88, myeloid differentiation protein 88; NEMO, NF-κB essential modifier; NF-κB, nuclear factor-κB; Nox4, NADPH oxidase; TLR4, Toll-like receptor 4; TRAF6, tumor necrosis factor receptor-associated factor 6. (From Puertollano, M.A. et al., *Curr Top Med Chem.*, 11, 1752, 2011.)

cell function, not only preserving integrity and functionality of lipids that constitute plasma membrane but also protecting cellular proteins and nucleic acids, and consequently for regulating signal transduction and gene expression in immune cells. The redox state of the cells may activate nuclear factor-κB (NF-κB), an inducible transcription factor that can rapidly regulate the expression of genes involved in inflammatory response (Schreck et al., 1991). The regulation of NF-κB by the oxidative stress status of the host can have a substantial effect on the host response to infection. A schematic representation of upregulation of inflammatory gene expression by the NF-κB pathway is illustrated in Figure 5.2.

The most important source of antioxidants that protect cells from oxidative stress is provided by nutrition. Dietary antioxidants constitute mainly free radical scavengers, and they act through different mechanisms and in different compartments: (i) they directly neutralize free radicals; (ii) they reduce the peroxide concentrations and repair oxidized membranes; (iii) they quench iron to decrease ROS production; and (iv) they neutralize ROS through lipid metabolism (short-chain free fatty acids and cholesteryl esters) (Parke, 1999).

DIETARY ANTIOXIDANTS AND HOST NATURAL RESISTANCE TO INFECTION

Natural antioxidants protect the body against the free radicals produced whenever the body undergoes the process of oxidation. As previously mentioned, immune system cells are particularly sensitive to oxidative stress, which occurs when an imbalance develops because of high ROS levels and/or low antioxidant levels. Thus, increased oxidative stress induced by a dietary deficiency in antioxidant nutrients would be expected to affect the host immune response against infection by infectious microorganisms. Hence, oxidative stress has been implicated in the pathogenesis of several microbial, parasitic, and viral infections, including hepatitis, influenza, and acquired immunodeficiency syndrome (AIDS) (Semba and Tang, 1999; Peterhans, 1997).

In the state of inflammation and infection, the antimicrobial activity of activated neutrophils and macrophages involves ROS generation. Moreover, under these circumstances, endothelial NO synthase (NOS) is uncoupled, resulting in reduced NO and increased O_2 production leading to systemic oxidative stress (Strand et al., 2000).

The presence of inadequate antioxidant defenses is responsible for the existence of oxidative stress in the cells. This is due to changes in the presence of antioxidant enzymes such as superoxide dismutase and catalase, or a reduction in vitamins C and E, and reduced glutathione. These actions may commonly occur during sepsis. Therefore, cells of the immune system are responsible for the generation of ROS in response to foreign pathogens. However, immune cells are especially sensitive not only to the presence of ROS from the microbicidal activity but also to external ROS. To avoid the immunosuppressive action that oxidative stress exerts, immune cells have a high content of antioxidants such as vitamins, which exert a protective role against oxidation of molecules present in the cells as polyunsaturated fatty acids (Bendich and Machlin, 1988). Thus, nutrients that affect the antioxidant status have important effects on immune function. The intake of vitamins and trace elements with antioxidant activity are essential for proper immune system activity (Wintergerst et al., 2007; Knight, 2000; Hughes, 2000). Table 5.1 summarizes the important role of selected vitamins and trace elements on immune system functions, and Table 5.2 represents the most important studies focused on the effect of vitamins and trace elements on host resistance to microorganisms.

TABLE 5.2
Antioxidants and Immune Functions

Dietary Antioxidants (Exogenous)	Types of Dietary Antioxidants	Immunological Effects
1. Trace Elements		
	Selenium	Increases lymphocyte proliferation, expression of IL-2R, and NK cell function. Se supplementation is involved in enhancing Th1-type immune responses to a greater extent than Th2-type responses. Deficiency promotes loss of immunocompetence (both cell-mediated immunity and B-cell function may be impaired)
	Copper	Adequate intake supports a Th1 response. Excessive supplementation reduces the activity of phagocytic cells. Deficiency reduces antibody production, phagocytic activity, T-cell proliferation, and B-cell numbers
	Zinc	Cytosolic defense against oxidative stress. Increases phagocytosis, NK cell activity, and DTH and antibody response. Augments cytotoxic CD8$^+$ T lymphocytes
	Iron	Differentiation and proliferation of T lymphocytes, NK cells, monocytes, and macrophages. Deficiency reduces cytotoxic activity of phagocytes and proliferation of Th1 cells, IL-2 production, phagocytic activity, and immunoglobulin levels
2. Vitamins		
	β-Carotene	Increases mitogen-induced lymphocyte proliferation, cell-mediated cytotoxicity, and NK cell activity. By contrast, it does not affect DTH, IL-2 production, and lymphocyte subsets
	Vitamin C	Increases neutrophil chemotaxis, NK cell activity, and T-lymphocyte proliferation. Augments cytokine production and immunoglobulin synthesis
	Vitamin E	Deficiency reduces lymphocyte proliferation and phagocyte functions while supplementation in healthy individuals increases lymphocyte proliferation, IL-2 production, NK cell activity, and phagocytic functions

Source: Puertollano, M.A. et al., *Curr Top Med Chem.*, 11, 1752, 2011.
Note: DTH, delayed type hypersensitivity; IL-2R, interleukin-2 receptor; NK, natural killer.

VITAMINS AND HOST RESISTANCE TO INFECTION

Dietary antioxidants are vital for proper immune system function. Among the most studied include vitamin C, vitamin E, and β-carotene. Vitamins C and E at high doses both exert a protective role by reducing the adverse effects of oxidative stress in sepsis. Vitamin C plays an important function particularly against oxidative stress in leukocytes. Vitamin C acts as an important reducer (powerful electron donor that reacts with O_2 and OH radicals); however, it is also involved in the modulation of complex biochemical pathways central to the function of the immune cells. Likewise, vitamin E is the major antioxidant present in the cell membranes. This vitamin is essential for the maintenance of adequate immune response to infection, especially in inflammatory cells. Finally, β-carotene is a potent quencher of singlet oxygen and acts as an antioxidant in biologically relevant systems, and it also affects several aspects of human immune system functions. Table 5.3 illustrates different studies determining the effects of vitamins on host resistance to infection.

Vitamin C

Vitamin C or ascorbic acid is defined as the major water-soluble cytosolic chain-breaking antioxidant that plays an important role in the host defense against oxidative damage, especially in leukocytes. In addition, vitamin C provides important antioxidant protection to plasma lipids and lipid membranes and can neutralize phagocyte-derived oxidants released extracellularly, preventing oxidant-mediated tissue damage especially in sites of infection (Frei et al., 1989; Anderson and Lukey, 1987). Indeed, a number of investigations have reported that vitamin C levels are decreased in plasma and leukocytes in patients with common cold or pneumonia, but moderate intake of ascorbic acid had no apparent effect on the duration or severity of the common cold, although it decreases the frequency of common cold (Sasazuki et al., 2006) and pneumonia (Hemila, 1997; Hemila and Douglas, 1999). In this context, it is important to underline other experimental observations that demonstrate a reduction of plasma ascorbate in subjects with human immunodeficiency virus (HIV) infection (Allard et al., 1998). In addition, high intakes of vitamin C were associated with a lower risk of progression to AIDS in an observational study, reducing the severity of HIV progression (Tang et al., 1993).

A number of results from studies *in vitro* and *in vivo* (in humans and other species) underline the functional significance of vitamin C in infection resistance. *In vitro* and *in vivo* studies demonstrate that low levels of ascorbic acid increases the susceptibility to candidiasis (Anderson and Theron, 1979; Rogers et al., 1983). A recent study has determined that the administration of both vitamins C and E together with antimicrobial therapy promotes and effective eradication of *Helicobacter pylori* (Sezikli et al., 2009; Zojaji et al., 2009).

Vitamin E

Vitamin E is an important lipid-soluble antioxidant that protects against free radical–initiated lipid peroxidation, and it constitutes the major chain-breaking lipid-soluble antioxidant that diminishes damage to lipid membranes due to the formation of ROS during infections. Vitamin E is involved in an increased resistance against infectious microorganisms, indicating that higher vitamin E intake induces a Th1 cytokine–mediated response and suppresses the Th2 response, offering protection against the

TABLE 5.3
Vitamin Effect on Host Resistance to Infection

Vitamins	Microorganisms	Effects	Humans (H) or Animals (A)	References
Vitamin A	HIV	Reduction of this vitamin in serum	H	Baum et al., 1995
	HIV	Dietary and supplemental intake delays AIDS progression	H	Tang et al., 1993
β-Carotene	HIV	Increases the number of NK cells but does not affect CD4+ population	H	Garewal et al., 1992
	HIV	Reduces T CD4+ subset and lowers mortality	H	Nimmagadda et al., 1996
Vitamin C	Common cold	Reduction of the duration and severity of symptoms. However, these conclusions have absolutely not been clarified	H	Hemila, 1996; Sasazuki et al., 2006
	Candida albicans	Inability of macrophages to eliminate the pathogen. Increases the susceptibility to microorganisms in ex vivo studies	In vitro; A	Anderson and Theron, 1979; Rogers et al., 1983
	Helicobacter pylori	High doses have an inhibitory effect on bacterial colonization. Increased antimicrobial activity in the presence of classic treatment	H	Sezikli et al., 2009; Zojaji et al., 2009

Vitamin E	Influenza virus	Supplementation resulted in significantly lower viral titer on 2, 5, and 7 days postinfection, as well as an increase of IL-2 and IFN-γ production	A	Han et al., 2000; Hayek et al., 1997
	Herpes simplex virus	Adequate levels limited herpes simplex virus encephalitis. Deficiencies impaired the course of infection, whereas supplementation did not affect the progression of virus	A	Sheridan and Beck, 2008
	Trypanosoma cruzi	Deficiency was associated with a reduction of T- and B-cell counts	A	Carvalho et al., 2006
	Common cold	Supplementation reduced the incidence rate of common colds but did not affect the duration of this infection	H	Meydani et al., 2004
	HIV	Reduction of viral load at 3 months of intervention	H	Allard et al., 1998
	HIV	Normalization and restoration of immune parameters after treatment with 160 IU/L	A	Wang et al., 1994
	Hepatitis B	HBeAg seroconversion after vitamin E treatment	H	Gerner et al., 2008

Source: Puertollano, M.A. et al., 2013. Natural antioxidants and resistance to infection. In: *Bioactive Food as Dietary Interventions for Arthritis and Related Inflammatory Diseases*, Watson, R.R. and Preedy, V.R., Eds. San Diego: Academic Press, 157–174.

intracellular growth of microorganisms such as viruses and bacteria (Meydani et al., 2005). Vitamin E participates in the increase of lymphocyte proliferation, IL-2 production, NK cell activity, and phagocytic functions by alveolar macrophages.

The investigation in mice treated with 160 IU/L liquid diet of vitamin E demonstrated normalization of immune parameters that are altered after HIV infection (Wang et al., 1994). Irrespective of the studies carried out in murine models, studies in humans are limited to aged subjects. A double-blind, placebo-controlled investigation determined a favorable effect on the incidence and severity of acute respiratory tract infections in the elderly after daily multivitamin–mineral supplementation at physiological doses and 200 mg of vitamin E (Graat et al., 2002). Overall, vitamin E supplementation was able to reduce the incidence rate of common colds; however, a nonstatistically significant reduction in the duration of colds was also reported (Meydani et al., 2004). Supplemental vitamin E (200 IU/day for 4 months) improved cell-mediated immunity among free-living US adults >65 years old compared with placebo (Meydani et al., 1997); however, a Dutch study did not find any effect of multivitamins on infection risk, and an adverse effect of vitamin E supplements on acute respiratory symptoms was observed among free-living elderly Dutch individuals (Graat et al., 2002).

β-Carotene

β-Carotene is the predominant source of the essential nutrient vitamin A. In fact, β-carotene has traditionally been considered as a source of vitamin A with this exclusive function. However, several studies have shown that carotenoids can enhance immune functions independently of any provitamin A activity. β-Carotene has been related to increased numbers of CD4+ cells (Fryburg et al., 1995). For this reason, it has been applied as an immune-enhancing agent in the treatment of HIV infection. Similarly, β-carotene is able to increase NK cell number without affecting the CD4+ population in HIV-infected patients (Santos et al., 1996, 1997). Taking into account that septic patients exhibit inadequate concentrations of β-carotene (Ribeiro Nogueira et al., 2009), different studies have determined that low concentrations of serum vitamin A and β-carotene in HIV-infected patients decrease CD4+ lymphocyte counts and increase mortality. Therefore, HIV-infected individuals who ingest moderately increased amounts of dietary β-carotene have a diminished risk of dying or developing AIDS (Nimmagadda et al., 1998).

TRACE ELEMENTS AND HOST RESISTANCE TO INFECTION

Immune cells, as the other cell types of an organism, require an adequate supply of trace elements for the structure and function of metalloproteins that contribute to maintain processes such as (i) energy production (copper for cytochrome c oxidase in the mitochondrial electron-transport chain), (ii) protection against ROS (as cofactors for enzymes with antioxidant activity), and (iii) protection against infection (trace elements are also necessary for the activity of defense mechanism). In general, trace elements (e.g., selenium, copper, and zinc) do not act directly as antioxidants but are critical components of the antioxidant enzymes (catalase, superoxide dismutase, and glutathione peroxidase [GPx]). Table 5.4 presents different studies determining the effects of vitamins on host resistance to infection.

Selenium

Selenium is an important antioxidant trace element participating in redox regulation and constituting a part of some antioxidant defense systems (selenium-dependent GPx, thioredoxin reductase, and selenoprotein P). Therefore, selenium is involved in protection against oxidative stress, and it firmly contributes to membrane integrity and protection against DNA damage. The participation of selenium as an integral part of the selenoenzyme GPx provided a mechanism by which this element could exert its biological functions. The selenoenzyme GPx detoxifies damaging organic hydroperoxides, as well as H_2O_2, which are produced during oxidative metabolism (Foster and Sumar, 1997). A lack of GPx produces a damage of lysosomal membranes by lipid hydroperoxides, leading to the release of various hydrolytic enzymes into the plasma (Reddanna et al., 1989).

The actions of selenium on the modulation of the immune system are multiple. Thus, selenium increases lymphocyte proliferation, expression of the high-affinity IL-2R, cytolytic T-lymphocyte tumor destruction, and NK cell function in humans (Kiremidjian-Schumacher et al., 1994), enhancing resistance to infections through modulation of interleukin production and subsequently the Th1/Th2 response (Baum et al., 2000a). A deficiency in selenium has been described to affect the immune system and to have an effect on the ability to control the infection (Harbige, 1996; Kukreja and Khan, 1998). Thus, selenium deficiency is involved in a higher host susceptibility to *Cryptosporidium parvum* infection (Wang et al., 2009b). Likewise, selenium deficiency in rats and mice has been shown in *in vitro* studies to alter the ability of neutrophils and peritoneal macrophages to eliminate *Candida albicans*. For other studies that have been conducted investigating the relation between selenium and different bacterial infections, deficiency of this trace element increases the persistence of *Listeria monocytogenes* in the intestine and mesentery lymphoid nodules (Wang et al., 2009a). By contrast, the removal of species such as *Salmonella typhimurium* and *Staphylococcus aureus* is not related to selenium deficiency (Boyne and Arthur, 1986; Boyne et al., 1986).

Changes in the intracellular environment that are induced by alterations in micronutrient status can directly influence viral virulence and can cause immune system dysfunction. Thus, selenium deficiency is able to promote the mutation of a virulent strain of coxsackievirus in the heart to a strain that causes myocarditis, when the virus is passed from the selenium-deficient to a nutritionally adequate host. This pathology is an endemic disease in China, which is called Keshan disease, a cardiomyopathy characterized by necrotic lesions throughout the myocardium accompanied by cellular infiltration and calcification. Indeed, the administration of selenium to individuals from deficient areas is able to prevent the disease. An important experience with Se-deficient and Se-adequate mice that were infected with a benign amyocarditic strain of coxsackievirus B3 (CVB3/0) demonstrated that the Se-adequate mice did not develop myocarditis when infected with the amyocarditic strain of the virus, whereas the Se-deficient animals developed a moderate level of myocarditis with similarities to that seen in humans (Heyland et al., 2005). In the same way, Se-deficient mice were more susceptible to influenza virus infection than Se-adequate mice (Beck et al., 2001), and selenium has been demonstrated to

TABLE 5.4

Trace Element Effect on Host Resistance to Infection

Trace Elements	Microorganisms	Effects	Humans (H) or Animals (A)	References
Selenium	Cryptosporidium parvum	Increased host susceptibility in selenium-deficient animals	A	Wang et al., 2009
	Trichinella spiralis	Supplementation played an important role in the treatment of parasitoses	A	Gabrashanska et al., 2010
	Candida albicans, Salmonella typhimurium, and Staphylococcus aureus	Deficiency impaired neutrophil and macrophage functionality to eliminate C. albicans without affect to neutrophil in the elimination of S. typhimurium or S. aureus	A	Boyne and Arthur, 1986; Boyne et al., 1986
	Listeria monocytogenes	Deficiency impaired systemic innate immune response to L. monocytogenes infection	A	Wang et al., 2009
	Coxsackievirus B	Coxsackievirus B mutated to a cardiotoxic form in selenium-deficient hosts (Keshan disease)	A and H	Beck et al., 1994
	Influenza virus	Selenium-deficient animals were more susceptible to influenza virus infection	A	Beck et al., 2001
	Hepatitis B or C viruses	Reduced the risk of hepatocarcinoma caused by virus infection	H	Yu et al., 1999
	HIV	Low plasma selenium levels were associated with a significant increase of death risk, as well as mycobacterial infections	H	Baum et al., 1997; Shor-Posner et al., 2002
Copper	Salmonella typhimurium	Deficiency produced higher mortality rates than in control animals	A	Newberne et al., 1968
	Trypanosoma lewisi	Copper deficiency was responsible for causing severe depression in the primary and secondary antibody responses	A	Crocker et al., 1992

Zinc	Listeria monocytogenes	Zinc-deficient animals showed thymic atrophy, reduced DTH, and impaired lymphocyte response	A	Carlomagno et al., 1986
	Salmonella enteritidis	Increased in vitro phagocytosis but did not affect the number of mononuclear cells	A	Kidd et al., 1994
	Mycobacterium tuberculosis	Zinc-deficient animals had fewer circulating T cells and reduced tuberculin hypersensitivity	A	McMurray et al., 1990
	Candida albicans	Increased host resistance against this pathogen because it potentiated T-lymphocyte and macrophage functions	A	Singh et al., 1992
	Trypanosoma cruzi	Increased peritoneal macrophages, as well as IFN-γ and NO production after zinc supplementation	A	Brazao et al., 2008
	Plasmodium falciparum	Reduction of morbidity after zinc supplementation	H	Shankar et al., 2000
	HIV	Increase of CD4+ counts and a reduction of opportunistic infections	H	Mocchegiani and Muzzioli, 2000
	Pneumonia	Reduction of incidence. Supplementation with zinc and selenium significantly increased the humoral response in elderly individuals after vaccination, and increased the number of patients without respiratory infections	H	Girodon et al., 1999; Fischer Walker and Black, 2004
	Common cold	No evidence of effective action	H	Marshall, 1999
Iron	Salmonella typhimurium	Severe deficiencies enhanced defenses against infection	A	Baggs and Miller, 1973
	Streptococcus pneumoniae	Severe deficiencies increased mortality	A	Chu et al., 1976

Source: Puertollano, M.A. et al., 2013. Natural antioxidants and resistance to infection. In: *Bioactive Food as Dietary Interventions for Arthritis and Related Inflammatory Diseases*, Watson, R.R. and Preedy, V.R., Eds. San Diego: Academic Press, 157–174.

be protective against infections caused by either hepatitis B or hepatitis C viruses because it reduces the risk of hepatocarcinoma promoted by these viruses (Yu et al., 1997, 1999). Selenium also plays a critical role in HIV-infected patients, in whom there has been a decrease in plasma levels of selenium together with a loss in the population of CD4 T cells (Look et al., 1997).

Iron

Iron deficiency has been considered the most common micronutrient deficiency in the world, particularly in the tropics. Cellular iron alters the proliferation and activation of lymphocytes and NK cells; modulates proliferation and differentiation of T cells, monocytes, and macrophages; interacts with cell-mediated immune response; and modulates cytokine activities. Iron accumulation has been shown to increase infection rates, whereas low iron concentrations are associated with an impaired immune system because critical immune cells such as macrophages are unable to produce microbial killing enzymes such as hydroxy radicals. However, iron deficiency may be protective against malaria and *Yersinia* infections, whereas ion overload may predispose to infection by supplying necessary amounts of iron for the development and growth of bacteria (Keush, 1990) or enhancing the rate of progression of HIV disease and decreasing survival (Cunnigham-Rundles et al., 2000).

It is important to note the existence of a protein called natural resistance associated macrophage protein-1, which is located in the membrane of the phagolysosome of macrophages, monocytes, and neutrophils, and has the function of transporting divalent metals, including Fe^{2+}, providing protection against intracellular microorganisms such as *Leishmania*, *Mycobacterium*, and *Salmonella* (Bellamy, 1999). In fact, experimental studies *in vitro* and animal studies suggest that the growth of intracellular organisms such as plasmodia, mycobacteria, and invasive *Salmonella* may be enhanced by iron therapy. By contrast, iron deficiency could have a protective effect against malaria, HIV, and tuberculosis (Oppenheimer, 2001). Effects of iron deficiencies are early known. Although iron exerts important modulatory effects on the immune system, a clinically important relation between states of iron deficiency and susceptibility to infection remains controversial.

Zinc

Zinc is an important antioxidant that plays an essential function in immune protection, particularly in the elderly. The contribution of zinc is crucial for the activity of superoxide dismutase and participates in T-cell division, maturation, and differentiation. Zinc deficiency results in a marked atrophy of the thymus involving an increase in lymphopenia. Zinc is crucial for normal development and adequate function of cells mediating nonspecific immunity, such as NK cells and neutrophils. Similarly, zinc deficiency affects the development of acquired immunity by preventing several functions of T lymphocytes, such as activation, Th1 cytokine production, and B-lymphocyte functions such as immunoglobulin G production. It is important to note that zinc deficiencies are characterized by an increased susceptibility to a diverse variety of infectious agents, including *Listeria monocytogenes* (Carlomagno et al., 1986), *Salmonella enteritidis* (Kidd et al., 1994), *Mycobacterium tuberculosis* (McMurray et al., 1990), and herpes simplex virus (Feiler et al., 1982).

In patients with AIDS, a zinc deficiency has been observed, and a disease progression as well as a depressed mitogenic response has been described (Bogden et al., 1990). However, these changes were partially reversible by zinc supplementation (Falutz et al., 1988). In contrast, an important study reported that zinc supplementation in patients with HIV induces a more rapid progression of the disease (Tang et al., 1996), probably due to an excessive zinc administration. Hence, these observations indicate the need to carefully consider therapeutic options, and immune status should be evaluated after identifying a beneficial role of zinc supplementation in these patients (Baum et al., 2000b). A recent review reports that low zinc status impairs immune function, impairs resistance to pathogens, and is associated with increased incidence and duration of pneumonia, resulting in augmented use and duration of antimicrobial treatment and increased mortality in the elderly (Barnett et al., 2010).

Copper

Copper deficiency impairs both the innate and acquired immunity, suppressing the proliferation of activated T cells and the production of proinflammatory cytokines (IL-1, IL-2, TNF); reducing phagocytic activities and the number of mature neutrophils in peripheral blood (Prohaska and Failla, 1993); and decreasing mononuclear phagocytic activities, which compromises the innate immune defense system and contributes to greater susceptibility to infection (Percival, 1995).

Although copper deficiency has been related with the reduction of several parameters in certain animal studies, human studies have reported inconclusive results. Indeed, copper supplementation has increased the numbers of neutrophils in peripheral blood and reduced the incidence of respiratory tract infections in infants recovering from marasmus, who were neither anemic nor neutropenic (Castillo-Duran et al., 1983). On the other hand, a recent study has demonstrated that a high intake of copper reduces some parameters of immune functions against the Beijing strain of influenza virus. These results indicate that under highly controlled conditions, long-term high copper intake affects several indices of immune function (Turnlund et al., 2004).

OTHER NATURAL ANTIOXIDANTS CONTAINED IN FOODS: A BRIEF DESCRIPTION

Polyphenols are bioactive compounds present in fruits and vegetables characterized by the presence of multiples of phenol structural units. In plants, polyphenols, besides providing color and flavor, have a defense function against ultraviolet radiation, pathogens, and other damage (Korkina et al., 2008). Polyphenols are separated from essential nutrients because a deficiency state has not been detected; nevertheless, these phytochemicals play an important biological role. Nowadays, a number of studies have shown that polyphenols are natural compounds with an interesting range of biological effects, including anti-inflammatory (González-Gallego et al., 2010), antioxidant (Izzi et al., 2012), cardiovascular (Andriantsitohaina et al., 2012), anticancer (Spagnuolo et al., 2012), and immunomodulatory actions (Clarke and Mullin, 2008).

Despite the strong evidence about the effect of polyphenols on the immune system, the mechanisms implied in these actions are not fully understood currently. One of the main theories is focused on the effect of polyphenols on epigenetic mechanisms such as DNA methylation, histone modifications, and posttranscriptional regulation by microRNAs. The epigenetic mechanisms are implied in numerous immune processes such as T- and B-cell differentiation, transcriptional control of *Foxp3* gene expression (leading to differentiation of CD4[+] cells into T regulatory cells [Tregs]), macrophage activation, and production of proinflammatory cytokines (reviewed in Cuevas et al., 2013). Recent studies have shown that polyphenols may act by modifying these epigenetic mechanisms in immune cells. In this sense, epigallocatechin-3-gallate (EGCG), the major polyphenol in green tea, have been shown, in an *in vitro* model, to increase Foxp3 and IL-10 in T cells. Interestingly, the same study showed an increase in the Treg subpopulation in different immune organs, with functionally active cells, in mice fed with this polyphenol (Wong et al., 2011). Recently, an intervention study has revealed that consumption of cocoa, a rich source of dietary polyphenols, decreases the DNA methylation in peripheral leukocytes (Crescenti et al., 2013). In the next paragraphs, the main dietary polyphenols and the effects on immune function and resistance to infection will be described.

Hydroxytyrosol (3,4-dihydroxyphenyl ethanol) has been shown to exert a protective effect against intestinal pathologies whose etiology has been related to ROS generation, in particular those characterized by changes in epithelium permeability such as inflammatory diseases (Manna et al., 1997). This dietary antioxidant may be found in olive oil, which is an important source of vitamins (e.g., α-tocopherols) and polyphenolic antioxidants, and has a balanced ratio of monounsaturated and polyunsaturated fatty acids. Olive oil has beneficial effects on human health, and it is implicated in the resolution, attenuation, or prevention of diverse pathologies. Among them, olive oil is characterized by modulating immune system functions (Puertollano et al., 2007, 2010), and it is involved in the prevention of cellular oxidative stress and inflammation due mainly to the presence of antioxidants (De la Puerta et al., 2009). Indeed, recent studies have shown the ability of hydroxytyrosol to prevent oxidative stress and DNA damage in human peripheral blood mononuclear cells (Ilavarasi et al., 2011). These regulatory functions in the immune system appear to be involved in an increase of host resistance to microorganisms after administration of diets containing olive oil (Puertollano et al., 2010). Studies *in vitro* have suggested that phenolic components from olive oil possess radical scavenging activity at least as strong as that of other relevant dietary antioxidants, such as ascorbic acid and α-tocopherol (Visioli et al., 1998a). Phenolic components from olive oil such as oleuropein added to murine macrophages together with a bacterial lipopolysaccharide increase the functional activity of macrophages in the production of the bactericidal and cytostatic factor NO (Visioli et al., 1998b). In addition, data from animal studies have suggested that oleuropein may act as an anti-*Toxoplasma* compound, evidencing the action of this polyphenol on infection resistance of animals infected with this parasite (Jiang et al., 2008).

Traditionally, green tea consumption has been related to a positive effect on human health, such as toxin elimination and improvement of resistance to infection. Green tea, the most ancient beverage in the world, has a high content of polyphenols, most of them catechins, which include epicatechin, epigallocatechin, epicatechin-3-gallate, and EGCG, the most abundant compound in tea (Kanwar et al., 2012). Catechins appear to be involved in the immunomodulating activities of tea. Indeed, several investigations have revealed that tea polyphenols are capable of modulating proinflammatory signals in certain *in vitro* and *in vivo* models, suggesting that green tea may be considered as an adjuvant treatment in some inflammatory disorders (Pajonk et al., 2006; Varilek et al., 2001). Regarding antimicrobial effects, green tea has been shown to inhibit the growth of bacteria responsible for upper respiratory tract infections (Hamilton-Miller, 1995; Yam et al., 1997). In addition, tea polyphenols and extracts delay or inhibit the growth of a wide variety of pathogenic strains of Enterobacteriaceae (Yam et al., 1997), without affecting lactobacilli growth. More recently, numerous investigations have pointed out the possible role of tea flavonoids in HIV type 1 (HIV-1) infection, proposing tea polyphenols as a promising adjuvant treatment in the prevention and treatment of this viral disease (Zhao et al., 2012). An interesting study has shown that EGCG targets semen-derived enhancer of virus infection, an important infectivity factor of HIV during sexual transmission, for degradation. This property may be useful in a concomitant treatment with antiretroviral drugs (Hauber et al., 2009). Other investigations have proposed that EGCG modifies the attachment of HIV-1-gp120 to the CD4 molecule, inhibiting HIV-1 infectivity in human CD4$^+$ T lymphocytes (Nance et al., 2009), and may act as reverse transcriptase inhibitor (Li et al., 2011).

Another main dietary polyphenol is resveratrol. Resveratrol is the main polyphenol contained in red wine and grapes and has shown a relevant immunomodulatory activity (Gao et al., 2001; Falchetti et al., 2001). Although the exact mechanism by which resveratrol exerts immunomodulatory activity has not clearly been defined, it appears to inhibit cell proliferation, cell-mediated cytotoxicity, and cytokine production (Docherty et al., 2004) through the inhibition of NF-κB activation (Gao et al., 2001). In addition, resveratrol is able to modulate T-cell differentiation (Petro, 2011). As a result of its immunomodulatory properties, it has been demonstrated that resveratrol protects mice from infection with herpes simplex viruses (Docherty et al., 2004, 2005) and exerts antiviral activity against varicella-zoster virus *in vitro* (Docherty et al., 2006). Another study has revealed that resveratrol has an antiviral activity against Epstein–Barr virus, inhibiting viral particle production, ROS generation, and activity of transcription factors such as NF-κβ and Ap1 (De Leo et al., 2012). These antimicrobial effects may be attributed, at least in part, to the potent antioxidant and anti-inflammatory effect of this polyphenol. In this way, in an *in vitro* model of lung infection by *Pseudomonas aeruginosa*, resveratrol reduced ROS generation, ICAM-1, and human β-defensin-2 expression, and upregulated GPx, protecting the cells against the deleterious effects caused by an exacerbated oxidative stress and inflammation produced by *P. aeruginosa* infection (Cerqueira et al., 2013).

Finally, recent researches are focusing on the effect of cocoa on the immune system. Cocoa flavonoids, including catechins and procyanidins, have been shown to be able to modulate different mechanisms of the immune system such as secretion of cytokine and other inflammatory molecules in different *in vitro* studies (reviewed in Perez-Cano et al., 2013). Different studies from this laboratory have pointed out that a cocoa diet is able to modify the different lymphocyte subsets. Concretely, these authors found that cocoa promotes T-cell maturation in thyme, increases B cells in the spleen, and increases the percentage of TCRγδ$^+$ cells in Peyer's patches in rats fed with a cocoa-rich diet, suggesting a positive effect on immune system maturation (Ramiro-Puig et al., 2007a,b, 2008).

REFERENCES

Allard, J.P., Aghdassi, E., Chau, J. et al. 1998. Effects of vitamin E and C supplementation on oxidative stress and viral load in HIV-infected subjects. *AIDS.* 12(13): 1653–1659.

Anderson, R. and Lukey, F.T. 1987. A biological role for ascorbate in the selective neutralisation of extracellular phagocyte-derived oxidants. *Ann NY Acad Sci.* 498: 229–247.

Anderson, R. and Theron, A. 1979. Effects of ascorbate on leucocytes: Part III. *In vitro* and *in vivo* stimulation of abnormal neutrophil motility by ascorbate. *S Afr Med J.* 56(11): 429–433.

Andriantsitohaina, R., Auger, C., Chataigneau, T. et al. 2012. Molecular mechanisms of the cardiovascular protective effects of polyphenols. *Br J Nutr.* 108(9): 1532–1549.

Baggs, R.B. and Miller, S.A. 1973. Nutritional iron deficiency as a determinant of host resistance in the rat. *J Nutr.* 103(11): 1554–1560.

Baker, K.R. and Meydani, M. 1994. Beta-carotene in immunity and cancer. *J Optim Nutr.* 3: 39–50.

Barnett, J.B., Hamer, D.H. and Meydani, S.N. 2010. Low zinc status: A new risk factor for pneumonia in the elderly? *Nutr Rev.* 68(1): 30–37.

Baum, M.K., Miguez-Burbano, M.J., Campa, A. and Shor-Posner, G. 2000a. Selenium and interleukins in persons infected with human immunodeficiency virus type 1. *J Infect Dis.* 182 Suppl 1: S69–S73.

Baum, M.K., Shor-Posner, G. and Campa, A. 2000b. Zinc status in human immunodeficiency virus infection. *J Nutr.* 130(5S Suppl): 1421S–1423S.

Baum, M.K., Shor-Posner, G., Lu, Y. et al. 1995. Micronutrients and HIV-1 disease progression. *AIDS.* 9(9): 1051–1056.

Beck, M.A., Kolbeck, P.C., Rohr, L.H., Shi, Q., Morris, V.C. and Levander, O.A. 1994. Benign human enterovirus becomes virulent in selenium-deficient mice. *J Med Virol.* 43(2): 166–170.

Beck, M.A., Nelson, H.K., Shi, Q. et al. 2001. Selenium deficiency increases the pathology of an influenza virus infection. *FASEB J.* 15(8): 1481–1483.

Bellamy, R. 1999. The natural resistance-associated macrophage protein and susceptibility to intracellular pathogens. *Microbes Infect.* 1(1): 23–27.

Bendich, A. and Machlin, L.J. 1988. Safety of oral intake of vitamin E. *Am J Clin Nutr.* 48(3): 612–619.

Bogden, J.D., Baker, H., Frank, O. et al. 1990. Micronutrient status and human immunodeficiency virus (HIV) infection. *Ann N Y Acad Sci.* 587: 189–195.

Boyne, R. and Arthur, J.R. 1986. The response of selenium-deficient mice to *Candida albicans* infection. *J Nutr.* 116(5): 816–822.

Boyne, R., Arthur, J.R. and Wilson, A.B. 1986. An *in vivo* and *in vitro* study of selenium deficiency and infection in rats. *J Comp Pathol.* 96(4): 379–386.

Brazao, V., Del Vecchio Filipin, M., Caetano, L.C., Toldo, M.P., Caetano, L.N. and do Prado, J.C., Jr. 2008. Trypanosoma cruzi: The effects of zinc supplementation during experimental infection. *Exp Parasitol.* 118(4): 549–554.

Carlomagno, M.A., Coghlan, L.G. and McMurray, D.N. 1986. Chronic zinc deficiency and listeriosis in rats: Acquired cellular resistance and response to vaccination. *Med Microbiol Immunol.* 175: 271–280.

Carvalho, L.S., Camargos, E.R., Almeida, C.T. et al. 2006. Vitamin E deficiency enhances pathology in acute Trypanosoma cruzi-infected rats. *Trans R Soc Trop Med Hyg.* 100(11): 1025–1031.

Castillo-Duran, C., Fisberg, M., Valenzuela, A., Egana, J.I. and Uauy, R. 1983. Controlled trial of copper supplementation during the recovery from marasmus. *Am J Clin Nutr.* 37: 898–903.

Cerqueira, A.M., Khaper, N., Lees, S.J. and Ulanova, M. 2013. The antioxidant resveratrol down-regulates inflammation in an *in-vitro* model of *Pseudomonas aeruginosa* infection of lung epithelial cells. *Can J Physiol Pharmacol.* 91(3): 248–255.

Chandra, R.K. 1999. Nutrition and immunology: From the clinic to cellular biology and back again. *Proc Nutr Soc.* 58(3): 681–683.

Chu, S.W., Welch, K.J., Murray, E.S. and Hegsted, D.M. 1976. Effect of iron deficiency on the susceptibility of *Streptococcus pneumoniae* in the rat. *Nutr Rep Int.* 14: 605–609.

Clarke, J.O. and Mullin, G.E. 2008. A review of complementary and alternative approaches to immunomodulation. *Nutr Clin Pract.* 23(1): 49–62.

Crescenti, A., Solà, R., Valls, R.M. et al. 2013. Cocoa consumption alters the global DNA methylation of peripheral leukocytes in humans with cardiovascular disease risk factors: A randomized controlled trial. *PLoS One.* 8(6): e65744.

Crocker, A., Lee, C., Aboko-Cole, G. and Durham, C. 1992. Interaction of nutrition and infection: Effect of copper deficiency on resistance to Trypanosoma lewisi. *J Natl Med Assoc.* 84(8): 697–706.

Cuevas, A., Saavedra, N., Salazar, L.A. and Abdalla, D.S. 2013. Modulation of immune function by polyphenols: Possible contribution of epigenetic factors. *Nutrients.* 5: 2314–2332.

Cunningham-Rundles, S., Giardina, P.J., Grady, R.W., Califano, C., McKenzie, P. and De Sousa, M. 2000. Effect of transfusional iron overload on immune response. *J Infect Dis.* 182 Suppl 1: S115–S121.

De la Puerta, R., Marquez-Martin, A., Fernandez-Arche, A. and Ruiz-Gutierrez, V. 2009. Influence of dietary fat on oxidative stress and inflammation in murine macrophages. *Nutrition.* 25(5): 548–554.

De Leo, A., Arena, G., Lacanna, E., Oliviero, G., Colavita, F. and Mattia, E. 2012. Resveratrol inhibits Epstein Barr virus lytic cycle in Burkitt's lymphoma cells by affecting multiple molecular targets. *Antiviral Res.* 96(2): 196–202.

De Pablo, M.A. and Alvarez de Cienfuegos, G. 2000. Modulatory effects of dietary lipids on immune system functions. *Immunol Cell Biol.* 78(1): 31–39.

Docherty, J.J., Fu, M.M., Hah, J.M., Sweet, T.J., Faith, S.A. and Booth, T. 2005. Effect of resveratrol on herpes simplex virus vaginal infection in the mouse. *Antiviral Res.* 67(3): 155–162.

Docherty, J.J., Smith, J.S., Fu, M.M., Stoner, T. and Booth, T. 2004. Effect of topically applied resveratrol on cutaneous herpes simplex virus infections in hairless mice. *Antiviral Res.* 61(1): 19–26.

Docherty, J.J., Sweet, T.J., Bailey, E., Faith, S.A. and Booth, T. 2006. Resveratrol inhibition of varicella-zoster virus replication in vitro. *Antiviral Res.* 72(3): 171–177.

Falchetti, R., Fuggetta, M.P., Lanzilli, G., Tricarico, M. and Ravagnan, G. 2001. Effects of resveratrol on human immune cell function. *Life Sci.* 70(1): 81–96.

Falutz, J., Tsoukas, C. and Gold, P. 1988. Zinc as a cofactor in human immunodeficiency virus-induced immunosuppression. *JAMA.* 259(19): 2850–2851.

Fischer Walker, C. and Black, R.E. 2004. Zinc and the risk for infectious disease. *Annu Rev Nutr.* 24: 255–275.

Feiler, L.S., Smolin, G., Okumoto, M. and Condon, D. 1982. Herpetic keratitis in zinc-deficient rabbits. *Invest Ophthalmol Vis Sci.* 22: 788–795.

Foster, L.H. and Sumar, S. 1997. Selenium in health and disease: A review. *Crit Rev Food Sci Nutr.* 37: 211–228.

Frei, B., England, L. and Ames, B.N. 1989. Ascorbate is an outstanding antioxidant in human blood plasma. *Proc Natl Acad Sci U S A.* 86(16): 6377–6381.

Fryburg, D.A., Mark, R.J., Griffith, B.P., Askenase, P.W. and Patterson, T.F. 1995. The effect of supplemental beta-carotene on immunologic indices in patients with AIDS: A pilot study. *Yale J Biol Med.* 68(1–2): 19–23.

Gabrashanska, M., Teodorova, S.E., Petkova, S., Mihov, L., Anisimova, M. and Ivanov, D. 2010. Selenium supplementation at low doses contributes to the antioxidant status in Trichinella spiralis-infected rats. *Parasitol Res.* 106(3): 561–570.

Gao, X., Xu, Y.X., Janakiraman, N., Chapman, R.A. and Gautam, S.C. 2001. Immunomodulatory activity of resveratrol: Suppression of lymphocyte proliferation, development of cell-mediated cytotoxicity, and cytokine production. *Biochem Pharmacol.* 62(9): 1299–1308.

Garewal, H.S., Ampel, N.M., Watson, R.R., Prabhala, R.H. and Dols, C.L. 1992. A preliminary trial of beta-carotene in subjects infected with the human immunodeficiency virus. *J Nutr.* 122(3S): 728–732.

Gerner, P., Posselt, H.G., Krahl, A. et al 2008. Vitamin E treatment for children with chronic hepatitis B: A randomized placebo controlled trial. *World J Gastroentero.* 14(47): 7208–7213.

Girodon, F., Galan, P., Monget, A.L. et al. 1999. Impact of trace elements and vitamin supplementation on immunity and infections in institutionalized elderly patients: A randomized controlled trial. MIN. VIT. AOX. geriatric network. *Arch Intern Med.* 159(7): 748–754.

González-Gallego, J., García-Mediavilla, M.V., Sánchez-Campos, S. and Tuñón, M.J. 2010. Fruit polyphenols, immunity and inflammation. *Br J Nutr.* 104 Suppl 3: S15–S27.

Graat, J.M., Schouten, E.G. and Kok, F.J. 2002. Effect of daily vitamin E and multivitamin-mineral supplementation on acute respiratory tract infections in elderly persons: A randomized controlled trial. *JAMA.* 288: 715–721.

Gruner, S., Volk, H.D., Falck, P. and Von Baehr, R. 1986. The influence of phagocytic stimuli on the expression of HLA-DR antigens; role of reactive oxygen intermediates. *Eur J Immunol.* 16(2): 212–215.

Hamilton-Miller, J.M. 1995. Antimicrobial properties of tea (*Camellia sinensis* L.). *Antimicrob Agents Chemother.* 39(11): 2375–2377.

Han, S.N., Wu, D., Ha, W.K. et al. 2000. Vitamin E supplementation increases T helper 1 cytokine production in old mice infected with influenza virus. *Immunology.* 100(4): 487–493.

Harbige, L.S. 1996. Nutrition and immunity with emphasis on infection and autoimmune disease. *Nutr Health.* 10(4): 285–312.

Hauber, I., Hohenberg, H., Holstermann, B., Hunstein, W. and Hauber, J. 2009. The main green tea polyphenol epigallocatechin-3-gallate counteracts semen-mediated enhancement of HIV infection. *Proc Natl Acad Sci U S A.* 106(22): 9033–9038.

Hayek, M.G., Taylor, S.F., Bender, B.S. et al. 1997. Vitamin E supplementation decreases lung virus titers in mice infected with influenza. *J Infect.* 176(1): 273–276.

Hemila, H. 1996. Vitamin C supplementation and common cold symptoms: Problems with inaccurate reviews. *Nutrition.* 12(1): 804–809.

Hemila, H. 1997. Vitamin C intake and susceptibility to pneumonia. *Pediatr Infect Dis J.* 16(9): 836–837.

Hemila, H. and Douglas, R.M. 1999. Vitamin C and acute respiratory infections. *Int J Tuberc Lung Dis.* 3(9): 756–761.

Heyland, D.K., Dhaliwal, R., Suchner, U. and Berger, M.M. 2005. Antioxidant nutrients: A systematic review of trace elements and vitamins in the critically ill patient. *Intensive Care Med.* 31(3): 327–337.

Hughes, D.A. 2000. Dietary antioxidants and human immune function. *Nutr Bull.* 25: 35–41.

Ilavarasi, K., Kiruthiga, P.V., Pandian, S.K. and Devi, K.P. 2011. Hydroxytyrosol, the phenolic compound of olive oil protects human PBMC against oxidative stress and DNA damage mediated by 2,3,7,8-TCDD. *Chemosphere.* 84(7): 888–893.

Izzi, V., Masuelli, L., Tresoldi, I. et al. 2012. The effects of dietary flavonoids on the regulation of redox inflammatory networks. *Front Biosci.* 17: 2396–2418.

Jiang, J.H., Jin, C.M., Kim, Y.C., Kim, H.S., Park, W.C. and Park, H. 2008. Anti-toxoplasmosis effects of oleuropein isolated from *Fraxinus rhychophylla*. *Biol Pharm Bull*. 31(12): 2273–2276.

Kanwar, J., Taskeen, M., Mohammad, I., Huo, C., Chan, T.H. and Dou, Q.P. 2012. Recent advances on tea polyphenols. *Front Biosci*. 4: 111–131.

Keusch, G.T. 1990. Micronutrients and susceptibility to infection. *Ann N Y Acad Sci*. 587: 181–188.

Kidd, M.T., Qureshi, M.A., Ferket, P.R. and Thomas, L.N. 1994. Dietary zinc-methionine enhances mononuclear-phagocytic function in young turkeys. Zinc-methionine, immunity, and *Salmonella*. *Biol Trace Elem Res*. 42: 217–229.

Kiremidjian-Schumacher, L., Roy, M., Wishe, H.I., Cohen, M.W. and Stotzky, G. 1994. Supplementation with selenium and human immune cell functions. II. Effect on cytotoxic lymphocytes and natural killer cells. *Biol Trace Elem Res*. 41(1–2): 115–127.

Klasing, K.C. and Leshchinsky, T.V. 2000. Interactions between nutrition and immunity. In: *Nutrition and Immunity*, Gershwin, M.E., German, S., and Keen, C.L., Eds. Totowa: Humana Press Inc., 363–373.

Knight, J.A. 2000. Review: Free radicals, antioxidants, and the immune system. *Ann Clin Lab Sci*. 30(2): 145–158.

Korkina, L.G., Pastore, S., De Luca, C. and Kostyuk, V.A. 2008. Metabolism of plant polyphenols in the skin: Beneficial versus deleterious effects. *Curr Drug Metab*. 9(8): 710–729.

Kukreja, R. and Khan, A. 1998. Effect of selenium deficiency and its supplementation on DTH response, antibody forming cells and antibody titre. *Indian J Exp Biol*. 36(2): 203–205.

Li, S., Hattori, T. and Kodama, E.N. 2011. Epigallocatechin gallate inhibits the HIV reverse transcription step. *Antivir Chem Chemother*. 21(6): 239–243.

Look, M.P., Rockstroh, J.K., Rao, G.S., Kreuzer, K.A., Spengler, U. and Sauerbruch, T. 1997. Serum selenium versus lymphocyte subsets and markers of disease progression and inflammatory response in human immunodeficiency virus-1 infection. *Biol Trace Elem Res*. 56(1): 31–41.

Manna, C., Galletti, P., Cucciolla, V., Moltedo, O., Leone, A. and Zappia, V. 1997. The protective effect of the olive oil polyphenol (3,4-dihydroxyphenyl)-ethanol counteracts reactive oxygen metabolite-induced cytotoxicity in Caco-2 cells. *J Nutr*. 27(2): 286–292.

Marshall, I. 1999. Zinc for the common cold. *Cochrane Database Syst Rev*. [Online], vol. 2, pp. CD001364. doi: 10.1001/14651858.

McMurray, D.N., Bartow, R.A., Mintzer, C.L. and Hernandez-Frontera, E. 1990. Micronutrient status and immune function in tuberculosis. *Ann N Y Acad Sci*. 587: 59–69.

Meydani, S.N., Han, S.N. and Wu, D. 2005. Vitamin E and immune response in the aged: Molecular mechanisms and clinical implications. *Immunol Rev*. 205: 269–284.

Meydani, S.N., Leka, L.S., Fine, B.C. et al. 2004. Vitamin E and respiratory tract infections in elderly nursing home residents: A randomized controlled trial. *JAMA*. 292: 828–836.

Meydani, S.N., Meydani, M., Blumberg, J.B. et al. 1997. Vitamin E supplementation and *in vivo* immune response in healthy elderly subjects. A randomized controlled trial. *JAMA*. 277: 1380–1386.

Mishra, V. 2007. Oxidative stress and role of antioxidant supplementation in critical illness. *Clin Lab*. 53(3–4): 199–209.

Mocchegiani, E., Muzzioli, M., and Giacconi, R. 2000. Zinc, metallothioneins, immune responses, survival and ageing. Review. PubMed PMID: 11707929. *Biogerontology* 1(2): 133–143.

Nance, C.L., Siwak, E.B. and Shearer, W.T. 2009. Preclinical development of the green tea catechin, epigallocatechin gallate, as an HIV-1 therapy. *J Allergy Clin Immunol*. 123(2): 459–465.

Newberne, P.M., Hunt, C.E. and Young, V.R. 1968. The role of diet and the reticuloendothelial system in the response of rats to Salmonella typhilmurium infection. *Brit J Exp Pathol*. 49(5): 448–457.

Nimmagadda, A., O'Brien, W.A. and Goetz, M.B. 1998. The significance of vitamin A and carotenoid status in persons infected by the human immunodeficiency virus. *Clin Infect Dis.* 26: 711–718.

Oppenheimer, S.J. 2001. Iron and its relation to immunity and infectious disease. *J Nutr.* 131(2S–2): 616S–633S; discussion 633S–635S.

Pajonk, F., Riedisser, A., Henke, M., McBride, W.H. and Fiebich, B. 2006. The effects of tea extracts on proinflammatory signaling. *BMC Med.* 4: 28.

Parke, D.V. 1999. Nutritional antioxidants in disease prevention mechanism of action. In: *Antioxidants in Humans Health and Disease*, Basu, T., Temple, N. and Garg, M., Eds. New York: CABI Publisher.

Percival, S.S. 1995. Neutropenia caused by copper deficiency: Possible mechanisms of action. *Nutr Rev.* 53(3): 59–66.

Peterhans, E. 1997. Oxidants and antioxidants in viral diseases: Disease mechanisms and metabolic regulation. *J Nutr.* 127(5 Suppl): 962S–965S.

Petro, T.M. 2011. Regulatory role of resveratrol on Th17 in autoimmune disease. *Int Immunopharmacol.* 11(3): 310–318.

Prohaska, J.R. and Failla, M.L. 1993. Cooper and immunity. In: *Human Nutrition: A Comprehensive Treatise*, Klurfield, D.M., Ed. New York: Plenum Press, 309–332.

Puertollano, M.A., Puertollano, E., Alvarez de Cienfuegos, G. and de Pablo, M.A. 2007. Significance of olive oil in the host immune resistance to infection. *Br J Nutr.* 98 Suppl 1: S54–S58.

Puertollano, M.A., Puertollano, E., Alvarez de Cienfuegos, G. and de Pablo, M.A. 2010. Olive oil and immune resistance to infectious microorganisms. In: *Olive Oil and Immune Resistance to Infectious Microorganism in Olive and Olive Oil in Health Disease and Prevention*, Preedy, V.R. and Watson, R.R., Eds. Oxford: Academic Press, 1039–1047.

Puertollano, M.A., Puertollano, E., Contreras-Moreno, J. et al. 2013. Natural antioxidants and resistance to infection. In: *Bioactive Food as Dietary Interventions for Arthritis and Related Inflammatory Diseases*, Watson, R.R. and Preedy, V.R., Eds. San Diego: Academic Press, 157–174.

Puertollano, M.A., Puertollano, E., de Cienfuegos, G.Á. and de Pablo, M.A. 2011. Dietary antioxidants: Immunity and host defense. *Curr Top Med Chem.* 11(14): 1752–1766.

Ramiro-Puig, E., Pérez-Cano, F.J., Ramírez-Santana, C. et al. 2007a. Spleen lymphocyte function modulated by a cocoa-enriched diet. *Clin Exp Immunol.* 149(3): 535–542.

Ramiro-Puig, E., Pérez-Cano, F.J., Ramos-Romero, S. et al. 2008. Intestinal immune system of young rats influenced by cocoa-enriched diet. *J Nutr Biochem.* 19(8): 555–565.

Ramiro-Puig, E., Urpí-Sardà, M., Pérez-Cano, F.J. et al. 2007b. Cocoa-enriched diet enhances antioxidant enzyme activity and modulates lymphocyte composition in thymus from young rats. *J Agric Food Chem.* 55(16): 6431–6438.

Reddanna, P., Whelan, J., Burgess, J.R. et al. 1989. The role of vitamin E and selenium on arachidonic acid oxidation by way of the 5-lipoxygenase pathway. *Ann N Y Acad Sci.* 570: 136–145.

Ribeiro Nogueira, C., Ramalho, A., Lameu, E., Da Silva Franca, C.A., David, C. and Accioly, E. 2009. Serum concentrations of vitamin A and oxidative stress in critically ill patients with sepsis. *Nutr Hosp.* 24(3): 312–317.

Rogers, T.J., Adams-Burton, K., Mallon, M. et al. 1983. Dietary ascorbic acid and resistance to experimental renal candidiasis. *J Nutr.* 113(1): 178–183.

Santos, M.S., Leka, L.S., Ribaya-Mercado, J.D. et al. 1997. Short- and long-term beta-carotene supplementation do not influence T cell-mediated immunity in healthy elderly persons. *Am J Clin Nutr.* 66(4): 917–924.

Santos, M.S., Meydani, S.N., Leka, L. et al. 1996. Natural killer cell activity in elderly men is enhanced by beta-carotene supplementation. *Am J Clin Nutr.* 64(5): 772–777.

Sasazuki, S., Sasaki, S., Tsubono, Y., Okubo, S., Hayashi, M. and Tsugane, S. 2006. Effect of vitamin C on common cold: Randomized controlled trial. *Eur J Clin Nutr.* 60(1): 9–17.

Shankar, A.H., Genton, B., Baisor, M. et al. 2000. The influence of zinc supplementation on morbidity due to Plasmodium falciparum: A randomized trial in preschool children in Papua New Guinea. *Am J Trop Med Hyg.* 62(2S): 663–669.

Sheridan, P.A. and Beck, M.A. 2008. The immune response to herpes simplex virus encephalitis in mice is modulated by dietary vitamin E. *J Nutr.* 138(1): 130–137.

Schreck, R., Rieber, P. and Baeuerle, P.A. 1991. Reactive oxygen intermediates as apparently widely used messengers in the activation of the NF-kappaB transcription factor and HIV-1. *EMBO J.* 10(8): 2247–2258.

Scrimshaw, N.S. and SanGiovanni, J.P. 1997. Synergism of nutrition, infection, and immunity: An overview. *Am J Clin Nutr.* 66(2): 464S–477S.

Semba, R.D. and Tang, A.M. 1999. Micronutrients and the pathogenesis of human immunodeficiency virus infection. *Br J Nutr.* 81(3): 181–189.

Sezikli, M., Cetinkaya, Z.A., Sezikli, H. et al. 2009. Oxidative stress in *Helicobacter pylori* infection: Does supplementation with vitamins C and E increase the eradication rate? *Helicobacter.* 14(4): 280–285.

Shor-Posner, G., Miguez, M.J., Pineda, L.M. et al. 2002. Impact of selenium status on the pathogenesis of mycobacterial disease in HIV-1-infected drug users during the era of highly active antiretroviral therapy. *J Acquir Immune Defic Syndr.* 29(2): 169–173.

Singh, K.P., Zaidi, S.I., Raisuddin, S., Saxena, A.K., Murthy, R.C. and Ray, P.K. 1992. Effect of zinc on immune functions and host resistance against infection and tumor challenge. *Immunopharmacol. Immunotoxicol.* 14(4): 813–840.

Spagnuolo, C., Russo, M., Bilotto, S., Tedesco, I., Laratta, B. and Russo, G.L. 2012. Dietary polyphenols in cancer prevention: The example of the flavonoid quercetin in leukemia. *Ann N Y Acad Sci.* 1259: 95–103.

Strand, O.A., Leone, A., Giercksky, K.E. and Kirkeboen, K.A. 2000. Nitric oxide indices in human septic shock. *Crit Care Med.* 28(8): 2779–2785.

Takeda, K., Kaisho, T. and Akira, S. 2003. Toll-like receptors. *Annu Rev Immunol.* 21: 335–376.

Tang, A.M., Graham, N.M. and Saah, A.J. 1996. Effects of micronutrient intake on survival in human immunodeficiency virus type 1 infection. *Am J Epidemiol.* 143(12): 1244–1256.

Tang, A.M., Graham, N.M., Kirby, A.J., McCall, L.D., Willett, W.C. and Saah, A.J. 1993. Dietary micronutrient intake and risk of progression to acquired immunodeficiency syndrome (AIDS) in human immunodeficiency virus type 1 (HIV-1)-infected homosexual men. *Am J Epidemiol.* 138(11): 937–951.

Turnlund, J.R., Jacob, R.A., Keen, C.L. et al. 2004. Long-term high copper intake: Effects on indexes of copper status, antioxidant status, and immune function in young men. *Am J Clin Nutr.* 79: 1037–1044.

Valko, M., Leibfritz, D., Moncol, J., Cronin, M.T., Mazur, M. and Telser, J. 2007. Free radicals and antioxidants in normal physiological functions and human disease. *Int J Biochem Cell Biol.* 39: 44–84.

Varilek, G.W., Yang, F., Lee, E.Y. et al. 2001. Green tea polyphenol extract attenuates inflammation in interleukin-2-deficient mice, a model of autoimmunity. *J Nutr.* 131(7): 2034–2039.

Visioli, F., Bellomo, G. and Galli, C. 1998a. Free radical-scavenging properties of olive oil polyphenols. *Biochem Biophys Res Commun.* 247(1): 60–64.

Visioli, F., Bellosta, S. and Galli, C. 1998b. Oleuropein, the bitter principle of olives, enhances nitric oxide production by mouse macrophages. *Life Sci.* 62(6): 541–546.

Wang, C., Wang, H., Luo, J. et al. 2009a. Selenium deficiency impairs host innate immune response and induces susceptibility to *Listeria monocytogenes* infection. *BMC Immunol.* 10: 55.

Wang, C., Wu, Y., Qin, J., Sun, H. and He, H. 2009b. Induced susceptibility of host is associated with an impaired antioxidant system following infection with *Cryptosporidium parvum* in Se-deficient mice. *PLoS One.* 4(2): e4628.

Wang, Y., Huang, D.S., Liang, B. and Watson, R.R. 1994. Nutritional status and immune responses in mice with murine AIDS are normalized by vitamin E supplementation. *J Nutr.* 124: 2024–2032.

Wintergerst, E.S., Maggini, S. and Hornig, D.H. 2007. Contribution of selected vitamins and trace elements to immune function. *Ann Nutr Metab.* 51(4): 301–323.

Wolowczuk, I., Verwaerde, C., Viltart, O. et al. 2008. Feeding our immune system: Impact on metabolism. *Clin Dev Immunol.* 2008: 639–803.

Wong, C.P., Nguyen, L.P., Noh, S.K., Bray, T.M., Bruno, R.S. and Ho, E. 2011. Induction of regulatory T cells by green tea polyphenol EGCG. *Immunol Lett.* 139(1–2): 7–13.

Yam, T.S., Shah, S. and Hamilton-Miller, J.M. 1997. Microbiological activity of whole and fractionated crude extracts of tea (*Camellia sinensis*), and of tea components. *FEMS Microbiol Lett.* 152(1): 169–174.

Yoneyama, M., Kikuchi, M., Matsumoto, K. et al. 2005. Shared and unique functions of the DExD/H-box helicases RIG-I, MDA5, and LGP2 in antiviral innate immunity. *J Immunol.* 175: 2851–2858.

Yu, M.W., Horng, I.S., Hsu, K.H., Chiang, Y.C., Liaw, Y.F. and Chen, C.J. 1999. Plasma selenium levels and risk of hepatocellular carcinoma among men with chronic hepatitis virus infection. *Am J Epidemiol.* 150(4): 367–374.

Yu, S.Y., Zhu, Y.J. and Li, W.G. 1997. Protective role of selenium against hepatitis B virus and primary liver cancer in Qidong. *Biol Trace Elem Res.* 56(1): 117–124.

Zhao, Y., Jiang, F., Liu, P., Chen, W. and Yi, K. 2012. Catechins containing a galloyl moiety as potential anti-HIV-1 compounds. *Drug Discov Today.* 17(11–12): 630–635.

Zojaji, H., Talaie, R., Mirsattari, D. et al. 2009. The efficacy of *Helicobacter pylori* eradication regimen with and without vitamin C supplementation. *Dig Liver Dis.* 41(9): 644–647.

6 Nutrient–Drug Interactions

Kathleen M. Gura

CONTENTS

Introduction 108
Factors That Affect Drug Pharmacokinetics 109
    Gastric Emptying and Intestinal Transit Time 109
    Presystemic Clearance 109
    Hepatic Metabolism 110
Basic Principles of Nutrient–Drug Interactions 112
Relation of Meal Timing and Drug Absorption 112
Drug and Nutrient Transport Systems 113
Interactions between Enteral Feedings and Medications Revisited 114
Effect of Malnutrition on Pharmacokinetic Parameters 115
Impact of Nutritional Status on Pharmacokinetic Properties 117
    Absorption 117
    Distribution 117
    Metabolism 118
    Clearance 118
    Impact of Kwashiorkor on Pharmacokinetics 119
    Drug Therapy in Marasmus 119
    Obesity 120
Influence of Dietary Manipulation on Pharmacokinetics 121
Influence of Specific Nutrients on Pharmacokinetics 134
    Carbohydrates 134
    Protein 134
    Dietary Fat 135
    Minerals 136
    Vegetables 136
    Drug and Grapefruit Juice Interactions 136
    Other Dietary Restrictions 137
    Effect of Beverage Type on Drug Bioavailability 137
    Parenteral Nutrition 138

Influence of Medications on Nutrient Status 138
    Nutrient Transport 138
    Nutrient Absorption... 138
    Nutrient Metabolism 138
    Medication-Associated Fluid and Electrolyte Disturbances........................... 139
    Glucose... 140
    Fat.. 140
Gastrointestinal Complications.. 142
    Alterations in Appetite 142
Examples of Drug–Nutrient Interactions in Specific Infectious
Disease Processes.. 144
    Tuberculosis 144
    Human Immunodeficiency Virus.. 144
Conclusion 145
References.. 145

INTRODUCTION

The nutritional status of a patient and the constituents of their diet can significantly affect the pharmacodynamic (e.g., affinities to receptors or tissues) and pharmacokinetic (i.e., absorption, distribution, metabolism, transport, and elimination) properties of drugs.[1] Gastrointestinal motility, blood flow, gastric secretions, and enzymatic activity, which affect biotransformation and disposition of drugs, can all be influenced by a variety of nutritional components (Figure 6.1). The extent of these effects, however, is extremely variable and patient specific, confounded by many other factors, and oftentimes unpredictable. Periods of increased caloric demand (i.e., during

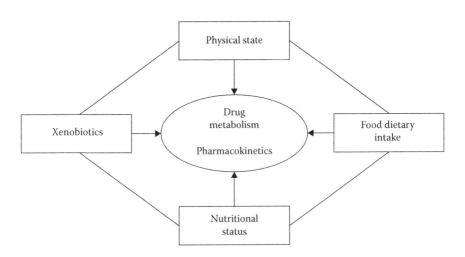

FIGURE 6.1 Relation between nutritional factors and drug therapy.

growth, pregnancy, and lactation) increase the susceptibility to drug-induced nutrient deficiencies. Failure to identify and address the impact of a drug–nutrient interaction can result in serious consequences. For example, the absorption of an orally administered antibiotic can be reduced, leading to treatment failure. Conversely, patients could develop drug toxicity if a nutrient inhibits enzymes in the gut that detoxify the medication. When developing a therapeutic plan, it is important that the practitioner considers the interactions that can occur between nutritional status, disease state, and drug action, and even patient age. By definition, *pharmacodynamics* is the study of the biochemical and clinical effects of drugs and the mechanisms of their action, including the correlation of actions and effects of drugs with their chemical structure, as well as the effects on the actions of another drug or nutrient. In contrast, the quantitative description of drug disposition is termed *pharmacokinetics.* This refers to the exposure of drugs in the body over a period of time, including the processes of absorption, distribution in tissues, metabolism, and elimination. This chapter will review how nutrition affects drug therapy with a particular emphasis on anti-infective agents.

FACTORS THAT AFFECT DRUG PHARMACOKINETICS

Differences in body composition are an important consideration when determining the pharmacokinetics of a given medication. Before reaching the systemic circulation and the sites of action, both nutrients and drugs delivered through the gastrointestinal tract must go through an absorption phase. Once absorbed, the compounds go from the gastrointestinal lumen into the hepatic portal vein and subsequently to the systemic circulation through a series of complex processes, including the dissolution of the solid dosage form, the passage of the chyme along the gastrointestinal tract (i.e., gastric emptying and intestinal transit), passive diffusion, active transport, and presystemic metabolism. Each of these processes alone may affect the pharmacokinetics of the drug.

Gastric Emptying and Intestinal Transit Time

The oral route continues to be the most widely used route of medication administration. As a result, intraluminal pH in different areas of the gastrointestinal tract can affect medication stability, dissolution rate of solid dosage forms, and even the extent of drug absorption in some cases. With the exception of a few acidic drugs (e.g., aspirin), maximal absorption of most drugs and nutrients take place in the small bowel. Taken together, both gastric emptying and intestinal transit time have a significant impact on the rate and magnitude of the oral absorption of the drugs and certain nutrients.

Presystemic Clearance

The removal of orally ingested compounds before reaching the systemic circulation is known as presystemic clearance (i.e., first-pass effect). Presystemic effect occurs primarily in the intestine and the liver; the stomach has only a minor role.[2] Type III alcohol dehydrogenase, for example, is present in the gastric mucosa and is responsible for the activation of some biogenic amines and steroids.

Many active transport proteins and drug-metabolizing enzymes are present in the intestinal epithelial tissues. For example, cytochrome P450 (CYP) 3A4 isoenzyme is present in the small bowel and is responsible for the oral bioavailability of a large number of medications. Induction or inhibition of the enzyme in the gut by nutrients can affect the oral bioavailability of drugs. Certain nutrients are known to affect the enzymatic activity of intestinal CYP3A4 and change the pharmacokinetics of the target drugs. Grapefruit juice is a classic example of an intestinal CYP3A4 inhibitor whose mechanism of action is further discussed later.[2] Water-soluble vitamin E (D-α-tocopheryl polyethylene glycol succinate) has also been found to increase the oral absorption of cyclosporine.[3] The primary mechanism appears to involve inhibition of an intestinal efflux protein, P-glycoprotein (P-gp), instead of intestinal CYP enzymes.[4]

HEPATIC METABOLISM

The metabolism of a drug involves further steps once it has been absorbed from the gastrointestinal tract. As drugs are metabolized, they first undergo biotransformation (i.e., phase I metabolism), which results in the formation of a more polar compound by oxidation, reduction, hydroxylation, etc. This results in either an activation of the drug or a deactivation. The second phase (i.e., phase II reaction) is a synthetic process, involving conjugation of the polar compound with endogenous molecules such as glucuronic acid, sulfate, glutathione, glycine, and acetate, resulting in a more hydrophilic compound that is more suitable for excretion into bile or urine.[5] It is important to point out that some drugs do not have to go through phase I metabolism before undergoing phase II metabolism. Lorazepam, for example, undergoes phase II metabolism (glucuronidation) by UDP-glucuronosyltransfersae (UGT) 2B7 without any phase I reaction. The resultant conjugated metabolite is then excreted renally. An enzyme system responsible for the metabolism of most nutrients and drugs is the CYP enzyme superfamily, principally located in the endoplasmic reticulum of the hepatocytes and enterocytes, which is somewhat unique in its ability to use a wide range of substrates.

The maturation of phase I and phase II enzymes varies among individuals. Limited studies suggest that fetal and neonatal CYP, the most important phase I enzyme in metabolizing drugs and biogenic amines and steroids, has about 50% to 70% of its adult counterpart and continues to mature throughout childhood. Whereas some children may have fully matured CYP enzyme activities as early as 6 months of age, it may take up to 12 months for others.[6] Similarly, N-demethylation of diazepam, a CYP2C19-mediated pathway, is also significantly slower in infants. There is no well-documented dietary factor known to promote the maturation of these enzymes during the prenatal period and infancy. Table 6.1 describes the impact of various nutrients on phase I/mixed function oxygenase metabolism.

TABLE 6.1

Impact of Nutrients on Phase I/Mixed Function Oxygenase Metabolism

Nutrient	Effect on Metabolism (↓ or ↑)	Proposed Mechanism
Macronutrients		
Carbohydrates	Excess: ↓	May be due to ↓ protein or inhibition of CYP450 through ↓ in supporting enzyme components
Fats	High intake of saturated fatty acids: ↓	Decreased CYP activity may be due to requirement of PUFAs in the B-position of phosphatidylcholine (lecithin), which is an essential component of the CYP system
	High intake of PUFAs: ↑ activity and induction of CYP enzymes	
	Deficiency: ↓	
	Excess: ↑	
Protein	Deficiency: ↓ rate of metabolism	↓ Protein synthesis
	Excess: ↑ rate of metabolism	↓ Synthesis of other elements (i.e., hormones) involved in enzyme induction
Micronutrients		
Ascorbic acid	Deficiency: ↓	Alterations in CYP450 and CYP450 reductase through changes in expression of specific CYP isoenzymes depending on deficiency or excess state
	Excess: ↑ CYP450 activity	
Iron	Deficiency: ↑↓	↑ Lipid peroxidation may lead to damage to the integrity of the system
	Excess: ↑ microsomal lipid peroxidation	
Pyridoxine	Deficiency: ↓	Impaired protein synthesis ↓ synthesis of heme
Riboflavin	Deficiency ↑↓ depending on severity	↓ Reductase activity but ↑ CYP450 activity such that drug metabolism may be altered (↑↓)
Thiamine	Deficiency: ↑ CYP450 activity	↑ Activity of specific CYP450 isoenzymes and perhaps other enzymes in deficiency due to an unknown mechanism
	Excess: ↓ (both reductase and CYP450)	Excess may be due to decreased substrate binding
Vitamin E	Deficiency: ↓	May be due to a reduction in antioxidative mechanisms (e.g., protection of the lecithin component; thus, the activities of CYP450 and reductase are unaffected)

Source: Adapted from Raiten DJ, *Am J Clin Nutr*, 94, 1697S, 2011.

BASIC PRINCIPLES OF NUTRIENT–DRUG INTERACTIONS

By definition, a nutrient–drug interaction is one that is the result of a chemical, physical, physiological, or pathological relation between a medication and a nutrient.[7] They are clinically relevant if the interaction affects the therapeutic response to the medication: either by increasing (and thus increasing the risk of toxicity) or decreasing (and thereby increasing the risk of treatment failure) the bioavailability of the drug.

There are four basic classifications of drug–food interactions that are based on their nature and mechanism.[8]

1. Type I *ex vivo* bioinactivations—These are interactions that occur between the drug and the nutrient, usually in the delivery device, through biochemical or physical reactions. Examples include complexation, hydrolysis, neutralization, oxidation, and precipitation. These interactions are most commonly seen with drugs and nutrients administered intravenously or through feeding tubes.
2. Type II—These interactions modify the bioavailability of the medication and affect absorption. The causative agent may alter the function of the enzymes (i.e., type A interaction) or transport systems that are responsible for drug biotransformation (i.e., type B interaction).
3. Type III—These interactions are involved in the systemic disposition of the drug and occur after the drug or nutrient has been absorbed from the gastrointestinal tract into the systemic circulation. This can result in changes in tissue distribution, transport, or penetration to a specific organ or tissue.
4. Type IV—In this type of interaction, the elimination or clearance of the drug or nutrient is affected. It may modify either the renal or enterohepatic elimination process.

RELATION OF MEAL TIMING AND DRUG ABSORPTION

The impact of concurrent meal intake and oral drug absorption is an example of a type II interaction. Both the rate and extent of drug absorption can be changed (Table 6.2). In most instances, food will stimulate both gastric and intestinal secretions, thus improving drug dissolution and aiding in its absorption. In the case of high-fat meals, the intestinal uptake of highly lipophilic drugs is improved owing to the release of bile salts triggered by the dietary fat. Furthermore, dietary fat can stimulate the release of cholecystokinin, which decreases gastric motility, thus increasing the contact time between the drug and the intestine and can potentially increase drug absorption. In some instances, this interaction is used for therapeutic benefit. For example, the antibiotics erythromycin ethylsuccinate and cefuroxime should both be taken with food to maximize their absorption.

Conversely, the composition of some foods may hinder drug absorption through binding. In such cases, the medication should be taken on an empty stomach (i.e., 1 h before or 2 h after a meal) to allow for maximal absorption. These include protease inhibitors such as indinavir and antibiotics such as ampicillin, ciprofloxacin,

---

TABLE 6.2
Examples of Anti-Infectives Whose Absorption Is Affected by Food

Drug Absorption Reduced/Delayed by Food	Drug Absorption Enhanced by Food
Ampicillin	Albendazole
Azithromycin	Atazanavir
Cefaclor	Atovaquone
Cefixime	Cefuroxime
Cephalexin	Clarithromycin
Ciprofloxacin	Clofazimine
Dapsone	Efavirenz
Didanosine	Etravirine
Doxycycline	Erythromycin estolate
Dirithromycin	Erythromycin ethylsuccinate
Erythromycin stearate	Ganciclovir
Famciclovir	Griseofulvin
Indinavir	Hydroxychloroquine
Isoniazid	Itraconazole
Metronidazole	Ivermectin
Naficillin	Ketoconazole
Nalidixic acid	Mebendazole
Penicillin G or V	Nelfinavir
Rifampin	Nitrofurantoin
Tetracycline	Rilpivirine
Voriconazole	Ritonavir
	Saquinavir
	Tenofovir
	Tipranavir
	Valganciclovir
	Zalcitabine

Source: Adapted from Gura KM. Drug–nutrient interactions. In: Hendricks KM, Duggan C, editors. *Manual of Pediatric Nutrition* (5th ed.). Hamilton, ON: BC Decker, pp. 545–85, 2013.

---

doxycycline, and tetracycline. In some instances, the dosage form of the antibiotic will determine if such meal timing is necessary. For example, the azalide antibiotic azithromycin, when the capsule form is administered in the fed state, exhibits a negative food effect in which there is lower azithromycin bioavailability in comparison to the tablet form.[9] The rationale for this phenomenon is that azithromycin capsules disintegrate more slowly than the tablet form in the fed stomach, resulting in more contact time with gastric acid and allowing significantly more descladinose azithromycin, an acid-degradation product, to form.

DRUG AND NUTRIENT TRANSPORT SYSTEMS

As previously discussed, oral drug absorption across the gastrointestinal tract is highly dependent on its lipophilic properties and its affinity for membrane transporters. Given that most drugs are absorbed in the small intestine, transport proteins present in the enterocytes play an essential role in facilitating the absorption of many drugs.[10] Although most transport proteins facilitate absorption by increasing the intraluminal uptake of compounds, some transporters efflux molecules already absorbed in the cytoplasm of the enterocyte back into the intestinal lumen, which decrease the bioavailability of some compounds. This is believed to be an intrinsic protective mechanism by the host to minimize xenobiotic exposure. P-gp is a representative of this type of efflux system.[11] P-gp belongs to the family of adenosine triphosphate binding cassette (ABC) transporters and is an efflux protein widely distributed in normal tissues, including the intestinal epithelium, renal tubule, liver, and blood–brain barrier. Hepatic transporters are membrane proteins that facilitate nutrient and drug transport into the cell through uptake transporters or pump out toxic entities through canalicular transporters.[12] Certain foods, in particular fruits and vegetables, contain photochemicals that have the potential to alter drug absorption. Recent studies suggest that phytochemicals can serve as substrates and modulators of specific members of the superfamily of ABC transporting proteins (i.e., P-gp, MRP1, MRP2, and BCRP). For example, isothiocyanates, a class of chemotherapeutic agents derived from cruciferous vegetables (i.e., broccoli, cabbage, and watercress) may influence the pharmacokinetics of substrates of these transporters and interact with ABC efflux transporters.[13] The two most important limiting factors in regulating the oral bioavailability of drugs are CYP3A4 and P-gp.[14] CYP3A4 is thought to be responsible for the metabolism of >50% of all medications.[15]

INTERACTIONS BETWEEN ENTERAL FEEDINGS AND MEDICATIONS REVISITED

Enteral nutrition and food intake are common causes of drug–nutrient interactions and are classic examples of type I *ex vivo* bioinactivations. In patients unable to swallow, enteral feeding is the preferred method of providing nutrition support and also allows easy access for administering medications. However, enteral feeding formulas have been implicated in numerous drug–nutrient interactions.[16] Moreover, in patients with chronic medical conditions receiving tube feedings, nutrient deficiencies are a concern as multiple medications and complicated feeding regimens can result in decreased intake due to feedings being held or due to drug interactions.[17] For example, when given with enteral feedings, the oral absorption of fluoroquinolone antibiotics and tetracycline is decreased.[16] Chelation of divalent and trivalent cations by milk formulas, dairy products, and fluoroquinolones, among others, is an important cause for drug–nutrient interactions.[18]

Unlike medications given through the oral route, whenever a medication is delivered by the feeding tube, tube placement and device characteristics must also be considered. Medications may adhere to the sides of the feeding tube, and thus not be delivered to the patient, or may obstruct the tube in the case of an oral solid not properly pulverized and diluted before administration. In some instances, medications are best absorbed in the "fasted" state, requiring that feedings be held so as to optimize absorption. Intragastric administration of a medication may delay gastric-emptying rates. Administering solid dosage forms of medications (e.g., crushed tablets) to patients with nasojejunal, nasoduodenal feeding, or jejunostomy tubes present an additional challenge as these devices bypass the stomach where medications are dissolved and diluted with gastric contents. Owing to the narrow bore of the devices and direct administration of medication into the small intestine, liquid dosage forms of medications (e.g., oral liquid, suspension, syrup) must be used. However, when administering oral dosage forms, several factors should be considered, including the osmolality of the drug, its viscosity, and particle size. Dumping can result when a hypertonic medication is not diluted before administration into the small bowel. The osmolality of stomach secretions is approximately 300 mOsm/kg, and many liquid medications exceed this value significantly, resulting in an osmotic-induced diarrhea if given in its undiluted state. When an undiluted hypertonic medication is administered, gastric-emptying rates are altered, resulting in a flux of water and electrolytes into the small bowel, overwhelming its absorptive capacity. Proper dilution of the medication can prevent this flux as well as improve drug and nutrient absorption. Furthermore, if the feeding tube does terminate in the jejunum, the pH must also be considered to assure optimal dissolution of certain dosage forms occurs.

EFFECT OF MALNUTRITION ON PHARMACOKINETIC PARAMETERS

A patient's nutritional status is capable of modifying the pharmacologic effect of a medication. Both undernutrition and obesity can alter drug pharmacokinetics and pharmacologic responses substantially by causing functional and structural alterations in organs that directly affect drug disposition.[19] Malnutrition can affect the absorption, distribution, metabolism, and elimination of a drug that can ultimately affect its therapeutic or toxic response. Interindividual and intraindividual variations in the pharmacokinetic responses to a medication can further complicate interpreting the real impact of altered nutritional status on drug disposition. The variation can be 3- to >20-fold, depending on genetic (e.g., genetic polymorphism) and environmental factors, patient variables, and underlying disease.[19] The pathologic changes seen in malnutrition can affect the pharmacokinetics of drugs in all phases of disposition within the body, suggesting that the degree of malnutrition can determine the body's response to a particular drug. The integrity of the intestinal mucosa is dependent on a continuous intake of adequate nutrition, as the turnover of enterocytes in the small intestine takes 2–3 days, and in the colonocytes of the large intestine 3–5 days.[20] Even short-term malnutrition can potentially have a negative impact on drug absorption and metabolism, a risk that increases significantly in patients who go without food for >5 days, owing to a decline in mucosal integrity. Physiologic changes of protein–energy malnutrition (PEM) may result in alterations in the absorptive capacity of the gastrointestinal tract, body fluid status, cardiac output, glomerular filtration rate (GFR), and plasma protein concentrations, as well as hormonal and metabolic changes. Therapeutic drug levels may be altered as a result of malnutrition-associated tissue receptor alterations.[21] The risk of toxicities owing to a drug or its metabolites appears to be greater in malnourished patients, with a subsequent risk of morbidity or mortality. This suggests that close therapeutic drug monitoring and dose adjustments are imperative in malnourished patients. Drugs with narrow therapeutic indices or narrow dose–response curves (i.e., gentamicin) are particularly responsible, as even small changes in absorption can become significant.[22]

Relatively little is known about the handling of drugs in malnourished patients, although the combination of malnutrition and accompanying disease (typically infection) is a common problem in many parts of the world. It is possible that the high morbidity or mortality, a characteristic of malnutrition, may be enhanced by adverse drug reactions.[23]

Starvation can even increase the risk of antimicrobial resistance. Bacteria encounter a variety of stresses in their natural environments, including, in the case of pathogens, their hosts. These stresses produce a myriad of adaptive responses that not only protect bacteria from the offending stress but also result in changes in the cell that affect innate antimicrobial susceptibility. Thus, exposure to nutrient starvation/limitation (nutrient stress) can affect bacterial susceptibility to a number of antimicrobials through their initiation of stress responses that positively influence recruitment of resistance determinants or promote physiological changes that compromise antimicrobial activity.[24] Antibiotics generally preferentially kill rapidly replicating bacteria, and it has been suggested that reduced growth and metabolic activity associated with starvation or nutrient-limited growth environments might account for resistance under those conditions.[25] An example of nutritional stress is protein–calorie malnutrition resulting in amino acid deprivation, which activates the stringent response.[26] Activated by a variety of nutritional stresses (e.g., iron deficiency, hypophosphatemia, carbon source, or fatty acid deficiencies), the stringent response-mediated increase in guanosine pentaphosphate (ppGpp) has a number of effects on bacterial cell physiology and affects antimicrobial susceptibility.[27,28] For example, limited protein intake (i.e., deprivation of amino acids) and the stringent response are linked to diminished penicillin susceptibility in *Escherichia coli* relA mutants unable to synthesize ppGpp, which are more susceptible to penicillin-dependent lysis during amino acid deprivation. Presumably, plsB is a ppGpp target and ppGpp-dependent inhibition of phospholipid biosynthesis interferes with membrane-associated steps in peptidoglycan biosynthesis, thereby promoting penicillin resistance. ppGpp inhibition of cell wall synthesis has been described in other bacteria (i.e., *Streptomyces coelicolor*, *Bacillus subtilis*, and *Mycobacterium tuberculosis*) where it is also linked to reduced β-lactam susceptibility.[28] ppGpp is also linked to resistance to other antimicrobials. *Escherichia coli* mutants deficient in ppGpp production are more susceptible to trimethoprim, gentamicin, and polymyxin B.[29,30] Increased ppGpp accumulation in mutant *E. coli* is also linked to increased resistance and increased survivability in the presence of fluoroquinolones.[31] Antimicrobials (i.e., mupirocin, vancomycin, penicillin) have been reported to stimulate ppGpp accumulation; however, this has not been correlated with any increases in antimicrobial resistance except in the case *Enterococcus faecalis*, where a mutant unable to synthesize ppGpp showed increased susceptibility to vancomycin.[32] Recent evidence illustrates that both ppGpp and the stringent response are linked to resistance to several antimicrobials in nutrient-starved biofilm cells of *Pseudomonas aeruginosa*.[33] Nguyen et al. report that nutrient-limited planktonic and biofilm cells that are defective in the genes for ppGpp production are less resistant to antimicrobials than their wild-type counterparts, with ppGpp-deficient biofilm cells showing increased susceptibility to several classes of antimicrobials, including aminoglycosides (e.g., gentamicin), β-lactams (e.g., meropenem), cationic antimicrobial peptides (e.g., colistin), and fluoroquinolones (e.g., ofloxacin).[33] The mechanism of cell killing is related to the production of hydroxyl radicals (·OH).[34] The stringent response promotes antimicrobial resistance by increasing antioxidant defenses and by limiting 4-hydroxy-2-alkylquinoline synthesis, both of which serve to improve the oxidative killing of cells upon exposure to antimicrobials. These results suggest that starved, nongrowing cells may be at a greater risk from oxidative stress/killing and to avoid it they adapt, thereby providing protection from the oxidative killing by bactericidal antimicrobials.

Even the type of nutrient starvation can affect the type and severity of antimicrobial resistance that results. One study of the effects of nutrient deprivation on antibiotic resistance in *E. coli* showed that phosphate starvation promoted a transient increase in ofloxacin resistance, whereas amino acid starvation was linked to transient resistance to both ofloxacin and ampicillin, and the combination of amino acid and glucose starvation led to prolonged resistance to ampicillin and ofloxacin.[35] Similarly, decreased magnesium intake may also affect antimicrobial susceptibility in a number of bacteria.[36] For example, in *Salmonella*, the response to decreased magnesium intake is mediated by the PhoPQ two-component system, where PhoQ, a sensor kinase, senses the nutrient limitation and activates the PhoP response regulator to upregulate a variety of target genes that ultimately promote adaptation to this nutrient stress.[37] Similarly, in the case of *P. aeruginosa*, there are several reports of PhoQ and pmrB mutations responsible for PXB and colistin resistance.[24]

IMPACT OF NUTRITIONAL STATUS ON PHARMACOKINETIC PROPERTIES

ABSORPTION

Little research has been done on the effect of malnutrition on drug absorption. Mehta et al. reported that the absorption rate of acetaminophen disposition in children with PEM remained constant and was not altered in malnutrition.[38] This contrasts with work by Raghuram and colleagues, which indicated that tetracycline absorption was significantly reduced in subjects with malnutrition and pellagra but not in patients with vitamin B complex deficiency or in those with severe anemia.[39]

DISTRIBUTION

The important serum proteins that bind to drug molecules and biogenic amines and lipids include albumin, α1-acid glycoprotein, sex hormone–binding proteins, and lipoproteins. Only free, unbound drug molecules are pharmacologically active. Drugs can distribute into various body compartments such as the intracellular fluids, extravascular space, lean body tissue, and adipose tissue. Alterations in body composition, particularly the presence of edema, can influence the plasma clearance of drug by changing the medication's volume of distribution.[40] Many drugs, once in the systemic circulation, become bound to plasma protein, such as albumin, globulins, and lipoproteins. These binding proteins play an important role in the intravascular transport of the drugs to the target organs. In the bloodstream, drugs that are not bound to plasma proteins are free and are able to exert their pharmacologic response.

Malnutrition can alter the concentration of plasma proteins as well as the rate of tissue protein synthesis. The extent of drug–protein binding depends on the physicochemical properties of the medication and the concentration of plasma bind proteins. In malnutrition, albumin and lipoprotein synthesis is reduced, whereas globulin and α1-acid glycoprotein synthesis is increased.[41] Drugs extensively bound to α1-acid glycoprotein, such as propranolol, have a decreased percentage of drug unbound in malnutrition, resulting in a less active drug available to exert a therapeutic response. Other drugs, such as metronidazole, have no significant change in volume of distribution between malnourished and well-fed individuals.[42] In the case of parenteral penicillin, no significant difference in C_{max} was noted when penicillin was administered intramuscularly to malnourished versus eutrophic individuals, suggesting that the rate of penicillin absorption from the muscle mass to the systemic circulating is unchanged. On the other hand, in patients with marasmus and kwashiorkor, there was a trend toward a lower volume of distribution for penicillin, suggesting that overdosing could be a concern in some individuals if the typical dosing strategies are employed.[43]

METABOLISM

In chronic starvation, the body is able to adapt and various processes are altered to protect or maintain enzyme activities.[44] In fact, in chronic starvation, enzyme activity may even increase. In the starved state, oxidation is dominant and conjugation and biotransformation of aromatic compounds are decreased.[45] Endocrine tissue is typically affected in semistarvation as many hormones serve as substrates for drug-metabolizing enzymes.[46] For example, elevations in free cortisol are often seen in malnutrition, which may enhance the metabolism of contraceptive steroids in malnourished women, thus increasing the risk of contraceptive failure in that population.[46]

CLEARANCE

Malnutrition can also affect the hepatic clearance of medications. Protein deprivation or malnutrition may result in a reduction in cardiac function with a subsequent decreased perfusion of the liver and kidneys.[47] Hepatic drug clearance is determined by three independent factors: hepatic blood flow, the amount of free fraction of the drug in blood, and hepatic clearance of the unbound drug. Diminished hepatic blood flow can reduce the clearance of drugs with high extraction ratios (i.e., drugs in which the hepatic clearance of the unbound fraction depends on hepatic blood flow but not on changes in protein binding). Presystemic metabolism can become altered. Increases in the unbound fraction of a drug owing to hypoalbuminemia provide more available drug for metabolism, resulting in higher clearance (i.e., rate of drug removal from the body) and lower serum concentrations.[47]

The kidney is extensively involved in drug elimination. Renal elimination includes the processes of glomerular filtration, active tubular secretion, and passive tubular excretion. Drugs or their metabolites that are primarily filtered and excreted renally may be affected by nutritional status. The GFR, renal blood flow, and renal tubular function can all be increased by dietary protein.[48] PEM is associated with decreased GFR and renal blood flow.[48] When renal perfusion is reduced, less drug is available to be filtered by the tubules. However, as plasma protein binding is similarly reduced, free drug becomes available for renal excretion, thus further reducing plasma drug concentrations. Drugs exhibiting decreased renal elimination in severely malnourished patients include aminoglycosides, cefoxitin, penicillins, and tetracyclines.[19]

Refeeding an undernourished patient can often increase the systemic clearance of a medication, dictating a dose adjustment be done to maintain efficacy. The protein component of enteral or parenteral nutrition appears to be the major macronutrient enhancing systemic clearance of affected drugs in patients transitioned from the "unfed" to the "fed" state. In their study investigating the pharmacokinetics of metronidazole in severely malnourished children, Lares-Asseff and associates confirmed this finding.[40] On the basis of the clearance data, they recommended that the daily maintenance doses for pediatric patients with severe malnutrition should be 60% less of the usual pediatric dose to achieve and maintain adequate therapeutic plasma levels of metronidazole.

IMPACT OF KWASHIORKOR ON PHARMACOKINETICS

Kwashiorkor is associated with edema because of increases in total body water, extracellular fluid volume, and plasma volume, and a decrease in intracellular water.[49] It is thought that low protein intake results in a negative nitrogen balance that leads to decreased drug metabolism, whereas in patients receiving adequate total calories but with less than optimal protein intake, drug metabolism is not significantly affected.[50]

DRUG THERAPY IN MARASMUS

Unlike kwashiorkor, marasmus can be considered as an adaptation to insufficient energy intake. There is decreased total body water and intracellular water, and increased extracellular fluid and plasma volume.[19] In malnourished patients, gentamicin, which distributes predominantly to extracellular fluids, has an increased volume of distribution in comparison with well-nourished patients.[51] Conversely, in patients treated with metronidazole, a medication that also has a large volume of distribution, no difference in volume of distribution was observed between those who were malnourished and those who were nutritionally rehabilitated.[42] A pharmacokinetic study by Treluyer and colleagues focused on the impact of PEM on quinine metabolism.[52] Metabolism of quinine is increased in patients with global malnutrition, suggesting that the dosing interval should be reduced in these individuals to obtain the same therapeutic quinine levels compared with well-nourished patients.

In summary, normal or increased drug metabolism occurs in mild to moderate cases of malnutrition, whereas decreased metabolism is seen in severe cases of malnutrition. Given the unique needs of the malnourished ill child, special guidelines have been created for the use of antimicrobial agents.[53] A recent systematic review of antibiotic use in children with severe acute malnutrition (SAM) has attempted to validate these guidelines.[19] On the basis of the evidence to date, the authors support the use of broad-spectrum antibiotics in this population. However, well-designed randomized controlled trials are needed to address whether routine use of antibiotics is required in patients with uncomplicated SAM and those with SAM and human immunodeficiency virus (HIV) infection.

OBESITY

Obesity (body mass index ≥95th percentile for age and sex) results in altered body composition in which there is both an increased proportion and absolute amount of adipose tissue, as well as increase in lean body mass, blood volume, cardiac output, and organ size. Obesity is linked with physiological changes that can affect the pharmacokinetic parameters of many medications; however, for most drugs, dosing recommendations do not take into account the need for dosage adjustments.

There appears to be no difference in albumin binding of drugs, although increases in both CYP2E1 activity and phase II conjugation activity have been observed.[54] Nevertheless, the increase in CYP2E1 activity appears to be downregulated with weight loss.[55] Increased abdominal fat can also lead to increased intra-abdominal pressure and affect gastric emptying. Drug distribution depends on body composition and may be altered in obese patients. Absorption of drugs evaluated to date appears to be unchanged owing to obesity, although the data are limited. Severely obese patients who have undergone bariatric surgery for weight loss are more likely to experience altered drug absorption that may affect the clinical responses to therapy. Generally speaking, malabsorption of drugs is more likely to occur with the primary malabsorptive procedures such as jejunoileal bypass and pancreatobiliary diversion.[55] A commonly performed surgical procedure for weight loss is the Rouxen-Y gastric bypass (RYGB), which is a primary restrictive procedure with a mild malabsorptive component. Studies aimed at investigating the impact of RYGB on pharmacokinetics are very limited. The lipophilicity of a drug determines the extent to which obesity influences the volume of distribution and ultimately whether dosing should be based on actual or adjusted body weight. In severely obese patients, modest increases in volume of distribution have also been observed with aminoglycosides and vancomycin.[54] This suggests that an adjusted body weight rather than actual body weight should be used to avoid toxicity. However, the most accurate approach to adjust for the excess body mass is unknown and appears to be variable depending on the characteristics of individual compounds. Therapeutic drug monitoring is recommended to optimize therapy.

Although the protein binding of acidic drugs is unchanged, the free fraction of basic drugs may be decreased with obesity.[54] Likewise, changes in hepatic drug clearance are variable. Phase I reactions and phase I acetylation appear to be unaffected by obesity; however, the phase II glucuronidation and sulfation pathways are heightened. Obesity may also affect the systemic clearance of highly extracted drugs such as aminoglycosides.[56] Both glomerular filtration and tubular secretion appear to be increased.

Aminoglycosides are distributed within the extracellular fluid compartment. Early dosing guidelines recommended that initial dosing be based on ideal body weight as it was thought that the drug distributed only into lean body mass. Schwartz and colleagues, however, have since shown that when the volume of distribution is corrected for total body weight, it is considerably smaller when compared with normal-weight subjects.[56] The distribution of aminoglycosides into excess body weight is estimated to be about 40% of that distributed into ideal body tissue. The authors concluded that initial doses of aminoglycosides in obese patients be calculated by adding 40% of the excess weight to the patient's ideal body weight, with subsequent dosage adjustments being determined by serum drug levels and clinical status.

INFLUENCE OF DIETARY MANIPULATION ON PHARMACOKINETICS

Modifying the intake of specific foods may affect the clinical response to a medication (Table 6.3). Individuals at particular risk to an adverse event due to a drug–nutrient interaction include those with a chronic condition requiring the use of multiple drugs, those requiring specialized nutritional support, or those with some evidence of malnutrition.

Several dietary factors can alter the rate of drug metabolism. Both food and fluids can change the rate and extent of drug absorption. These alternations in response may occur as a result of the effects on gastric pH, gastric-emptying time, intestinal motility, and mesenteric and hepatic portal blood flow or biliary flow, or the activities of the enzymes and transport proteins in the gut.[57] Direct physicochemical interactions with dietary components can also alter the absorption of susceptible agents.[58] Interactions such as solubilization of the drug in dietary fat, binding of the medication with metal ions, or adsorption of the drug to insoluble dietary components may occur.

Dietary changes can alter the activity and expression of hepatic drug-metabolizing enzymes.[59] This can lead to alteration in the systemic elimination kinetics of medications metabolized by these enzymes, although the impact of this change is typically minimal.[59] The rate of drug metabolism can be accelerated by the drugs themselves or by a variety of dietary factors, such as protein supplementation or inclusion of charcoal-broiled meats or cruciferous vegetables in the diet.[60] Large quantities of polycyclic aromatic hydrocarbons contained in charcoal broiled beef were found to be responsible for hepatic enzyme induction. Conversely, high-carbohydrate, low-protein diets and various vitamin and mineral deficiencies can reduce levels of drug-metabolizing enzymes and consequently the rate of drug metabolism so that the serum drug concentrations decline much more slowly, resulting in increased drug potency.[61]

In general, as discussed above, when orally administered medications are taken with meals, the rate, rather than the extent, of absorption is more significantly affected. Food affects drug absorption by enhancing gastric blood flow in conjunction with delayed gastric emptying or by altering dissolution. Food can increase, decrease, or have no effect on the absolute systemic availability of a medication.[62] Concomitant food ingestion reduces the absorption of drugs such as ampicillin, penicillin, and isoniazid.[19] Conversely, food may actually enhance the absorption of other medications, such as griseofulvin. Table 6.2 lists medications whose absorption is altered by food. In most cases, altering the rate of absorption of a drug alone without affecting the total amount absorbed should not affect its efficacy.

TABLE 6.3
Examples of Drug–Nutrient Interactions

	Nutritional Considerations	Possible Gastrointestinal Side Effects	Comments/Recommendations
		Antibiotics	
General	Decreased synthesis of vitamin K by gut microflora; depletion of gut microflora can also lead to dysbiosis that can alter the digestion and absorption of nutrients; some antibiotics are folate and B12 antagonists	N/V/D, lactase deficiency	
Aminoglycosides	Increased urinary excretion of potassium and magnesium; may also deplete sodium and calcium	Decreased appetite, N/V, increased salivation	
Amoxicillin/clavulanic acid (Augmentin®)		N/V/D, incidence of diarrhea higher with Augmentin vs. amoxicillin alone	Take with food to reduce gastrointestinal (GI) upset
Cephalosporins	Possible nephrotoxicity with vitamin K deficiency	GI mucosa damage, V/D	
Chloramphenicol (Chloromycetin®)	Decreased protein synthesis: increased need for riboflavin, B6, B12	V/D, stomatitis, enterocolitis, glossitis	Take on an empty stomach
Clindamycin (Cleocin®)		N/V/D, esophagitis, pseudomembranous colitis	Take with a full glass of water to avoid esophageal irritation
Clofazimine (Lamprene®)	Food increases the extent of absorption	Constipation, abdominal pain, N/V/D, anorexia, GI bleeding, dysgeusia	Administer with meals or milk to maximize absorption
Dapsone	Do not administer with alkaline foods or antacids (may decrease dapsone absorption)	Vomiting, anorexia, abdominal pain	

Drug	Interaction	Adverse effects	Recommendations
Linezolid (Zyvox®)	Concurrent use of linezolid and foods or beverages containing large quantities of tyramine may result in a significant pressor response	N/D, dyspepsia, oral moniliasis, tongue discoloration, localized abdominal pain, constipation, pseudomembranous colitis	Patients receiving linezolid and tyramine-containing foods or beverages should be monitored for significant blood pressure increases. Avoid foods containing large amounts of tyramine (aged cheese, sour cream, red wine) (<100 mg/meal).
Macrolides: azithromycin, clarithromycin, erythromycin	Rate and extent of GI absorption may be altered depending on the formulation. Azithromycin: Food does not affect bioavailability of the tablet formulation, immediate-release oral suspension, or the 1 g suspension regimen; however, extended release suspension ↑ absorption when given with a high-fat meal. Clarithromycin: Food delays rate, but not extent of absorption. Extended release: Food increases clarithromycin AUC by ~30% relative to fasting conditions. Erythromycin serum levels may be altered if taken with food (formulation dependent)	Abdominal pain, cramping, N/V/D, stomatitis, dyspepsia	Do not crush enteric coated or delayed release products. Azithromycin: Immediate-release suspension and tablet may be taken without regard to food; extended release suspension should be taken on an empty stomach (at least 1 h before or 2 h after a meal). Clarithromycin: immediate-release tablets and oral suspension may be given with or without meals, may be taken with milk. Extended release tablets should be taken with food. Erythromycin: avoid milk and acidic beverages 1 h before or after a dose; administer after food to decrease GI discomfort
Metronidazole (Flagyl®)	Food decreases peak drug concentration	N/V/D, metallic taste, xerostomia, furry tongue	Disulfiram—reaction with alcohol
Neomycin (Mycifradin®)	Decreased absorption of fat; MCT; vitamins A, D, K, B12; sodium; glucose; lactose; sucrose; xylose. May also deplete β-carotene, calcium, iron, magnesium, potassium	N/V/D, colitis, candidiasis, inactivation of bile salts, GI mucosal damage, decreased activity of disaccharidases, lipase inhibition	

(continued)

TABLE 6.3 (Continued)
Examples of Drug–Nutrient Interactions

	Nutritional Considerations	Possible Gastrointestinal Side Effects	Comments/Recommendations
Penicillins	Increased urinary potassium excretion; may inactivate B6; food ↓ drug absorption	Decreased appetite, diarrhea	Administer with water on an empty stomach (1 h before or 2 h after meals); may take with food to ↓ GI upset
Quinolones	Dairy foods, mineral supplements, calcium-fortified juices decrease drug concentrations; may increase caffeine concentrations	N/V/D, GI bleeding, abdominal pain, anorexia, pseudomembranous colitis, dyspepsia	Administer 2 h after meals, may take with food to ↓ GI upset
Sulfonamides	Decreased synthesis of folic acid, B vitamins, vitamin K; decreased iron absorption; increased urinary excretion of vitamin C; presence of food delays but does not ↓ absorption	Decreased appetite, N/V, stomatitis, pseudomembranous colitis, abdominal pain	Avoid large amounts of vitamin C or acidifying agents (cranberry juice) to prevent crystalluria
Tetracyclines	Chelate divalent ions; decreased absorption of calcium, iron, magnesium, zinc, amino acids; increased urinary excretion of vitamin C; absorption of tetracycline hydrochloride ↓ by 50% when taken with milk/dairy products	N/V/D, anorexia, stomatitis, glossitis, antibiotic-associated pseudomembranous colitis, esophagitis, oral candidiasis	Take on empty stomach 1 h before/2 h after dose; avoid milk/dairy products, polyvalent ions with 2–3 h of dose; doxycycline and minocycline may be given without regard to meals but best to avoid concurrent administration with milk/dairy products
Trimethoprim (Trimpex®, TMP)	Decreased folate concentrations	N/V, epigastric distress	Leucovorin may be given until normal hematopoeisis is restored

Antifungals

Drug	Interaction	Adverse effects	Recommendations
Amphotericin B (Fungizone®)	Possible nephrotoxicity with increased urinary excretion of potassium and magnesium	Decreased appetite, N/V, steatorrhea, diarrhea with oral formulation	Monitor potassium, magnesium, supplementation usually necessary
Caspofungin (Cancidas®)		N/V/D, abdominal pain, anorexia, mucosal inflammation	
Fluconazole (Diflucan®)	Food delays time of peak absorption but has no effect on total amount of drug absorbed	Mild–moderate GI upset (N/V/D), abdominal pain	
Flucytosine (Ancoban®)	Food ↓ rate but not extent of absorption; magnesium or aluminum salts delay rate of absorption	N/V/D, enterocolitis	May take with food
Griseofulvin (Grisactin®, Fulvicin®)	High-fat foods ↑ absorption rate	N/V/D, oral thrush	Give with fatty meals to ↑ absorption as well as avoid GI upset
Itraconazole (Sporanox®)	Food ↑ absorption of capsule formulation; hypochlorhydria may ↓ absorption; grapefruit juice ↓ itraconazole AUC by 30%; absorption ↑ when taken with a cola beverage	N/V/D, abdominal pain, anorexia	Take capsules with food; take oral solution on an empty stomach
Ketoconazole (Nizoral®)	Food ↑ rate and extent of absorption; administration with an acidic beverage (cola, citrus juice) enhances absorption	N/V/D, abdominal discomfort, GI bleeding	Take with food to ↓ GI upset
Micafungin (Mycamine®)		N/V/D, mucosal inflammation, constipation, anorexia, dyspepsia	
Posaconazole (Noxafil®)	Adequate posaconazole absorption from the GI tract and subsequent plasma concentrations are dependent on food for efficacy	N/V/D, anorexia, abdominal pain, constipation, dyspepsia	Must be administered during or within 20 min of a full meal or oral liquid nutritional supplement; alternatively, may be given with an acidic carbonated beverage
Voriconazole (VFEND®)	High-fat meals reduce extent of absorption	N/V, anorexia, constipation, abdominal pain	Take 1 h before or 1 h after meals

(continued)

TABLE 6.3 (Continued)
Examples of Drug–Nutrient Interactions

	Nutritional Considerations	Possible Gastrointestinal Side Effects	Comments/Recommendations
Anthelmintics			
Albendazole (Albenza®)	Bioavailability increased when taken with a fatty meal	N/V, abdominal pain	
Ivermectin (Stromectol®)	Bioavailability ↑ 2.5-fold when administered after a high-fat meal	N/D	Take on an empty stomach with water
Mebendazole (Vermox®)	Food ↑ drug absorption	N/V/D, abdominal pain	Administer with food
Antimalarials			
Artemether and lumefantrine (Coartem®)		N/V, abdominal pain, anorexia	Administer with a full meal for best absorption. Patients should be encouraged to take with a meal as soon as food can be tolerated. Patients who remain averse to food during treatment should be closely monitored as the risk of recrudescence increases.
Chloroquine phosphate (Aralen®)		N/V/D, anorexia, stomatitis, weight loss	Take with food to ↓ GI upset; bitter taste may be masked by mixing with chocolate syrup
Hydroxychloroquine (Plaquenil®)	Food increases bioavailability	N/V/D, anorexia, abdominal cramps	Take with food to ↓ GI upset
Primaquine phosphate		N/V, abdominal cramps, anorexia	Take with food to ↓ GI upset; drug has bitter taste
Pyrimethamine (Daraprim®)	↓ Serum folate concentrations	Anorexia, abdominal cramps, V/D, atrophic glossitis	Take with meals to ↓ GI upset; leucovorin may be given until normal hematopoieisis is restored

Drug		
Sulfadoxine and pyrimethamine (Fansidar®)	Anorexia, gastritis, glossitis, V/D	↓ Serum folate concentrations	Take with meals; leucovorin may be given until normal hematopoiesis is restored

Antiprotozoals

Drug	Adverse effects	Interaction	Recommendation
Atovaquone (Mepron®)	N/V/D, abdominal pain, constipation, anorexia	Food increases bioavailability	Patients who cannot take with meals or have chronic diarrhea or GI problems at risk for drug malabsorption and treatment failure
Nitazoxanide (Alinia®)	N/V/D, abdominal pain	Food increases AUC	Administer with food
Antiretrovirals			
Amprenavir (Agenerase®)	N/V/D, taste disorders	High-fat meals may decrease AUC; product contains vitamin E to improve bioavailability; may increase risk of bleeding if vitamin K deficient or on concomitant anticoagulant therapy	Fat redistribution and accumulation has been reported
Atazanavir (Reyataz®)	N/V/D	Bioavailability ↑ when taken with food	Administer with food; may cause redistribution of fat (e.g., buffalo hump, peripheral wasting with increased abdominal girth, cushingoid appearance)
Fosamprenavir (Lexiva®)	N/V/D; abdominal pain. May cause transaminase elevations, hepatitis, and/or exacerbate pre-existing hepatic dysfunction	Tablets may be taken with or without food. Adults should take oral suspension without food; however, children should take oral suspension with food	Take tablets with food if taken with ritonavir. May be administered without regard to food if not taken with ritonavir. Adults should take oral suspension without food; however, children should take oral suspension with food
May cause redistribution of fat (e.g., buffalo hump, peripheral wasting with increased abdominal girth)

(continued)

TABLE 6.3 (Continued)
Examples of Drug–Nutrient Interactions

	Nutritional Considerations	Possible Gastrointestinal Side Effects	Comments/Recommendations
Indinavir (Crixivan®)	↓ Absorption when given with high amounts of protein or fatty foods; grapefruit juice ↓ AUC by 26%	N/V/D, abdominal pain, metallic taste	Ensure adequate hydration; take on empty stomach; if GI upset is a problem, take with light meals or other liquids
Lopinavir and ritonavir (Kaletra®)	Solution should be taken with food. Tablet may be taken with or without food	N/V/D, abdominal pain, altered taste, weight loss	Solution: Administer with food; if using didanosine, take didanosine 1 h before or 2 h after lopinavir/ritonavir. Tablet: May be taken with or without food. Swallow whole, do not break, crush, or chew. May be taken with didanosine when taken without food
Nelfinavir (Viracept®)	Food ↑ absorption	N/V/D, abdominal pain, anorexia, dyspepsia epigastric pain, mouth ulceration, GI bleeding, pancreatitis	Powder formulation contains 11.2 mg phenylalanine per gram powder; do not administer with acidic foods or juices (results in bitter taste)
Ritonavir (Norvir®)	Food ↑ absorption; may cause avitaminosis	N/V/D, taste perversion, abdominal pain, pancreatitis	Administer with food to ↑ absorption; liquid formulations tastes unpleasant, reserve use for tube-fed patients or mix with chocolate milk or nutritional supplement
Saquinavir (Fortovase®, Invirase®)	High-fat meals maximize bioavailability; grapefruit juice ↑ saquinavir levels	N/V/D, abdominal discomfort, stomatitis	Take within 2 h of a full meal; high-calorie/high-fat meals ↑ AUC and C_{max} more than low-calorie/low-fat meals

Drug			
Tipranavir (Aptivus®)	Coadministration with ritonavir is required. Administer with ritonavir capsules or solution without regard to meals; administer with ritonavir tablets with meals	N/V/D, abdominal pain, weight loss, dehydration, taste perversion	Capsule contains dehydrated ethanol. Oral solution formulation contains vitamin E; additional vitamin E supplements should be avoided
			May cause redistribution of fat (e.g., buffalo hump, peripheral wasting with increased abdominal girth, Cushingoid appearance). May cause facial wasting
Abacavir (Ziagen®)	Food does not affect AUC	N/V/D, anorexia, pancreatitis	Fat redistribution and accumulation has been reported
Didanosine (Videx®)	May alter GI absorption of various nutrients due to prolonged GI transient time. Food may decrease oral bioavailability by 50%	N/V, constipation, xerostomia, dry throat, dysphagia	Buffered powder for oral solution is inactivated in acidic juices/fluids
Emtricitabine (Emtriva®)	May be administered with or without food	N/V/D, abdominal discomfort, gastroenteritis,	May cause redistribution of fat
Lamivudine (Epivir®, 3TC)	Food may ↓ rate of absorption and peak serum concentrations, but does not significantly change the AUC	N/V/D, feeding problems, abdominal discomfort, pancreatitis, anorexia, stomatitis	May cause fat redistribution and accumulation
Stavudine (Zerit®, d4T)	Food ↓ peak serum concentrations by 45%, bioavailability not changed	N/V/D, abdominal pain, anorexia, pancreatitis	Take without regard to food
Tenofovir disoproxil fumarate (Viread®)	High-fat meals ↑ oral bioavailability	N/V/D, flatulence, anorexia, pancreatitis	Administer with meals to improve absorption
Zalcitabine (Hivid®, ddC)	Food ↓ rate and extent of absorption; AUC ↓ by 14%	N/V/D, oral/esophageal ulcers, dysphagia, anorexia, abdominal pain, constipation, pancreatitis, weight loss, anemia	Take on empty stomach

(continued)

TABLE 6.3 (Continued)
Examples of Drug–Nutrient Interactions

	Nutritional Considerations	Possible Gastrointestinal Side Effects	Comments/Recommendations
Zidovudine (Retrovir®, AZT, ZDV)	Folate/B12 deficiency increases zidovidine associated myelosuppression; rate of absorption and peak serum concentration may ↓ when taken with food	N/V/D, anorexia	May take with food; take capsules while in upright position to ↓ risk of esophageal ulceration; syrup is strawberry flavored
Delavirdine (Rescriptor®)	Patients with achlorhydria should take the drug with an acidic beverage	N/V/D, abdominal pain	May be taken without regard to meals. Patients with achlorhydria should take the drug with an acidic beverage; 200 mg tablets should be taken intact. May cause fat redistribution and accumulation
Efavirenz (Sustiva®)	High-fat/high-caloric meals ↑ AUC and peak concentration and may ↑ adverse effects	N/V/D, abdominal pain	Take with water on an empty stomach preferred, tastes peppery (grape jelly may be used to improve taste). Tablets should not be broken. Some clinicians recommend opening capsules and adding to liquid or food for patients that cannot swallow capsules; however, no pharmacokinetic data are available and this is not recommended
Etravirine (Intelence®)	Food increases absorption of etravirine by ~50%	N/D	Central redistribution of body fat. Take after meals. May disperse tablets in glass of water; stir well before drinking and rinse glass several times to ensure administration of complete dose

Drug		Adverse effects	Comments
Nevirapine (Viramune®)	Can be given without regard to food	N/V/D, abdominal pain	Central redistribution of body fat. Extended release tablets must be swallowed whole and not crushed, chewed, or divided.
Rilpivirine (Edurant™)	Administer with a normal- to high-caloric meal. Absorption increased by ~40% when taken with a normal to high-caloric meal. Administration with a protein supplement drink alone does not increase absorption	Abdominal discomfort/pain, appetite decreased, N/V/D	May cause redistribution of fat
Enfurvitide (Fuzeron®)		D/N, weight loss, abdominal pain, appetite decreased, pancreatitis, anorexia, xerostomia	
Maraviroc (Selzentry®)	Absorption of maraviroc is somewhat reduced with ingestion of a high-fat meal; however, maraviroc can be given with or without food	Abdominal pain, altered appetite, constipation	
Integrase Inhibitor			
Raltegravir (Isentress®)	May be administered without regard to meals; however, clinically insignificant variability in absorption exists depending on meal type	N/D	May be taken without regard to meals. Some products may contain phenylalanine
Antitubercular Agents			
Cycloserine (Seromycin®)	B6 antagonist; ↓ absorption of calcium, magnesium, vitamin B12; decreased folate utilization and vitamin K synthesis; may increase B12 and folate requirements		Some neurotoxic effects may be prevented or lessened by pyridoxine supplementation. May be administered without regard to meals
Ethambutol (Myambutol®)	May deplete copper and zinc	N/V, abdominal pain, anorexia	Take with food to ↓ GI upset
Ethionamide (Trecator®)	Neurotoxic effects may be prevented or relieved by the coadministration of pyridoxine	N/V/D, abdominal pain, anorexia, excessive salivation, metallic taste, stomatitis, weight loss	May be taken with or without meals

(continued)

TABLE 6.3 (Continued)
Examples of Drug–Nutrient Interactions

	Nutritional Considerations	Possible Gastrointestinal Side Effects	Comments/Recommendations
Rifabutin (Mycobutin®)	High-fat meal may decrease the rate but not extent of drug absorption	N/V/D, anorexia, dyspepsia, abdominal pain, dysgeusia, flatulence	Take with food to ↓ GI upset
Rifampin	Food may decrease or delay amount of drug absorbed	N/V/D, anorexia, stomatitis	Take on empty stomach
Antivirals			
Acyclovir (Zovirax®)	Food does not appear to affect absorption	N/V/D	May administer with food
Amantadine (Symmetrel®)		N/V/D, xerostomia, anorexia, constipation	
Cidofovir (Vistide®)		N/V/D, anorexia	
Famciclovir (Famvir®)	Rate of absorption and/or conversion to penciclovir and peak concentration are ↓ with food, bioavailability not affected	N/V/D, constipation, anorexia, abdominal pain	May take with food to ↓ GI upset
Ganciclovir (Cytovene®)	High-fat meal ↑ AUC	N/V/D, pancreatitis	Administer with food; do not open capsules or crush tablets
Oseltamivir (Tamiflu®)	May be administered without regard to meals; take with food to improve tolerance. Capsules may be opened and mixed with sweetened liquid (e.g., chocolate syrup).	N/V/D, pseudomembranous colitis	Administer with food to ↓ GI upset
Valacyclovir (Valtrex®)	May administer with or without food	N/V/D, abdominal pain	May be taken with or without food Administer with food to ↓ GI upset

Drug	Interaction	GI/Adverse effects	Recommendation
Valganciclovir (Valcyte®)	Coadministration with a high-fat meal increased AUC by 30%	N/V/D, abdominal pain, constipation, dyspepsia, ↓ appetite	Take with food
Miscellaneous Anti-Infective Agents			
Clofazimine (Lamprene®)	Food ↑ extent of absorption	N/V/D, abdominal pain; constipation; bowel obstruction, GI bleeding, dysgeusia	Administer with meals/milk to maximize absorption
Fuazolidine (Furoxone®)	Large doses or prolonged therapy ↑ risk of hypertensive effects if taken with tyramine containing foods	N/V/D	Avoid tyramine-containing foods
Methenamine (Hiprex®, Mandelamine®)	Foods/diets that alkalinize urine pH > 5.5 ↓ activity of methenamine; cranberry juice can be used to acidify urine and ↑ activity of methenamine	N/V/D, abdominal cramping, anorexia, stomatitis	Administer with food
Nalidixic acid (NegGram®)	Food delays absorption	N/V/D, abdominal pain	Suspension is raspberry flavored
Nitrofurantoin (Furadantin®, Macrodantin®)	Food ↑ total amount absorbed. Cranberry juice or other urine acidifiers enhance drug action	N/V, anorexia, pancreatitis	Administer with food or milk
Pentamidine (Pentam®)		N/V/D; metallic taste, pancreatitis, anorexia, dyspepsia, xerostomia	

Source: Adapted from Gura KM. Drug–nutrient interactions. In: Hendricks KM, Duggan C, editors. Manual of Pediatric Nutrition (5th ed.). Hamilton, ON: BC Decker, pp. 545–585, 2013.

The composition of the meal will alter splanchnic blood flow. Blood flow can be slightly reduced by a liquid glucose meal and doubled by a high-protein liquid meal.[63] The significance of this effect on splanchnic flow is important for those medications with high hepatic extraction. Continued meal intake, especially with high-fat-content foods, will also slow the rate of gastric emptying, which may subsequently cause a delay in drug absorption from the gastrointestinal tract. Changes in gastric emptying are related not only to the physicochemical properties of the drug but also to the type of meal itself. Hot meals, highly viscous solutions, or those rich in fat have the most significant effect in decreasing gut motility.[64] Melander and colleagues reviewed the impact of food on the presystemic clearance of drugs.[63] They observed that meals commonly enhanced presystemic clearance of lipophilic basic drugs (e.g., amitriptyline, propranolol) but rarely altered the clearance of drugs that were lipophilic acids (e.g., salicylic acid, penicillin). Alternatively, food may reduce the presystemic clearance of some lipophilic basic drugs through transient, complex effects on splanchnic–hepatic blood flow. Moreover, repeated intake of specific nutrients (e.g., protein) and food contaminants (e.g., aromatic hydrocarbons) can enhance presystemic drug clearance by enzyme induction.

INFLUENCE OF SPECIFIC NUTRIENTS ON PHARMACOKINETICS

Until recently, the concept that dietary substances could significantly alter medication response by affecting intestinal transporter and metabolizing enzymes was viewed as irrelevant. This misconception was based on the premise that drug absorption was a passive process and the role of the intestine in drug elimination was minimal.[65] Since the report of the interaction between grapefruit juice and several medications was first described, this commonly held belief has changed, and the role of the diet on drug performance has been reevaluated.[66]

CARBOHYDRATES

There is conflicting evidence on the role of carbohydrates on drug metabolism. It is known that diets high in carbohydrates may induce the expression of several lipogenic and glycolytic hepatic enzymes.[67] Others suggest that carbohydrates have little impact on drug metabolism.[66] Animal studies by Sonawane et al. suggest that dietary carbohydrates and fat may significantly influence the hepatic drug-metabolizing enzymes.[67] It has been hypothesized that these changes may occur owing to alteration in the phospholipid composition of endoplasmic reticulum or by limiting the supply of cofactor(s) necessary for optimal functioning of CYP and UGT.

PROTEIN

Medications that undergo extensive first-pass effect can have enhanced bioavailability after a high-protein meal owing to enhanced hepatic blood flow. High-extraction drugs can then rapidly pass through the liver, allowing higher drug concentrations in the systemic circulation.[64,66] Decreases in dietary protein reduces creatinine clearance and renal plasma flow.[68] In situations where there is low protein intake, careful attention is needed to avoid toxicity secondary to delayed drug clearance.

Specific dietary proteins can also affect medication response. One classic example is the interaction between the monoamine oxidase inhibitor (MAO-I) drug class and the amino acid tyramine that is contained in aged cheeses, pickled/smoked meats, fermented foods, and red wines. Tyramine is an indirect sympathomimetic amine that releases norepinephrine from the adrenergic neurons, resulting in a significant pressor response. Normally, tyramine is metabolized by the enzyme monoamine oxidase before any significant increases in blood pressure occur. If the enzyme is blocked, however, severe and potentially fatal increases in blood pressure can occur when tyramine-rich foods are ingested. Although MAO-Is are not used routinely as antidepressants, other medications, such as isoniazid and the oxazolidinone antibiotic linezolid, also possess MAO-I properties. Patients should avoid ingesting large amounts of tyramine while being treated with these medications.[69]

Dietary protein also affects the renal tubular transport of certain compounds. The binding of dietary proteins to a drug may underscore changes in bioavailability after a protein meal. For example, ciprofloxacin when taken with milk or other dairy products not only undergoes complexation with calcium but also adsorbs to the surface of proteins, which further decreases the absorbable amount of ciprofloxacin and may increase the chance of treatment failure or resistance.[70] The authors hypothesize that the casein component present in milk has a more pronounced effect on the amount of absorbable ciprofloxacin.

Dietary Fat

Lipids are an essential part of cell membrane structure and are involved in many of the normal enzymatic activities located within the cell membrane.[57] Low-fat diets or those deficient in essential fatty acids decrease the activity of the enzyme systems responsible for nutrient metabolism.[71] After consumption of a high-fat meal, plasma free fatty acid levels become elevated, increasing the potential to become bound to plasma albumin and subsequently displace albumin-bound drugs, thus increasing the risk of drug toxicity.[72] Dietary fats along with food-stimulated secretions (e.g., bile salts) may facilitate the solubilization and dispersion of lipophilic compounds. This contributes to a reduction in the extent of first-pass metabolism due to enhanced splanchnic blood flow. High-fat diets have been associated with the induction of CYP2E1.[73] The type of fat determines the extent to which this enzyme is upregulated. Poly-unsaturated fats (PUFAs) such as corn and menhaden oils appear to have the greatest influence in comparison with lard or olive oils. This can result in enhanced peroxidation of the PUFA substrates and contribute to free radical production. The rate of gastric emptying is also influenced by the fat content of a meal. Fat delays gastric emptying to a greater degree than does protein or carbohydrate.[74]

The effect of dietary fat on drug absorption, however, depends on the location of the drug absorption, either portal or lymphatic.[71] For medications absorbed through the lymphatic system, dietary fat enhances the absorption of the dissolved drug while poorly bioavailable lipophilic drugs absorbed by the portal route (thus bypassing the lymphatic system) have their absorption enhanced by improved drug dissolution. On the other hand, lipophilic medications having good bioavailability are less likely to be affected by a high-fat meal. Fatty meals do not appear to affect the absorption of hydrophilic medications.

MINERALS

In most instances, mineral deficiencies (i.e., iodine, magnesium, potassium, and zinc) have been associated with a decrease in drug oxidation and drug clearance.[5] For reasons that are not fully apparent, low dietary intake of iron has been associated with an increase in some CYP functions and a decrease in other degradative activities. Foods fortified with multivalent minerals, such as calcium, are presenting a new challenge. For example, any medication carrying a warning to avoid milk, dairy products, or nutritional supplements can be affected by calcium-fortified orange juice.[75] As a class, antibiotics are the most susceptible to chelation and adsorption by fortified cereals, calcium-fortified orange juice, or protein supplements. Patients need to be counseled that consuming fortified foods may decrease the clinical efficacy, thereby increasing the risk of treatment failure.

VEGETABLES

Drug response may also be affected by diets rich in fruits and vegetables. Both serve as sources of trace minerals that are contained in metalloenzymes, including several antioxidants. Many plants contain flavonoids, isothiocyanates, and allyl sulfides that are potent modulators of the cytochrome monooxygenase system.[76]

The modulation of a variety of metabolic pathways is associated with phytochemicals found in cruciferous vegetables, citrus juices, spices, dietary supplements, and herbs. There are five major families of phytochemicals: alkaloid, carotenoids (e.g., β-carotene, lycopene), nitrogen compounds, phenolics (e.g., flavonoids, coumarins, tannins), and sulfur compounds (e.g., isothiocyanates, allylic sulfur).[77] Vegetables and fruits can influence a variety of enzymatic pathways. Typically, induction of these enzyme systems is rapid and plateaus within 5 days of continued daily ingestions of the food with the enzyme-inducing capacity.[78]

DRUG AND GRAPEFRUIT JUICE INTERACTIONS

Bailey and his colleagues discovered that grapefruit juice, which was used as a taste-masking agent for alcohol, caused a 2- to 3-fold increase in oral absorption of the calcium channel blocker felodipine.[2] This interaction is the classic example of a drug–nutrient interaction exclusively caused by inhibition of intestinal CYP3A4. Oral absorption pharmacokinetic studies of CYP3A4 substrates have demonstrated that grapefruit juice increased the oral bioavailability of these agents. The plasma half-lives of most of the drugs studied were not affected, suggesting that the systemic clearance or hepatic metabolism of these drugs was unchanged by grapefruit juice, as this interaction occurs in the enterocytes and not in the hepatocytes. Furthermore, repeated consumption of grapefruit juice inhibits not only the intestinal CYP3A4 activity but also the expression of this gene in the enterocytes. As grapefruit juice inhibits intestinal CYP3A4 expression and thus decreases the presystemic metabolism of certain drugs, the bioavailability of the affected agents will remain increased until the expression of the CYP3A4 gene returns to baseline. This suggests that simply separating the administration time between grapefruit juice and the potential interacting drugs cannot prevent this interaction.

Grapefruit products also interact with uptake transporters such as organic anion-transporting polypeptides (OATPs).[79] OATPs are uptake transporters distributed in the brain, kidney, liver, and small intestine. OATPs are expressed on the apical surface of enterocytes within the small intestine, facilitating in the intestinal absorption of orally administered medications. Nutrients able to alter OATP activity can affect the bioavailability of a drug that relies on influx transport systems for its intestinal absorption. This decrease in oral bioavailability among OATP1A2 substrates by flavonoids in grapefruit (naringin) affects both hydrophilic and renally excreted drugs such as ciprofloxacin, more than lipophilic agents. Medications with greater polarity are eliminated mainly by excretion and are more dependent on uptake transporters rather than passive diffusion. Thus, OATP1A2 substrates, which are excreted renally unchanged, may undergo significant decrease in oral bioavailability if given concurrently with orange or grapefruit juice.[80] As the aforementioned example illustrates, the clinical significance of these interactions depends on the pharmacokinetic as well as toxicity profiles of the co-administered medication. Rather than empirically reducing the dose of the affected drugs to avoid toxicity, it is more advisable to suggest that patients avoid grapefruit juice if they are taking an interacting drug since the magnitude of interaction is inconsistent among individuals and difficult to predict.

OTHER DIETARY RESTRICTIONS

In addition to caloric restriction, restriction of other dietary components can also affect drug response. For example, patients receiving aminoglycosides, amphotericin B, cisplatin, or radiocontrast media in conjunction with a low sodium diet have an increased risk for hemodynamic nephrotoxic and ischemic acute renal failure.[81]

EFFECT OF BEVERAGE TYPE ON DRUG BIOAVAILABILITY

"Beverages" refer to any drinkable liquid other than plain water. They are typically classified as alcoholic, caffeinated, fruit/vegetable juices milk-based, or mineral waters. Depending on the type of fluid that is taken, drug absorption may be affected.[82] Mixing drugs with fruit juices or other beverages to mask their taste may affect absorption due to changes in gastric pH, which in turn can affect dissolution of solid dosage forms and formulations with a pH-sensitive coating. Dairy products decrease the absorption of tetracyclines and reduce their bioavailability due to the formation of insoluble chelates between the drug and the calcium present in the beverage. Soft drinks, such as colas, may decrease drug absorption for a variety of reasons. The phosphoric acid and sugar present in these drinks can slow gastric emptying, and the tendency to serve them chilled may also reduce the rate of blood flow within the intestines. Moreover, the carbonation may increase mixing and possibly motility. Interestingly, the acidic pH of cola beverages can be used to optimize clinical responses of both ketoconazole and itraconazole when administered as solid dosage forms in patients with gastric hypochlorhydria, such as those with AIDS gastropathy.[83] Acidic beverages improve the dissolution of tablets and capsules, and thus can improve and stabilize oral bioavailability if these drugs are ones that are poorly soluble at higher pH.

PARENTERAL NUTRITION

The lack of oral nutrient intake during parenteral nutrition often leads to mucosal atrophy along with a reduction in gastric biliary, pancreatic, and intestinal secretions. Bacterial overgrowth can result in a progressive decline in intestinal function due to impaired motility and depressed enzyme activity. Both may alter the rate and extent of absorption of specific nutrients as well as various drugs. Decreases in nutrient absorption include fat, iron, peptides, and vitamins A and B12, as well as drugs such as chloramphenicol, chloroquine, tetracycline, and rifampin.[84]

INFLUENCE OF MEDICATIONS ON NUTRIENT STATUS

NUTRIENT TRANSPORT

Medications can also affect the uptake of nutrients. Hirano et al. describe the impact of five fluoroquinolones on L-carnitine transport, finding that each inhibited its transport, which may potentially be responsible for the toxicity of this drug class to the fetus.[85]

NUTRIENT ABSORPTION

There are also secondary mechanisms that can interfere with nutrient absorption. The direct systemic effect of a medication on one nutrient may have secondary effects on another nutrient. For example, isoniazid and cimetidine inhibit the hydroxylation of vitamin D in the liver and kidney, whereas barbiturates promote the breakdown of vitamin D metabolites, each resulting in a functional deficiency of vitamin D and secondary to impaired calcium absorption.[86] Similarly, neomycin, colchicine, and para-aminosalicylic acid may damage intestinal mucosa and destroy intestinal villi and microvilli, resulting in an inhibition of brush border enzymes and intestinal transport systems.[87]

NUTRIENT METABOLISM

Drugs may affect nutrient metabolism by several methods. They may inhibit the essential intermediary metabolism of a nutrient, usually a vitamin, or promote the catabolism of the nutrient. Medications with these properties may be used therapeutically, as in the case of coumarin anticoagulants. In other cases, this may be an unwanted side effect, as in the case of pyridoxine antagonism seen in isoniazid use. Isoniazid use can result in pyridoxine deficiency by the inhibition of pyridoxal kinase. Isoniazid depletes pyridoxine stores and consequently the neurotransmitter γ-aminobutyric acid (GABA), resulting in seizures. In the event of an isoniazid overdose, administration of pyridoxine can eliminate the resulting seizures and metabolic acidosis.[88]

Many medications induce drug metabolism enzymes, which leads to enhanced activity of these enzymes, thus increasing the demand for their vitamin cofactor. In the case of chronic drug therapy with a corresponding marginal nutrient intake, signs of vitamin deficiency can result. For example, patients treated with cephalosporin antibiotics may develop hemorrhagic states secondary to drug-induced vitamin K deficiency.[89] Cephalosporins block the vitamin K reductase, which is necessary for vitamin K activation.[90] They may also block carboxylation of vitamin K–dependent peptides to yield γ-carboxyglutamic acid residues that are required for calcium binding in the conversion of vitamin K–dependent proenzymes to their active state, which are needed in the coagulation cascade.[90]

MEDICATION-ASSOCIATED FLUID AND ELECTROLYTE DISTURBANCES

Several widely used anti-infectives can affect electrolyte balance, as summarized in Table 6.3. Renal wasting of potassium, resulting in hypokalemia, has been associated with amphotericin B and antipseudomonal penicillins.[84] Conversely, potassium-sparing diuretics (e.g., spironolactone), angiotensin-converting enzyme inhibitors (e.g., enalapril), heparin, and trimethoprim can cause hyperkalemia.[91] A variety of mechanisms are involved. Trimethoprim has weak diuretic properties with potassium-sparing activity. The impact of medications on phosphorus balance is important in patients receiving nutritional support as the synthesis of new cells increases the need for phosphorus. Patients already at risk for refeeding syndrome are particularly susceptible to the effects of drugs known to decrease available phosphorus stores.[92] Drugs such as antacids and sucralfate can alter the absorption of phosphorus from the gastrointestinal tract by binding to dietary phosphate, thus preventing its absorption. Conversely, patients with renal dysfunction are at risk for development of hyperphosphatemia due to the inherent phosphate content present in the phospholipid emulsifiers in intravenous fat emulsion or clindamycin phosphate injection.[91] In addition, medications such as isoniazid can inhibit the hepatic and/or renal hydroxylation of vitamin D, leading to impaired calcium absorption.[86] Hypomagnesemia as a result of renal wasting can occur in patients treated with loop diuretics, thiazide diuretics, amphotericin B, aminoglycosides, cisplatin, or cyclosporine.[93] Renal wasting of magnesium is also common in patients on prolonged courses of high doses of aminoglycosides.[94] Aminoglycosides can inhibit the proximal tubular transport of magnesium in the kidney, predisposing patients with already low magnesium intake to hypomagnesemia.[94] If left untreated, hypomagnesemia will ultimately lead to hypocalcemia. Magnesium deficiency can induce a transient hypoparathyroidism by reducing the secretion of parathyroid hormone (PTH), and a blunted PTH response. This results in an inhibition of the hypocalcemic feedback loop.[93] Treatment for hypocalcemia induced by hypomagnesemia involves correcting the hypomagnesemia first and then managing the magnesium losses. In some cases, calcium supplementation may be unnecessary.[93]

GLUCOSE

Patients with diabetes mellitus or others with insulin resistance (e.g., severe infections, catabolic stress) are susceptible to the effects of medications known to affect glucose metabolism. Hyperglycemia occurs in approximately 20% of patients treated with pentamidine.[95] Moreover, protease inhibitors have been recognized as a cause of hyperglycemia.[96] Table 6.4 lists some of the more common medications that alter glucose metabolism or response.

Hypoglycemia is the most common metabolic abnormality associated with pentamidine therapy.[97] The mechanism responsible for this adverse effect may involve a direct cytolytic effect on pancreatic beta cells, resulting in insulin release and hypoglycemia and a subsequent insulin deficiency owing to loss of β-cell function.[98] Eventually, however, pentamidine-induced pancreatic β-cell damage may lead to insulin deficiency and result in hyperglycemia, although this is considerably less frequent than hypoglycemia.[99]

FAT

In patients in whom no other causes of dyslipidemia exist, drug-induced lipoprotein abnormalities must be considered (Table 6.5). Some of the most common causes of secondary dyslipidemia are medications. When a drug is used for a short period only, practitioners need to be aware of the effects on the patient's baseline lipoprotein

TABLE 6.4
Medications That Alter Glucose Metabolism/Response

Medication	Response
Amprenavir	Hyperglycemia
Chloroquine	Hypoglycemia
Clofazimine	Hyperglycemia
Didanosine	Hyperglycemia
Emtricitabine	Hyperglycemia
Ethionamide	Hypoglycemia
Etravirine	Hyperglycemia
Fosamprenavir	Hyperglycemia
Indinavir	Hyperglycemia
Lamivudine	Hyperglycemia
Micofungin	Hyper/hypoglycemia
Nelfinavir	Hyperglycemia
Pentamidine	Hyper/hypoglycemia
Posaconazole	Hyperglycemia
Quinine	Hypoglycemia
Ritonavir	Hyperglycemia
Saquinavir	Hyperglycemia
Valganciclovir	Hyperglycemia
Zalcitabine	Hyperglycemia

TABLE 6.5
Medications Associated with Dyslipidemia

Medication	Total Lipids	Total Cholesterol	Triglycerides	Low-Density Lipoprotein	High-Density Lipoprotein	Very Low-Density Lipoprotein
Abacavir			↑			
Amprenavir		↑	↑			
Atazanavir		↑				
Didanosine			↑			
Efavirenz		↑	↑		↑	
Entricitabine			↑			
Etravirine		↑	↑	↑		
Fluconazole		↑	↑			
Fosamprenavir		↑	↑			
Idinavir			↑			
Itraconazole			↑			
Miconazole (IV)	↑	↑				
Nelfinavir	↑					
Nevirapine			↑		↑	
Rilpivirine		↑	↑	↑		
Risperidone			↑			
Ritonavir		↑	↑			
Tipranavir		↑	↑			

Source: Adapted from Gura KM. Drug–nutrient interactions. In: Hendricks KM, Duggan C, editors. *Manual of Pediatric Nutrition* (5th ed.). Hamilton, ON: BC Decker, pp. 545–585, 2013.

profile versus the chance that an underlying dyslipidemia has been exacerbated. Drugs used chronically may be more problematic as they may predispose the patient to atherosclerosis.[100]

Protease inhibitors interfere with some proteins involved in fat metabolism (i.e., cytoplasmic retinoic acid–binding protein type 1).[101] Protease inhibitor binding to low-density lipoprotein receptor–related proteins (LRPs) impairs hepatic chylomicron uptake and triglyceride clearance by the endothelial LRP–lipoprotein lipase complex. The resulting hyperlipidemia contributes to central fat deposition and insulin resistance.[101] Protease inhibitors may also disrupt steroid hormone production, leading to lipodystrophy.[102]

GASTROINTESTINAL COMPLICATIONS

Many medications can adversely affect the function of the gastrointestinal tract. Most are minor and resolved over time without any specific intervention. Others, however, can be significant and result in severe gastrointestinal illness (e.g., colitis, esophagitis) that can negatively affect the tolerance to an oral or tube-fed diet. Drug-induced esophagitis can occur with such antibiotics as doxycycline and tetracycline.[103] Typically, "pill esophagitis" occurs in adolescents who drink inadequate amounts of fluid with their medications, or patients with left atrial enlargement or cardiomegaly as the heart impinges on the esophagus, thus increasing the transit time of the medication in the esophagus. Administering the problematic drug with plenty of water or switching to the liquid formulation of the medication often helps alleviate the situation.

ALTERATIONS IN APPETITE

Impairment of nutritional status secondary to medication use often results in drug-induced nutritional deficiencies in those instances in which the medication results in appetite suppression and decreased food intake. Often these signs and symptoms of nutrient deficiencies are nonspecific and may mimic those of other diseases and conditions.

Drugs can reduce food intake through a variety of mechanisms. Drugs that affect appetite (Table 6.6) may do so by either a central or peripheral effect, including loss of appetite, inducing sedation, or evoking adverse response when food is ingested.[104] The primary effect typically centers on appetite suppression, a centrally acting mechanism that includes the catecholaminergic, dopaminergic, serotoninergic, and endorphin modulators, which may all act to suppress appetite.[104] Peripherally acting mechanisms that can indirectly suppress appetite include those agents that inhibit gastric emptying or bulking agents. A secondary response may also occur when an adverse response to food caused by the drug results in a loss of appetite. The emetic center, located within the brain stem, is easily stimulated by the action of many drugs. These include drugs that cause nausea and vomiting, a loss of taste, stomatitis, and hepatoxic agents.[105] Altered taste perception can also lead to a decrease in nutrient intake. Medications such as metronidazole have all been linked with causing taste perversions. Taste is regulated by chemosensory nerves that respond to stimulation

TABLE 6.6
Examples of Medications That Decrease Appetite

Abacavir
Amantadine
Aminoglycosides
Artemether and lumefantrine
Atovaquone
Caspofungin
Cidofovir
Chloroquine
Clofazimine
Dapsone
Enfurvitide
Ethionamide
Ethambutol
Griseofulvin
Hydroxychloroquine
Indinavir
Itraconazole
Lamivudine
Lopinavir and Ritonavir
Metronidazole
Micafungin
Nelfinavir
Nitrofurantoin
Penicillins
Pentamidine
Posaconazole
Primaquine
Quinolones
Rifabutin
Rifampin
Rilpivirine
Ritonavir
Stavudine
Tenofovir
Tetracycline
Tipranavir
Valganciclovir
Voriconazole
Zalcitabine
Zidovudine

Source: Adapted from Gura KM. Drug–nutrient interactions. In: Hendricks KM, Duggan C, editors. *Manual of Pediatric Nutrition* (5th ed.). Hamilton, ON: BC Decker, pp. 545–585, 2013.

chemicals by direct receptor binding, opening ion channels, or through secondary messenger channels using nucleotides or phosphorylated inositol.[106] Medications that disrupt these cellular processes can cause a loss or distortion of taste. Similarly, dry mouth due to reduced saliva production can alter ion concentrations between saliva and plasma that results in decreased taste sensation. Another way in which medications can cause anorexia is through depletion of various nutrients. Drugs known to deplete folate, such as phenytoin, sulfasalazine, and trimethoprim, can result in weight loss and anorexia.[107]

EXAMPLES OF DRUG–NUTRIENT INTERACTIONS IN SPECIFIC INFECTIOUS DISEASE PROCESSES

TUBERCULOSIS

One of the leading causes of death due to infection is tuberculosis.[108] Effective treatment of patients with this condition is crucial. This includes adhering to medication regimens and minimizing any drug–nutrient or drug–food interactions. Failure to do so can result in treatment failures, disease relapse, and the development of drug-resistant tuberculosis. Noncompliance with these multidrug regimens is often due to the gastrointestinal side effects that accompany these therapies in the initial weeks of therapy (e.g., anorexia, nausea, vomiting, and abdominal pain). The Centers for Disease Control and Prevention, the Infectious Disease Society of America, and the American Thoracic Society all recommend that these medications best be taken with meals if gastrointestinal intolerance persists.[109] Others, however, recommend that the bioavailability of both rifampin and isoniazid are reduced when taken with food and may lead to treatment failure.[110] The C_{max} and AUC of isoniazid are reduced 69% and 43%, respectively, when administered with a high-fat meal.[111] Similarly, in comparison with the fasted state, the absorption of rifampin is reduced, with the mean C_{max} and AUC reduced 29% and 16%, respectively.[112] Ethambutol, pyrazinamide, and ethionamide are less likely to be affected by the presence of food.[113] Food also delays the absorption of the second-line antitubercular agent cycloserine/teridone by 3.5 times along with a 35% reduction in maximum blood levels.[114] Conversely, food can increase the absorption of para-aminosalicylic acid and clofazimine.[114,115]

In addition to altered bioavailability when taken with food, isoniazid can also interact with scombroid fish, cheeses, or red wine that have high histamine and/or tyramine content.[116] Isoniazid indirectly inhibits the metabolism of tyramine and histamine and may predispose patients to histamine poisoning (e.g., headache, palpitations, sweating) or tyramine intoxication (e.g., hypertension).

HUMAN IMMUNODEFICIENCY VIRUS

Patients infected by HIV, especially those who abuse drugs, may be particularly prone to developing nutritional deficiencies secondary to drug–nutrient interactions.[117] The relation between antiretroviral therapies (ARTs) and nutrition has been an important factor in the effectiveness of these agents in the prevention and treatment of HIV and its comorbidities. A 2005 World Health Organization report provided recommendations for the nutritional care of individuals with HIV and AIDS with special emphasis on drug–nutrient interactions.[118] The authors noted that certain foods such as garlic and African potato altered the bioavailability of ARTs and that complementary and alternative "traditional" medicines also affected the efficacy of ARTs and patient compliance. Table 6.3 lists the common drug–nutrient interactions seen with ARTs.

Certain ARTs affect nutrient utilization. For example, protease inhibitors, such as ritonavir and nelfinavir, can alter lipid metabolism, resulting in hypertriglyceridemia and elevated cholesterol levels. In other instances, protease inhibitors have been associated with changes in carbohydrate metabolism, leading to insulin resistance.[119] Interestingly, the initiation of antiretroviral therapy in HIV-infected children with marasmus can precipitate the onset of kwashiorkor.[120] Several mechanisms have been proposed. It is thought that some immune competence is necessary to develop the edema associated with kwashiorkor. Second, immune reconstitution inflammatory syndrome may occur soon after ART is started. Lastly, the edema that results may be due to refeeding syndrome that may be the result of ART-associated appetite stimulation. It may also be simply a manifestation of ART toxicity in severely malnourished children. Current guidelines recommend initial therapeutic feedings for HIV-infected children with severe malnutrition, followed by 50–100% increased energy intake for the first 6–10 weeks of ART.[121]

Macronutrients can also affect the bioavailability of many ARTs. The absorption of the antiviral agent zidovudine is affected by dietary fat. When administered orally with a high-fat meal, its absorption is reduced in comparison with when the drug is taken in the fasted state.[72] It is recommended that zidovudine be taken on an empty stomach to achieve peak serum concentrations and minimize the risk of treatment failure.

CONCLUSION

The human diet is highly heterogeneous in its composition, method of preparation, quantity, and time of consumption. These variations may alter the body's responses to drugs. Consequently, pharmacokinetic and pharmacodynamic responses as a result of diet vary widely in subjects according to age, sex, culture, genetic makeup, and economic status. Even within the same individual, seasonal variations will occur that influence dietary habits and ultimately drug-related effects. Although each factor may play a small role by itself, a much larger synergistic effect could occur when combined with other dietary genetic and environmental factors. By limiting medication use to as short a period as possible and with periodic reassessment of treatment options, we can potentially minimize the risks associated with drug–nutrient interactions.

REFERENCES

1. Waler-Sack I, Klotz U. Influence of diet and nutritional status on drug metabolism. *Clin Pharmacokinet* 1996;31:47–64.
2. Lown KS, Bailey DG, Fontana RJ, Janardan SK, Adair CH, Fortlage LA, Brown MB, Guo W, Watkins PB. Grapefruit juice increases felodipine oral availability in humans by decreasing intestinal CYP3A protein expression. *J Clin Invest* 1997;99:2545–53.

3. Pan S, Lopez RR, Sher LS, Hoffman AL, Podesta LG, Makowka L, Rosenthal P. Enhanced oral cyclosporine absorption with water-soluble vitamin E after liver transplantation. *Pharmacotherapy* 1996;16:59–65.
4. Chan L, Humma LM, Schriever CA, Fahsingbauer LA, Dominguez CP, Baum CL. Vitamin E formulation affects digoxin absorption by inhibiting P-glycoprotein (P-gp) in humans. *Clin Pharmacol Ther* 2004;75(2):P95.
5. Guengerich FR. Influence of nutrients and other dietary materials on cytochrome P450 enzymes. *Am J Clin Nutr* 1995;61:651S–8S.
6. Stewart CF, Hampton EM. Effect of maturation on drug disposition in pediatric patients. *Clin Pharm* 1987;6:548–64.
7. Santos CA, Boullata JI. An approach to evaluating drug–nutrient interactions. *Pharmacotherapy* 2005;25(12):1789–800.
8. Rodríguez-Fragoso L, Martínez-Arismendi JL, Orozco-Bustos D, Reyes-Esparza J, Torres E, Burchiel SW. Potential risks resulting from fruit/vegetable–drug interactions: Effects on drug-metabolizing enzymes and drug transporters. *J Food Sci* 2011;76(4):R112–24.
9. Curatolo W, Foulds G, Labadie R. Mechanistic study of the azithromycin dosage-form-dependent food effect. *Pharm Res* 2010;27(7):1361–6.
10. Reuss L. One-hundred years of inquiry: The mechanism of glucose absorption in the intestine. *Annu Rev Physiol* 2000;62:939–46.
11. Kim RB. Drugs as P-glycoprotein substrates, inhibitors, and inducers. *Drug Metab Rev* 2002;34:47–54.
12. Li P, Wang GJ, Robertson TA, Roberts MS. Liver transporters in hepatic drug disposition: An update. *Curr Drug Metab* 2009;10(5):482–98.
13. Ito K, Kusuhara H, Sugiyama Y. Effects of intestinal CYP3A4 and P-glycoprotein on oral drug absorption—Theoretical approach. *Pharm Res* 1999;16:225–31.
14. Kimura Y, Ito H, Ohnishi R, Hatano T. Inhibitory effects of polyphenols on human cytochrome P450 3A4 and 2C9 activity. *Food Chem Toxicol* 2010;48(1):429–35. Epub October 31, 2009.
15. Chan L-N. Drug–nutrient interactions in transplant recipients. *JPEN J Parenter Enteral Nutr* 2001;25:132–41.
16. Skelton JA, Havens PL, Werlin SL. Nutrient deficiencies in tube-fed children. *Clin Pediatr (Phil)* 2006;45(1):37–41.
17. Penod LE, Allen JB, Cabacungan LR. Warfarin resistance and enteral feedings: 2 Case reports and a supporting *in vitro* study. *Arch Phys Med Rehabil* 2001;82:1270–3.
18. Wright DH, Pietz SL, Konstantinides FN, Rotschafer JC. Decreased *in vitro* fluoroquinolone concentrations after admixture with an enteral feeding formulation. *JPEN J Parenter Enteral Nutr* 2000;24(1):42–8.
19. Lazzerini M, Tickell D. Antibiotics in severely malnourished children: Systematic review of efficacy, safety and pharmacokinetics. *Bull World Health Organ* 2011;89(8):594–607. Epub May 2011.
20. McCabe BJ. Prevention of food–drug interactions with special emphasis on older adults. *Curr Opin Clin Nutr Metab Care* 2004;7(1):21–6.
21. Erikson M, Catz C, Yaffe S. Effect of weanling malnutrition upon hepatic drug metabolism. *Biol Neonate* 1975;27:339–51.
22. Khan AM, Ahmed T, Alam NH, Chowdhury AK, Fuchs GJ. Extended-interval gentamicin administration in malnourished children. *J Trop Pediatr* 2006;52(3):179–84. Epub August 26, 2005.
23. O'Doherty DS, O'Malley WE, Denckla MB. Oral absorption of diphenylhydantoin as measured by gas liquid chromatography. *Trans Am Neurol Assoc* 1969;94:318–9.
24. Poole K. Bacterial stress responses as determinants of antimicrobial resistance. *J Antimicrob Chemother* 2012;67(9):2069–89. Epub May 22, 2012.

25. Eng RH, Padberg FT, Smith SM, Tan EN, Cherubin CE. Bactericidal effects of antibiotics on slowly growing and nongrowing bacteria. *Antimicrob Agents Chemother* 1991;35:1824–8.
26. Chatterji D, Ojha AK. Revisiting the stringent response, ppGpp and starvation signaling. *Curr Opin Microbiol* 2001;4:160–5.
27. Sharma UK, Chatterji D. Transcriptional switching in *Escherichia coli* during stress and starvation by modulation of sigma activity. *FEMS Microbiol Rev* 2010;34:646–57.
28. Wu J, Long Q, Xie J. (p)ppGpp and drug resistance. *J Cell Physiol* 2010;224:300–4.
29. Kusser W, Ishiguro EE. Involvement of the relA gene in the autolysis of *Escherichia coli* induced by inhibitors of peptidoglycan biosynthesis. *J Bacteriol* 1985;164:861–5.
30. Wang G, Hosaka T, Ochi K. Dramatic activation of antibiotic production in *Streptomyces coelicolor* by cumulative drug resistance mutations. *Appl Environ Microbiol* 2008;74(9): 2834–40. doi: 10.1128/AEM.02800-07. Epub February 29, 2008.
31. Rodionov DG, Ishiguro EE. Dependence of peptidoglycan metabolism on phospholipid synthesis during growth of *Escherichia coli*. *Microbiology* 1996;142(Pt 10):2871–7.
32. Abranches J, Martinez AR, Kajfasz JK, Chávez V, Garsin DA, Lemos JA. The molecular alarmone (p)ppGpp mediates stress responses, vancomycin tolerance, and virulence in *Enterococcus faecalis*. *J Bacteriol* 2009;191:2248–56.
33. Nguyen D, Joshi-Datar A, Lepine F, Bauerle E, Olakanmi O, Beer K, McKay G et al. Active starvation responses mediate antibiotic tolerance in biofilms and nutrient-limited bacteria. *Science* 2011;334:982–6.
34. Dwyer DJ, Kohanski MA, Collins JJ. Role of reactive oxygen species in antibiotic action and resistance. *Curr Opin Microbiol* 2009;12:482–9.
35. Fung DK, Chan EW, Chin ML, Chan RC. Delineation of a bacterial starvation stress response network which can mediate antibiotic tolerance development. *Antimicrob Agents Chemother* 2010;54:1082–93.
36. Groisman EA, Kayser J, Soncini FC. Regulation of polymyxin resistance and adaptation to low-Mg^{2+} environments. *J Bacteriol* 1997;179:7040–5.
37. Kato A, Groisman EA. The PhoQ/PhoP regulatory network of *Salmonella enterica*. *Adv Exp Med Biol* 2008;631:7–21.
38. Mehta S, Nain CK, Yadav D, Sharma B, Mathur VS. Disposition of acetaminophen in children with protein calorie malnutrition. *Int J Clin Pharmacol Ther Toxicol* 1985;23:311–5.
39. Raghuram TC, Krishnaswamy K. Tetracycline absorption in malnutrition. *Drug Nutr Interact* 1981;1(1):23–9.
40. Lares-Asseff I, Cravioto J, Santigo P, Perex-Ortiz B. Pharmacokinetics of metronidazole in severely malnourished and nutritionally rehabilitated children. *Clin Pharmacol Ther* 1992;51:42–50.
41. Singh BN. Effects of food on clinical pharmacokinetics. *Clin Pharmacokinet* 1999;37:213–55.
42. Bolme P, Gebre-Ab T, Hadgu P, Meeuwisse G, Stintzing G. Absorption and elimination of penicillin in children with malnutrition. *Ethiop Med J* 1980;18(4):151–7.
43. Krishnaswamy K. Nutrients/non-nutrients and drug metabolism. *Drug Nutr Interact* 1985;4:235–47.
44. Fishman J, Bradlow HL. Effect of malnutrition on the metabolism of sex hormones in man. *Clin Pharmacol Ther* 1977;22:721–7.
45. Mandl J, Bánhegyi G, Kalapos MP, Garzó T. Increased oxidation and decreased conjugation of drugs in the liver caused by starvation. Altered metabolism of certain aromatic compounds and acetone. *Chem Biol Interact* 1995;96(2):87–101.
46. Prasad KVS, Rao BSN, Sivakumar B, Prema K. Pharmacokinetics of norethindrone in Indian women. *Contraception* 1979;20:77–90.
47. Park GD, Spector R, Kitt TM. Effect of dietary protein on renal tubular clearance of drugs in humans. *Clin Pharmacokinet* 1989;17:441–51.
48. Alleyne GA. The effect of severe protein calorie malnutrition on renal function of Jamaican children. *Pediatrics* 1967;39:400–11.

49. Lares-Asseff I, Flores-Perez J, Juarez-Olguin H, Ramírez-Lacayo M, Loredo-Abdalá A, Carbajal-Rodríguez L. Influence of nutritional status on the pharmacokinetics of acetylsalicylic acid and its metabolites in children with autoimmune disease. *Am J Clin Nutr* 1999;69:318–24.

50. Zarowtiz B, Pilla A, Popovich J. Expended gentamicin volume of distribution in patients with indicators of malnutrition. *Clin Pharm* 1990;9:40–4.

51. Naran RK, Mehta S, Mathur BS. Pharmacokinetics study of antipyrine in malnourished children. *Am J Clin Nutr* 1977;30:1979–82.

52. Treluyer JM, Roux A, Mugnier C, Flouvat B, Lagardère B. Metabolism of quinine in children with global malnutrition. *Pediatr Res* 1996;40:558–63.

53. World Health Organization. *Management of Severe Malnutrition: A Manual for Physicians and Other Senior Health Workers.* Geneva: WHO, 1999.

54. Blouin RA, Kolpek JH, Mann HJ. Influences of obesity on drug disposition. *Clin Pharm* 1987;6:706–14.

55. Emery MG, Fisher JM, Chien JY, Kharasch ED, Dellinger EP, Kowdley KV, Thummel KE. CYP2E1 activity before and after weight loss in morbidly obese subjects with nonalcoholic fatty liver disease. *Hepatology* 2003;38(2):428–35.

56. Schwartz SN, Pazin GJ, Lyon JA, Ho M. A controlled investigation of the pharmacokinetics of gentamicin and tobramycin in obese patients. *J Infect Dis* 1978;138:499–505.

57. Evans AM. Influence of dietary components on the gastrointestinal metabolism and transport of drugs. *Ther Drug Monit* 2000;22:131–6.

58. Fleisher D, Li C, Zhou Y, Pao LH, Karim A. Drug, meal and formulation interactions influencing drug absorption after oral administration. Clinical implications. *Clin Pharmacokinet* 1999;36:233–54.

59. Ioannides C. Effect of diet and nutrition on the expression of cytochrome P450. *Xenobiotica* 1999;29:109–54.

60. Kappas A, Alvares AP, Anderson KE, Pantuck EJ, Pantuck CB, Chang R, Conney AH. Effect of charcoal broiled beef on antipyrine and theophylline metabolism. *Clin Pharmacol Ther* 1978;23:445–50.

61. Kappas A, Anderson KE, Conney AH, Alvares AP. Influence of dietary protein and carbohydrate on antipyrine and theophylline metabolism in man. *Clin Pharmacol Ther* 1976;20:643–53.

62. Schwartz JG, McMahan CA, Green GM, Phillips WT. Gastric emptying in Mexican Americans compared to non-Hispanic whites. *Dig Dis Sci* 1995;40:624–30.

63. Melander A, Danielson K, Schersten B, Wahlin E. Enhancement of the bioavailability of propranolol and metoprolol by food. *Clin Pharmcol Ther* 1977;22:108–12.

64. Vessell ES. Complex effects of diet on drug disposition. *Clin Pharmacol Ther* 1984;36:285–96.

65. Bailey DG, Spence JD, Munoz C, Arnold JM. Interaction of citrus juices with felodipine and nifedipine. *Lancet* 1991;337:268–9.

66. Williams L, David JA, Lowenthal DT. The influence of food on the absorption and metabolism of drugs. *Med Clin North Am* 1993;77:815–29.

67. Sonawane BR, Coates PM, Yaffe SJ, Koldovsky O. Influence of dietary carbohydrates (alpha-saccharides) on hepatic drug metabolism in male rats. *Drug Nutr Interact* 1983;2:7–16.

68. Anderson KE. Influences on diet and nutrition on clinical pharmacokinetics. *Clin Pharmacokinet.* 1988;14:325–46.

69. Rumore MM, Roth M, Orfanos A. Dietary tyramine restriction for hospitalized patients on linezolid: An update. *Nutr Clin Pract* 2010;25(3):265–9.

70. Pápai K, Budai M, Ludányi K, Antal I, Klebovich I. *In vitro* food–drug interaction study: Which milk component has a decreasing effect on the bioavailability of ciprofloxacin? *J Pharm Biomed Anal* 2010;52(1):37–42.

71. Zimmerman JJ, Ferron GM, Lim HK, Parker V. The effect of a high-fat meal on the oral bioavailability of the immunosuppressant sirolimus (rapamycin). *J Clin Pharmacol* 1999;39(11):1155–61.

72. Unadkat JD, Collier AC, Crosby SS, Cummings D, Opheim KE, Corey L. Pharmacokinetics of oral zidovudine (azidothymidine) in patients with AIDS when administered with and without a high fat meal. *AIDS* 1990;4:229–32.

73. Ghose R, Omoluabi O, Gandhi A, Shah P, Strohacker K, Carpenter KC, McFarlin B, Guo T. Role of high-fat diet in regulation of gene expression of drug metabolizing enzymes and transporters. *Life Sci* 2011;89(1–2):57–64.

74. Clegg ME, McKenna P, McClean C, Davison GW, Trinick T, Duly E, Shafat A. Gastrointestinal transit, post-prandial lipaemia and satiety following 3 days high-fat diet in men. *Eur J Clin Nutr* 2011;65(2):240–6.

75. Wallace AW, Victory JM, Amsden GW. Lack of bioequivalence when levofloxacin and calcium-fortified orange juice are coadministered to healthy volunteers. *J Clin Pharmacol* 2003;43(5):539–44.

76. Lampe JW. Health effects of vegetables and fruit: Assessing mechanisms of action in human experimental studies. *Am J Clin Nutr* 1999;70(3 Suppl):475S–490S.

77. Won CS, Oberlies NH, Paine MF. Mechanisms underlying food–drug interactions: Inhibition of intestinal metabolism and transport. *Pharmacol Ther* 2012;136(2):186–201.

78. Pantuck EJ, Pantuck CB, Anderson KE, Wattenberg LW, Conney AH, Kappas A. Effect of Brussels sprouts and cabbage on drug conjugation. *Clin Pharmacol Ther* 1984;35:161–9.

79. Bailey DG, Dresser GK, Leake BF, Kim RB. Naringin is a major and selective clinical inhibitor of organic anion-transporting polypeptide 1A2 (OATP1A2) in grapefruit juice. *Clin Pharmacol Ther* 2007;81(4):495–502.

80. Bailey DG. Fruit juice inhibition of uptake transport: A new type of food–drug interaction. *Br J Clin Pharmacol* 2010;70(5):645–55.

81. Bennett WM. Drug interactions and consequences of sodium restriction. *Am J Clin Nutr* 1997;65(2 Suppl):678S–81S.

82. Walravens J, Brouwers J, Spriet I, Tack J, Annaert P, Augustijns P. Effect of pH and comedication on gastrointestinal absorption of posaconazole: Monitoring of intraluminal and plasma drug concentrations. *Clin Pharmacokinet* 2011;50(11):725–34.

83. Wimberley SL, Haug MT 3rd, Shermock KM, Qu A, Maurer JR, Mehta AC, Schilz RJ, Gordon SM. Enhanced cyclosporine–itraconazole interaction with cola in lung transplant recipients. *Clin Transplant* 2001;15(2):116–22.

84. Brown RO, Dickerson RN. Drug–nutrient interactions. *Am J Manag Care* 1999;5(3):345–52.

85. Hirano T, Yasuda S, Osaka Y, Asari M, Kobayashi M, Itagaki S, Iseki K. The inhibitory effects of fluoroquinolones on L-carnitine transport in placental cell line BeWo. *Int J Pharm* 2008;351(1–2):113–8.

86. Gura KM, Couris RR. Drug-induced bone disease. *US Pharmacist* 2002;27:HS43–57.

87. Dobbins WO 3rd, Herrero BA, Mansbach CM. Morphologic alterations associated with neomycin induced malabsorption. *Am J Med Sci* 1968;255:63–77.

88. Romero JA. Kuczler FJ Jr. Isoniazid overdose: Recognition and management. *Am Fam Physician* 1998;57:749–52.

89. Reddy J, Bailey RR. Vitamin K deficiency developing in patients with renal failure, treated with cephalosporin antibiotics. *N Z Med J* 1980;92:378–9.

90. New example of vitamin K–drug interaction (editorial). *Nutr Rev* 1984;42:161–3.

91. Velazquez H, Perazella MA, Wright FR, Ellison DH. Renal mechanism of trimethoprim-induced hyperkalemia. *Ann Intern Med* 1993;119:296–301.

92. Brown GR, Greenwood JK. Drug- and nutrition-induced hypophosphatemia: Mechanisms and relevance in the critically ill. *Ann Pharmacother* 1994;28:626–32.

93. al-Ghamdi SM, Cameron EC, Sutton RA. Magnesium deficiency: Pathophysiologic and clinical overview. *Am J Kidney Dis* 1994;24:737–52.

94. Shetty AK, Rogers NI, Mannick EE, Aviles DH. Syndrome of hypokalemic metabolic alkalosis and hypomagnesemia associated with gentamicin therapy: Case reports. *Clin Pediatr* 2000;39:529–33.
95. Pandit MK, Burke J, Gustafson AB, Minocha A, Peiris AN. Drug-induced disorders of glucose tolerance. *Ann Intern Med* 1993;118:529–39.
96. Kaufman MG, Simionatto C. A review of protease inhibitor-induced hyperglycemia. *Pharmacotherapy* 1999;19:114–7.
97. Shen M, Orwoll ES, Conte JE Jr, Prince MJ. Pentamidine-induced pancreatic beta-cell dysfunction. *Am J Med* 1989;86(6 Pt 1):726–8.
98. O'Brien JG, Dong BJ, Coleman RL, Gee L, Balano KB. A 5-year retrospective review of adverse drug reactions and their risk factors in human immunodeficiency virus-infected patients who were receiving intravenous pentamidine therapy for *Pneumocystis carinii* pneumonia. *Clin Infect Dis* 1997;24:854–9.
99. Coyle P, Carr AD, Depczynski BB, Chisholm DJ. Diabetes mellitus associated with pentamidine use in HIV-infected patients. *Med J Aust* 1996;165:587–8.
100. Henkin J, Como JA, Oberman A. Secondary dyslipidemia: Inadvertent effects of drugs in clinical practice. *JAMA* 1992;267:961–8.
101. Korach M, Leclercq P, Peronnet F, Leverve X. Metabolic response to a C-glucose load in human immunodeficiency virus patients before and after antiprotease therapy. *Metab Clin Exp* 2002;51:307–13.
102. Jain RG, Furfine ES, Pedneault L, White AJ, Lenhard JM. Metabolic complications associated with antiretroviral therapy. *Antiviral Res* 2001;51:151–77.
103. Bonavina L, Demeester TR, McChesney L, Schwizer W, Albertucci M, Bailey RT. Drug-induced esophageal strictures. *Ann Surg* 1987;206:173–83.
104. Halford JC, Blundell JE. Pharmacology of appetite suppression. *Prog Drug Res* 2000;54:25–58.
105. Leong RW, Chan FK. Drug-induced side effects affecting the gastrointestinal tract. *Expert Opin Drug Sat* 2006;5(4):585–92.
106. Knudsen L, Weismann K. Taste dysfunction and changes in zinc and copper metabolism during penicillamine therapy for generalized scleroderma. *Acta Med Scand* 1978;204:75–9.
107. Dreizen S, McCredie KB, Keating MJ, Andersson BS. Nutritional deficiencies in patients receiving cancer chemotherapy. *Postgrad Med* 1990;87:163–7.
108. Dye C. Global epidemiology tuberculosis. *Lancet* 2006;367:938–9.
109. Lin MY, Lin SJ, Chan LC, Lu YC. Impact of food and antacids on the pharmacokinetics of anti-tuberculosis drugs: Systematic review and meta-analysis. *Int J Tuberc Lung Dis* 2010;14(7):806–18.
110. Yew WW. Clinically significant interactions with drugs used in the treatment of tuberculosis. *Drug Saf* 2002;25(2):111–33.
111. Melander A, Danielson K, Hanson A, Jansson L, Rerup JC, Scherstén B, Thulin T, Wåhlin E. Reduction of isoniazid bioavailability in normal men by concomitant intake of food. *Acta Med Scand* 1976;200:93–7.
112. Polasa K, Krishnaswamy K. Effect of food on bioavailability of rifampicin. *J Clin Pharmacol* 1983;23(10):433–7.
113. Arbex MA, Varella Mde C, Siqueira HR, Mello FA. Antituberculosis drugs: Drug interactions, adverse effects, and use in special situations. Part 1: First-line drugs. *J Bras Pneumol* 2010;36(5):626–40.
114. Arbex MA, Varella Mde C, Siqueira HR, Mello FA. Antituberculosis drugs: Drug interactions, adverse effects, and use in special situations. Part 2: Second line drugs. *J Bras Pneumol* 2010;36(5):641–56.

115. Nix DE, Adam RD, Auclair B, Krueger TS, Godo PG, Peloquin CA. Pharmacokinetics and relative bioavailability of clofazimine in relation to food, orange juice and antacid. *Tuberculosis (Edinb)* 2004;84(6):365–73.
116. Kaneko T, Ishigatsubo Y. Isoniazid and food interactions—Fish, cheese, and wine. *Intern Med* 2005;44(11):1120–1.
117. Baum MK, Shor-Posner G, Zhang G, Lai H, Quesada JA, Campa A, Jose-Burbano M, Fletcher MA, Sauberlich H, Page JB. HIV-1 infection in women is associated with severe nutritional deficiencies. *J Acquir Immune Defic Syndr Hum Retrovirol* 1997;16(4):272–8.
118. Raiten DJ, Grinspoon S, Arpadi S. *Nutritional Considerations in the Use of ART in Resource-Limited Settings.* Geneva, Switzerland: World Health Organization, 2005.
119. Gelato MC. Insulin and carbohydrate dysregulation. *Clin Infect Dis* 2003;36(2 Suppl):S91–5.
120. Amadi B, Kelly P, Mwiya M, Mulwazi E, Sianongo S, Changwe F, Thomson M et al. Intestinal and systemic infection, HIV, and mortality in Zambian children with persistent diarrhea and malnutrition. *J Pediatr Gastroenterol Nutr* 2001;32(5):550–4.
121. World Health Organization. *Guidelines for an Integrated Approach to the Nutritional Care of HIV-Infected Children (6 Months-14 Years).* Geneva: WHO Press, 2009.

7 HIV and Micronutrient Supplementation

Elaine A. Yu, Julia L. Finkelstein,
and Saurabh Mehta

CONTENTS

Introduction 153
Methods 154
Results 154
   Mortality 155
   HIV Progression, Transmission, and Related Indicators 155
      HIV Progression 155
      Transmission 163
      Birth Outcomes 165
      Hematological Indicators 165
      Other Clinical Morbidities and Assessments 167
Discussion 171
References 173

INTRODUCTION

There are 35 million people living with human immunodeficiency virus (HIV) infection globally, according to the latest 2012 estimates (Joint United Nations Program on HIV/AIDS [UNAIDS]) [1]. Transnational and domestic initiatives on HIV prevention, diagnostics, and provision of antiretroviral drugs have rapidly expanded, yet significant challenges remain in improving the effectiveness of these efforts. Although the number of individuals receiving antiretroviral therapy (ART) tripled in the last 5 years, 66% of individuals in middle- and low-income countries living with HIV and eligible for ART under the 2013 World Health Organization (WHO) treatment guidelines are not receiving treatment [1].

Over the past several decades, the dynamic interrelatedness between immunity and nutrition has been established in a large body of literature, including *in vitro* [2–4] and epidemiological studies [5,6]. This evidence includes substantial work on evaluating the association between HIV and nutritional status [7]. However, there is limited understanding about the impacts of nutritional interventions on clinical morbidity and mortality, as well as related biological and immunological responses, among individuals with HIV infection [8–11]. Importantly, despite the increasing availability and accessibility of ART and highly active ART (HAART), interactions between HIV treatment and nutritional status remain largely undefined.

This review focuses on randomized control trials (RCTs) with micronutrient (multiple, single) interventions among adults and children living with or exposed to HIV/AIDS, as earlier reviews have comprehensively summarized the observational evidence on this topic [12]. While the effects of ART were of interest, we included studies regardless of how current or past ART treatment status was reported.

METHODS

We searched PubMed with "HIV" or "AIDS" as search terms, and the following additional terms sequentially: "micronutrient, multiple micronutrient supplement, supplement, multivitamin, vitamin; vitamins A, B1, B2, B6, B12, C, D, E, K; retinol, thiamine, riboflavin, pyridoxine, cobalamin, tocopherol; iodine, folate, zinc, selenium, iron." This search was restricted to RCTs published from March 1, 2008, to May 28, 2013, in English. Inclusion screening criteria included randomized study regimen involving micronutrients and a control arm; HIV infection and/or exposure status of study participants; and outcomes related to morbidity and mortality. Additional studies cited by these reports were included if relevant. We extracted RCTs from a previous comprehensive review on HIV/AIDS and nutrition, which considered studies published before March 2008 [13]. We included studies that directly compared patients living with and without HIV, reported results specific to a strata of individuals with HIV, or assessed micronutrients in fortified foods.

RESULTS

Broadly, the articles included in this review (Figure 7.1) were among

1. Patients living with HIV and receiving ART (including those initiating or already receiving stable treatment)
2. Patients living with HIV but not receiving ART (owing to lack of availability or pre-ART disease stage)
3. Individuals living with HIV and variable or unspecified past or current ART treatments
4. Children (<18 years) living with or exposed to HIV with mothers living with HIV

These studies were published between 1995 and 2012; only 13.0% of studies were published before 2000 (n = 9) and 43.5% of studies were published after 2009 (n = 30). Seven of eight studies among patients with HIV initiating or on ART were published beginning in 2006. More than 70% of studies included individuals living in Africa (n = 50), including Tanzania (40.6%), South Africa (8.7%), Zambia (5.8%), Uganda (5.8%), Kenya (5.8%), Malawi (4.3%), and Zimbabwe (1.4%). In other

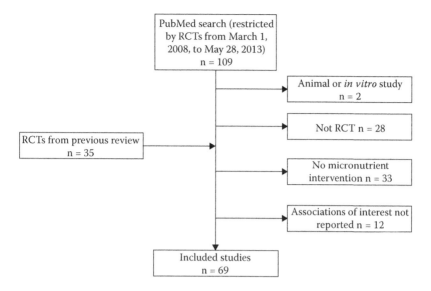

FIGURE 7.1   Study selection flow diagram.

studies, study participants resided in the United States, Canada, Thailand, Peru, and France. Approximately half the studies included children infected with or exposed to HIV; only a subset of these studies also reported maternal outcomes. Sample populations widely ranged from 19 [14] to 4495 study participants [15]. More than 65% of studies were placebo controlled; other control treatment regimens included nonfortified macronutrients, standard (recommended daily allowance [RDA]) micronutrient dosages, or no supplementation.

MORTALITY

Eighteen trials with micronutrient interventions considered mortality (excluding AIDS-related deaths; see "AIDS-Related Deaths" in "HIV Progression, Transmission, and Related Indicators") among adults and children with HIV infection or exposure (Table 7.1).

HIV PROGRESSION, TRANSMISSION, AND RELATED INDICATORS

HIV Progression

AIDS-Related Deaths

ART Naïve   In a TOV study among ART-naive pregnant women with HIV (n = 1078), receiving vitamins (vitamins B, C, and E) was associated with decreased risk of death from AIDS (RR 0.73, 95% CI 0.51–0.04, p = .09) [16]. In contrast, vitamin A supplementation was not associated with reduced risk of AIDS-related death over the follow-up period [16].

TABLE 7.1
Effects of Micronutrient Interventions on Mortality[a] among Adults and Children with HIV Infection and Exposure

	Multiple Micronutrients		Single Micronutrients		
	Supplementation		Vitamin A	Zinc	Selenium
ART	Isanaka et al. 2012 [17]	↔ (vs. standard dose)	Austin et al. 2006 [18] → HR 3.15, 95% CI 1.10–8.98 (placebo vs. vitamin A)		
	Kelly et al. 1999 [19]	↔ (vs. placebo)			
No ART	Jiamton et al. 2003 [20]	→ HR 0.37, 95% CI 0.13–1.06 (p = .052) among those with CD4 <200 × 10^6 cells/L (vs. placebo)			Kupka et al. 2008 [21] ↔ p = .96 (vs. placebo)
		→ HR 0.26, 95% CI 0.07–0.97 (p = .03) among those with CD4 <100 × 10^6 cells/L (vs. placebo)			
Unspecified or heterogeneous ART	Kelly et al. 2008 [22]	→ p = .029 (vs. placebo)		Baum et al. 2010 [23] ↔ (vs. placebo)	
Children	Kawai et al. 2010 [24]	→ RR 0.68, 95% CI 0.47–0.97 among girls (vs. no multivitamins)	Humphrey et al. 2006 [15] ↔ Among infants with HIV at birth (vs. placebo)	Fawzi et al. 2005 [25] ↔ (vs. placebo)	Kupka et al. 2008 [21] ↑ RR 1.58, 95% CI 0.95–2.63 (p = .08; vs. placebo)

Kawai et al. 2010 [24]	↕	among boys (vs. no multivitamins)	Humphrey et al. 2006 [15]	↓	28% decrease in risk (p = .010 among infants uninfected at birth and infected at 6 weeks (vs. placebo)	Srinivasan et al. 2012 [26]	→	Among children with severe pneumonia (vs. placebo)
Duggan et al. 2012 [27]	↕	(vs. no multivitamins)	Semba et al. 2005 [28]	↑	2-fold increase (p < = .05) among infants uninfected at birth and 6 weeks (vs. placebo)			
Ndeezi et al. 2010 [29]	↕	(vs. RDA dose)	Fawzi et al. 1999 [30]	↓	RR 0.37, 95% CI 0.14–0.95 (vs. placebo)			
Kawai et al. 2010 [31]	↕	(vs. RDA dose)		↓	92% decrease risk in diarrhea-related death (95% CI 51–100%, p = .01; vs. placebo)			
Chilenje Infant Growth, Nutrition Infection Study Team 2010 [32]	↕	(fortified vs. not fortified macronutrient)	Semba et al. 2005 [28]	↓	RR 0.54, 95% CI 0.30–0.98 (p = .044; vs. placebo)			

a Excluding AIDS-related mortality.

Children   A Tanzanian study randomized 687 children (aged 6 months to 5 years) admitted to a hospital with pneumonia to receive vitamin A (400,000 IU; 200,000 IU for infants) or placebo [30]. Treatment regimens were received at baseline, 4 months, and 8 months after hospital discharge [30]. Vitamin A reduced AIDS-related deaths (RR 0.28, 95% CI 0.08–1.04, p = .06) when deaths from AIDS among children not living with HIV were excluded [30].

Disease Stage Changes

ART   Among 3418 patients with HIV initiating HAART in Dar es Salaam, the effects of high- and standard-dose multivitamin regimens for 24 months were similar in terms of HIV progression [17].

ART Naïve   In a Tanzanian study among 1078 ART-naive pregnant women with HIV, multivitamins (vitamins B, C, and E) reduced HIV progression to WHO stage IV (RR 0.50, 95% CI 0.28–0.90, p = .02) and progression to ≥ stage III (RR 0.72, 95% CI 0.58–0.90, p = .003), compared with placebo [16]. In contrast, vitamin A and placebo groups showed similar HIV disease progression [16].

HIV Viral Load, Infected Cells, DNA, and RNA

ART   In one study among 3418 nonpregnant adults with HIV and who were initiating HAART, high-dose multivitamins (vitamins B complex, C, and E) for 24 months did not affect plasma viral load, relative to a standard dose [17]. Similarly, in a study among adults with HIV, body mass index (BMI) <18.5, and who were initiating ART, multiple micronutrient food fortification did not affect HIV viral load (as a secondary outcome) compared with the control group (receiving a corn–soy blend) [33].

ART Naïve   Currently available studies on the effects of multiple micronutrient supplements on HIV viral load reported disparate associations (negative [16], null [20,34,35]). Among 1078 ART-naïve pregnant women with HIV, multivitamins (vitamins B complex, C, and E) were associated with lower HIV viral load [16]. Three studies among ART-naïve individuals with HIV were heterogeneous, in terms of multiple micronutrient regimens and supplementation periods; yet, all found no effects on HIV viral loads in blood [20,34] and breast milk samples [35], as well as proviral load in breast milk [35]. Separately, in a study among 400 nonpregnant ART-naïve Kenyan women with HIV-1, multivitamins with selenium increased HIV-1-infected vaginal cells and HIV-1 RNA in vaginal secretions compared with women with placebo [34].

Receiving vitamin A and β-carotene supplements was associated with increased prevalence of viral load detection (51.3%) in breast milk among women with HIV, compared with those who did not receive vitamin A (44.8%, p = .02) [35]. In contrast, three studies reported no effects of vitamin A supplementation on HIV viral load in blood [16,36] and breast milk [35], or proviral load in breast milk [35].

Zinc supplements were not observed to affect HIV viral load [37]. One study assessed the effects of selenium on HIV viral loads of 913 pregnant Tanzanian women with HIV, among whom HAART was not common [21]. Study participants received daily oral supplements (200 µg selenomethionine) from pregnancy (12–27 weeks' gestational age) until 6 months postpartum [21]. Viral load did not differ by treatment group [21].

Heterogeneous or Unspecified ART   Two studies reported no effects of vitamin A on plasma HIV viral loads of individuals with HIV [38,39]. In a trial among 120 injection drug users with HIV, study participants received a single dose of vitamin A (200,000 IU equivalent to 60 mg retinol) or placebo [39]. Plasma HIV viral load did not differ between treatment arms at 2 and 4 weeks [39]. In a study among Kenyan women with HIV-1 (n = 400), there were no differences in plasma HIV-1 viral load of those who received daily oral vitamin A (10,000 IU retinyl palmitate) for 6 weeks compared with the placebo group [38]. HIV-1 DNA prevalence or HIV-1 RNA quantity in vaginal secretions were similar between treatment arms [38]. Separately in a study among 231 adults with HIV and low plasma zinc (<0.75 mg/L at baseline), random assignments of elemental zinc (12 mg women, 15 mg men) or placebo study regimens for 18 months resulted in similar HIV viral loads [23].

Children   In one study among children with HIV, vitamin A (200,000 IU) or placebo was administered on the first 2 days of the trial; on day 14, influenza vaccine was administered [40]. Children who received vitamin A had a lower mean HIV viral load 2 weeks after vaccination, compared with the placebo group [40]. Among youth with HIV, bimonthly oral vitamin D supplements (100,000 IU cholecalciferol) and calcium (1 g/day) did not affect HIV viral load, compared with placebo [41]. In a South African trial among 96 children with HIV-1, daily oral zinc supplementation (10 mg elemental zinc as sulfate) or placebo was randomly assigned [42]. At 6 months after treatment initiation, there were no significant differences in mean log_{10} HIV-1 viral load between study arms [42].

T-Lymphocyte Subsets

ART   In studies among patients with HIV who were initiating or on ART treatment, micronutrient interventions did not influence T-lymphocyte subsets, including CD4 T cells (Table 7.2) [17,19]. A study among 3418 Tanzanian adult patients with HIV found no effect of a high-dose daily oral multivitamin (vitamins B complex, C, and E), compared with the standard-dose supplementation, for 24 months on CD4 count [17]. Patients with HIV serum antibodies and persistent diarrhea (>1 month) were recruited from a hospital in Ndola, Zambia, which provided drugs and food [19]. All patients received albendazole, and either a daily micronutrient supplement (vitamins A, C, E, selenium, zinc) or placebo for 2 weeks [19]. CD4 counts did not differ between treatment arms [19].

In Malawi, a study compared the effects of a multiple micronutrient-fortified spread and control (corn–soy blend) and found no differences in CD4 counts among adults with HIV and low BMI (<18.5) [33]. Another study among Canadian patients with HIV on HAART found no statistical differences in CD4 cells/µmol between different study regimens of fortified yogurts (micronutrient, probiotics, both) [43].

ART Naïve   Studies in Tanzania, Kenya, Zambia, Thailand, and the United States assessed the effects of micronutrient interventions (multivitamins, vitamin A, zinc,

TABLE 7.2
Effects of Micronutrient Interventions on CD4+ T Cells among Adults and Children with HIV Infection and Exposure

| | Multiple Micronutrients | | Single Micronutrients | | | |
	Supplementation	Fortification	Vitamin A	Vitamin D	Zinc	Selenium
ART	Isanaka et al. 2012 [17] ↔ (vs. standard dose) Kelly et al. 1999 [19] ↔ (vs. placebo)	Ndekha et al. 2009 [33] ↔ (vs. nonfortified macronutrient control) Hemsworth et al. 2012 [43] ↔ (vs. nonfortified macronutrient control)				
No ART	Fawzi et al. 2004 [16] ↑ +48 cells/mm³ (95% CI 10–85, p = .01; vs. placebo) McClelland et al. 2004 [34] ↑ +23 cells/µL, p = .03 (vs. placebo) Fawzi et al. 1998 [44] ↑ p = .01 (vs. no multivitamins) Jiamton et al. 2003 [20] ↔ (vs. placebo)		Humphrey et al. 1999 [36] ↔ (vs. placebo) Fawzi et al. 2004 [16] ↔ (vs. placebo) Fawzi et al. 1998 [44] ↔ (vs. no vitamin A)		Fawzi et al. 2005 [25] ↔ (vs. placebo)	Kupka et al. 2008 [21] ↔ (vs. placebo)

	Baeten et al. 2002 [38]	↔	(vs. placebo)
	Semba et al. 1998 [39]	↔	(vs. placebo)
	Coodley et al. 1996 [46]	↔	(vs. placebo)
	Bang et al. 2012 [45]	↔	(vs. placebo)
	Baum et al. 2010 [23]	↑	Relative Rate of low CD4 count (<200 cells/mm³): 0.24, 95% CI 0.10–0.56, p < .002 (vs. placebo)
	Kakalia et al. 2011 [47]	↔	(vs. no supplement)
	Arpadi et al. 2009 [41]	↔	(vs. placebo)
	Bobat et al. 2005 [42]	↔	(vs. placebo)
Unspecified or heterogeneous ART	Kelly et al. 2008 [22]	↔	(vs. placebo)
Children	Ndeezi et al. 2010 [29]	↔	(2× RDA vs. RDA)

selenium) on T-cell subsets among individuals with HIV but not receiving ART [16,20,21,25,34,36,44]. Three studies found positive associations between multiple micronutrient supplements and T-cell subsets, including CD4 [16,34,44], CD8 [34,44], and CD3 [16,44]. Two TOV studies included pregnant women with HIV who were followed up from 12 to 27 weeks' gestational age to postpartum. Relative to the placebo group, T-cell subsets were higher among the multivitamin group at delivery [44] and during the postpartum follow-up (at 2- and 4-year time points; over the entire period) [16]. In a study among nonpregnant ART-naïve women with HIV-1 in Mombasa, a 6-week micronutrient supplementation was associated with higher CD4 (+23 cells/µL, p = .03) and CD8 counts (+74 cells/µL, p = .005) [34]. However, it should be noted that T-lymphocyte subsets were a secondary outcome in this study.

A study among 481 Thai patients with HIV but not receiving ART at baseline reported no effects of multivitamin supplementation for 48 weeks on CD4 cell counts, relative to those in the placebo group [20]. The micronutrient supplement consisted of doses higher than the RDA, and was consumed twice daily [20]. In three studies, vitamin A supplementation was not observed to affect CD4 [16,36,44], CD8 [16,36,40], and CD3 [36,44] T-cell subsets. A randomized trial with a single-dose vitamin A supplementation (300,000 IU) and placebo study regimens among women with HIV seroconversion (n = 40) observed no differences in T-lymphocyte subsets (CD4, CD8, CD3, CD45) or activation markers (CD4-DR, CD4-38, CD8-DR, CD8-38) at any assessed time point during 8 weeks of follow-up [36]. An RCT with daily oral zinc supplementation (25 mg) from pregnancy to 6 weeks after delivery observed no effects on CD4, CD8, and CD3 counts [25]. In a Tanzanian study, daily oral selenium supplement (200 µg selenomethionine) taken from pregnancy to 6 months postpartum did not affect CD4 T cells among 913 pregnant women with HIV [21].

Heterogeneous or Unspecified ART   In studies involving individuals with HIV infections and unspecified or variable ART, micronutrient interventions were not observed to affect T-cell counts. In a cluster-randomized crossover trial among adults in a region of Zambia with poor nutritional status, study participants received either a daily multiple micronutrient tablet (15 micronutrients) or placebo [22]. Multivitamins did not influence CD4 count, which was a secondary study outcome [22]. Several vitamin A studies varied significantly in terms of forms, doses, frequencies, and durations of interventions (including 60 mg β-carotene three times daily for 3 months [46]; 10,000 IU retinyl palmitate once daily for 6 weeks [38]; one single high dose of 60 mg retinol equivalent [200,000 IU] with a 4-week follow-up period [39]). Vitamin A supplements were not observed to affect T-lymphocyte subsets [46], including CD4 [38,39] and CD8 cells [38]. A study with two vitamin D supplementation treatments (0.5–1.0 µg calcitriol, 1200 IU [30 µg] cholecalciferol; or 1200 IU cholecalciferol) or placebo among patients with HIV reported no differential effects on T-lymphocyte subsets, including CD4, CD8, and CD3 [45]. Among adults with HIV and low plasma zinc (<0.75 mg/L), zinc supplementation (12 mg women, 15 mg men) for 18 months reduced the risk of immunological failure (defined as CD4 T-cell count <200 cells/mm^3) by 4-fold (relative rate 0.24, 95% CI 0.10–0.56, p < .002), adjusting for age, sex, food insecurity, baseline CD4 cell count, viral load, and ART [23].

Children In studies among youth with HIV exposure or infection, no effects of several micronutrient interventions (multivitamins, zinc, vitamin D) were observed on CD4 lymphocytes [29,41,42,47].

Transmission

Children

Several RCTs considered the effects of maternal micronutrient supplementation during pregnancy, delivery, or early infancy on vertical HIV transmission to infants [24,34,48–51]. All involved the recruitment and enrollment of pregnant mothers with HIV residing in Africa (Tanzania, Malawi, South Africa), and assessment of infants at birth and in early childhood.

Three studies in Tanzania involved a two-by-two factorial design of micronutrient supplements from pregnancy (12–27 weeks' gestational age) through lactation. HIV transmission in infants was assessed at different time points, including birth [49], 6 weeks [49], and 2 years of age [48]. At birth, supplements were not associated with infant HIV infection or death (multivitamins: RR 0.98, 95% CI 0.76–1.27, p = .89; vitamin A: RR 1.01, 95% CI 0.78–1.31, p = .95) [49]. At 6 weeks, among infants uninfected at birth, supplements also did not affect HIV status (multivitamins: RR 1.04, 95% CI 0.65–1.66, p = .88; vitamin A: RR 1.30, 95% CI 0.80–2.09, p = .29) [49]. At 24 months, multivitamins did not affect the overall mother-to-child transmission (MTCT) risk (p = .76) [48]. Among live births, vitamin A supplements increased the risk of MTCT (RR 1.38, 95% CI 1.09–1.76, p = .009) up to 24 months [48]. This increased risk was not modified by infant sex [24].

A study in Malawi randomized pregnant women with HIV to receive a daily oral vitamin A supplement (3 mg retinol equivalent) or no vitamin A from 18 to 28 weeks' gestational age to delivery [50]. All women received iron and folate [50]. Infant HIV status at 6 weeks (p = .76) and 24 months (p = .21) did not differ by treatment group [50]. In Durban, a study among 728 pregnant women with HIV randomly assigned vitamin A supplements (daily dose of 5000 IU retinyl palmitate and 30 mg β-carotene during third trimester; 200,000 IU retinyl palmitate at delivery) or placebo as study regimens [51]. Among 632 children with available HIV infection status data, no differences in MTCT were observed by 3 months of age between treatment groups [51].

Another study in Dar es Salaam randomly assigned 400 pregnant women with HIV daily oral zinc supplements (25 mg) or placebo from their first prenatal visit until 6 weeks after delivery. No differences between treatment arms were observed on infant HIV status at birth or 6 weeks postpartum [37].

Anthropometry

ART In a study among 3418 patients with HIV initiating HAART, there were no differences between the effects of randomized daily oral multivitamins (vitamins B complex, C, and E) in high or standard RDA doses on BMI [17]. However, BMI was not a primary outcome in this trial [17]. A study in Malawi reported that a fortified macronutrient spread increased BMI and fat-free body mass among adults with HIV and low BMI (<18.5) at baseline, compared with a control group (receiving corn–soy blend) [33].

ART Naïve   In Tanzania, 1078 women with HIV infections were randomly assigned to one of four treatment arms in a two-by-two factorial design [52]. Multiple micronutrient supplements were protective against the risk of a first episode of a mid-upper arm circumference (MUAC) <22 cm (relative risk [RR] 0.66, 95% CI 0.47–0.94, p = .02) over the entire follow-up period (median of 5.3 years) [52]. Multivitamins did not affect BMI or weight [52]. In contrast, in a study among 400 pregnant women with HIV-1, zinc supplementation was associated with increased risk of low MUAC (<22 cm; RR 2.7, 95% CI 1.1–6.4, p = .03) and an average 4 mm lower MUAC during the second trimester (p = .02) [37].

Heterogeneous or Unspecified ART   A study involving a lipid-based nutrient supplement among mothers with HIV and their infants for 28 weeks found less weight loss among women, adjusting for ART and baseline BMI [53]. A second study involved Tanzanian patients with tuberculosis (TB) who were provided a multivitamin fortified or nonfortified biscuit every day during the initial 60 days of anti-TB treatment [54]. Among patients with HIV–TB coinfections, reduced weight gain was observed (p = .002); among patients with TB (and no HIV) infections, increased weight (p = .07) and handgrip strength were observed [54]. A South African study included breast-feeding women with HIV infections who were randomized to received fortified food ("Sibusiso ready food supplement") or nonfortified food [55]. No effects of the supplement on anthropometry or BMI of mothers or infants were observed [55]. However, among a small subgroup of women with low BMI, fortified foods were protective against lean body mass loss (p = .03) [55].

Children   Multiple micronutrient interventions (including supplements and fortified foods) consumed by mothers with HIV showed limited effects on anthropometric assessments of their offspring. Multivitamin supplements (in multiple RDA dosages) randomly assigned to infants [29] and mothers [31] did not affect weight, compared with a standard RDA dosage. Among mothers with HIV, birth weights of infants with HIV did not differ by treatment group (multivitamins vs. no multivitamins); however, among uninfected infants, multivitamins were associated with a mean 94 g increased birth weight (p = .02) [49]. Micronutrient food fortification of mothers and children showed no effects on child anthropometry indicators [55], including length-for-age Z (LAZ) score [32,56], length [57], weight [57], weight-for-age score [56], head circumference [57], MUAC [57], and skinfold thicknesses (subscapular, triceps [57]). However, a study with random assignment of a multiple micronutrient–fortified porridge observed reduced stunting (LAZ <–2) among breast-fed infants exposed to HIV, compared with controls [32].

In a trial among 255 children (6 weeks to 5 years) with TB, study participants were randomly assigned daily oral multivitamins or placebo during the initial 8 weeks of anti-TB treatment [58]. Among a subset of children with HIV (6 months to 3 years; n = 48), multivitamin supplements were associated with a greater height increase relative to the placebo group (p = .01, p for interaction by age group = .01) [58].

In another study, vitamin A supplement or placebo was randomly assigned to 687 Tanzanian children (6–60 months) who were admitted to a hospital with pneumonia [59]. The vitamin A supplement was administered in four doses (200,000 IU/dose; 100,000 IU/dose if <12 months) on days 1 and 2, as well as months 4 and 8 after hospital discharge [59]. Among children (6–18 months) with HIV, vitamin A supplements increased length at month 4, compared with the placebo group; this association was not observed among uninfected children [59]. In a study in Malawi among 697 pregnant women with HIV, daily doses of either vitamin A (3 mg retinol equivalent) with iron and folate, or only iron and folate were provided as study regimens [50]. Infants of women who received vitamin A were higher in mean birth weight (2895 ± 31 g), compared with those with mothers in the placebo group (2805 ± 32 g, p = .05) [50].

Separately, in a Tanzanian study, among 400 pregnant women with HIV, daily oral zinc supplements (25 mg) or placebo were randomly assigned and received from enrollment (12–27 weeks' gestation) until 6 weeks after delivery [25]. No effects on birth weight were observed [25]. In another Dar es Salaam study among 913 pregnant women with HIV, daily oral selenium supplements (200 μg selenomethionine) consumed for the same duration appeared marginally associated with reduced low birth weight (LBW) risk (RR 0.71, 95% CI 0.49–1.05, p = .09) [21].

Birth Outcomes

RCT studies among children with HIV exposure or infection observed protective and null effects of micronutrient interventions on LBW, small for gestational age (SGA), and preterm delivery. Mothers with HIV who prenatally received multivitamin supplements (vitamins B complex, C, and E) [24,44] or vitamin A [50] were less likely to have LBW offspring; one study observed effects only among girls (RR 0.39, 95% CI 0.22–0.67) [24]. Multivitamin supplements (multiple vs. single RDA dose) [31], vitamin A [44], and selenium [21] also were not observed to affect LBW risk.

Women with HIV who received multivitamin supplements (vitamin B complex, C, and E) during pregnancy had infants with reduced SGA risk [44]. Other studies also showed that multivitamins (multiple vs. single RDA dose) [31], as well as vitamin A [44], and selenium [21] received were not associated with the risk of SGA birth.

Studies in Dar es Salaam and Durban among pregnant women with HIV observed that multivitamins [44] and vitamin A [51] were associated with reduced risk of preterm delivery. In contrast, no effects of multivitamins (multiple vs. single RDA dose) [31], vitamin A [44], and selenium [21] on pretermity were reported by other studies. Maternal zinc supplementation (25 mg) during pregnancy did not affect gestational duration compared with placebo [25].

Hematological Indicators

Hemoglobin and Anemia

ART   In a study among 3418 patients with HIV and initiating HAART, high and standard RDA dose multivitamin supplements (vitamins B complex, C, and E) did not differentially affect hemoglobin concentrations [17]. It should be noted that hemoglobin was a secondary outcome in this study.

ART Naïve   Among 1078 pregnant women with HIV but not on ART treatment in Dar es Salaam, daily multivitamin supplements (vitamins B complex, C, and E) were associated with higher hemoglobin concentrations (0.33 g/dL), compared with women who did not receive multivitamins (p = .07) [60]. Vitamin A and β-carotene supplements did not affect hemoglobin, relative to women who did not receive the treatment (0.07 g/dL, p = .68) [60]. Separately, in a Tanzanian study among 400 women with HIV, zinc supplementation (25 mg) and placebo were both associated with increased hemoglobin between treatment initiation (pregnancy) until 6 weeks postpartum [25]. Zinc was associated with a reduced hemoglobin increase, compared with placebo (p = .03) [25].

The effects of daily oral selenium supplements were assessed in an RCT among 915 pregnant Tanzanian women who received either treatment (200 μg selenomethionine) or placebo from pregnancy (12–27 weeks' gestational age) until 6 months postpartum [61]. No effects of selenium on hemoglobin concentrations were observed (mean difference 0.05 g/dL, 95% CI −0.07 to 0.16 g/dL) [61].

Among Kenyan adults with HIV but who had not progressed to stage IV or clinical AIDS, a daily food supplement, alone or with a micronutrient capsule (including 30 mg iron), was randomly assigned to study participants [62]. Compared with those in the food-only group, increased ferritin was observed in men and women receiving multivitamins; no effects were observed on hemoglobin [62]. Among a subset of participants without inflammation, hemoglobin increased (p = .019) but ferritin was not affected [62].

Children   In a Tanzanian study, mothers with HIV who received multivitamins (vitamins B complex, C, and E) during pregnancy had infants with reduced risk of anemia [62]. Children of mothers who received multivitamins were less likely to have severe microcytic anemia (RR 0.60, 95% CI 0.42–0.85, p = .004), compared with children with mothers who did not receive multivitamins [62]. Risks of microcytic hypochromic anemia (RR 0.70, 95% CI 0.51–0.95, p = .02) and macrocytic anemia (RR 0.37, 95% CI 0.18–0.79, p = .01) were decreased in the multivitamins-only group, relative to the placebo group [62].

Among pregnant women with HIV receiving iron and folate, study participants were randomly assigned to receive or not receive vitamin A (3 mg retinol equivalent) from 18 to 28 weeks' gestation to delivery. Anemia was less prevalent among infants of vitamin A group mothers, compared with the control (23.4% vs. 40.6%, p < .001) [50]. Daily zinc supplement (10 mg elemental zinc as sulfate) for 6 months among children with HIV (n = 96) did not affect hemoglobin [42].

Micronutrient Concentrations

ART   Among study participants with HIV and persistent diarrhea, who received either multivitamins (vitamins A, C, and E; selenium; zinc) or placebo for 2 weeks, there were no differences in serum concentrations of vitamins A and E between treatment groups [17]. Vitamin D supplements were observed to increase serum 25-hydroxyvitamin D (25(OH)D) [41,63–65].

ART Naïve   In Dar es Salaam, among 626 pregnant women with HIV who received vitamin A supplements (with β-carotene) during pregnancy, concentrations of retinol, β-carotene, and α-carotene in breast milk were higher at delivery, compared with those who did not receive vitamin A and β-carotene (all p < .0001) [66]. Multivitamin supplements reduced retinol and γ-tocopherol concentrations in breast milk but did not affect α- or δ-tocopherol [66]. Daily food supplement with or without multivitamins (including 15 mg zinc) did not affect plasma zinc, although inflammation was observed to impair plasma zinc increases [67].

Heterogeneous or Unspecified ART   Among adults with HIV and diarrhea (≥7 days), zinc supplementation (50 mg twice daily) for 14 days reduced zinc deficiency, compared with those in the placebo group [68].

Children   A supplement with 14 multiple micronutrients for 6 months significantly increased vitamin B12 and folate concentrations among 847 Ugandan children (1–5 years) with HIV [69]. No differences were observed in the control group (who received six multivitamins per standard of care) [69]. Relative to children with HIV randomized to receive no supplements, two levels of vitamin D supplementation (5600 and 11,200 IU/week) both increased serum 25(OH)D (p = .0002, p < .001) [47]. Similarly, studies among children with HIV observed vitamin D supplementation associated with increased vitamin D sufficiency (≥30 ng/mL [2]; ≥20 ng/mL [70]).

Other
ART   Among 3418 individuals with HIV initiating HAART at seven clinics in Dar es Salaam, a high-dose multivitamin supplement for 24 months increased alanine transaminase concentrations, compared with a standard-dose supplement [17].

ART Naïve   Daily oral zinc supplements (25 mg) between 12 and 27 weeks' gestational age until 6 weeks postpartum reduced changes in red blood cell count and packed cell volume (both p < .01) after delivery among women (n = 400) with HIV, compared with those who received placebo [25].

Heterogeneous or Unspecified ART   In a pilot study among 52 patients with HIV and CD4 cell counts <400/mm³, two supplement groups of daily selenium (250 µg L-selenomethionine) and vitamin A (50,000 IU provitamin A) for 1 year both showed improved oxidative stress markers [71].

Children   A study among children with HIV involved two doses of vitamin A (200,000 IU) or placebo at baseline and day 1, followed by influenza vaccine administration on day 14. Compared with the placebo, vitamin A did not appear to affect vaccine serologic responses [40].

Other Clinical Morbidities and Assessments
Diarrhea
RCTs considering the effects of micronutrient interventions either reported protective or no effects on diarrhea among adults with HIV, and children with HIV exposure or infection.

ART   In one Ndola study, patients with HIV and persistent diarrhea were randomized to receive either micronutrients (vitamins A, C, and E; selenium; zinc) or placebo along with albendazole for 2 weeks [19]. Time with diarrhea did not differ by treatment group [19].

ART Naïve   A study among 915 pregnant Tanzanian women found reduced risk of diarrhea associated with receiving daily selenium supplement (200 μg selenomethionine) from pregnancy (12–27 weeks' gestational age) until 6 months postpartum, compared with those who received placebo treatments (RR 0.60, 95% CI 0.42–0.84) [60].

Heterogeneous or Unspecified ART   A study among 231 adults with HIV and low plasma zinc (<0.75 mg/L) at baseline reported that zinc supplementation for 18 months reduced diarrhea rate (OR 0.4, 95% CI 0.18–0.98, p = .02) relative to placebo [23]. A study involving zinc supplementation (15 mg twice daily for 14 days) found no effects on diarrhea persistence [68] and cessation [68].

Children   In TOV studies, dyads of mothers with HIV and their offspring in Tanzania, women received one of four treatment regimens from pregnancy until after delivery [16,44,72]. Mothers with multivitamins (vitamins B complex, C, and E) had infants with reduced risk of diarrhea during the first 2 years of life, compared with those with mothers not receiving multivitamins (RR 0.83, 95% CI 0.71–0.98, p = .03) [73]. No differences by sex were found [24]. Vitamin A did not affect diarrhea risk [73].

In Dar es Salaam, infants of mothers with HIV were randomly assigned to receive daily oral multiple multivitamins (vitamins B complex, C, and E; n = 1193) or placebo (n = 1194) from 6 weeks to 24 months of age [27]. On the basis of the maternal report, diarrhea incidence was similar between treatment arms (RR 0.97, 95% CI 0.87–1.10, p = .64) [27].

In another study, 687 Tanzanian children (6–60 months) hospitalized for pneumonia received vitamin A supplements at baseline, 4 months, and 8 months [74]. Among a small subset of children (n = 37) with HIV, there was a marginally statistically significant association between vitamin A and acute diarrhea risk, relative to those with placebo [74].

Two studies assessed micronutrient supplement interventions among Ugandan children with HIV. One study was among 181 children with HIV who were enrolled at 6 months of age, and received either vitamin A supplement (60 mg retinol equivalent) or placebo every 3 months between 15 and 36 months of age [28]. This trial was not completed as planned because of the implementation of a new policy; the median follow-up after age 15 months was 17.8 months (interquartile range 11.1–21.0) [28]. Vitamin A was protective against chronic diarrhea, compared with placebo (OR 0.48, 95% CI 0.19–1.18, p = .11) [28]. In a second study, 847 children with HIV received either a standard dose (one RDA of six multivitamins) or higher dose (2-fold RDA supplement of 14 multivitamins) for 6 months [75]. Diarrhea incidence did not differ by treatment group, but was lower among those receiving HAART [75].

One research team assessed the effects of vitamin A and zinc supplements on diarrhea among children in South Africa with HIV exposure or infection. In one trial, 118 infants of mothers with HIV received either six doses of vitamin A (50,000

IU at 1 and 3 months of age; 100,000 IU at 6 and 9 months; 200,000 IU at 12 and 15 months) or placebo [76]. HIV status was available for only 85 children [76]. Vitamin A was associated with reduced diarrhea-related morbidity among children with HIV (OR 0.51, 95% CI 0.27–0.99); no effects were observed among uninfected children [76]. Separately, another study randomly assigned daily oral zinc (10 mg) or placebo as treatment regimens for 6 months among 96 children with HIV [42]. Zinc supplements were protective against the risk of watery diarrhea, compared with placebo (p = .001) [42].

Chronic Diseases and Long-Term Health Outcomes

ART   One study in Ohio (United States) was among 45 individuals with low baseline serum 25(OH)D ($\leq$20 ng/mL) and HIV but on stable ART. Treatment (4000 IU vitamin D3 daily) or placebo study regimens were randomly assigned and received for 12 weeks [65]. No effects on altered flow-mediated brachial artery dilation were observed between study arms [65].

RCTs assessing the effects of niacin and chromium supplementation focused on dyslipidemia, which is commonly observed among patients with HIV on ART. Two studies involving niacin supplementation both found that high-density lipoprotein-cholesterol (HDL-C) levels improved (increased) among participants with HIV who received niacin supplements and were on ART, although supplementation differed [14,77]. In one study, adults (n = 19) with HIV and low HDL-C received extended-release niacin (ERN) every night for 12 weeks (initially 500 mg/night; increasing to 1500 mg/night by week 8 for the last 4 weeks) [14]. Among those receiving ERN, flow-mediated dilation of brachial arteries also differed significantly from controls (p = .05) [14]. In the second study, adult patients (n = 191) with HIV and hypertriglyceridemia received a 24-week randomized treatment of (i) ERN (gradually increasing from one to four pills [500 mg] per night), low-saturated-fat diet, exercise; or (ii) fenofibrate (145 mg/night), niacin, low-saturated-fat diet, exercise [77]. In addition to improving HDL-C (p = .03), niacin also reduced the total cholesterol-to-HDL-C ratio (p = .005–.01) and doubled adiponectin levels [77]. In combination with diet, exercise, and fenofibrate, niacin was more beneficial in decreasing triglycerides, increasing HDL-C, and reducing non-HDL-C and total cholesterol-to-HDL-C ratio [77].

A Canadian study randomized individuals with HIV to receive either chromium nicotinate (400 µg/day; n = 23) or placebo (n = 23) for 16 weeks [78]. Individuals in the chromium group showed decreased homeostasis model of assessment (HOMA-IR), insulin, and body composition (total body fat mass, trunk fat mass) [78].

ART Naïve   Among 1078 ART-naïve pregnant women with HIV, the effects of multivitamins (20 mg thiamine, 20 mg riboflavin, 25 mg B6, 50 µg B12, 500 mg C, 30 mg E, 0.8 mg folic acid) and vitamin A supplement (30 mg β-carotene and 5000 IU preformed vitamin A) on hypertension during pregnancy were assessed [79]. Multivitamins were associated with reduced hypertension risk (systolic blood pressure $\geq$140 mm Hg or diastolic blood pressure $\geq$90 mm Hg; RR 0.62, 95% CI 0.40–0.94, p = .03), compared with those with no multivitamins [79]. Vitamin A was not observed to affect hypertension [79].

HIV-Exposed Children   Among 327 Tanzanian children of women with HIV, the effects of maternal micronutrient supplementation during pregnancy and lactation on child development were assessed by Bayley's Scales of Development at 6, 12, and 18 months of age [80]. Multivitamins (vitamins B complex, C, and E) increased the mean score of Psychomotor Development Index and reduced risk of development delay on the motor scale, but did not affect the Mental Development Index [80]. No effects were associated with vitamin A treatment [80].

In a study among 59 children (6–16 years) with HIV infection and receiving ART, receiving vitamin D (100,000 IU cholecalciferol bimonthly) and calcium (1 g/day) or placebo for 2 years was compared [63]. No effects of vitamin D were observed on bone health outcomes, including total-body bone mineral content, total-body bone mineral density, spine bone mineral content, and spine bone mineral density [63].

Other Clinical Indicators, Signs, and Symptoms

ART Naïve   In a study among 674 ART-naïve pregnant women with HIV, multivitamins increased the risks of any subclinical mastitis by 33% (p = .005) and severe subclinical mastitis by 75% (p = .0006), compared with women who received placebo [81]. Vitamin A and β-carotene were associated with a 45% increased risk of severe subclinical mastitis (p = .03) [81].

Heterogeneous or Unspecified ART   An RCT in Tanzania included adult patients with pulmonary TB (n = 416) and HIV–TB coinfections (n = 471) [82]. Among study participants with coinfections, micronutrients (vitamins A, B complex, C, and E; selenium) reduced TB recurrence risk by 63% (95% CI 8–85%, p = .02) [82].

Children   In Dar es Salaam, RCT among infants of mothers with HIV, a study regimen was randomly assigned between 6 weeks and 24 months of age. Children who received daily oral multiple multivitamins (n = 1193) or placebo (n = 1194) had similar records of hospitalizations and unscheduled clinic visits [27]. Multivitamin group children were less likely to have fever (p = .02) and vomit (p = .007) [27]. Another RCT evaluated the effects of a daily oral multiple micronutrient supplementation (vitamins A, B complex, C, D, and E; folic acid; copper; iron; zinc) versus placebo among children (4–24 months) with HIV who were hospitalized for diarrhea or pneumonia [83]. Hospitalization duration was reduced among children receiving multivitamins from enrollment until discharge, compared with the placebo group (p < .05) [83].

One study randomly assigned vitamin A (baseline at hospital; 4 and 8 months after discharge) or placebo study regimens to 687 Tanzanian children (6–60 months) hospitalized for pneumonia [74]. Vitamin A was associated with increased risk of cough and rapid respiratory rate (OR 1.67, 95% CI 1.17–2.36, p = .004) [74]. Risk of respiratory tract infection was elevated among children not infected with HIV, but not among children with HIV (p = .07 for interaction) [74].

In a study among 99 children (6–24 months) with HIV and previous hospitalizations, daily multivitamin supplements were associated with increased amounts of food eaten per kilogram of body weight, compared with a placebo group [84].

DISCUSSION

The majority of trials involving multiple and single micronutrient interventions among adults and children with HIV infection or exposure reported either protective or null associations with improved health outcomes. However, there were exceptions showing associations between micronutrients and adverse effects on indicators related to morbidity and mortality among individuals with HIV. Notably, vitamin A supplementation appears to increase mortality and vertical transmission risks.

Protective effects of multiple micronutrients on health outcomes among individuals with HIV were observed. Multiple micronutrient supplementation among adults with HIV were associated with reduced mortality risks among adults [16,20,22] and their infants [24]. Among infants alive and not infected with HIV at 6 weeks of age, multivitamins decreased transmission risk [48]. Studies found that multiple micronutrients increased CD4 counts [22,44] and reduced viral load [16]. Among adults, multiple micronutrient–fortified foods were associated with increased BMI [33], reduced weight gain [54], and lean body mass loss [55]. A study among breastfed infants who received micronutrient-fortified foods observed increased LAZ [32]. Multiple micronutrient supplements were associated with positive effects on MUAC among adults [52], and height among children [58].

However, a number of studies also showed no effects of multiple micronutrients on mortality (adult [17,19,24,31], child [27,29,32] supplementation), HIV viral and proviral load in blood and breast milk [17,20,33–35], CD4 T cells (from supplements [16,17,19,20,29,34,44] and fortified foods), HIV vertical transmission [48,49], and anthropometry (adults [17,52] and children [29,31,49,56,57]). One study reported adverse effects from multiple micronutrients on increased HIV-1-infected vaginal cells and HIV-1 RNA in vaginal secretions [34].

Disparate associations between vitamin A supplementation and health outcomes among adults and children with HIV infection or exposure were observed. A study found that maternal supplementation of vitamin A during pregnancy and lactation was associated with increased MTCT among infants who were alive and not infected with HIV at 6 weeks of age [48]; however, the risk was not modified by sex [24]. Both increased [15,18] and decreased [15,28,30] mortality risks from vitamin A supplements were reported. One study found increased viral load detection in breast milk of women with HIV [35], although a separate study showed reduced viral load among children who were simultaneously administered influenza vaccine [40]. Vitamin A supplements received by children were associated with beneficial effects on anthropometry [59]. However, several studies also observed null effects of vitamin A supplementation on mortality [15,16,24], HIV viral load [16,38,39,44], CD4 counts (including individuals receiving no ART [16,36,44], unspecified or heterogeneous ART [38,39,46]), and anthropometry [52].

Only a limited number of RCTs considered the effects of zinc, vitamin D, selenium, niacin, or chromium supplements on health outcomes among individuals with HIV. Zinc supplements generally did not affect many assessed outcomes (mortality [23,25], HIV viral load [23,39,42], CD4 lymphocytes [25,42], HIV vertical transmission [47], and infant birth weight [25]) with the exception of two studies that reported protective effects on mortality [26] and CD4 counts [23]. Three studies, including two among youth [41,47], showed no effects of vitamin D on CD4 lymphocytes [45]. Selenium supplements for pregnant women with HIV resulted in null effects on maternal mortality, HIV viral loads, and CD4 counts, but increased fetal deaths and reduced LBW risks [21]. Generally, micronutrient supplements were associated with correspondingly increased blood concentrations.

Comparisons between results were significantly limited by the extensive heterogeneity of exposures and outcomes across studies. Variability in study interventions included dosage (single or multiple RDA doses; mega doses), single or joint administration with other micronutrients or macronutrients, duration (ranged from weeks to years), frequency (three times daily, once daily, weekly, monthly), recipient (mother vs. infant in MTCT studies), and control group. Baseline characteristics of study populations differed widely, in terms of health (nutritional status, drug treatment regimens, other morbidities, WHO HIV disease stage), sociodemographic factors, and geographic regions. Some studies were among specific subpopulations (such as lactating women, injection drug users, children hospitalized for pneumonia or diarrhea, patients with severe infections), and therefore have accordingly limited external generalizability. ART treatments were heterogeneous at baseline (e.g., initiating, already on ART), and often reflective of the conventional treatment and drug management for specific study populations at the time of the study.

Despite efforts to address gaps in literature, a number of questions still remain, including

1. Are there effective micronutrient supplementation interventions that affect health outcomes among adults and children with HIV infection and exposure? What are the efficacious dosages, in terms of frequency, timing (relative to pregnancy, and other clinical treatments), needs of recipients (infant, mother), and means of delivery (in combination with other micronutrients or macronutrients, alone)?
2. How are higher-risk subgroups, such as infants of mothers with HIV, affected by micronutrient supplementations? To what extent does timing of HIV infection in MTCT matter?
3. Do ART and nutritional status interact? Are different stages of treatment differentially modified by nutritional status?

Especially in limited-resource contexts with dual burdens of disease from HIV and poor nutrition, relatively low-cost micronutrient interventions are potentially beneficial adjuncts to HIV/AIDS management and treatment. Furthermore, identifying and defining any potential risks relating to nutritional interventions is critical, particularly in the context of vertical transmission of HIV and interactions with ART. In spite of this, the relation between micronutrient interventions among populations with HIV infection and exposure remains unclear. As a number of gaps in literature are evident, additional RCTs with adequate sample sizes and intervention duration are necessary in order to confirm or elucidate current findings, particularly in distinguishing intervention effects from differences in study design and baseline status of participants.

REFERENCES

1. Joint United Nations Program on HIV/AIDS (UNAIDS), *UNAIDS Report on the Global AIDS Epidemic 2013*. 2013, UNAIDS: Geneva, Switzerland.
2. Chandra, R.K., Nutrition and the immune system: An introduction. *Am J Clin Nutr*, 1997. **66**(2): p. 460S–3S.
3. Chandra, R.K., Nutrition and immunology: From the clinic to cellular biology and back again. *Proc Nutr Soc*, 1999. **58**(3): p. 681–3.
4. Kudsk, K.A., Current aspects of mucosal immunology and its influence by nutrition. *Am J Surg*, 2002. **183**(4): p. 390–8.
5. Keusch, G.T., The history of nutrition: Malnutrition, infection and immunity. *J Nutr*, 2003. **133**(1): p. 336S–40S.
6. Scrimshaw, N.S., C.E. Taylor, and J.E. Gordon, Interactions of nutrition and infection. *Monogr Ser World Health Organ*, 1968. **57**: p. 3–329.
7. Mangili, A. et al., Nutrition and HIV infection: Review of weight loss and wasting in the era of highly active antiretroviral therapy from the nutrition for healthy living cohort. *Clin Infect Dis*, 2006. **42**(6): p. 836–42.
8. Grobler, L. et al., Nutritional interventions for reducing morbidity and mortality in people with HIV. *Cochrane Database Syst Rev*, 2013. **2**: p. CD004536.
9. Irlam, J.H. et al., Micronutrient supplementation in children and adults with HIV infection. *Cochrane Database Syst Rev*, 2005. (4): p. CD003650.
10. Irlam, J.H. et al., Micronutrient supplementation in children and adults with HIV infection. *Cochrane Database Syst Rev*, 2010. (12): p. CD003650.
11. Siegfried, N. et al., Micronutrient supplementation in pregnant women with HIV infection. *Cochrane Database Syst Rev*, 2012. **3**: p. CD009755.
12. Mehta, S. and W. Fawzi, Effects of vitamins, including vitamin A, on HIV/AIDS patients. *Vitam Horm*, 2007. **75**: p. 355–83.
13. Finkelstein, J.L. et al., HIV/AIDS and Nutrition in the HAART era: Programmatic implications for HIV/AIDS care and treatment in resource-limited settings, in *From the Ground Up: Building Comprehensive HIV/AIDS Care Programs in Resource-Limited Settings*, R.G. Marlink and S.J. Teitelman, Editors. 2009, Elizabeth Glaser Pediatric AIDS Foundation: Washington, DC.
14. Chow, D.C. et al., Short-term effects of extended-release niacin on endothelial function in HIV-infected patients on stable antiretroviral therapy. *AIDS*, 2010. **24**(7): p. 1019–23.
15. Humphrey, J.H. et al., Effects of a single large dose of vitamin A, given during the postpartum period to HIV-positive women and their infants, on child HIV infection, HIV-free survival, and mortality. *J Infect Dis*, 2006. **193**(6): p. 860–71.
16. Ndekha, M.J. et al., Supplementary feeding with either ready-to-use fortified spread or corn–soy blend in wasted adults starting antiretroviral therapy in Malawi: Randomised, investigator blinded, controlled trial. *BMJ*, 2009. **338**: p. b1867.
17. Fawzi, W.W. et al., A randomized trial of multivitamin supplements and HIV disease progression and mortality. *N Engl J Med*, 2004. **351**(1): p. 23–32.
18. Austin, J. et al., A community randomized controlled clinical trial of mixed carotenoids and micronutrient supplementation of patients with acquired immunodeficiency syndrome. *Eur J Clin Nutr*, 2006. **60**(11): p. 1266–76.
19. Kelly, P. et al., Micronutrient supplementation in the AIDS diarrhoea-wasting syndrome in Zambia: A randomized controlled trial. *AIDS*, 1999. **13**(4): p. 495–500.
20. Isanaka, S. et al., Effect of high-dose vs standard-dose multivitamin supplementation at the initiation of HAART on HIV disease progression and mortality in Tanzania: A randomized controlled trial. *JAMA*, 2012. **308**(15): p. 1535–44.

21. Jiamton, S. et al., A randomized trial of the impact of multiple micronutrient supplementation on mortality among HIV-infected individuals living in Bangkok. *AIDS*, 2003. **17**(17): p. 2461–9.
22. Kupka, R. et al., Randomized, double-blind, placebo-controlled trial of selenium supplements among HIV-infected pregnant women in Tanzania: Effects on maternal and child outcomes. *Am J Clin Nutr*, 2008. **87**(6): p. 1802–8.
23. Kelly, P. et al., Micronutrient supplementation has limited effects on intestinal infectious disease and mortality in a Zambian population of mixed HIV status: A cluster randomized trial. *Am J Clin Nutr*, 2008. **88**(4): p. 1010–7.
24. Kawai, K. et al., Sex differences in the effects of maternal vitamin supplements on mortality and morbidity among children born to HIV-infected women in Tanzania. *Br J Nutr*, 2010. **103**(12): p. 1784–91.
25. Srinivasan, M.G. et al., Zinc adjunct therapy reduces case fatality in severe childhood pneumonia: A randomized double blind placebo-controlled trial. *BMC Med*, 2012. **10**: p. 14.
26. Chilenje Infant Growth, Nutrition Infection Study Team, Micronutrient fortification to improve growth and health of maternally HIV-unexposed and exposed Zambian infants: A randomised controlled trial. *PLoS One*, 2010. **5**(6): p. e11165.
27. Semba, R.D. et al., Effect of periodic vitamin A supplementation on mortality and morbidity of human immunodeficiency virus-infected children in Uganda: A controlled clinical trial. *Nutrition*, 2005. **21**(1): p. 25–31.
28. Kawai, K. et al., A randomized trial to determine the optimal dosage of multivitamin supplements to reduce adverse pregnancy outcomes among HIV-infected women in Tanzania. *Am J Clin Nutr*, 2010. **91**(2): p. 391–7.
29. Ndeezi, G. et al., Effect of multiple micronutrient supplementation on survival of HIV-infected children in Uganda: A randomized, controlled trial. *J Int AIDS Soc*, 2010. **13**: p. 18.
30. Fawzi, W.W. et al., A randomized trial of vitamin A supplements in relation to mortality among human immunodeficiency virus-infected and uninfected children in Tanzania. *Pediatr Infect Dis J*, 1999. **18**(2): p. 127–33.
31. Fawzi, W.W. et al., Trial of zinc supplements in relation to pregnancy outcomes, hematologic indicators, and T cell counts among HIV-1-infected women in Tanzania. *Am J Clin Nutr*, 2005. **81**(1): p. 161–7.
32. Duggan, C. et al., Multiple micronutrient supplementation in Tanzanian infants born to HIV-infected mothers: A randomized, double-blind, placebo-controlled clinical trial. *Am J Clin Nutr*, 2012. **96**(6): p. 1437–46.
33. Villamor, E. et al., Zinc supplementation to HIV-1-infected pregnant women: Effects on maternal anthropometry, viral load, and early mother-to-child transmission. *Eur J Clin Nutr*, 2006. **60**(7): p. 862–9.
34. Baeten, J.M. et al., Vitamin A supplementation and human immunodeficiency virus type 1 shedding in women: Results of a randomized clinical trial. *J Infect Dis*, 2002. **185**(8): p. 1187–91.
35. Semba, R.D. et al., Vitamin A supplementation and human immunodeficiency virus load in injection drug users. *J Infect Dis*, 1998. **177**(3): p. 611–6.
36. Hanekom, W.A. et al., Effect of vitamin A therapy on serologic responses and viral load changes after influenza vaccination in children infected with the human immunodeficiency virus. *J Pediatr*, 2000. **136**(4): p. 550–2.
37. Arpadi, S.M. et al., Effect of bimonthly supplementation with oral cholecalciferol on serum 25-hydroxyvitamin D concentrations in HIV-infected children and adolescents. *Pediatrics*, 2009. **123**(1): p. e121–6.
38. Bobat, R. et al., Safety and efficacy of zinc supplementation for children with HIV-1 infection in South Africa: A randomised double-blind placebo-controlled trial. *Lancet*, 2005. **366**(9500): p. 1862–7.

39. Hemsworth, J.C., S. Hekmat, and G. Reid, Micronutrient supplemented probiotic yogurt for HIV-infected adults taking HAART in London, Canada. *Gut Microbes*, 2012. **3**(5): p. 414–9.

40. Fawzi, W.W. et al., Randomised trial of effects of vitamin supplements on pregnancy outcomes and T cell counts in HIV-1-infected women in Tanzania. *Lancet*, 1998. **351**(9114): p. 1477–82.

41. Bang, U. et al., Correlation of increases in 1,25-dihydroxyvitamin D during vitamin D therapy with activation of CD4+ T lymphocytes in HIV-1-infected males. *HIV Clin Trials*, 2012. **13**(3): p. 162–70.

42. Coodley, G.O. et al., Beta-carotene in HIV infection: An extended evaluation. *AIDS*, 1996. **10**(9): p. 967–73.

43. Kakalia, S. et al., Vitamin D supplementation and CD4 count in children infected with human immunodeficiency virus. *J Pediatr*, 2011. **159**(6): p. 951–7.

44. McClelland, R.S. et al., Micronutrient supplementation increases genital tract shedding of HIV-1 in women: Results of a randomized trial. *J Acquir Immune Defic Syndr*, 2004. **37**(5): p. 1657–63.

45. Fawzi, W.W. et al., Randomized trial of vitamin supplements in relation to vertical transmission of HIV-1 in Tanzania. *J Acquir Immune Defic Syndr*, 2000. **23**(3): p. 246–54.

46. Fawzi, W.W. et al., Randomized trial of vitamin supplements in relation to transmission of HIV-1 through breastfeeding and early child mortality. *AIDS*, 2002. **16**(14): p. 1935–44.

47. Kumwenda, N. et al., Antenatal vitamin A supplementation increases birth weight and decreases anemia among infants born to human immunodeficiency virus-infected women in Malawi. *Clin Infect Dis*, 2002. **35**(5): p. 618–24.

48. Baum, M.K. et al., Randomized, controlled clinical trial of zinc supplementation to prevent immunological failure in HIV-infected adults. *Clin Infect Dis*, 2010. **50**(12): p. 1653–60.

49. Coutsoudis, A. et al., Randomized trial testing the effect of vitamin A supplementation on pregnancy outcomes and early mother-to-child HIV-1 transmission in Durban, South Africa. South African Vitamin A Study Group. *AIDS*, 1999. **13**(12): p. 1517–24.

50. Villamor, E. et al., Vitamin supplements, socioeconomic status, and morbidity events as predictors of wasting in HIV-infected women from Tanzania. *Am J Clin Nutr*, 2005. **82**(4): p. 857–65.

51. Kayira, D. et al., A lipid-based nutrient supplement mitigates weight loss among HIV-infected women in a factorial randomized trial to prevent mother-to-child transmission during exclusive breastfeeding. *Am J Clin Nutr*, 2012. **95**(3): p. 759–65.

52. PrayGod, G. et al., Daily multi-micronutrient supplementation during tuberculosis treatment increases weight and grip strength among HIV-uninfected but not HIV-infected patients in Mwanza, Tanzania. *J Nutr*, 2011. **141**(4): p. 685–91.

53. Kindra, G., A. Coutsoudis, and F. Esposito, Effect of nutritional supplementation of breastfeeding HIV positive mothers on maternal and child health: Findings from a randomized controlled clinical trial. *BMC Public Health*, 2011. **11**: p. 946.

54. Flax, V.L. et al., Use of lipid-based nutrient supplements by HIV-infected Malawian women during lactation has no effect on infant growth from 0 to 24 weeks. *J Nutr*, 2012. **142**(7): p. 1350–6.

55. Filteau, S. et al., Provision of micronutrient-fortified food from 6 months of age does not permit HIV-exposed uninfected Zambian children to catch up in growth to HIV-unexposed children: A randomized controlled trial. *J Acquir Immune Defic Syndr*, 2011. **56**(2): p. 166–75.

56. Mehta, S. et al., A randomized trial of multivitamin supplementation in children with tuberculosis in Tanzania. *Nutr J*, 2011. **10**: p. 120.

57. Villamor, E. et al., Vitamin A supplements ameliorate the adverse effect of HIV-1, malaria, and diarrheal infections on child growth. *Pediatrics*, 2002. **109**(1): p. E6.

58. Kupka, R. et al., Effect of selenium supplements on hemoglobin concentration and morbidity among HIV-1-infected Tanzanian women. *Clin Infect Dis*, 2009. **48**(10): p. 1475–8.
59. Mburu, A.S. et al., The influence and benefits of controlling for inflammation on plasma ferritin and hemoglobin responses following a multi-micronutrient supplement in apparently healthy, HIV+ Kenyan adults. *J Nutr*, 2008. **138**(3): p. 613–9.
60. Villamor, E. et al., Effect of vitamin supplements on HIV shedding in breast milk. *Am J Clin Nutr*, 2010. **92**(4): p. 881–6.
61. Fawzi, W.W. et al., Multivitamin supplementation improves hematologic status in HIV-infected women and their children in Tanzania. *Am J Clin Nutr*, 2007. **85**(5): p. 1335–43.
62. Arpadi, S.M. et al., Effect of supplementation with cholecalciferol and calcium on 2-y bone mass accrual in HIV-infected children and adolescents: A randomized clinical trial. *Am J Clin Nutr*, 2012. **95**(3): p. 678–85.
63. Havens, P.L. et al., Serum 25-hydroxyvitamin D response to vitamin D3 supplementation 50,000 IU monthly in youth with HIV-1 infection. *J Clin Endocrinol Metab*, 2012. **97**(11): p. 4004–13.
64 Longenecker, C.T. et al., Vitamin D supplementation and endothelial function in vitamin D deficient HIV-infected patients: A randomized placebo-controlled trial. *Antivir Ther*, 2012. **17**(4): p. 613–21.
65. Webb, A.L. et al., Effect of vitamin supplementation on breast milk concentrations of retinol, carotenoids and tocopherols in HIV-infected Tanzanian women. *Eur J Clin Nutr*, 2009. **63**(3): p. 332–9.
66. Mburu, A.S. et al., The influence of inflammation on plasma zinc concentration in apparently healthy, HIV+ Kenyan adults and zinc responses after a multi-micronutrient supplement. *Eur J Clin Nutr*, 2010. **64**(5): p. 510–7.
67. Carcamo, C. et al., Randomized controlled trial of zinc supplementation for persistent diarrhea in adults with HIV-1 infection. *J Acquir Immune Defic Syndr*, 2006. **43**(2): p. 197–201.
68. Ndeezi, G. et al., Multiple micronutrient supplementation improves vitamin B(1)(2) and folate concentrations of HIV infected children in Uganda: A randomized controlled trial. *Nutr J*, 2011. **10**: p. 56.
69. Havens, P.L. et al., Vitamin D3 decreases parathyroid hormone in HIV-infected youth being treated with tenofovir: A randomized, placebo-controlled trial. *Clin Infect Dis*, 2012. **54**(7): p. 1013–25.
70. Constans, J. et al., One-year antioxidant supplementation with beta-carotene or selenium for patients infected with human immunodeficiency virus: A pilot study. *Clin Infect Dis*, 1996. **23**(3): p. 654–6.
71. Fawzi, W.W. et al., Rationale and design of the Tanzania vitamin and HIV infection trial. *Control Clin Trials*, 1999. **20**(1): p. 75–90.
72. Humphrey, J.H. et al., Short-term effects of large-dose vitamin A supplementation on viral load and immune response in HIV-infected women. *J Acquir Immune Defic Syndr Hum Retrovirol*, 1999. **20**(1): p. 44–51.
73. Fawzi, W.W. et al., Effect of providing vitamin supplements to human immunodeficiency virus-infected, lactating mothers on the child's morbidity and CD4+ cell counts. *Clin Infect Dis*, 2003. **36**(8): p. 1053–62.
74. Fawzi, W.W. et al., Vitamin A supplements and diarrheal and respiratory tract infections among children in Dar es Salaam, Tanzania. *J Pediatr*, 2000. **137**(5): p. 660–7.
75. Ndeezi, G. et al., Multiple micronutrient supplementation does not reduce diarrhoea morbidity in Ugandan HIV-infected children: A randomised controlled trial. *Paediatr Int Child Health*, 2012. **32**(1): p. 14–21.

76. Coutsoudis, A. et al., The effects of vitamin A supplementation on the morbidity of children born to HIV-infected women. *Am J Public Health*, 1995. **85**(8 Pt 1): p. 1076–81.
77. Balasubramanyam, A. et al., Combination of niacin and fenofibrate with lifestyle changes improves dyslipidemia and hypoadiponectinemia in HIV patients on antiretroviral therapy: Results of "heart positive," a randomized, controlled trial. *J Clin Endocrinol Metab*, 2011. **96**(7): p. 2236–47.
78. Aghdassi, E. et al., In patients with HIV-infection, chromium supplementation improves insulin resistance and other metabolic abnormalities: A randomized, double-blind, placebo controlled trial. *Curr HIV Res*, 2010. **8**(2): p. 113–20.
79. Merchant, A.T. et al., Multivitamin supplementation of HIV-positive women during pregnancy reduces hypertension. *J Nutr*, 2005. **135**(7): p. 1776–81.
80. McGrath, N. et al., Effect of maternal multivitamin supplementation on the mental and psychomotor development of children who are born to HIV-1-infected mothers in Tanzania. *Pediatrics*, 2006. **117**(2): p. e216–25.
81. Arsenault, J.E. et al., Vitamin supplementation increases risk of subclinical mastitis in HIV-infected women. *J Nutr*, 2010. **140**(10): p. 1788–92.
82. Villamor, E. et al., A trial of the effect of micronutrient supplementation on treatment outcome, T cell counts, morbidity, and mortality in adults with pulmonary tuberculosis. *J Infect Dis*, 2008. **197**(11): p. 1499–505.
83. Mda, S. et al., Short-term micronutrient supplementation reduces the duration of pneumonia and diarrheal episodes in HIV-infected children. *J Nutr*, 2010. **140**(5): p. 969–74.
84. Mda, S. et al., Improved appetite after multi-micronutrient supplementation for six months in HIV-infected South African children. *Appetite*, 2010. **54**(1): p. 150–5.

8 Tuberculosis and Human Nutrition

Kee Thai Yeo and Anna Mandalakas

CONTENTS

Introduction... 179
Effect of Malnutrition on TB 180
  Malnutrition and the Risk for TB... 180
    Undernutrition and the Risk for TB 181
    Obesity, Diabetes Mellitus, and Risk for TB.. 184
  Malnutrition and Effects on TB Testing... 186
    Effects on TST... 186
    Effects on IFN-γ Release Assays 187
Effects of TB on Human Nutrition 188
  Effects on Macronutrients 188
    Protein–Energy Malnutrition and Mechanisms of Wasting 188
    Potential Mediators of Wasting 190
    Evidence for Nutritional Supplementation for Treatment of Wasting.......... 193
  Micronutrients and TB 198
    Macrominerals.. 198
    Vitamins.. 198
    Trace Elements 208
Conclusion 209
References... 210

INTRODUCTION

The interaction between tuberculosis (TB) and nutrition in humans has long been recognized. Malnutrition is thought to modulate the risk for the development of active TB. Patients with TB may then develop wasting and micronutrient deficiency. Figure 8.1 summarizes this complex malnutrition–TB–malnutrition interaction between different nutritional factors and TB. *In vitro* and animal studies of protein–energy malnutrition and micronutrient deficiency have demonstrated dysfunctions in the innate and adaptive immune systems against *Mycobacterium tuberculosis* (MTb). This is thought to be the mechanism behind the increased risk for the development of active TB in patients with evidence of undernutrition. This immune dysfunction is also thought to explain the strong association between diabetes mellitus (DM) and TB. These interactions have important implications in populations with high

179

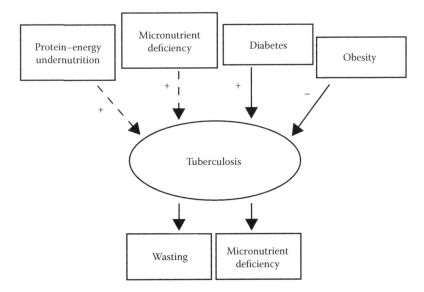

FIGURE 8.1 Malnutrition–TB–malnutrition interaction. A combination of nutritional–metabolic conditions predisposes and protects against the development of active TB. In return, TB has been shown to lead to wasting, alteration of body composition, and micronutrient deficiency. Solid arrows indicate a stronger association compared with broken ones.

incidence of undernutrition, DM, and latent TB infection (LTBI). This is in contrast with the reduced risk of TB in persons with obesity and increased body mass index (BMI). Several studies have shown an inverse dose response of TB risk with increasing BMI; however, the mechanism of this association is not fully understood.

TB is the classic disease known to cause wasting, leading to it being known as consumption. Studies of TB patients have shown alterations in body composition as a result of changes in protein, fat, and micronutrient metabolism. Some of these alterations are notably persistent and may have long-term effects. This may all lead to reduction in physical abilities and potential losses in productivity and financial earnings. Multiple mediators and factors have been proposed to be involved in the manifestation of malnutrition as a result of TB. There have also been numerous trials studying the effects of nutritional supplementation as an adjunct to standard TB treatment. This chapter will review the literature about the complex interaction between TB and nutrition, while summarizing the evidence concerning the effects of nutritional supplementation on TB outcomes, and highlight clinical implications and research opportunities.

EFFECT OF MALNUTRITION ON TB

MALNUTRITION AND THE RISK FOR TB

Research demonstrates that nutritional status is inversely associated with the risk of developing TB; as BMI increases, the individual's risk of TB decreases. Together with DM, nutritional status may be important in modulating the incidence of active TB in populations where a broad spectrum of nutritional states occurs.

Undernutrition and the Risk for TB

Undernutrition is recognized as a significant risk factor in the development of active TB. This association is supported by observations made in historical reports of TB incidence during the world wars and analyses of national databases [1–5]. Data from animal models and *in vitro* studies are compelling in demonstrating the impairment of both innate and adaptive immunity due to poor nutrition, and the consequent increased risk of developing TB. The known effects of protein malnutrition and micronutrient deficiency on the human immune system have also been used to explain the observed association between undernutrition and the increased risk of TB.

Animal Studies

There is a substantial body of evidence linking malnutrition and incidence of TB in animal models. Experiments in the guinea pig and mouse TB models suggest that chronic protein–energy malnutrition has significant effects on the innate and adaptive immune systems' responses against MTb [6]. The results of these experiments point to defects in T-cell function by the inability to form mature granulomas and the diminished production of protective cytokines [7–10]. The efficacy of bacille Calmette–Guerin (BCG) vaccination in these undernourished mice was also profoundly reduced compared with normal mice [11]. Macrophages suppressed T cells further by the production of suppressive factors, including transforming growth factor-β (TGF-β) [12,13]. As a result, undernourished mice were shown to suffer from higher mycobacterial burden and a higher rate of mortality [14].

Human Studies

Despite compelling evidence from animal models, the available human data are not conclusive. Review of available evidence attempting to establish the link between undernutrition and TB has revealed many inherent methodological issues and confounders [15,16]. Studies of TB and undernutrition typically occur in settings with complex social factors that are difficult to control and are independently recognized as risk factor for TB, including overcrowding, poor housing, poor health-care access, and social upheavals. These studies also do not account for the temporal link between the onset of undernutrition and the development of TB. Timing is critical in making the causal association between poor nutrition and the subsequent development of TB. It is also important to recognize that studies have focused on the relation between poor nutrition and the risk of developing active TB. Most studies do not attempt to distinguish the association between undernutrition states and the risk of developing primary TB infection or LTBI.

Ecological Studies

Early studies on the interaction between nutrition and TB were composed of ecological studies and observations. These studies did not attempt to make any distinction between deficiencies of macronutrients or micronutrients and were confounded by settings riddled with complex social situations. Classic examples of this include observations that during the two world wars, higher TB incidence was noted in populations with poorer and more restricted diet [1,2,4]. Observations were also made that the incidence of TB varied regionally as a function of food production, where regions rich in food production had diminished incidence of TB despite ongoing occupation and hostilities [2]. One study noted that supplementation of diet decreased TB mortality although improvements in housing and hygiene were unsuccessful [17]. The increase of food in Denmark in 1917 on account of reduced export due to intensification of the war was associated with a decrease in TB death rate despite increasing rates in surrounding countries [5]. Despite methodological limitations, these studies suggest that nutritional status of the population was associated with TB incidence as well as mortality and morbidity.

Case Series

The effect of nutritional derangement on the risk of TB was also illustrated in several case series that demonstrated an increased risk of TB following gastric and intestinal bypass surgery [18–20]. This association was first recognized in the 1940s when bypass surgeries were performed for the treatment of peptic ulcer disease as well as morbid obesity. Pulmonary TB was the most commonly reported cause of death after partial gastrectomy in many series. In a prospective study of a cohort of postgastrectomy patients, Thorn and colleagues identified a high number of incident pulmonary TB cases that occurred during the follow-up period in adult men with normal chest x-ray (CXR) before surgery [19]. The risk of incident TB was 14 times higher in patients who were <15% of their expected standard weight before surgery compared with those with standard weight. In this study, approximately one-third of all men and women who developed pulmonary TB after surgery had evidence of prior pulmonary TB infection on CXR, indicating that the postgastrectomy episode of TB was due to a reactivation or reinfection with TB.

Case–Control and Cohort Studies

Several case–control studies attempted to measure the association between TB and nutrition [21–24]. The sequence of cause and effect is difficult to discern from these studies. Owing to the lack of nutritional assessment of participants before the development of TB, it is difficult to determine the contribution of malnutrition to the development of TB. A number of cohort studies have also attempted to measure the relation between nutrition and TB. In a follow-up study of participants of BCG vaccine trials, Comstock and Palmer noted that TB incidence was 2.2 times higher in children with limited subcutaneous fat (0–4 mm) than those with 10 mm of fat [25]. Cegielski and colleagues studied the impact of undernutrition on TB incidence by analyzing data from the first US National Health and Nutrition Examination Survey (NHANES-1) Epidemiologic Follow-up Study (NHEFS) [3]. The NHANES-1 is a cross-sectional survey on a sample of the US population carried out between 1971 and 1975. The NHEFS consists of adult subjects of NHANES-1 who were followed longitudinally until 1992. Incident cases of TB were determined from interviews, medical records, and death certificates. Analysis of these data indicated that persons with low BMI (<18.5 kg/m^2), little subcutaneous fat (<5th percentile of study population for right triceps and subscapular skinfold thicknesses), or low skeletal muscle

(<5th percentile for cross-sectional area of right mid-upper arm muscle) had between 5.5- and 12.5-fold higher risk of TB than persons with normal nutritional status. Low albumin levels were also associated with increased risk of TB. A longitudinal study of a random sample of US Navy recruits found that the risk of developing TB was strongly associated with decreased weight for height [26]. An extension of this study with more recruits found that TB developed three times more often in men who were 10% or more below their ideal body weight compared with those who were 10% or more above it [27].

Micronutrients

The effect of micronutrient deficiency on the incidence of TB has also been studied. In 1949, 194 black families with known active TB exposure and nutritional status were enrolled into a trial of micronutrient supplementation and its effect on the incidence of TB [28]. Families were matched by income, crowding, and food habits and alternately allocated to receive multivitamin and mineral supplementation or no supplementation. Isoniazid preventive therapy (IPT) was not provided. After a 5-year follow-up period, it was noted that micronutrient supplementation substantially reduced the risk of TB among the family contacts of individuals with active TB. The risk of TB in the control group was a 2.8 times greater than the risk of the intervention group.

The role of vitamin D on TB has also been studied extensively [29]. In a study of sub-Saharan African immigrants in Australia, an association between vitamin D deficiency and LTBI was found, where individuals with LTBI had significantly lower mean 25-hydroxyvitamin D3 ($25(OH)D_3$) level compared with those without [30]. This difference was present when LTBI was detected by either the tuberculin skin testing (TST) or the newer interferon-γ (IFN-γ) release assays (IGRAs). A subsequent household contact cohort study in Pakistan noted about a 5-fold increase in the risk of developing active TB in contacts with vitamin D deficiency [31]. These findings suggest that adequate vitamin D stores may play a role in preventing initial TB infection and subsequent development of active TB disease [30–32].

Vitamin D exerts its actions through the vitamin D receptor (VDR), a nuclear hormone receptor. Polymorphisms in the *VDR* gene may influence the activity of receptor and subsequent downstream effects. Differences in this polymorphism may be associated with susceptibility to TB infection and disease [33,34]. There are four VDR polymorphisms that have been studied widely—*Fok*I, *Taq*I, *Apa*I, and *Bsm*I. These four polymorphisms have been associated with modulation of risk to TB infection, decreased vitamin D levels, and response to antimycobacterial therapy [34–36]. Specific VDR polymorphisms may predominate in certain populations and may also be associated with sex [37,38]. A recent meta-analysis of 23 studies measuring associations between TB and VDR polymorphisms found significant associations between *Fok*I and *Bsm*I polymorphisms and TB in the Asian population but not among Africans or South Americans [34]. The inconsistencies seen between populations may be related to environmental factors affecting TB susceptibility, including sunlight exposure as well as the diverse genetic background.

The association between undernutrition and the purported increased risk of TB is based on limited human evidence. Animal studies indicate that impairment in innate and humoral immunity as a result of protein–energy malnutrition contributes to the increased risk of TB. Results from human studies are complicated by many inherent methodological issues and confounders. Only a handful of longitudinal studies have attempted to establish the timing of undernutrition and subsequent development of TB. The role of micronutrient deficiency such as vitamin D also needs to be considered as they have been shown to modulate the risk of TB infection and disease. Taken as a whole, these results suggest that undernutrition may contribute to the development of active TB and warrant clinical vigilance in undernourished populations who should be prioritized for inclusion in IPT programs when indicated.

Obesity, Diabetes Mellitus, and Risk for TB

Obesity

The link between obesity and TB has been increasingly reported in the literature. Several epidemiologic studies from Scandinavia and the United States have suggested a link between increased BMI and decreased risk of TB [3,27,39]. Analysis of the NHEFS data from the United States indicated that individuals who were overweight, had thick fat or large muscles, had one-third to one-fifth the risk of TB compared with those with normal nutritional status [3]. A study of Finnish elderly men examining the risk of TB to vitamin C intake noted that increased BMI was associated with protection against TB [40]. Men with BMI between 23 and 27 kg/m^2 had a relative risk of 0.48 (95% CI, 0.34–0.68) compared with those with low BMI (<23 kg/m^2). Relative risk reduction was even greater in individuals with BMI >27 kg/m^2 at 0.29 (0.19–0.44).

The obesity dose–response relation was also noted in two other cohort studies [41,42]. Leung and colleagues described the potential links between obesity and TB in a cohort of elderly patients in Hong Kong [41]. Obesity (>30 kg/m^2) and overweight status (25–30 kg/m^2) by BMI were associated with a significantly lower risk of developing clinically active and culture-confirmed pulmonary TB compared with those with normal BMI (18.5–<25 kg/m^2). Even after exclusion and adjustment for possible confounding variables, including DB, smoking status, regular alcohol intake, malignancies, weight loss, and hospital admissions, the association remained statistically significant. A linear dose–response relation was noted with a 10% risk reduction of active TB for each unit increase above a BMI of 18.5. Human immunodeficiency virus (HIV) positivity was not systemically evaluated in this study, as the study population was known to have a very low prevalence of HIV infection. A subsequent prospective cohort study by Hanrahan and colleagues evaluated the effect of BMI on TB incidence and all-cause mortality in a cohort of South African HIV-positive patients [42]. Similar to the Leung et al. study, it showed a significant protective effect of increased BMI on the incidence of TB and all-cause mortality after adjustment for CD4 count as well as HAART (highly active antiretroviral therapy) use. A systematic review of six studies conducted by Lonnroth and colleagues confirms the dose–response relation described previously between BMI and TB incidence [43]. The combined analysis notes a reduction in TB incidence of 13.8% (13.4–14.2) for every unit of increase in BMI in the 18.5–30 kg/m^2 range.

The evidence for the protective effect of obesity on the risk of active TB is very compelling, although the underlying mechanism for the protection conferred by obesity remains unknown. Nutritional differences may be important in modulating this effect. Higher protein and energy stores may translate to more robust immune abilities. Also, higher micronutrient levels and differences in immune–metabolic factors such as leptins may also be important in this regard.

Diabetes Mellitus

The association of TB and DM has been recognized for thousands of years. Medical texts from all regions of the world have described the frequent occurrence of DM with TB. Root described that "in the latter half of the 19th century the diabetic patient appeared doomed to die of pulmonary TB if he succeeded in escaping coma" [44]. After the emergence and increased availability of antimycobacterial therapy in most industrialized countries, the association became less important as TB was no longer prevalent in areas where DM was present.

With the increasing prevalence of DM in low- to middle-income countries, the importance of the association between TB and DM has reemerged. DM affected an estimated 366 million people globally in 2011; this number is expected to increase to 552 million by 2030 [45]. An estimated 80% of diabetic patients worldwide live in low- to middle-income countries, with a predominance of cases coming from the Southeast Asia and the Western Pacific region. Recognizing the increasing overlap between DM and TB, there is significant concern that the incidence of TB may increase.

Several *in vitro* studies in mice and human cells have supported the association between DM and impairment of innate and adaptive immunity against TB. In a study of experimental DM in mice, chronic infection with MTb resulted in a higher load of mycobacteria and an increased expression of inflammatory cytokines compared with euglycemic controls [46,47]. Diabetic mice were shown to have an initial delay in the recruitment of IFN-γ-producing T cells in the lung, a delay in the presentation of MTb antigens to the lymph nodes, and an initial reduction in the expression of certain chemokines. Another study also noted reduction in T helper 1 (Th1)-related cytokines and nitric oxide (NO) in diabetic mice that could contribute to the altered host defenses against MTb [48].

In human cells, high levels of insulin have been shown to be associated with a decrease in Th1 immunity [49]. Production of these Th1 cytokines were notably impaired in *ex vivo* studies of human cells of individuals with DM compared with normal controls [50]. Neutrophil function and macrophage function were also found to be impaired, with reduced chemotaxis, phagocytosis, and oxidative killing potential in diabetic individuals [51,52]. The roles of micronutrient deficiency, pulmonary angiopathy, and renal insufficiency have been implicated. Changes in cough threshold, alterations in bronchociliary function, and reduced bronchial reactivity may occur as a result of tissue protein glycosylation and autonomic neuropathy [53]. This has been postulated to lead to increased sputum stagnation and reduced clearance of bacterial load.

Jeon and Murray conducted a systematic review and meta-analysis of 13 studies that associated DM with active TB [54]. This included three prospective cohort studies and eight case–control studies contributing to 17,698 TB cases under review. The pooled analysis from the prospective cohort studies illustrated that individuals with DM have an approximately 3-fold risk of developing active TB compared with individuals without DM. Increased risk were seen in younger, high-TB-incidence, and non–North American populations. In the same analysis, odds ratios from the combined case–control studies ranged from 1.16 to 7.83. These results were also corroborated by an earlier review of nine studies that found a statistically significant association between DM and TB [55]. They noted a 1.5- to 7.8-fold increased risk of developing TB in diabetics compared with nondiabetic controls. The different strengths of association noted in these studies likely reflect geographic/ethnic differences in DM severity, transmission dynamics, age distribution, and socioeconomics as well as study methods.

A recent systematic review assessed the yield of screening diabetic persons for TB and the yield of screening TB patients for DM [56]. Twelve studies were found that evaluated the presence of TB in patients with DM. The prevalence of active TB among people with DM ranged from 1.7% to 36%. TB was more common in those who were insulin dependent compared with those with mild diabetes. In settings where TB prevalence is <25 per 100,000 persons, at least 1000 people with DM would need to be screened to detect an additional case of TB (number needed to screen = 1000). As the TB incidence increases in the population, the number needed to screen diminishes. In India (estimated TB incidence = 283/100,000), screening 90–350 people with DM would detect one additional case of TB. In the 18 studies reviewed that screened TB patients for DM, DM incidence was higher in TB patients than in the baseline population. Several studies of oral glucose tolerance tests in patients with TB have shown higher rates of glucose intolerance compared with controls [57,58]. Nevertheless, there is no definitive evidence to prove that TB increases the risk of DM. Increased DM detection could potentially result from expanded medical care related to TB. However, data from these studies collectively highlight the clinical importance of screening TB patients for DM and screening diabetic patients for TB. There are suggestions that TB severity may increase in diabetics. This is evidenced by findings of increased lung cavitation, increased treatment failure, and increased mortality [59–63]. Baker and colleagues conducted a systematic review of 33 studies to summarize the current evidence for the impact of DM on TB outcomes. There was an increased relative risk of death during TB therapy—1.89 (95% CI,1.52–2.36) among 23 unadjusted studies and 4.95 (95% CI, 2.69–9.10) among the four studies that adjusted for potential confounders [64]. DM also was associated with an increased risk of TB relapse—relative risk 3.89 (2.43–6.23).

In summary, there is consistent evidence for an increased risk of active TB among individuals with underlying diabetes. Data from both basic and epidemiologic studies indicate that diabetes may influence the development, clinical course, and treatment of patients with TB. The attributable risk for DM in the development of TB is comparable to that of HIV/acquired immunodeficiency syndrome (AIDS). Although HIV/AIDS is a stronger risk factor for TB, it is a less prevalent condition compared with DM. The current epidemic of DM in middle- to low-income countries with high prevalence of TB heralds a potential public health threat.

MALNUTRITION AND EFFECTS ON TB TESTING

Effects on TST

TST has been traditionally relied on for diagnosing persons with LTBI. It is a measure of cell-mediated immunity in the form of a delayed-type hypersensitivity (DTH) reaction to purified protein derivate (PPD), which is a crude mixture of antigens that has components of MTb, *Mycobacterium bovis*, BCG, and nontuberculous mycobacteria (NTM). This test has limitations with regard to sensitivity and specificity. It is influenced by immunodeficiency, BCG vaccination status, NTM infection, and malnutrition status. It is also subject to the technical ability and inter-reader variability in the administration and interpretation of the test.

Studies have related undernutrition states, such as low protein stores and micronutrient deficiencies, to increased false-negative TST tests in the presence of TB. Data from adults have shown a significant inverse relation between measures of protein deficiency such as low albumin levels and low corrected arm muscle area with that of TST measurements in patients with TB [65,66]. Pelly and colleagues also showed that anergy secondary to protein deficiency may be TST antigen specific, as protein-deficient patients were able to respond to *Candida* and tetanus antigens [66]. Older studies of malnourished children have also demonstrated similar effects on TST [67–71]. These studies showed that (i) children who had the least response to TST were the ones with evidence of protein deficiency, and (ii) improved nutritional status was positively correlated with increments in mean size of induration.

Studies on micronutrient deficiency and supplementation have demonstrated notable effects on DTH skin testing [72,73]. Investigators have focused on zinc as it is thought to be important in modulating cutaneous responses [74,75]. A study of zinc supplementation in children demonstrated an augmentation of TST response (increase in the number of positive reactions and size of the induration) compared with placebo controls [74]. The use of zinc cream has also been shown to augment skin test finding, especially in zinc-deficient individuals. In a randomized, doubled-blinded trial of topical zinc application to TST sites, low zinc plasma level was found to be predictive of negative TST results, and this was reversed by topical zinc supplementation at the site of inoculation [75]. Topical zinc supplementation was also shown to have no effect on individuals with adequate concentrations of zinc.

Effects on IFN-γ Release Assays

A more recent alternative to the TST to aid in the diagnosis of LTBI is the IGRAs. These *in vitro* T-cell-based assays are dependent on the production of IFN-γ by sensitized T cells upon reexposure to mycobacterial antigens. Two types of IGRAs are commercially available—the ELISA-based Quantiferon (QFT) tests and the ELISPOT-based T-Spot.TB (T-Spot TB) assays. These tests have several advantages over TST, including increased specificity owing to the use of antigens encoded within the MTb genome that are not found in BCG and most NTM. However, because of the reliance on cell-mediated immune responses, the sensitivity may be decreased in immunocompromised populations.

Malnutrition is known to interfere with T-cell responses as well as IFN-γ production [14,76]. There is limited evidence supporting the association between malnutrition and IGRA response. Several pediatric studies have found a decreased sensitivity in the presence of malnutrition. Thomas and colleagues reported an increase in indeterminate results in children who were undernourished and with helminth infections [77]. One recent study reported that the QFT test may be less sensitive in HIV-infected children with evidence of chronic malnutrition [78]. After controlling for degree of TB exposure, BCG vaccination, and prior TB episodes, it was found that HIV-infected children were less likely to be QFT positive as the degree of chronic malnutrition progresses, compared with nutritionally matched HIV-uninfected peers. This association was not observed with the T-Spot TB assay, suggesting that this assay may be less affected by chronic malnutrition although this could be due to the limited sample size in this study.

Even as IGRAs are becoming widely accepted as the preferred test for diagnosing MTb infection, there are limited data to guide the interpretation of IGRAs in patients with malnutrition and HIV infection. IGRAs should be interpreted with caution in patients with malnutrition, especially those with HIV infection. Similar to the TST, a negative IGRA does not rule out TB or LTBI.

EFFECTS OF TB ON HUMAN NUTRITION

EFFECTS ON MACRONUTRIENTS

The link between TB and the development of malnutrition has been recognized for centuries as illustrated by historical disease names including "phthisis" and "consumption," both terms describing the wasting that typically accompanies TB. Multiple studies in developed and developing economies have demonstrated significant nutritional depletion upon diagnosis of TB, as well as continued nutritional derangement through the course of disease [21–23,79,80]. The wasting phenomenon in TB is notably more severe in populations with high rates of malnutrition as well as HIV infection [80,81].

Studies on TB patients have shown alterations in protein, fat, and micronutrient metabolism leading to changes in body composition and micronutrient deficiency. The malnutrition that accompanies TB is thought to be mediated through inadequate intake of nutrients due to anorexia, and altered nutrient metabolism as well as changes in the immune–endocrine–metabolic systems as a result of chronic inflammation. Wasting and changes in body composition may have effects on physical function as well as mortality [82–86]. Although body weight increases during antimycobacterial therapy, changes in body composition may occur and persist for months [87]. Studies of nutritional supplementation of both macronutrients and micronutrients, in addition to TB therapy, have yielded varying results.

Protein–Energy Malnutrition and Mechanisms of Wasting

It is reported that up to two-thirds of patients with TB present with cachexia and wasting [88]. The mechanism by which this occurs is poorly understood. It is thought to be due to a combination of decreased energy intake and alterations in energy expenditure and metabolism in response to the chronic inflammation of TB. In conditions where wasting is due to inadequate nutrient intake, the body typically responds by several metabolic changes, including reduced energy expenditure, preferential utilization of fat, and the conservation of vital tissues and protein. However, these responses are thought to be altered in conditions of chronic inflammation. Increase in energy expenditure as well as changes in protein metabolism are noted to occur. Protein breakdown is increased, resulting in increased nitrogen excretion.

This eventually leads to depletion of whole body protein and vital lean tissues in the body.

Studies of body composition and energy expenditure in TB patients have revealed different patterns of metabolic response as would be expected in chronic inflammatory states. Macallan and colleagues showed that patients presenting with active TB did not have increased energy expenditure or accelerated whole body protein turnover compared with controls without TB [89]. In a body composition study of adult male Asian patients presenting with active pulmonary TB, the proportion of lean mass reduction was consistent with reduction of energy intake as the primary contributor toward TB-associated wasting [86]. This study of body composition measured by dual-energy x-ray absorptiometry (DEXA) and bioelectrical impedance analysis also showed that lean tissue depletion in TB patients typically occurs in the limbs rather than the trunk. Fat composition was also altered with depletion of fat mass in the trunk compared with the limbs. The significant depletion of skeletal muscle in TB patients compared with controls was reflected in decreased physical function (decreased grip strength and timed stands).

There may also be sex differences in the pattern of wasting. A study of 944 adults in Uganda found that changes in body composition in men and women differed with TB disease [90]. Compared with controls without TB, men waste both fat and body cell mass, where women predominantly waste body fat. HIV infection did not seem to influence the effect of the nutritional status of these patients. This sex difference may be related to differences in fat metabolism as well as hormonal influences.

Anabolic block is also believed to contribute to the pathophysiology of wasting in TB. This is a condition where amino acid intake is diverted to oxidation and exertion. Excess energy is deposited as fat rather than lean tissue, while the breakdown of body protein continues [91]. Macallan and colleagues conducted a study in India to investigate the pathophysiology of wasting using ^{12}C-labeled leucine [89]. They compared whole body protein metabolism in TB subjects with anthropometrically matched persons who were chronically undernourished (BMI < 18.5) and a group of well-nourished Indian controls (BMI > 20). They noted that a lesser proportion of amino acid ingested by TB patients was used for protein synthesis, with an increase in protein oxidation compared with the other two groups. The mechanism of this block is still to be elucidated but is thought to be mediated by cytokines and hormone. Several studies have also shown that, as nutrition improves in TB patients, the weight gained is predominantly due to gain in fat mass [92,93].

There is evidence to show that the effect of metabolic changes in TB disease can be prolonged, even after recovery from the disease. Several longitudinal studies have consistently shown that the weight of TB patients tends to remain lower than that of controls even after 6 months of successful chemotherapy [21,88,92,94]. While this may represent differences in socioeconomic status and nutritional intake, there is evidence for persistent alterations in the body composition in these patients. In a longitudinal study conducted in England, Schwenk and colleagues studied the changes in fat and protein stores in a cohort of patients with pulmonary TB receiving standard antimycobacterial therapy [92]. Using a combination of anthropometric measurements, DEXA, and dilution methods, they were able to assess the different body compartments. Despite clinical recovery in these patients, the improvement in weight was correlated to the accumulation of fat but not with protein mass. Strikingly, this pattern of protein and fat metabolism was noted even after 6 months of therapy.

Potential Mediators of Wasting

Proinflammatory cytokines and certain gastrointestinal hormones are critical factors in the immune–endocrine–metabolic changes that lead to the development of TB-associated wasting. A number of these factors have been proposed to be involved in the pathogenesis of wasting in patients with TB, including leptin, ghrelin, peptide YY, tumor necrosis factor-α (TNF-α), interleukin (IL)-6, and IFN-γ (Table 8.1). These factors are involved in the regulation of energy expenditure, appetite, and immunity. However, the distinction between maladaptive responses in TB versus compensatory mechanisms is difficult to discern. Accurate and reliable measurement of these factors is challenging because of the pulsatile nature of their secretion.

Leptin

Leptin is a 16-kDa product from the *ob/ob* gene and is involved in the cross-regulation between nutritional status and immune responses. This hormone is produced in adipocytes and binds to receptors in the hypothalamus. Concentrations of leptin have been shown to be proportional to fat mass [95,96]. It is known to suppress appetite and increase energy expenditure [97,98]. Leptin is also involved in the proinflammatory response and modulation of immune responses [99,100].

Leptin has been proposed to be involved in the development of anorexia and wasting in chronic inflammatory states such as TB. However, studies of leptin levels in patients presenting with active TB have yielded conflicting results, including elevated [101,102], unchanged [94], or decreased [88,95,96,103] levels. Many investigators did not find a conclusive correlation between leptin levels and anorexia. Furthermore, the link between leptin levels and that of proinflammatory cytokines remain unclear, as some studies have found no association [94,95] and others have found an inverse relation between leptin levels and cytokines [96]. Differences in body composition, inflammatory conditions, and immunological state may all contribute to the effects and function of leptin in TB. On the basis of these studies, there does not seem to be a clear and direct relation between anorexia, wasting, and leptin.

Ghrelin

Ghrelin is a 28-amino-acid peptide hormone that is produced by the endocrine cells of the stomach. It stimulates food intake and reduces fat utilization by acting through vagal afferent pathways to increase feeding, promote gastric emptying, and decrease energy consumption [104]. This peptide has also been shown to have anti-inflammatory properties [104]. It decreases proinflammatory cytokine concentrations and muscle breakdown in inflammatory states. It has also been shown to protect against cytokine-mediated anorexia and is elevated in patients with cachexia resulting from cancer, anorexia nervosa, and chronic obstructive pulmonary disease [105].

Measurement of ghrelin in patients presenting with active TB have yielded differing results. A study of adult pulmonary TB patients in the pretreatment phase from Bolivia observed significantly higher levels of ghrelin compared with controls [88]. They also noted a negative correlation of ghrelin with body fat mass as well as BMI. Levels were

TABLE 8.1

Summary of Factors Studied in the Pathogenesis of Wasting in Patients with Tuberculosis

Factors	Source	Known Effects	Results from Human Nutrition-Related Studies
Leptin	Adipose tissue	Suppresses appetite and increases energy expenditure; thought to be involved in immune regulation by stimulating proinflammatory cytokine and the proliferation, differentiation, and activation of hematopoietic cells.	Levels of leptin have been associated with fat mass and sex. Studies have shown conflicting results about baseline leptin levels in PTB patients—some reporting increases, decreases, or no changes.
Ghrelin	Endocrine cells of the stomach	Stimulates food intake, promotes gastric emptying, reduces fat utilization; stimulates production of growth hormone; thought to decrease proinflammatory cytokines and muscle breakdown in inflammatory states.	Baseline ghrelin levels in PTB patients found to be elevated in one study and have no difference in another. Lower ghrelin levels were also found in malnourished patients compared with well-nourished ones.
Peptide YY	Distal small intestine and large intestine	Decreases appetite and food intake.	High baseline PYY at baseline was found in one study of PTB patients. It was associated with poor weight gain, appetite, body fat, and lower BMI. Levels normalized during TB therapy.
TNF-α	Produced mainly by monocytes/macrophages	Known as cachectic factor; some studies showed correlation with levels of leptin in a dose-dependent manner. Involved in regulation of immune response.	TNF-α is elevated at baseline in patients with active TB and decreases with treatment. Low BMI <18.5 was associated with high concentration of TNF-α. Increased TNF-α is also associated with early clinical deterioration seen in the treatment of severe tuberculosis.
IFN-γ	T cells, NK cells	Plays a central role in immunity to MTb.	Elevated at baseline in PTB patients, also higher in patients with anorexia and malaise. Reduced IFN-y production by PBMCs is a marker of severe disease.
IL-6	Produced mainly by monocytes/macrophages	Proinflammatory cytokine; production is thought to be influenced by TNF-α.	IL-6 found to be higher at baseline in PTB patients and even during treatment. Cavitation, anorexia, and anemia were shown to be associated with high concentration of IL-6. BMI <18.5 was also associated with higher IL-6.

normalized by 30 days of antimycobacterial therapy. This is contrasted with the finding of Kim and colleagues who noted lower ghrelin levels in malnourished adult Korean patients with active TB compared with those in the well-nourished group [94]. There was no correlation found with anorexia, weight loss, or TB severity.

Protein YY

Protein YY (PYY) is a hormone that is secreted by the distal small intestine and large intestine that inhibits appetite through the hypothalamus. Elevated PYY is linked with decreased appetite and food intake. PYY has been associated with malabsorptive disorders such as inflammatory bowel disease, celiac sprue, anorexia nervosa, and cancer [106–109]. In a study of adult Bolivian TB patients, Chang and colleagues found PYY level to be a strong predictor of appetite and body fat [88]. High PYY concentrations corresponded to low BMI and poor appetite. This hormone also normalized rapidly during treatment.

TNF-α

TNF-α is a cytokine produced predominantly by monocytes and macrophages. It is also known as a cachectic factor [110]. Systemic TNF-α and its soluble receptor have been shown to be significantly increased in patients with untreated and severe TB [94,101]. This association was also found in individuals who were malnourished [94] and also those with low BMI [101]. In mice studies, TNF-α administration results in a rapid and dose-dependent increase in the levels of serum leptin and expression of leptin mRNA in adipose tissue in mice [111]. This correlation has been shown to be true in humans in the active infection stage of the disease.

The immune functions of TNF-α have been shown to be divergent, acting as a "double-edged sword." Local TNF-α is key in the formation of granuloma and in NO-dependent killing of intracellular mycobacteria [112]. However, TNF-α has also been shown to contribute to killing of host cells and have been associated with clinical deterioration in patients undergoing treatment for severe TB [110,113].

IL-6

IL-6 is a cytokine that has both proinflammatory and anti-inflammatory properties. IL-6 is a principal stimulator of the production of a number of acute phase proteins [114]. It is produced by a number of cells, especially macrophages. In patients with TB, IL-6 is found to be higher at baseline and even during antimycobacterial treatment [115,116]. Anorexia, low BMI < 18.5, and anemia were associated with high concentrations of IL-6 in patients with TB [103,115–117].

IFN-γ

IFN-γ is a cytokine that is important for innate and adaptive immunity against viral and intracellular organisms. It is typically produced by T cells and natural killer (NK) cells. In mouse models, IFN-γ has been shown to be necessary for the control of MTb. In humans, individuals with mutations in the IFN-γ receptor are prones to mycobactrerial infection. The mean IFN-γ serum level has been shown to be significantly elevated in patients with active TB, particularly in those with anorexia and malaise [116].

More research is needed to further our understanding of the pathophysiology of wasting in TB and the potential mediators of this process. This knowledge could inform novel therapeutic approaches in conjunction with traditional TB therapy.

Evidence for Nutritional Supplementation for Treatment of Wasting

Since 2002, several randomized clinical trials have attempted to evaluate the effects of macronutrient supplementation on the clinical course of adult patients with TB (Table 8.2). They attempted to determine if the adjunctive provision of energy and protein to standard TB chemotherapy would counter the effects of wasting and improve TB outcomes. A few studies also provided micronutrient supplementation as part of this adjunct therapy. One study evaluated the effects of increased cholesterol on clinical outcomes related to pulmonary TB.

With regard to body weight and composition, the results were inconclusive. Three studies from India, Timor-Leste, and Singapore found significant improvements in weight and changes in body composition, whereas two others from India and Tanzania did not find significant changes [93,118–121]. Paton and colleagues found a mean increase of 8% of patient's body weight after 6 weeks of supplementation compared with nonsupplemented controls [93]. Forty-six percent of this weight gain comprised increase in lean body tissue mass. Supplemented patients continued to show greater improvement of body weight during later follow-up, up to 6 months after completion of therapy. Interestingly, the pattern of change was skewed toward deposition of predominantly fat mass. A similar increase in mean body weight was also noted in the study from India (8.6%) by the end of the 3-month study [119]. The change in mass was accompanied by improvement in functional ability as assessed by improved grip strength. It is important to note that studies describing a positive effect on body weight and composition excluded patients with HIV infection.

There is also limited evidence of improved clinical resolution of TB disease by measurement of time to sputum culture conversion in patients supplemented by macronutrients. One small trial from India showed significant improvement in the time to clearance of mycobacteria from sputum in the group with nutritional supplementation. In another trial from Mexico, Perez-Guzman and colleagues supplemented pulmonary TB patients with a high-cholesterol diet [122]. They noted that a higher proportion of patients had sputum conversion in the cholesterol-supplemented group compared with the nonsupplemented group. Furthermore, sputum conversion from positive to negative occurred at a faster rate compared with the control group. The rationale behind cholesterol supplementation originates from previous studies showing low cholesterol levels in TB patients and an association between low cholesterol levels and increased mortality rates. *In vitro* studies have also shown cholesterol to be important in the ability of macrophages to phagocytose mycobacteria [123].

The current available evidence from the trials does not conclusively prove the benefit of macronutrient supplementation on weight, functional ability, and TB outcomes. Larger studies are needed to determine the potential utility of such nutritional supplementation on TB outcomes, TB adherence, and also the potential financial benefits of mitigating the effects of TB disease.

TABLE 8.2

Summary of Trials of Macronutrient Support in Patients with Pulmonary Tuberculosis

Investigators	Intervention	Participants	Methods	Main Outcomes	Notes
Paton N et al., Singapore	Group 1: increased nutrition with supplement counseling. Group 2: standard nutritional counseling.	36 included (19 intervention). All received standard combination ATT.	Nov 2000–Jul 2002. Inclusion: 18–65 years, fever/cough and sputum smear positive, BMI <20 kg/m² , started ATT within 2 weeks. Twenty-four-hour food recall at intake, patient given dietary plan and high-energy oral nutritional supplements. At 2–3 weeks, 24-h food recall and compliance review. At 6 weeks, supplement stopped if BMI > 20.	(1) Body composition by DXA: at 6 weeks, increase in body weight of supplement group 2.57 kg vs. 0.84 kg (p = .001); also lean mass 1.17 kg vs. 0.04 kg (p = .006). (2) Maximum grip strength: increase in supplement group 2.79 kg vs. −0.65 kg (p = .016).	HIV-positive patients excluded. Body weight still significantly higher at week 12; no difference of body weight and lean mass by week 24. Fat mass increased in both groups.
Perez-Guzman et al., Mexico	Group 1: cholesterol-rich diet. Group 2: normal diet (control).	21 included (10 intervention). All received short-course regimen during the 8-week study.	Mar 2001–Jan 2002. Inclusion: newly diagnosed patients with PTB with bacteriologic confirmation, 19–60 years. All patients received 2500-calorie diet in three meals; including cholesterol 800 mg/day (intervention) or 250 mg/day (control). Sputum smear + culture, blood work at baseline and weekly. Clinical symptoms monitored daily.	(1) Sputum culture conversion: faster in intervention group and proportion becoming negative at end of second week significantly greater (8 of 10 vs. 1 of 11, p = .002). (2) Median duration for sputum conversion faster (14 days for intervention vs. 28 days, p < .006).	HIV-positive, diabetes mellitus patients excluded. Higher percentage of cavitary lesions in intervention group (90% vs. 36%, p = .02). Similar daily dietary intake excluding cholesterol.

Martins N et al., Timor-Leste	Group 1: supplementary food. Group 2: nutritional advice (control).	265 included (136 intervention). All received antimycobacterial treatment.	Mar 2005–Nov 2005. Inclusion: newly diagnosed PTB (sputum smear test positive or no response to broad-spectrum antibiotics and CXR consistent with PTB), >18 years. Received food supplements.	(1) Clearance of bacilli from sputum or completion of 8 months therapy or both: no significant difference. (2) Adherence to ATT, clinical improvement, adverse events: in intensive phase, adherence lower in intervention group; weight gain significantly greater in intervention group at 2 months and end of therapy.	Civil conflict during the trial with significant default rate in both groups.
Jahnavi G and Sudha CH, India	Group 1: food supplement (target 35 kcal/d/kg). Group 2: normal diet (control).	100 included (50 intervention). All received DOTS antimycobacterial therapy.	Aug 2005–Dec 2005. Inclusion: fulfill all criteria: (1) active TB patients (positive sputum smear and cough/fever or positive culture from extrapulmonary site; (2) wasting (BMI <20 kg/m^2); (3) DOTS within past 2 weeks. Twenty-four-hour food recall at intake. Dietary plan and food supplement to intervention group. Body weight, height, BMI, grip strength, timed-stands test at intake and 3 months. Sputum samples at 2 months, 4 months, and completion.	(1) Body weight: significant increase with intervention (8.6% vs. 2.8%, p < .01). (2) Grip strength: significantly increased in intervention. (3) Sputum conversion: significantly higher in intervention at 2 months (97.2% vs. 80.6%, p = .04).	HIV-positive, diabetes mellitus patients excluded. Treatment completion rate significantly higher with intervention (98% vs. 82%, p = .03).

(continued)

TABLE 8.2 (Continued)
Summary of Trials of Macronutrient Support in Patients with Pulmonary Tuberculosis

Investigators	Intervention	Participants	Methods	Main Outcomes	Notes
Sudarsanam TD et al., India	Group 1: nutritional supplement. Group 2: normal diet (control).	103 included (51 intervention). All received DOTS antimycobacterial therapy.	Jan 2005–Nov 2005. Inclusion: >12 years, sputum positive or sputum negative with clinical and radiological evidence of PTB or culture/biopsy proven extrapulmonary TB, BMI <19 kg/m^2. Twenty-four-hour and 3-month diet recall at baseline and 2, 4, and 6 months. Dietary advice at baseline and food supplement to intervention group (6 months total supplementation). Height, weight, skinfold thickness, MUAC, and BIA were recorded at baseline and 6 months. Blood tests at baseline and 6 months. Sputum at baseline and 5 months.	(1) TB outcome—no statistical difference between groups. Patients with good outcomes gained more lean body mass regardless of supplementation. (2) Body composition and compliance—no statistical difference between groups.	22 were coinfected with HIV. Intervention group had poorer initial nutritional status. Micronutrient supplement also given.

Praygod G et al., Tanzania	Group 1: six energy–protein bars daily. Group 2: one energy–protein bar (control). Total duration of 60 days.	377 included (189 intervention). All received antimycobacterial therapy.	Apr 2006–Mar 2009. Inclusion: new or relapsed PTB coinfected patients (two sputum positive or one sputum and CXR suggestive of TB), >15 years. Weight, height, MUAC, triceps skinfold thickness at intake, 2 months, and 5 months. Handgrip strength at intake, 2 and 5 months.	(1) Weight gain at 2, 5, and 8 months: no significant difference. (2) Gain in arm fat, arm muscle, handgrip strength at 2 and 5 months: no significant differences found; marginal increase in hand grip at 5 months in intervention group (p = .07).	All given micronutrients within the biscuit bar. At 2 months, interaction between intervention and CD4 count, 1.9 kg higher weight gain for CD4 count >350 cells/μL. Similar compliance to ATT.

Note: ARV, antiretroviral; ATT, antituberculosis treatment; BIA, body impedance analysis; CXR, chest x-ray; DOTS, directly observed therapy; E, ethambutol; H, isoniazid; MDA, malondialdehyde; MMN, multiple micronutrient; MUAC, mid-upper arm circumference; PTB, pulmonary tuberculosis; R, rifampin; RDA, recommended daily allowance; Z, pyrazinamide.

MICRONUTRIENTS AND TB

Micronutrients are essential in the maintenance of the immune system and in the control of mycobacterial infection and disease. Several studies have demonstrated low levels of micronutrients in patients presenting with TB. Deficiencies in these micronutrients have also been shown to modulate the risk of the development and the severity of TB disease. Several randomized clinical trials have also been undertaken to study the effects of micronutrient supplementation on the TB outcomes, severity of disease, and mortality (Tables 8.3 and 8.4).

Macrominerals

Iron

There has been much attention focused on the processes underlying the reliance of MTb on iron. Evidence from mice and observations in human studies indicate that the host's iron status can influence the risk of infection [124]. Several studies have made the link between iron overload status and increased risk for TB. Analysis of a series of autopsies performed in South Africa in the 1920s found an association between high splenic iron overload and death from TB [125]. In a study from Zimbabwe, increased dietary iron was associated with a 3.5-fold increase in risk of developing TB after adjusting for HIV status and liver function [126]. There was also a trend toward increased mortality in patients with increased iron intake after adjustment. However, in this study, the presence of cirrhosis was not evaluated and iron status was estimated indirectly through history of dietary intake. In a Ghanaian study that examined anemic patients presenting with pulmonary TB, antimycobacterial treatment was associated with a decrease in inflammatory markers (erythrocyte sedimentation rate, C-reactive protein) and a significant rise in hemoglobin within 2 months of initiating treatment [127].

While anemia is a common finding in studies of patients with TB, the prevalence of iron deficiency in these patients is variable (32%–86%) [128,129] and dependent on geographic locale and local dietary practices [130–132]. Suppression of erythropoiesis is seen due to cytokine-mediated reduction of erythropoietin, reduced responsiveness to the hormone, and impaired mobilization of iron from macrophages [133–135]. Anemia has been associated with an increased risk of death in several studies of TB risk factors for mortality [84,136].

The evidence for the role of iron deficiency and anemia in TB disease had been explored in several studies. A recent randomized, placebo-controlled trial from Dar es Salaam, Tanzania, evaluated the potential effects of iron status on the progression of TB disease and death [132]. Low plasma ferritin was associated with increased risk of treatment failure at 1 month after initiation of antimycobacterial therapy and TB recurrence in patients who were HIV infected. After controlling for acute-phase response, high plasma ferritin was found to be associated with an increased risk of mortality.

Vitamins

Vitamin A

Vitamin A is essential for immunity, cellular differentiation, and maintenance of epithelial surfaces, growth, reproduction, and vision [137]. It has been shown to modulate lymphocyte proliferation and normal functioning of T cells, B cells, and

TABLE 8.3

Summary of Randomized Controlled Trials Involving Single or Combination Micronutrient Supplementation in Patients with Pulmonary Tuberculosis

Investigators	Intervention	Participants	Methods	Main Outcomes	Notes
Hanekom WA et al., Dec 1997, South Africa	Group 1: 200,000 IU vitamin A ×2 doses before ATT. Group 2: placebo.	85 children included (44 received vitamin A).	All received routine ATT. Mantoux skin test, CXR, plasma retinol, sputum for smear, and culture at baseline. Physical examination; nutritional status; CXR at baseline, 6 weeks, and 3 months.	(1) Clinical findings, CXR, nutritional status at 6 weeks and 3 months: no difference noted between groups. (2) Extrapulmonary TB was associated with low vitamin A (p = .04).	Excluded HIV-positive individuals; 53 of 85 (62%) had vitamin A <20 μg/dL.
Karyadi E et al., Apr 2002, Indonesia	Group 1: 5000 IU vitamin A and 15 mg zinc. Group 2: lactose placebo.	80 included (40 intervention). Inclusions: newly diagnosed PTB by sputum smear and culture, 15–55 years, consistent CXR.	Dec 1997–Dec 1998. All received EHRZ daily for 2 months, H and R three times per week for 4 months (DOTS). Clinical examination, CXR, sputum smear and culture, blood samples, measurements at baseline, 2 months, and 6 months after ATT.	(1) Sputum conversion: higher sputum negative in micronutrient group (p < .01). (2) CXR lesion: significant mean reduction in cavity size in micronutrient group; increase in retinol was correlated with reduction in lesion area after 6 months ATT (p = .02).	64% of the group are underweight at baseline. Retinol levels were significantly higher at 2 and 6 months in both groups, not zinc.
Armijos RX et al., May 2010, Mexico	Group 1: 5000 IU vitamin A and 50 mg zinc per day. Group 2: placebo.	39 included (20 intervention). Inclusions: PTB patients with positive sputum smear, 18–65 years.	Aug 2005–Jul 2006. All received EHRZ for 2 months, followed by H and R for 45 doses. Clinical examination; dietary recall at baseline, months 1–4, and month 6. Blood samples at baseline, 2 months, and 6 months.	Sputum conversion: more pronounced proportion of positive smear decreased in micronutrient group with significant differences between both groups after month 3.	Micronutrient group had a significant increase in plasma zinc levels compared with placebo; no difference for retinol.

(continued)

TABLE 8.3 (Continued)

Summary of Randomized Controlled Trials Involving Single or Combination Micronutrient Supplementation in Patients with Pulmonary Tuberculosis

Investigators	Intervention	Participants	Methods	Main Outcomes	Notes
Pakasi TA et al., Sep 2010, Indonesia	Group 1: 5000 IU vitamin A. Group 2: 15 mg zinc. Group 3: 5000 IU vitamin A and 15 mg zinc. Group 4: lactose placebo. Daily intake for 6 months.	300 included (76 zinc, 72 vitamin A, 66 vitamin A and zinc, 86 placebo). Inclusion: positive sputum smears, 15–55 years.	Jan 2004–Dec 2005. All received EHRZ daily for 2 months, followed by 3×/week H and R for 4 months Physical examination; CXR; blood samples; nutritional and food intake assessment at baseline, 2 months, and 6 months; weekly sputum examination (three samples).	(1) Sputum conversion time: combined vitamin A and zinc had shortest conversion; no statistical difference between groups at 2 and 6 months. (2) MUAC, BMI, skinfold thickness: significantly improved from baseline at 2 + 6 months. (3) Micronutrient status: significant improvement at 2 and 6 months in all groups.	HIV status not assessed; mean BMI 16.5 for population; 40% of population had cavities on CXR.
Visser ME et al., Nov 2010, South Africa	Group 1: single 200,000 IU vitamin A. Group 2: placebo sunflower oil. 15 mg zinc 5 days/week for 2 months.	154 included. Inclusion: 18–60 years, 2 positive sputum smear or 1 positive sputum smear, and suggestive CXR.	May 2005–Dec 2008. All received EHRZ for 5 days/ week. Clinical symptoms, Karnofsky score, anthropometry at baseline and 8 weeks. Dietary intake at baseline, week 2, and week 8. Sputum smears and cultures were collected every week for 8 weeks. CXR and blood samples at baseline.	(1) Time to culture detection: similar in both groups. (2) CXR: no difference on cavity resolution.	Significant increase of retinol over time; no significant change in serum zinc.

| Lawson L et al., Dec 2010, Nigeria | Group 1: 90 mg elemental zinc weekly. Group 2: 90 mg zinc and 5000 IU vitamin A. Group 3: placebo. | 350 included (117 zinc, 117 zinc and vitamin A, 116 placebo). Inclusions: ≥15 years, positive sputum smear. | Sep 2003–Jun 2005. All received EHRZ for 2 months, followed by H and E for 6 months (DOTS). Blood samples at enrolment. CXR at baseline, 2 months, and 6 months. Sputum weekly for first 8 weeks, then at 3, 4, 5, and 6 months. | (1) Time to sputum conversion: no difference in time to conversion compared with placebo for both interventions. (2) CXR score: No difference in improvement. (3) Mortality: No significant differences comparing individual groups; when both intervention arms combined, significant increase risk of mortality (p = .03). | No ARV during study. HIV seropositivity was 45%, with no difference between groups. 32% had BMI <18.5. |
| Seyedrezazadeh E et al., 2008, Iran | Group 1: vitamin E (140 mg) and selenium (200 µg). Group 2: placebo. | 35 included (17 intervention). Inclusions: newly diagnosed PTB based on sputum or culture, consistent CXR, and clinical presentation. | All received EHRZ daily for 2 months, followed H and R daily for 6 months. Blood samples for MDA and vitamin E | MDA levels: significantly decreased in groups supplemented with vitamin E and selenium (p = .01) after 2 months. | MDA is measure of lipid peroxidation. Vitamin E significantly increased in intervention compared with placebo. |

Note: ARV, antiretroviral; ATT, antituberculosis treatment; CXR, chest x-ray; DOTS, directly observed therapy; E, ethambutol; H, isoniazid; MDA, malondialdehyde; MMN, multiple micronutrient; MUAC, mid-upper arm circumference; PTB, pulmonary tuberculosis; R, rifampin; RDA, recommended daily allowance; Z, pyrazinamide.

TABLE 8.4
Summary of Randomized Controlled Trials Involving Multiple Micronutrients Supplementation in Patients with Pulmonary Tuberculosis

Investigators	Intervention	Participants	Methods	Main Outcomes	Notes
Range N et al., Sep 2005 and Apr 2006, Tanzania	2 × 2 factorial design. Randomized to daily zinc vs. placebo and then MMN vs. placebo.	499 included (246 zinc, 251 MMN). Inclusions: PTB by sputum smear and/or culture >15 years.	Aug 2001–Jul 2002. All received 4 ATT for 2 months (DOTS) and continuation for 6 months. Clinical examination at baseline. Sputum smear and culture at baseline and 2, 4, and 8 weeks, then every 6 months. Viral load and CD4 counts after 2 months. Weight at 7 months. Survival up to 8 months.	(1) Sputum culture conversion at 2, 4, and 8 weeks—no significant difference between zinc and placebo and MMN and placebo. (2) Mortality: no overall effect of Zn, MMN, or combined MMN and Zn; for HIV-infected patients, combined MMN and Zn significantly reduced mortality (70%).	No interaction between zinc and multimicronutrient. Multimicronutrient group had gained 0.8 kg more than placebo (p = .02).
Semba RD et al., Aug 2007, Malawi	Group 1: multimicronutrient. Group 2: placebo. Not stratified on HIV status.	1148 included (575 micronutrient). Inclusions: sputum smear positive, 18–60 years, no recent ATT or vitamin supplements.	Jun 1999–Feb 2005. All received EHRZ 3 days/week for 2 months, followed by 6 months H and E. Clinical examination at 2, 5, 8, 12, 16, 20, and 24 months. Micronutrient supplementation for 24 months.	Mortality: no significant difference between MMN and placebo groups among HIV-negative and HIV-positive groups.	Multivitamin at RDA levels, except higher vitamins E and C. At time of study, no local ARV program.
Villamor E et al., Jun 2008, Dar es Salaam, Tanzania	Stratified according to HIV status. Group 1: multimicronutrient. Group 2: placebo.	887 included (416 HIV negative—208 received MMN; 471 HIV positive—233 received MMN). Inclusions:	Apr 2000–Apr 2005. Stratified on the basis of HIV status to either micronutrient or placebo. All received EHRZ for 2 months, H and E for subsequent 6 months DOTS.	(1) Sputum culture conversion at 1 month after ATT: no significant difference between groups. (2) Mortality within 2 years: no significant difference between groups.	At time of study, ARV was unavailable. Supplementation caused significant reduction of risk for peripheral neuropathy,

	positive sputum smears, 18–65 years, Karnofsky score ≥ 40%.	Physician examination every 3 months. Clinic visit (+body composition) at baseline and monthly. Sputum smear and culture and blood samples at baseline and 1, 2, 5, 8, and 12 months.	(3) TB recurrence (1–8 months): those sputum negative by 1 month, micronutrient decreased risk by 45% (p = .02) for all patients, 63% reduction for HIV-positive patients.	extrapulmonary TB, and genital ulcers. No effect on nutritional parameters.
Mehta S et al., Oct 2011, Dar es Salaam, Tanzania	Group 1: MMN (vitamin B complex, C, and E). Group 2: placebo.	255 children with probably TB (6 weeks–5 years). 128 received MMN. Inclusion: TST ≥10 mm in HIV-uninfected, ≥5 mm in HIV-infected or CXR findings.	May 2005–Sep 2007. All received EHRZ for 2 months, followed by HR for 4 months (DOTS). Blood sample, HIV testing weight, height, length, MUAC, triceps skinfold thickness at baseline. Nurse or clinic visit every 2 weeks.	(1) Weight gain, length, MUAC, skinfold thickness: no significant differences between two groups. (2) Clearance of x-ray: no difference. (3) Mortality: no difference.	29% placebo and 39% MMN group were HIV infected. Median Hgb levels increased in MMN group by 2 months.
Praygod G et al., Feb 2011, Tanzania	Group 1: daily MMN. Group 2: placebo. Both given in form of protein–energy biscuit for 60 days.	865 included (433 MMN group). Inclusions: PTB diagnosed by sputum smear, >15 years.	Apr 2006–Mar 2009. All received standard ATT treatment for 6–8 months. Weight, MUAC, triceps skinfold thickness, handgrip strength at baseline, repeated at 2 and 5 months.	(1) Weight gain at 2 and 5 months: no significant overall difference between groups; significant increase weight in HIV-negative group by 5 months. (2) Arm fat, arm muscle, handgrip strength: no significant difference except at 2 months, increased handgrip strength in the MMN group specifically HIV negative group.	11% of HIV-positive patients were on ARV (27 of 245).

Note: ARV, antiretroviral; ATT, antituberculosis treatment; CXR, chest x-ray; DOTS, directly observed therapy; E, ethambutol; H, isoniazid; MMN, multiple micronutrient; MUAC, mid-upper arm circumference; PTB, pulmonary tuberculosis; R, rifampin; RDA, recommended daily allowance; Z, pyrazinamide.

macrophages. Vitamin A has an important role in inhibiting multiplication of virulent bacilli in cultured human macrophages [138]. Multiple studies have demonstrated deficiency of vitamin A at presentation of pulmonary TB disease, ranging from 32% to 90% of all patients [139–143]. A combination of both HIV and TB infections increases the likelihood of vitamin A deficiency more than with one infection alone [144]. The decrease in vitamin A levels seen in the pretreatment, acute phase of TB has been postulated to be due to decreased retinol-binding proteins [145] and related to increased excretion of vitamin A in the urine [146]. Vitamin A levels have been shown to increase and return to the reference range in patients at the end of antimycobacterial treatment.

The potential benefit of supplementation of vitamin A in patients with TB has been the subject of multiple randomized, double-blinded, placebo-controlled clinical trials (Table 8.3). They have included trials that have evaluated vitamin A by itself [140,147] and also in combination with zinc [142,148–150]. Trials of single supplementation with vitamin A have found no difference in the clinical status, CXR, or sputum conversion in patients with TB compared with the comparator placebo group. The results of studies with combined vitamin A and zinc supplementation on clinical course of TB have yielded varying results, with two studies showing an improvement in the time to sputum conversion [142,149] and three showing no difference [147,148,150].

As yet, the effect of vitamin A supplementation on the clinical course of pulmonary TB is inconclusive, and further understanding of the mechanism of vitamin A function and metabolism is needed. Several important factors may be the reasons for the differing conclusions of these trials, including different treatment regiments of vitamin A, differing baseline proportions of vitamin A deficiency, and differing daily intake.

Vitamin D

The properties of vitamin D in the management of TB have been recognized since the 1940s. Charpy and Dowling separately published on the use of vitamin D in the treatment of cutaneous TB [151]. The benefit of taking cod liver oil (rich in vitamin D) had also been known since the pre–antibiotic era. Additionally, the importance of sunlight has been appreciated throughout the history of TB treatment [152,153]. Vitamin D has been thought to have an important role in host immune defenses against MTb. The antimycobacterial properties of vitamin D has been shown *in vitro* [154,155].

The mechanism of vitamin D effect on TB is primarily mediated through 1,25(OH)D3. It is thought to induce the production of antimicrobial peptides and also enhance macrophage ability [156]. Studies have shown that binding of mycobacterial ligands to Toll-like receptor 2/1 combination upregulates VDR and the enzyme 1α-hydroxylase. This leads to the conversion of 25(OH)D3 to the bioactive 1,25(OH)D$_3$, also known as calcitriol. Calcitriol increases the expression of cathelicidin, which is cleaved to LL-37, a class of defensin–antimicrobial peptide that inhibits the growth of MTb [155,156]. *In vitro* studies have also shown that the antimycobacterial activity of IFN-γ-activated macrophages is enhanced with the addition of calcitriol [157–159]. This is thought to be associated with the induction of increased NO production by activated macrophages.

Studies of immigrants living in Australia, the United Kingdom, the United States, and Europe have found significantly low serum levels of vitamin D in active TB cases compared with healthy controls [35,160–164]. A meta-analysis of seven studies between 1985 and 2005 found that on average, patients presenting with TB have lower serum levels of 25(OH)D$_3$ than healthy controls matched on sex, age, ethnicity, diet, and geographic locations [165]. A summary of the effect size in this analysis proposed that the levels of 25 (OH) D3 in patients with TB were about 0.68 standard deviation (95% CI, 0.42–0.93) lower than controls. Differences in the risk of TB and its association with vitamin D levels have been attributed to differences in sun exposure, socioeconomic status, dietary intake, and lifestyle [32,33,165].

In several of these studies, the severity of TB disease (assessed radiographically) was inversely associated with levels of vitamin D [32,35]. Studies have also shown differences in vitamin D levels according to sex and differential risk for TB as a result. In a study from Vietnam, men with TB were found to have a higher percentage of vitamin D deficiency compared with controls; however, no such differences were detected in women with TB [166]. This was in contrast to a study in Pakistan that showed a higher rate of TB in women who had a significantly higher rate of vitamin D deficiency [31]. The sex differences in vitamin D levels and the higher susceptibility for TB may be related to socioeconomic status, exposure to sunlight, TB exposure, and cultural practices that may differ in respective populations. The effect of estrogen as a possible mediator of risk for TB remains to be defined [167].

Martineau et al. conducted a double-blinded, placebo-controlled randomized trial of vitamin D supplementation in a cohort of TB contacts in London, evaluating the effect of vitamin D on a functional whole blood assay, the BCG-lux assay [168]. A single dose of 2.5 mg of vitamin D significantly enhanced the ability of TB contacts to restrict BCG-lux luminescence. This is an indicator of the enhancement of the host's innate and acquired immune ability. There was no effect of vitamin D on antigen-stimulated IFN-γ responses to early secretory antigenic target-6 and culture filtrate protein 10. Supplementation with a single dose also corrected all patients with severe deficiency of 25(OH)D3.

Four randomized clinical trials have been conducted evaluating the impact of vitamin D supplementation on the clinical course of pulmonary TB (Table 8.5). All evaluated time to sputum conversion from positive to negative as one of the outcomes. Only one Indonesian study noted a significant improvement in the time to sputum conversion [169]. There was no effect reported on mortality and TBscore (a clinical score combining signs and symptoms to assess clinical outcomes) [170,171]. A recent study from Pakistan reported a significant improvement in weight gain, disease involvement by CXR, as well as the MTbs (MTb sonicate) antigen induced IFN-γ secretion in the intervention group [171]. The difference in results of these trials may be due to the vitamin D dosing strategy and the baseline vitamin levels in the population. Thus far, the proposed benefits of vitamin D on pulmonary TB as seen in epidemiologic studies and animal models have yet to be proven conclusively.

TABLE 8.5

Summary of Randomized, Double-Blinded, Placebo-Controlled Trials of Vitamin D Supplementation in Patients with Pulmonary Tuberculosis

Investigators	Methods	Participants	Intervention	Main Outcomes	Notes
Nursyam EW et al., Jan 2006, Jakarta, Indonesia	All received 2 months of EHRZ followed by 4 months H and R DOTS. Baseline blood samples. Clinical examination every 2 weeks. CXR at baseline and 6 months. Sputum smear at baseline, 6 weeks, and 8 weeks.	67 analyzed (34 intervention). Inclusion: new diagnosis of PTB, >15 years.	Group 1: 0.25 mg/day for 6 weeks. Group 2: placebo.	Sputum conversion: 34 of 34 (100%) in intervention vs. 25 of 33 (76.7%) (p = .002).	Baseline vitamin D not performed. Follow-up CXR on 36 of 67 patients—improvement in 87.5% in intervention vs. 65% in placebo.
Wejse C et al., Jan 2009, Guinea-Bissau	Nov 2003–Dec 2005. All received 2 months of EHRZ followed by 6 months H and E Sputum at 2, 4, and 6 weeks and 2, 5, and 8 months, Clinical examination at 2, 5, and 8 months.	365 analyzed (187 intervention). Inclusion: diagnosis of TB by sputum or WHO clinical criteria, >15 years.	Group 1: 100,000 IU cholecalciferol at enrollment, at 5 months, and at 8 months. Group 2: placebo vegetable oil.	(1) Clinical improvement by TBscore: similar in both groups. (2) All-cause mortality at 12 months: 30 of 187 died in the intervention and 24 of 178 died in the placebo group (p = .45).	Mean baseline vitamin D for study. 78.3 ng/ mL. Sputum conversion and weight gain not different between groups. No hypercalcemia.

Study	Methods	Sample/Inclusion	Intervention	Results	Conclusions
Martineau AR et al. Jan 2011, London, UK	Jan 2007–Jul 2009. All received EHRZ. Baseline clinical examination, CXR, sputum, and blood samples. Clinical review and sputum at 2, 4, 6, and 8 weeks after ATT. CXR at 8 weeks.	126 analyzed (62 intervention). Inclusion: newly diagnosed PTB and AFB-positive sputum, >18 years.	Group 1: 2.5 mg vitamin D_3 for four oral doses (first dose <7 days of TB therapy then 2, 4, and 6 weeks). Group 2: placebo miglyol oil.	Time from initiation of antimicrobial to sputum culture conversion: median 36 days in intervention, 43.5 days in placebo (p = .41).	75 of 126 had vitamin D <20 ng/mL. Vitamin D hastens sputum culture conversion in patients with the TT genotype of Taq1 VDR polymorphism.
Salahuddin N et al. (SUCCINT trial), Jan 2013, Karachi, Pakistan	Oct 2009–Jul 2010. All received 2 months of EHRZ followed by 6 months H and E (DOTS). Clinical examination and sputum examination at baseline and 1, 2, and 3 months; CXR and blood samples at baseline and 3 months; 25(OH)D_3 at baseline and 3 months.	259 analyzed (132 intervention. Inclusion: adults ≥16 years and smear-positive active PTB.	Group 1: 600,000 IU intramuscular vitamin D_3 for 2 doses 1 month apart. Group 2: normal saline.	(1) Mean weight gain: +3.75 kg in intervention vs. 2.61 kg in placebo (p = .009). (2) Improvement by CXR: 1.35 zones in intervention vs. 1.82 zones in placebo (p = .004). (3) Increased MTb antigen induced IFN-γ secretion with intervention in baseline deficient group (<20 ng/mL 25(OH)D_3).	Mean baseline vitamin D for study, 21.3 ng/mL. No significant differences in TBscore or sputum conversion at 1 and 3 months.

Note: ATT, antituberculosis treatment; CXR, chest x-ray; DOTS, directly observed therapy; E, ethambutol; H, isoniazid; PTB, pulmonary tuberculosis; R, rifampin; Z, pyrazinamide.

Vitamin E

Vitamin E is one of the most important lipophilic antioxidants and protects against oxidative stress, specifically lipid peroxidation [172–175]. Activation of lung macrophages in pulmonary TB is thought to be associated with free radical–associated injury, which results in diversion of vitamin E to the lungs. Patients with pulmonary TB have been reported to have decreased levels of antioxidants, increased reactive oxygen species, and increased levels of lipid peroxidation. Vitamin E has also been shown to improve immunologic functions, by increasing proliferation of lymphocytes as well as enhancing the production of IFN-γ. At the cellular level, vitamin E increased PPD-induced peripheral blood mononuclear cell (PBMC) proliferation in TB patients [176].

Prior studies have observed low levels of vitamin E in patients presenting with pulmonary TB compared with healthy controls [175–177]. In a study from South Africa, Plit and colleagues noted an association between persistent low levels of vitamin E with elevated levels of lipid peroxides despite antimycobacterial therapy for 6 months [175]. They postulate that TB was a primary contributor to chronic oxidative stress leading to altered levels of vitamin E and lipid peroxides.

Studies of vitamin E supplementation in other respiratory illnesses have reported conflicting results, ranging from a lack of benefit to increased risk [178,179]. In a Finnish cohort study of vitamin E and β-carotene supplementation, vitamin E was shown to have no impact on the incidence of TB [180]. However, in a subgroup analysis, the effect of vitamin E was significantly modified by the dietary intake of vitamin C and smoking status. Vitamin E intake (DL-α-tocopheryl acetate 50 mg/dL daily) increased the risk of reactivation of latent TB in participants with high dietary vitamin C intake and who were heavy smokers (>20 cigarettes/day). This analysis did not control for other potential TB risk factors, and the suggested deleterious effect of vitamin E in this specific population would need to be studied further.

Vitamin C

Ascorbic acid plays an important role in pulmonary antioxidant defense. It is a critical component in maintaining balance between oxidants and antioxidants in the lung. This has been studied together with other micronutrients such as vitamin E in the context of oxidative stress. Early studies found associations between low vitamin C levels in plasma with increased incidence of TB [181].

Several studies have evaluated the levels of vitamin C in pulmonary TB and noted decreased levels of vitamin C at the presentation of pulmonary TB disease [175,182, 183]. This decrease could be due to alterations in dietary habits or due to accelerated turnover as a response to increased oxidative stress [175]. Restoration of this vitamin to normal levels was seen after completion of antimycobacterial therapy. Studies of vitamin C intake did not find any significant effect on susceptibility to development of TB disease.

Trace Elements

Zinc

Zinc is important in proper functioning of B cells, T cells, neutrophils, and NK cells [184,185]. Zinc deficiency is known to cause thymic atrophy, impair proliferation of

T lymphocytes, and is associated with Th1/Th2 lymphocyte cytokine imbalances [184,186]. Phagocytosis and intracellular killing are also affected by zinc deficiency. Zinc supplementation in states of zinc deficiency has been shown to increase immune function [187]. Zinc also functions as an antioxidant and stabilizes cell membranes.

Studies on zinc concentrations in TB patients have shown significantly lower plasma zinc level than those without TB irrespective of nutritional status [128,143, 188]. Zinc levels are also associated with severity of pulmonary TB disease radiographically, with an inverse relation noted [189]. Deficiency of this trace element in TB is thought to be due to redistribution of zinc from plasma to other tissues, or a reduction in carrier and an increase in metallothionein protein transport to the liver [190].

In a study of childhood TB in India, Ray and colleagues compared the zinc levels of 50 children with TB, 10 malnourished children without TB, and 10 healthy children [188]. They found that plasma zinc levels were significantly lower in children with TB when compared with controls or malnourished children, irrespective of the manifestations of TB (disseminated, pulmonary, lymphadenitis, or central nervous system). Children with disseminated TB had the lowest levels of zinc. Successful antimycobacterial therapy was associated with significant improvement in levels of zinc in these children.

Randomized clinical trials involving zinc have included supplementation with zinc only, and in combination with vitamin A and with multimicronutrients. None of the trials involving a zinc-only arm revealed any differences in the clinical improvements of active pulmonary TB disease [147,150]. In combination with vitamin A, trials in Indonesia, Mexico, and Nigeria have conflicting results in terms of sputum conversion as well as CXR improvements [142,148–150]. A trial of multimicronutrient and zinc supplementation in Tanzania showed significant reduction in mortality of HIV coinfected patients [191].

Selenium

This essential trace element is important in immune processes and the clearance of mycobacteria. Studies have related a decrease of selenium to the development of TB disease in HIV-positive patients [192]. Low levels of selenium have been described in association with TB, and levels were improved by the completion of TB treatment [193].

Selenium is required by the antioxidant glutathione peroxidase and may have a role in decreasing oxidative stress in patients with active pulmonary TB. Studies of selenium supplementation in combination with vitamin E have showed improvement in levels of serum malondialdehyde, which is a marker of oxidative stress [194].

CONCLUSION

The interaction between TB and nutrition in humans is bidirectional. Malnutrition is a likely risk factor for TB, and patients with TB may subsequently develop wasting and nutritional deficits. The compelling evidence for immune dysfunction in animal studies of undernutrition leading to increased risk for active TB has not been as strongly demonstrated in human epidemiological studies. The evidence for the association between TB and DM is much more convincing. Patients with increased BMI have been shown to have a lower risk of developing active TB, although the mechanism of this interaction is not clear. The diagnostics tests for MTb infection, especially the TST, have also been shown to be affected by undernutrition and micronutrient deficiency (e.g., zinc). There is also some evidence for decreased sensitivity in IGRAs in patients with undernutrition and HIV infection.

Wasting has been synonymously known to occur with active TB disease. The mechanism of this phenomenon is still to be elucidated, although multiple hormones and factors have been investigated. Active disease has also been shown to have variable effects on micronutrients. Despite this, the benefits of nutritional supplementation on TB outcome and functional abilities have had varying results.

There is a need for more research to understand better the bidirectional effects of TB and nutrition. This is especially important in light of the ever-prevailing problems of undernutrition, as well as the increasing problems of DM and obesity. The effects of nutritional supplementation as an adjunct to TB therapy needs to be studied further as it may have potential benefits in terms of TB outcomes and also restoration of functional abilities and productivity.

REFERENCES

1. Leyton, G.B., Effects of slow starvation. *Lancet*, 1946. **2**(6412): 73–9.
2. Marche, J. and H. Gounelle, The relation of protein scarcity and modification of blood protein to tuberculosis among undernourished subjects. *The Milbank Memorial Fund Quarterly*, 1950. **28**(2): 114–26.
3. Cegielski, J.P., L. Arab, and J. Cornoni-Huntley, Nutritional risk factors for tuberculosis among adults in the United States, 1971–1992. *American Journal of Epidemiology*, 2012. **176**(5): 409–22.
4. Cochrane, A.L., Tuberculosis among prisoners of war in Germany. *British Medical Journal*, 1945. **2**(4427): 656–8.
5. Faber, K., Tuberculosis and nutrition. *Acta Tuberculosea Scandinavica*, 1938. **12**: 287–335.
6. McMurray, D.N. and R.A. Bartow, Immunosuppression and alteration of resistance to pulmonary tuberculosis in guinea pigs by protein undernutrition. *The Journal of Nutrition*, 1992. **122**(3 Suppl): 738–43.
7. Dai, G. and D.N. McMurray, Altered cytokine production and impaired antimycobacterial immunity in protein-malnourished guinea pigs. *Infection and Immunity*, 1998. **66**(8): 3562–8.
8. Mainali, E.S. and D.N. McMurray, Protein deficiency induces alterations in the distribution of T-cell subsets in experimental pulmonary tuberculosis. *Infection and Immunity*, 1998. **66**(3): 927–31.
9. Mainali, E.S., Adoptive transfer of resistance to pulmonary tuberculosis in guinea pigs is altered by protein deficiency. *Nutrition Research*, 1998. **18**(2): 309–17.
10. McMurray, D.N. et al., *Mycobacterium bovis* BCG vaccine fails to protect protein-deficient guinea pigs against respiratory challenge with virulent *Mycobacterium tuberculosis*. *Infection and Immunity*, 1985. **50**(2): 555–9.
11. Cohen, M.K. et al., Effects of diet and genetics on *Mycobacterium bovis* BCG vaccine efficacy in inbred guinea pigs. *Infection and Immunity*, 1987. **55**(2): 314–9.
12. McMurray, D.N., G. Dai, and S. Phalen, Mechanisms of vaccine-induced resistance in a guinea pig model of pulmonary tuberculosis. *Tubercle and Lung Disease: The Official*

Journal of the International Union against Tuberculosis and Lung Disease, 1999. **79**(4): 261–6.

13. Dai, G. and D.N. McMurray, Effects of modulating TGF-beta 1 on immune responses to mycobacterial infection in guinea pigs. *Tubercle and Lung Disease: The Official Journal of the International Union against Tuberculosis and Lung Disease*, 1999. **79**(4): 207–14.

14. Chan, J. et al., Effects of protein calorie malnutrition on tuberculosis in mice. *Proceedings of the National Academy of Sciences of the United States of America*, 1996. **93**(25): 14857–61.

15. Cegielski, J.P. and D.N. McMurray, The relationship between malnutrition and tuberculosis: Evidence from studies in humans and experimental animals. *The International Journal of Tuberculosis and Lung Disease: The Official Journal of the International Union against Tuberculosis and Lung Disease*, 2004. **8**(3): 286–98.

16. Gupta, K.B. et al., Tuberculosis and nutrition. *Lung India*, 2009. **26**(1): 9–16.

17. Munro, W.T. and I. Leitch, Diet and tuberculosis. *The Proceedings of the Nutrition Society*, 1945. **3**: 155–64.

18. Werbin, N., Tuberculosis after jejuno-ileal bypass for morbid obesity. *Postgraduate Medical Journal*, 1981. **57**(666): 252–3.

19. Thorn, P.A., V.S. Brookes, and J.A. Waterhouse, Peptic ulcer, partial gastrectomy, and pulmonary tuberculosis. *British Medical Journal*, 1956. **1**(4967): 603–8.

20. Bruce, R.M. and L. Wise, Tuberculosis after jejunoileal bypass for obesity. *Annals of Internal Medicine*, 1977. **87**(5): 574–6.

21. Onwubalili, J.K., Malnutrition among tuberculosis patients in Harrow, England. *European Journal of Clinical Nutrition*, 1988. **42**(4): 363–6.

22. Harries, A.D., J. Thomas, and K.S. Chugh, Malnutrition in African patients with pulmonary tuberculosis. *Human Nutrition. Clinical Nutrition*, 1985. **39**(5): 361–3.

23. Scalcini, M. et al., Pulmonary tuberculosis, human immunodeficiency virus type-1 and malnutrition. *Bulletin of the International Union against Tuberculosis and Lung Disease*, 1991. **66**(1): 37–41.

24. Harrison, B.D., P. Tugwell, and I.W. Fawcett, Tuberculin reaction in adult Nigerians with sputum-positive pulmonary tuberculosis. *Lancet*, 1975. **1**(7904): 421–4.

25. Comstock, G.W. and C.E. Palmer, Long-term results of BCG vaccination in the southern United States. *The American Review of Respiratory Disease*, 1966. **93**(2): 171–83.

26. Palmer, C.E., S. Jablon, and P.Q. Edwards, Tuberculosis morbidity of young men in relation to tuberculin sensitivity and body build. *American Review of Tuberculosis*, 1957. **76**(4): 517–39.

27. Edwards, L.B. et al., Height, weight, tuberculous infection, and tuberculous disease. *Archives of Environmental Health*, 1971. **22**(1): 106–12.

28. Downes, J., An experiment in the control of tuberculosis among negroes. *The Milbank Memorial Fund Quarterly*, 1950. **28**(2): 127–59.

29. Davies, P.D., The role of vitamin D in tuberculosis. *The American Review of Respiratory Disease*, 1989. **139**(6): 1571.

30. Gibney, K.B. et al., Vitamin D deficiency is associated with tuberculosis and latent tuberculosis infection in immigrants from sub-Saharan Africa. *Clinical Infectious Diseases: An Official Publication of the Infectious Diseases Society of America*, 2008. **46**(3): 443–6.

31. Talat, N. et al., Vitamin D deficiency and tuberculosis progression. *Emerging Infectious Diseases*, 2010. **16**(5): 853–5.

32. Grange, J.M. et al., A study of vitamin D levels in Indonesian patients with untreated pulmonary tuberculosis. *Tubercle*, 1985. **66**(3): 187–91.

33. Luong, K. and L.T. Nguyen, Impact of vitamin D in the treatment of tuberculosis. *The American Journal of the Medical Sciences*, 2011. **341**(6): 493–8.

34. Gao, L. et al., Vitamin D receptor genetic polymorphisms and tuberculosis: Updated systematic review and meta-analysis. *The International Journal of Tuberculosis and Lung Disease: The Official Journal of the International Union against Tuberculosis and Lung Disease*, 2010. **14**(1): 15–23.

35. Wilkinson, R.J. et al., Influence of vitamin D deficiency and vitamin D receptor polymorphisms on tuberculosis among Gujarati Asians in west London: A case–control study. *Lancet*, 2000. **355**(9204): 618–21.

36. Babb, C. et al., Vitamin D receptor gene polymorphisms and sputum conversion time in pulmonary tuberculosis patients. *Tuberculosis*, 2007. **87**(4): 295–302.

37. Fitness, J. et al., Large-scale candidate gene study of tuberculosis susceptibility in the Karonga district of northern Malawi. *The American Journal of Tropical Medicine and Hygiene*, 2004. **71**(3): 341–9.

38. Liu, W. et al., VDR and NRAMP1 gene polymorphisms in susceptibility to pulmonary tuberculosis among the Chinese Han population: A case–control study. *The International Journal of Tuberculosis and Lung Disease: The Official Journal of the International Union against Tuberculosis and Lung Disease*, 2004. **8**(4): 428–34.

39. Tverdal, A., Body mass index and incidence of tuberculosis. *European Journal of Respiratory Diseases*, 1986. **69**(5): 355–62.

40. Hemila, H. et al., Vitamin C and other compounds in vitamin C rich food in relation to risk of tuberculosis in male smokers. *American Journal of Epidemiology*, 1999. **150**(6): 632–41.

41. Leung, C.C. et al., Lower risk of tuberculosis in obesity. *Archives of Internal Medicine*, 2007. **167**(12): 1297–304.

42. Hanrahan, C.F. et al., Body mass index and risk of tuberculosis and death. *Aids*, 2010. **24**(10): 1501–8.

43. Lonnroth, K. et al., A consistent log-linear relationship between tuberculosis incidence and body mass index. *International Journal of Epidemiology*, 2010. **39**(1): 149–55.

44. Root, H., The association of diabetes and tuberculosis. *New England Journal of Medicine*, 1934. **210**: 1–13.

45. Federation, I.D. *IDF Diabetes Atlas*, 5th edn. 2012 [cited 2013 February 15]; Available from: http://www.idf.org/diabetesatlas.

46. Martens, G.W. et al., Tuberculosis susceptibility of diabetic mice. *American Journal of Respiratory Cell and Molecular Biology*, 2007. **37**(5): 518–24.

47. Vallerskog, T., G.W. Martens, and H. Kornfeld, Diabetic mice display a delayed adaptive immune response to *Mycobacterium tuberculosis*. *Journal of Immunology*, 2010. **184**(11): 6275–82.

48. Yamashiro, S. et al., Lower expression of Th1-related cytokines and inducible nitric oxide synthase in mice with streptozotocin-induced diabetes mellitus infected with *Mycobacterium tuberculosis*. *Clinical and Experimental Immunology*, 2005. **139**(1): 57–64.

49. Viardot, A. et al., Potential antiinflammatory role of insulin via the preferential polarization of effector T cells toward a T helper 2 phenotype. *Endocrinology*, 2007. **148**(1): 346–53.

50. Stalenhoef, J.E. et al., The role of interferon-gamma in the increased tuberculosis risk in type 2 diabetes mellitus. *European Journal of Clinical Microbiology & Infectious Diseases: Official Publication of the European Society of Clinical Microbiology*, 2008. **27**(2): 97–103.

51. Delamaire, M. et al., Impaired leucocyte functions in diabetic patients. *Diabetic Medicine: A Journal of the British Diabetic Association*, 1997. **14**(1): 29–34.

52. Rayfield, E.J. et al., Infection and diabetes: The case for glucose control. *The American Journal of Medicine*, 1982. **72**(3): 439–50.

53. Kant, L., Diabetes mellitus–tuberculosis: The brewing double trouble. *Indian Journal of Tuberculosis*, 2003. **50**(4): 183–4.
54. Jeon, C.Y. and M.B. Murray, Diabetes mellitus increases the risk of active tuberculosis: A systematic review of 13 observational studies. *PLoS Medicine*, 2008. **5**(7): e152.
55. Stevenson, C.R. et al., Diabetes and the risk of tuberculosis: A neglected threat to public health? *Chronic Illness*, 2007. **3**(3): 228–45.
56. Jeon, C.Y. et al., Bi-directional screening for tuberculosis and diabetes: A systematic review. *Tropical Medicine & International Health: TM & IH*, 2010. **15**(11): 1300–14.
57. Zack, M.B., L.L. Fulkerson, and E. Stein, Glucose intolerance in pulmonary tuberculosis. *The American Review of Respiratory Disease*, 1973. **108**(5): 1164–9.
58. Nichols, G.P., Diabetes among young tuberculous patients: A review of the association of the two diseases. *American Review of Tuberculosis*, 1957. **76**(6): 1016–30.
59. Mboussa, J. et al., Course of pulmonary tuberculosis in diabetics. *Revue de Pneumologie Clinique*, 2003. **59**(1): 39–44.
60. Fielder, J.F. et al., A high tuberculosis case-fatality rate in a setting of effective tuberculosis control: Implications for acceptable treatment success rates. *The International Journal of Tuberculosis and Lung Disease: The Official Journal of the International Union against Tuberculosis and Lung Disease*, 2002. **6**(12): 1114–7.
61. Shaikh, M.A. et al., Does diabetes alter the radiological presentation of pulmonary tuberculosis. *Saudi Medical Journal*, 2003. **24**(3): 278–81.
62. Restrepo, B.I. et al., Type 2 diabetes and tuberculosis in a dynamic bi-national border population. *Epidemiology and Infection*, 2007. **135**(3): 483–91.
63. Oursler, K.K. et al., Survival of patients with pulmonary tuberculosis: Clinical and molecular epidemiologic factors. *Clinical Infectious Diseases: An Official Publication of the Infectious Diseases Society of America*, 2002. **34**(6): 752–9.
64. Baker, M.A. et al., The impact of diabetes on tuberculosis treatment outcomes: A systematic review. *BMC Medicine*, 2011. **9**: 81.
65. Kardjito, T., M. Donosepoetro, and J.M. Grange, The Mantoux test in tuberculosis: Correlations between the diameters of the dermal responses and the serum protein levels. *Tubercle*, 1981. **62**(1): 31–5.
66. Pelly, T.F. et al., Tuberculosis skin testing, anergy and protein malnutrition in Peru. *The international Journal of Tuberculosis and Lung Disease: The Official Journal of the International Union against Tuberculosis and Lung Disease*, 2005. **9**(9): 977–84.
67. Lloyd, A.V., Tuberculin test in children with malnutrition. *British Medical Journal*, 1968. **3**(5617): 529–31.
68. Sinha, D.P. and F.B. Bang, Protein and calorie malnutrition, cell-mediated immunity, and B.C.G. vaccination in children from rural West Bengal. *Lancet*, 1976. **2**(7985): 531–4.
69. Satyanarayana, K. et al., Influence of nutrition on postvaccinial tuberculin sensitivity. *The American Journal of Clinical Nutrition*, 1980. **33**(11): 2334–7.
70. Kielmann, A.A. et al., The effect of nutritional status on immune capacity and immune responses in preschool children in a rural community in India. *Bulletin of the World Health Organization*, 1976. **54**(5): 477–83.
71. Koster, F.T. et al., Cellular immune competence and diarrheal morbidity in malnourished Bangladeshi children: A prospective field study. *The American Journal of Clinical Nutrition*, 1987. **46**(1): 115–20.
72. Golden, M.H. et al., Zinc and immunocompetence in protein–energy malnutrition. *Lancet*, 1978. **1**(8076): 1226–8.
73. Bogden, J.D. et al., Daily micronutrient supplements enhance delayed-hypersensitivity skin test responses in older people. *The American Journal of Clinical Nutrition*, 1994. **60**(3): 437–47.

74. Cuevas, L.E. et al., Effect of zinc on the tuberculin response of children exposed to adults with smear-positive tuberculosis. *Annals of Tropical Paediatrics*, 2002. **22**(4): 313–9.

75. Rao, V.B. et al., Zinc cream and reliability of tuberculosis skin testing. *Emerging Infectious Diseases*, 2007. **13**(7): 1101–4.

76. Haque, R. et al., Correlation of interferon-gamma production by peripheral blood mononuclear cells with childhood malnutrition and susceptibility to amebiasis. *The American Journal of Tropical Medicine and Hygiene*, 2007. **76**(2): 340–4.

77. Thomas, T.A. et al., Malnutrition and helminth infection affect performance of an interferon gamma-release assay. *Pediatrics*, 2010. **126**(6): e1522–9.

78. Mandalakas, A.M. et al., Detecting tuberculosis infection in HIV-infected children: A study of diagnostic accuracy, confounding and interaction. *The Pediatric Infectious Disease Journal*, 2013. **32**(3): e111–8.

79. Harries, A.D. et al., Nutritional status in Malawian patients with pulmonary tuberculosis and response to chemotherapy. *European Journal of Clinical Nutrition*, 1988. **42**(5): 445–50.

80. Kennedy, N. et al., Nutritional status and weight gain in patients with pulmonary tuberculosis in Tanzania. *Transactions of the Royal Society of Tropical Medicine and Hygiene*, 1996. **90**(2): 162–6.

81. Lucas, S.B. et al., Contribution of tuberculosis to slim disease in Africa. *BMJ*, 1994. **308**(6943): 1531–3.

82. Melchior, J.C. et al., Improved survival by home total parenteral nutrition in AIDS patients: Follow-up of a controlled randomized prospective trial. *Aids*, 1998. **12**(3): 336–7.

83. Lubart, E. et al., Mortality of patients hospitalized for active tuberculosis in Israel. *The Israel Medical Association Journal: IMAJ*, 2007. **9**(12): 870–3.

84. Sacks, L.V. and S. Pendle, Factors related to in-hospital deaths in patients with tuberculosis. *Archives of Internal Medicine*, 1998. **158**(17): 1916–22.

85. PrayGod, G. et al., Weight, body composition and handgrip strength among pulmonary tuberculosis patients: A matched cross-sectional study in Mwanza, Tanzania. *Transactions of the Royal Society of Tropical Medicine and Hygiene*, 2011. **105**(3): 140–7.

86. Paton, N.I. and Y.M. Ng, Body composition studies in patients with wasting associated with tuberculosis. *Nutrition*, 2006. **22**(3): 245–51.

87. Schwenk, A. and D.C. Macallan, Tuberculosis, malnutrition and wasting. *Current Opinion in Clinical Nutrition and Metabolic Care*, 2000. **3**(4): 285–91.

88. Chang, S.W. et al., Gut hormones, appetite suppression and cachexia in patients with pulmonary TB. *PloS One*, 2013. **8**(1): e54564.

89. Macallan, D.C. et al., Whole body protein metabolism in human pulmonary tuberculosis and undernutrition: Evidence for anabolic block in tuberculosis. *Clinical Science*, 1998. **94**(3): 321–31.

90. Mupere, E. et al., Body composition among HIV-seropositive and HIV-seronegative adult patients with pulmonary tuberculosis in Uganda. *Annals of Epidemiology*, 2010. **20**(3): 210–6.

91. Streat, S.J., A.H. Beddoe, and G.L. Hill, Aggressive nutritional support does not prevent protein loss despite fat gain in septic intensive care patients. *The Journal of Trauma*, 1987. **27**(3): 262–6.

92. Schwenk, A. et al., Nutrient partitioning during treatment of tuberculosis: Gain in body fat mass but not in protein mass. *The American Journal of Clinical Nutrition*, 2004. **79**(6): 1006–12.

93. Paton, N.I. et al., Randomized controlled trial of nutritional supplementation in patients with newly diagnosed tuberculosis and wasting. *The American Journal of Clinical Nutrition*, 2004. **80**(2): 460–5.

94. Kim, J.H. et al., Relation of ghrelin, leptin and inflammatory markers to nutritional status in active pulmonary tuberculosis. *Clinical Nutrition*, 2010. **29**(4): 512–8.
95. Schwenk, A. et al., Leptin and energy metabolism in pulmonary tuberculosis. *The American Journal of Clinical Nutrition*, 2003. **77**(2): 392–8.
96. van Crevel, R. et al., Decreased plasma leptin concentrations in tuberculosis patients are associated with wasting and inflammation. *The Journal of Clinical Endocrinology and Metabolism*, 2002. **87**(2): 758–63.
97. Ukkola, O., Peripheral regulation of food intake: New insights. *Journal of Endocrinological Investigation*, 2004. **27**(1): 96–8.
98. Sarraf, P. et al., Multiple cytokines and acute inflammation raise mouse leptin levels: Potential role in inflammatory anorexia. *The Journal of Experimental Medicine*, 1997. **185**(1): 171–5.
99. Lam, Q. and L. Lu, Role of leptin in immunity. *Cellular & Molecular Immunology*, 2007. **4**(1): 1.
100. Lord, G.M. et al., Leptin modulates the T-cell immune response and reverses starvation-induced immunosuppression. *Nature*, 1998. **394**(6696): 897–901.
101. Cakir, B. et al., Relation of leptin and tumor necrosis factor alpha to body weight changes in patients with pulmonary tuberculosis. *Hormone Research*, 1999. **52**(6): 279–83.
102. Yuksel, I. et al., The relation between serum leptin levels and body fat mass in patients with active lung tuberculosis. *Endocrine Research*, 2003. **29**(3): 257–64.
103. Santucci, N. et al., A multifaceted analysis of immune–endocrine–metabolic alterations in patients with pulmonary tuberculosis. *PloS One*, 2011. **6**(10).
104. Asakawa, A. et al., Ghrelin is an appetite-stimulatory signal from stomach with structural resemblance to motilin. *Gastroenterology*, 2001. **120**(2): 337–45.
105. Kamiji, M.M. and A. Inui, The role of ghrelin and ghrelin analogues in wasting disease. *Current Opinion in Clinical Nutrition and Metabolic Care*, 2008. **11**(4): 443–51.
106. Adrian, T.E. et al., Peptide YY abnormalities in gastrointestinal diseases. *Gastroenterology*, 1986. **90**(2): 379–84.
107. Wahab, P.J., W.P. Hopman, and J.B. Jansen, Basal and fat-stimulated plasma peptide YY levels in celiac disease. *Digestive Diseases and Sciences*, 2001. **46**(11): 2504–9.
108. Beck, A.L. et al., Peptide YY: A gut hormone associated with anorexia during infectious diarrhea in children. *The Journal of Pediatrics*, 2008. **153**(5): 677–82.
109. Misra, M. et al., Elevated peptide YY levels in adolescent girls with anorexia nervosa. *The Journal of Clinical Endocrinology and Metabolism*, 2006. **91**(3): 1027–33.
110. Mootoo, A. et al., TNF-alpha in tuberculosis: A cytokine with a split personality. *Inflammation & Allergy Drug Targets*, 2009. **8**(1): 53–62.
111. Zumbach, M.S. et al., Tumor necrosis factor increases serum leptin levels in humans. *The Journal of Clinical Endocrinology and Metabolism*, 1997. **82**(12): 4080–2.
112. Kaneko, H. et al., Role of tumor necrosis factor-alpha in *Mycobacterium*-induced granuloma formation in tumor necrosis factor-alpha-deficient mice. *Laboratory Investigation; A Journal of Technical Methods and Pathology*, 1999. **79**(4): 379–86.
113. Bekker, L.G. et al., Selective increase in plasma tumor necrosis factor-alpha and concomitant clinical deterioration after initiating therapy in patients with severe tuberculosis. *The Journal of Infectious Diseases*, 1998. **178**(2): 580–4.
114. Zhang, Y., M. Broser, and W.N. Rom, Activation of the interleukin 6 gene by *Mycobacterium tuberculosis* or lipopolysaccharide is mediated by nuclear factors NF-IL6 and NF-kappa B. *Proceedings of the National Academy of Sciences of the United States of America*, 1994. **91**(6): 2225–9.
115. Karyadi, E. et al., Cytokines related to nutritional status in patients with untreated pulmonary tuberculosis in Indonesia. *Asia Pacific Journal of Clinical Nutrition*, 2007. **16**(2): 218–26.

116. Verbon, A. et al., Serum concentrations of cytokines in patients with active tuberculosis (TB) and after treatment. *Clinical and Experimental Immunology*, 1999. **115**(1): 110–3.

117. van Lettow, M. et al., Interleukin-6 and human immunodeficiency virus load, but not plasma leptin concentration, predict anorexia and wasting in adults with pulmonary tuberculosis in Malawi. *The Journal of Clinical Endocrinology and Metabolism*, 2005. **90**(8): 4771–6.

118. PrayGod, G. et al., The effect of energy–protein supplementation on weight, body composition and handgrip strength among pulmonary tuberculosis HIV-co-infected patients: Randomised controlled trial in Mwanza, Tanzania. *The British Journal of Nutrition*, 2012. **107**(2): 263–71.

119. Jahnavi, G. and C.H. Sudha, Randomised controlled trial of food supplements in patients with newly diagnosed tuberculosis and wasting. *Singapore Medical Journal*, 2010. **51**(12): 957–62.

120. Martins, N., P. Morris, and P.M. Kelly, Food incentives to improve completion of tuberculosis treatment: Randomised controlled trial in Dili, Timor-Leste. *BMJ*, 2009. **339**: b4248.

121. Sudarsanam, T.D. et al., Pilot randomized trial of nutritional supplementation in patients with tuberculosis and HIV–tuberculosis coinfection receiving directly observed short-course chemotherapy for tuberculosis. *Tropical Medicine & International Health: TM & IH*, 2011. **16**(6): 699–706.

122. Perez-Guzman, C. et al., A cholesterol-rich diet accelerates bacteriologic sterilization in pulmonary tuberculosis. *Chest*, 2005. **127**(2): 643–51.

123. Gatfield, J. and J. Pieters, Essential role for cholesterol in entry of mycobacteria into macrophages. *Science*, 2000. **288**(5471): 1647–50.

124. Drakesmith, H. and A.M. Prentice, Hepcidin and the iron–infection axis. *Science*, 2012. **338**(6108): 768–72.

125. Gordeuk, V.R. et al., Associations of iron overload in Africa with hepatocellular carcinoma and tuberculosis: Strachan's 1929 thesis revisited. *Blood*, 1996. **87**(8): 3470–6.

126. Gangaidzo, I.T. et al., Association of pulmonary tuberculosis with increased dietary iron. *The Journal of Infectious Diseases*, 2001. **184**(7): 936–9.

127. Lawn, S.D. et al., Resolution of the acute-phase response in West African patients receiving treatment for pulmonary tuberculosis. *The International Journal of Tuberculosis and Lung Disease: The Official Journal of the International Union against Tuberculosis and Lung Disease*, 2000. **4**(4): 340–4.

128. Karyadi, E. et al., Poor micronutrient status of active pulmonary tuberculosis patients in Indonesia. *The Journal of Nutrition*, 2000. **130**(12): 2953–8.

129. Lee, S.W. et al., The prevalence and evolution of anemia associated with tuberculosis. *Journal of Korean Medical Science*, 2006. **21**(6): 1028–32.

130. Friis, H. et al., Acute-phase response and iron status markers among pulmonary tuberculosis patients: A cross-sectional study in Mwanza, Tanzania. *The British Journal of Nutrition*, 2009. **102**(2): 310–7.

131. Morris, C.D., A.R. Bird, and H. Nell, The haematological and biochemical changes in severe pulmonary tuberculosis. *The Quarterly Journal of Medicine*, 1989. **73**(272): 1151–9.

132. Isanaka, S. et al., Iron deficiency and anemia predict mortality in patients with tuberculosis. *The Journal of Nutrition*, 2012. **142**(2): 350–7.

133. Schaible, U.E. and S.H. Kaufmann, Iron and microbial infection. *Nature Reviews. Microbiology*, 2004. **2**(12): 946–53.

134. Means, R.T., Jr., Pathogenesis of the anemia of chronic disease: A cytokine-mediated anemia. *Stem Cells*, 1995. **13**(1): 32–7.

135. Weiss, G., C. Bogdan, and M.W. Hentze, Pathways for the regulation of macrophage iron metabolism by the anti-inflammatory cytokines IL-4 and IL-13. *Journal of Immunology*, 1997. **158**(1): 420–5.

136. Kourbatova, E.V. et al., Risk factors for mortality among adult patients with newly diagnosed tuberculosis in Samara, Russia. *The International Journal of Tuberculosis and Lung Disease: The Official Journal of the International Union against Tuberculosis and Lung Disease*, 2006. **10**(11): 1224–30.

137. Semba, R.D., Vitamin A, immunity, and infection. *Clinical Infectious Diseases: An Official Publication of the Infectious Diseases Society of America*, 1994. **19**(3): 489–99.

138. Crowle, A.J. and E.J. Ross, Inhibition by retinoic acid of multiplication of virulent tubercle bacilli in cultured human macrophages. *Infection and Immunity*, 1989. **57**(3): 840–4.

139. Rwangabwoba, J.M., H. Fischman, and R.D. Semba, Serum vitamin A levels during tuberculosis and human immunodeficiency virus infection. *The International Journal of Tuberculosis and Lung Disease: The Official Journal of the International Union against Tuberculosis and Lung Disease*, 1998. **2**(9): 771–3.

140. Hanekom, W.A. et al., Vitamin A status and therapy in childhood pulmonary tuberculosis. *The Journal of Pediatrics*, 1997. **131**(6): 925–7.

141. Ramachandran, G. et al., Vitamin A levels in sputum-positive pulmonary tuberculosis patients in comparison with household contacts and healthy 'normals.' *The International Journal of Tuberculosis and Lung Disease: The Official Journal of the International Union against Tuberculosis and Lung Disease*, 2004. **8**(9): 1130–3.

142. Karyadi, E. et al., A double-blind, placebo-controlled study of vitamin A and zinc supplementation in persons with tuberculosis in Indonesia: Effects on clinical response and nutritional status. *The American Journal of Clinical Nutrition*, 2002. **75**(4): 720–7.

143. Koyanagi, A. et al., Relationships between serum concentrations of C-reactive protein and micronutrients, in patients with tuberculosis. *Annals of Tropical Medicine and Parasitology*, 2004. **98**(4): 391–9.

144. Mugusi, F.M. et al., Vitamin A status of patients presenting with pulmonary tuberculosis and asymptomatic HIV-infected individuals, Dar es Salaam, Tanzania. *The International Journal of Tuberculosis and Lung Disease: The Official Journal of the International Union against Tuberculosis and Lung Disease*, 2003. **7**(8): 804–7.

145. Fleck, A., Clinical and nutritional aspects of changes in acute-phase proteins during inflammation. *The Proceedings of the Nutrition Society*, 1989. **48**(3): 347–54.

146. Ross, A.C., Vitamin A status: Relationship to immunity and the antibody response. *Proceedings of the Society for Experimental Biology and Medicine. Society for Experimental Biology and Medicine*, 1992. **200**(3): 303–20.

147. Pakasi, T.A. et al., Zinc and vitamin A supplementation fails to reduce sputum conversion time in severely malnourished pulmonary tuberculosis patients in Indonesia. *Nutrition Journal*, 2010. **9**: 41.

148. Visser, M.E. et al., The effect of vitamin A and zinc supplementation on treatment outcomes in pulmonary tuberculosis: A randomized controlled trial. *The American Journal of Clinical Nutrition*, 2011. **93**(1): 93–100.

149. Armijos, R.X. et al., Adjunctive micronutrient supplementation for pulmonary tuberculosis. *Salud Publica de Mexico*, 2010. **52**(3): 185–9.

150. Lawson, L. et al., Randomized controlled trial of zinc and vitamin A as co-adjuvants for the treatment of pulmonary tuberculosis. *Tropical Medicine & International Health: TM & IH*, 2010. **15**(12): 1481–90.

151. Dowling, G.B., S. Gauvain, and D.E. Macrae, Vitamin D in treatment of cutaneous tuberculosis. *British Medical Journal*, 1948. **1**(4548): 430–5.

152. Ellman, P. and K.H. Anderson, Calciferol in tuberculous peritonitis with disseminated tuberculosis. *British Medical Journal*, 1948. **1**(4547): 394.
153. Brincourt, J., Liquefying effect on suppurations of an oral dose of calciferol. *La Presse Medicale*, 1969. **77**(13): 467–70.
154. Crowle, A.J., E.J. Ross, and M.H. May, Inhibition by 1,25(OH)2-vitamin D3 of the multiplication of virulent tubercle bacilli in cultured human macrophages. *Infection and Immunity*, 1987. **55**(12): 2945–50.
155. Martineau, A.R. et al., IFN-gamma- and TNF-independent vitamin D-inducible human suppression of mycobacteria: The role of cathelicidin LL-37. *Journal of Immunology*, 2007. **178**(11): 7190–8.
156. Liu, P.T. et al., Cutting edge: Vitamin D-mediated human antimicrobial activity against *Mycobacterium tuberculosis* is dependent on the induction of cathelicidin. *Journal of Immunology*, 2007. **179**(4): 2060–3.
157. Rook, G.A. et al., The role of gamma-interferon, vitamin D3 metabolites and tumour necrosis factor in the pathogenesis of tuberculosis. *Immunology*, 1987. **62**(2): 229–34.
158. Rook, G.A. et al., Vitamin D3, gamma interferon, and control of proliferation of *Mycobacterium tuberculosis* by human monocytes. *Immunology*, 1986. **57**(1): 159–63.
159. Denis, M., Killing of *Mycobacterium tuberculosis* within human monocytes: Activation by cytokines and calcitriol. *Clinical and Experimental Immunology*, 1991. **84**(2): 200–6.
160. Ustianowski, A. et al., Prevalence and associations of vitamin D deficiency in foreign-born persons with tuberculosis in London. *Journal of Infection*, 2005. **50**(5): 432–7.
161. Martin, J.A. and D.B. Mak, Changing faces: A review of infectious disease screening of refugees by the Migrant Health Unit, Western Australia in 2003 and 2004. *The Medical Journal of Australia*, 2006. **185**(11–12): 607–10.
162. Skull, S.A. et al., Vitamin D deficiency is common and unrecognized among recently arrived adult immigrants from The Horn of Africa. *Internal Medicine Journal*, 2003. **33**(1–2): 47–51.
163. Nolan, C., S. Goldberg, and J. Wallace, Increase in African immigrants and refugees with tuberculosis—Seattle-King County, Washington, 1998–2001. *MMWR. Morbidity and Mortality Weekly Report*, 2002. **51**(39): 882–3.
164. Lopez-Velez, R., H. Huerga, and M.C. Turrientes, Infectious diseases in immigrants from the perspective of a tropical medicine referral unit. *The American Journal of Tropical Medicine and Hygiene*, 2003. **69**(1): 115–21.
165. Nnoaham, K.E. and A. Clarke, Low serum vitamin D levels and tuberculosis: A systematic review and meta-analysis. *International Journal of Epidemiology*, 2008. **37**(1): 113–9.
166. Ho-Pham, L.T. et al., Association between vitamin D insufficiency and tuberculosis in a Vietnamese population. *BMC Infectious Diseases*, 2010. **10**: 306.
167. Neyrolles, O. and L. Quintana-Murci, Sexual inequality in tuberculosis. *PLoS Medicine*, 2009. **6**(12): e1000199.
168. Martineau, A.R. et al., A single dose of vitamin D enhances immunity to mycobacteria. *American Journal of Respiratory and Critical Care Medicine*, 2007. **176**(2): 208–13.
169. Nursyam, E.W., Z. Amin, and C.M. Rumende, The effect of vitamin D as supplementary treatment in patients with moderately advanced pulmonary tuberculous lesion. *Acta Medica Indonesiana*, 2006. **38**(1): 3–5.
170. Wejse, C. et al., Vitamin D as supplementary treatment for tuberculosis: A double-blind, randomized, placebo-controlled trial. *American Journal of Respiratory and Critical Care Medicine*, 2009. **179**(9): 843–50.
171. Salahuddin, N. et al., Vitamin D accelerates clinical recovery from tuberculosis: Results of the SUCCINCT Study (Supplementary Cholecalciferol in recovery from tuberculosis). A randomized, placebo-controlled, clinical trial of vitamin D supplementation in patients with pulmonary tuberculosis'. *BMC Infectious Diseases*, 2013. **13**: 22.

172. Chow, C.K., Vitamin E and oxidative stress. *Free Radical Biology & Medicine*, 1991. **11**(2): 215–32.
173. Packer, L., Protective role of vitamin E in biological systems. *The American Journal of Clinical Nutrition*, 1991. **53**(4 Suppl): 1050S–5S.
174. Pryor, W.A., The antioxidant nutrients and disease prevention—What do we know and what do we need to find out? *The American Journal of Clinical Nutrition*, 1991. **53**(1 Suppl): 391S–3S.
175. Plit, M.L. et al., Influence of antimicrobial chemotherapy and smoking status on the plasma concentrations of vitamin C, vitamin E, beta-carotene, acute phase reactants, iron and lipid peroxides in patients with pulmonary tuberculosis. *The International Journal of Tuberculosis and Lung Disease: The Official Journal of the International Union against Tuberculosis and Lung Disease*, 1998. **2**(7): 590–6.
176. Hernandez, J. et al., Effect of exogenous vitamin E on proliferation and cytokine production in peripheral blood mononuclear cells from patients with tuberculosis. *The British Journal of Nutrition*, 2008. **99**(2): 224–9.
177. Madebo, T. et al., Circulating antioxidants and lipid peroxidation products in untreated tuberculosis patients in Ethiopia. *The American Journal of Clinical Nutrition*, 2003. **78**(1): 117–22.
178. Meydani, S.N. et al., Vitamin E and respiratory tract infections in elderly nursing home residents: A randomized controlled trial. *JAMA: The Journal of the American Medical Association*, 2004. **292**(7): 828–36.
179. Graat, J.M., E.G. Schouten, and F.J. Kok, Effect of daily vitamin E and multivitamin-mineral supplementation on acute respiratory tract infections in elderly persons: A randomized controlled trial. *JAMA: The Journal of the American Medical Association*, 2002. **288**(6): 715–21.
180. Hemila, H. and J. Kaprio, Vitamin E supplementation may transiently increase tuberculosis risk in males who smoke heavily and have high dietary vitamin C intake. *The British Journal of Nutrition*, 2008. **100**(4): 896–902.
181. Getz, H.R., E.R. Long, and H.J. Henderson, A study of the relation of nutrition to the development of tuberculosis; influence of ascorbic acid and vitamin A. *American Review of Tuberculosis*, 1951. **64**(4): 381–93.
182. Bakaev, V.V. and A.P. Duntau, Ascorbic acid in blood serum of patients with pulmonary tuberculosis and pneumonia. *The International Journal of Tuberculosis and Lung Disease: The Official Journal of the International Union against Tuberculosis and Lung Disease*, 2004. **8**(2): 263–6.
183. Awotedu, A.A., E.O. Sofowora, and S.I. Ette, Ascorbic acid deficiency in pulmonary tuberculosis. *East African Medical Journal*, 1984. **61**(4): 283–7.
184. Prasad, A.S., Effects of zinc deficiency on Th1 and Th2 cytokine shifts. *The Journal of Infectious Diseases*, 2000. **182**(Suppl 1): S62–8.
185. Shankar, A.H. and A.S. Prasad, Zinc and immune function: The biological basis of altered resistance to infection. *The American Journal of Clinical Nutrition*, 1998. **68**(2 Suppl): 447S–63S.
186. Ibs, K.H. and L. Rink, Zinc-altered immune function. *The Journal of Nutrition*, 2003. **133**(5 Suppl 1): 1452S–6S.
187. Abul, H.T. et al., Interleukin-1 alpha (IL-1 alpha) production by alveolar macrophages in patients with acute lung diseases: The influence of zinc supplementation. *Molecular and Cellular Biochemistry*, 1995. **146**(2): 139–45.
188. Ray, M., L. Kumar, and R. Prasad, Plasma zinc status in Indian childhood tuberculosis: Impact of antituberculosis therapy. *The International Journal of Tuberculosis and Lung Disease: The Official Journal of the International Union against Tuberculosis and Lung Disease*, 1998. **2**(9): 719–25.

189. Ghulam, H. et al., Status of zinc in pulmonary tuberculosis. *Journal of Infection in Developing Countries*, 2009. **3**(5): 365–8.
190. Gabay, C. and I. Kushner, Acute-phase proteins and other systemic responses to inflammation. *The New England Journal of Medicine*, 1999. **340**(6): 448–54.
191. Range, N. et al., The effect of micronutrient supplementation on treatment outcome in patients with pulmonary tuberculosis: A randomized controlled trial in Mwanza, Tanzania. *Tropical Medicine & International Health: TM & IH*, 2005. **10**(9): 826–32.
192. Shor-Posner, G. et al., Impact of selenium status on the pathogenesis of mycobacterial disease in HIV-1-infected drug users during the era of highly active antiretroviral therapy. *Journal of Acquired Immune Deficiency Syndromes*, 2002. **29**(2): 169–73.
193. Kassu, A. et al., Alterations in serum levels of trace elements in tuberculosis and HIV infections. *European Journal of Clinical Nutrition*, 2006. **60**(5): 580–6.
194. Seyedrezazadeh, E. et al., Effect of vitamin E and selenium supplementation on oxidative stress status in pulmonary tuberculosis patients. *Respirology*, 2008. **13**(2): 294–8.

9 Impact of Malaria and Parasitic Infections on Human Nutrition

Athis Rajh Arunachalam,
Vedanta S. Dariya, and Celia Holland

CONTENTS

Global Burden of Parasitic Infections 222
Global Burden of Malnutrition 224
    Protein–Energy Malnutrition (PEM) 225
    Iron Deficiency Anemia (IDA) 225
    Vitamin A Deficiency (VAD) 225
    Iodine Deficiency Disorders (IDD) 225
Malaria and Nutrition 225
    Introduction 225
    Nutrition 225
    Malaria—Case Definitions 227
Impact of PEM on Malaria 227
    Evidence from Animal Studies 228
    Evidence from Human Studies 228
Impact of Malaria on PEM 229
Malaria, Nutrition, and Immunity 230
Micronutrients and Malaria 231
Impact of Nutrient-Based Interventions on Malaria 231
Parasitic Infections Other than Malaria and Human Nutrition 232
    Nematodes 233
        Hookworm 233
        Ascariasis 233
        Trichuriasis 234
    Giardiasis 234
    Amoebiasis 234
    Leishmaniasis 234
Malnutrition, Parasitic Infections, and Immunity 235
Effects of Macronutrient and Micronutrient Deficiencies on Parasitic Infections 236

Protein–Energy Malnutrition 236
Micronutrients 236
   Zinc Deficiency and Parasitic Infections 236
   Selenium Deficiency and Parasitic Infections 237
   VAD and Parasitic Infections 237
Nutritional Interventional Programs and Parasitic Infections 237
Conclusions 238
References 238

GLOBAL BURDEN OF PARASITIC INFECTIONS

Nearly a third of the world's population, 2 billion people, are infected with soil-transmitted helminths, which include >270 million preschool and >600 million school-aged children [1]. Parasitic infections are widespread throughout the tropics and subtropics, particularly in developing countries where social and economic deprivation, poor hygienic conditions, malnutrition, and warm climates favor the spread of intestinal parasites. Infection with multiple parasite species (polyparasitism) also occurs not uncommonly [2]. Parasite infections contribute to malabsorption and chronic blood loss and, in children, lead to long-term effects on physical and cognitive development [3–5]. Malnutrition makes children more vulnerable to intestinal parasites, which in turn leads to even worse nutritional status, creating a synergistic relation that impairs growth and development. Young children are a

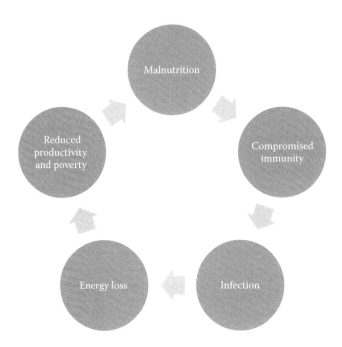

FIGURE 9.1 Relation between malnutrition, energy loss, and infection. (Modified from Schaible, U.E. and S.H. Kaufmann, *PLoS Med*, 4, e115, 2007.)

TABLE 9.1

Major Parasitic Diseases, Their Global Prevalence, and Potential Mechanisms of Nutritional Impairment

Illness	Parasitic Agent	Prevalence/Incidence	Disease Manifestations That Lead to Nutritional Impairment
		Protozoa	
Amoebiasis [6]	*Entamoeba histolytica*	Up to 100 million infections/year	Dysentery, colitis
Giardiasis [7–10]	*Giardia lamblia*	2%–7% of the population in developed and 20%–30% in developing countries	Acute and chronic diarrhea, steatorrhea, leading to fat and fat-soluble-vitamin malabsorption
Malaria [11–14]	*Plasmodium vivax, Plasmodium falciparum, Plasmodium ovale, Plasmodium malariae*	~200 million episodes of infection and ~600,000 deaths	Anorexia, fever, vomiting, hypercatabolic state, and anemia
Leishmaniasis [15–17]	*Leishmania donovani*	1.3 million new cases annually	Loss of appetite, asthenia, diarrhea
Trypanosomiasis [1]	*Trypanosoma cruzi*	8 million infected worldwide	Dilation of digestive tract (megaesophagus, megacolon) leading to dysphagia/odynophagia
		Soil-Transmitted Nematodes	
Ascariasis [18–20]	*Ascaris lumbricoides* (roundworm)	1.2 billion prevalence	Malabsorption of nutrients, vitamin A and C deficiency, bile duct obstruction, cholangitis and pancreatitis
Trichuriasis [21–23]	*Trichuris trichiura* (whipworm)	604 million prevalence	Heavy infections: dysentery, mild chronic form: growth retardation, asymptomatic infection: subtle impairment of nutritional status
Hookworm [23–25]	*Necator americanus, Ancylostoma duodenale*	576 million prevalence	Intestinal blood loss: iron deficiency and microcytic hypochromic anemia, intestinal inflammation
Strongyloidiasis [1,23]	*Strongyloides stercoralis* (thread worm)	30–100 million prevalence	Diarrhea, intestinal malabsorption

(continued)

TABLE 9.1 (Continued)
Major Parasitic Diseases, Their Global Prevalence, and Potential
Mechanisms of Nutritional Impairment

Illness	Parasitic Agent	Prevalence/Incidence	Disease Manifestations That Lead to Nutritional Impairment
Filarial Nematodes			
Lymphatic filariasis [1,23]	*Wuchereria bancrofti, Brugia malayi*	120 million prevalence	Fever, anorexia
Onchocerciasis (river blindness) [1,23]	*Onchocerca volvulus*	37 million prevalence	Blindness, skin nodules, and debilitating itching
Loiasis [23]	*Loa loa*	13 million prevalence	Local inflammation and Calabar swellings
Dracunculiasis [23]	*Dracunculus medinensis* (guinea worm)	0.01 million prevalence	Local inflammation and secondary joint disease
Platyhelminth Flukes/Trematodes			
Schistosomiasis [23]	*Schistosoma haematobium, Schistosoma mansoni, Schistosoma japonicum* (blood flukes)	207 million prevalence	Abdominal pain, diarrhea, bloody stools, intestinal inflammation, rarely hematuria
Food-borne trematodiases [1]	*Clonorchis sinensis* (liver fluke), *Paragonimus* spp. (lung flukes), *Fasciolopsis buski* (intestinal fluke)	56 million prevalence	Systemic inflammation and intestinal malabsorption
Platyhelminth Tapeworms/Cestodes			
Cysticercosis [1]	*Taenia solium* (pork tapeworm)	14–35 million prevalence	Diarrhea, nausea, abdominal pain

particularly vulnerable subset of patients given their underdeveloped immune systems. The relation between malnutrition, infections, and altered immune status is depicted in Figure 9.1 [26]. Commonly encountered parasitic infections and potential mechanisms of nutritional impairment are shown in Table 9.1.

GLOBAL BURDEN OF MALNUTRITION

According to World Health Organization (WHO) estimates in 2010, about 104 million children worldwide are underweight and undernutrition contributes to about one-third of all childhood deaths [27]. Malnutrition is responsible in some way for a little more than half (54%) of the 10.8 million deaths per year in children < 5 years old [28,29]. The four most important forms of malnutrition worldwide are discussed below.

PROTEIN–ENERGY MALNUTRITION (PEM)

In 2000, the WHO estimated that malnourished children numbered 181.9 million (32%) in developing countries, with about half the children in south-central Asia and Central Africa having growth retardation due to PEM.

IRON DEFICIENCY ANEMIA (IDA)

In developing countries, IDA may affect about 43% of women, 34% of men, and around 40% of school-aged children.

VITAMIN A DEFICIENCY (VAD)

Clinical VAD affects at least 2.8 million preschool children in >60 countries, and subclinical VAD is considered a problem for at least 251 million [30].

IODINE DEFICIENCY DISORDERS (IDD)

According to WHO estimates, >740 million people worldwide have iodine deficiency goiter [31]. IDD is the single most important preventable cause of brain damage. Salt iodization is currently the most widely used strategy to control and eliminate IDD.

MALARIA AND NUTRITION

INTRODUCTION

Malaria is one of the oldest and the most prevalent parasitic disease of humans. Malaria is caused by the *Plasmodia* species and is transmitted by the bite of female anopheles mosquitoes. The four *Plasmodia* species that infect human beings are *Plasmodium falciparum*, *P. vivax*, *P. malariae*, and *P. ovale*, of which *P. falciparum* and *P. vivax* cause the majority of infections and *P. falciparum* is responsible for most deaths. Malaria remains a significant cause of mortality and morbidity worldwide (Figure 9.2). The most severe cases of malaria are due to *P. falciparum* infection. The significance of malarial disease can be recognized by the fact that there were an estimated 216 million clinical episodes of infestation in 2010 and approximately 655,000 deaths. Most of the deaths related to malaria (86%) were in children [11].

NUTRITION

Nutrition plays a pivotal role in health, and malnutrition increases the susceptibility to a large number of infectious diseases [32–35]. Children and pregnant women,

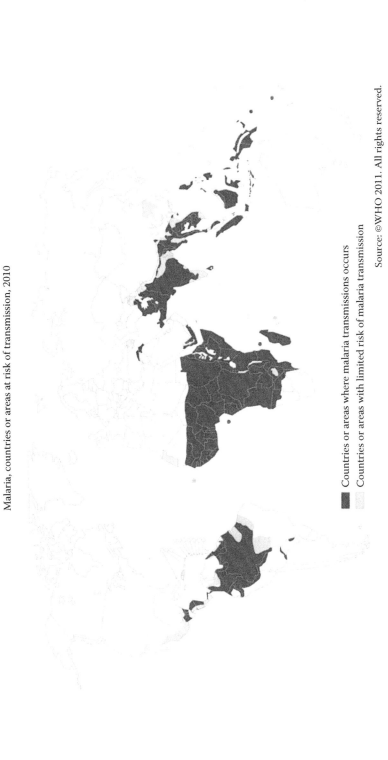

Malaria, countries or areas at risk of transmission, 2010

■ Countries or areas where malaria transmissions occurs

  Countries or areas with limited risk of malaria transmission

FIGURE 9.2 (**See color insert.**) Areas of high incidence of malaria. Note: This map is intended as a visual aid only and not as a definitive source of information about malaria endemicity. (From Global Malaria Programme: Information for travellers, 2011. Available at http://www.who.int/malaria/travellers/en/.)

who are typically affected by undernutrition, share the greatest burden of malarial illness [11]. On the basis of the prevalence of malnutrition published by the WHO, the regions with the highest prevalence of undernutrition are also the areas with a high incidence of malaria [36,37]. The interaction between malnutrition and malaria may contribute to a significant proportion of the disease burden globally. Despite malnutrition and malaria being major public health problems, there is a relative paucity of studies directly examining the influence of nutrition on the malarial burden. Although it seems intuitive that undernutrition increases the burden of malaria, studies over the last several decades have shown that the interaction between malaria and nutrition is not straightforward. This interrelation between malnutrition and malaria is generally viewed as synergistic, although several reports from the past have pointed to the contrary. Early studies showed a protective role of undernutrition [38–41], and recent studies indicate a decrease in malarial illness from nutritional supplementation [42–46]. A better understanding of the interplay between malaria and nutrition will improve our control strategies against this ancient enemy. In this chapter, we will explore the complex linkages between malaria and host nutritional status through a review of relevant studies conducted in animals and humans.

MALARIA—CASE DEFINITIONS

An important and very relevant end point in any clinical malaria study is to look for reduction in clinical episodes of malaria. However, precise definition of clinical malaria in research studies is difficult primarily for two reasons: (i) malarial symptoms are nonspecific and (ii) the incidence of parasitemia is high in asymptomatic population in endemic areas. The optimal definition of clinical malaria may differ with the age of the population and the geographical site, which makes it difficult to compare studies done in areas with different levels of malaria transmission [47–49].

A malarial episode is often defined as fever (axillary temperature $\geq 37.5°C$) with parasitemia (any level of parasite density). However, the case definition of malaria in studies has not been consistent. In some studies, malaria has been loosely defined as the mere presence of fever without microscopic confirmation of the malarial parasite. The distinction between mild and severe malaria is also not consistent; however, the case definition of severe malaria usually encompasses one of the clinical syndromes:

  i. Malaria with impaired consciousness (cerebral malaria)
 ii. Malaria with respiratory distress (severe anemia, pulmonary edema)
iii. Malaria with organ dysfunction (hypotension, severe jaundice, renal failure)

IMPACT OF PEM ON MALARIA

The interaction between nutrition and infection was recognized only after the 1950s. Quantitative and qualitative changes to host nutritional status can have significant influence on the dynamics of infectious diseases [50]. Pioneering studies by Scrimshaw and several others laid emphasis on the fact that the host nutritional status is as important as the infectious agent in influencing the course of a disease process [51–53]. Evidence from both animal and human studies has shown that the interplay of malaria and malnutrition is complex, and comprehending this complexity enhances our understanding of the disease process and implementation of intervention strategies.

EVIDENCE FROM ANIMAL STUDIES

Early animal experiments made an interesting conclusion that PEM has a protective effect on the severity of malarial illness. Monkeys and rats fed a protein-restricted diet were noted to have less *Plasmodium knowlesi* and *P. berghei* parasitemia [54–56]. A mechanistic insight on how malnutrition confers protection to malarial infection was suggested in studies of murine malaria. Malarial parasites were shown to inflict oxidative damage to infected erythrocytes [57]. It is likely that this oxidant stress is enhanced by the accompanying deficiency of antioxidants due to poor nutritional intake. This potentially could lead to enhanced lysis of infected cells, leading to parasite death and protection from the disease [58]. The above phenomenon was complemented by a study where vitamin E-deficient diet exerted a pronounced suppressive effect against the malarial parasite [59]. A recent study demonstrated that inhibition of α-*TTP* gene, responsible for regulation of host vitamin E concentration, resulted in resistance to malarial infection [60].

Despite the evidence that protein-restricted animals experienced less malarial morbidity and mortality, infected animals had impaired ability to clear infection [61], depressed cell-mediated immunity [62], and a strong relapse reaction [56]. Some studies also showed increased mortality in severely malnourished young rats [56]. In a recent study from Cornet et al., the influence of host nutritional status on infection dynamics and parasite virulence in a bird–malaria system was determined. Replication of the avian malaria parasite *Plasmodium relictum* was controlled well in hosts (canaries) who received a supplemented diet (protein and vitamin) and the avian populations exposed to reduced food availability were more susceptible to malaria parasites [63].

EVIDENCE FROM HUMAN STUDIES

Similar to animal studies, early human studies suggested a protective effect of malnutrition on malarial morbidity and mortality. The evidence came largely from autopsy reports and case–control studies [38,64]. Several aspects of these studies had methodological limitations such as lack of healthy control population for comparison, incomplete data analyses, lack of information on comorbid factors like socioeconomic status, and poor description of malnourished status of the study population [65]. Some of the early studies, which were conducted in famine environments, noted an increase in *P. falciparum* episodes in the postfamine refeeding phase [39,66]. It is possible that the biology of the famine-stricken population was different from the nonfamine-afflicted population with chronic malnutrition.

Studies exploring the association between malaria and growth in humans have shown inconsistent results. Several studies done in Africa indicate that malnutrition predisposes to infection [67–70]. In these studies, malnourished children were also reported to have increased mortality or neurologic sequelae when compared with normally nourished malarial patients. However, other studies found no association [71,72], lower risk of malaria in severely stunted children [73], or a greater risk of malaria in children with better height-for-age z-scores [74]. As part of a large cross-sectional study in the remote northern Ghana region, two cross-sectional surveys, one in the rainy season and the other in the dry season, involving ~2000 children showed that being underweight increased the risk of malaria by approximately 70% [75].

A prospective study conducted in rural Gambia noted that 51% of stunted children at baseline (chronic undernutrition) had increased episodes of *P. falciparum* infection when compared with 38% of children who were not stunted (relative risk [RR] 1.35) [76]. In this study, wasting (weight-for-height z-score < 2 SD) and undernutrition (weight-for-age z-score < 2 SD) were not associated with malaria. A prospective study conducted in Uganda also showed a strong association between malaria and stunting [13]. In a study done in children aged 6–30 months in Burkina Faso, mortality was significantly associated with both acute malnutrition (wasting) and chronic malnutrition (stunting) but an association between malaria and malnutrition could not be demonstrated [77]. Several hospital-based studies conducted in Gambia [35], Madagascar [78], Nigeria [64], Tanzania [79], and Ghana [80] showed increased case-fatality rates in malnourished children admitted with severe falciparum malaria when compared with well-nourished children with severe malaria. A similar conclusion was derived after a systematic review of all cohort and case–control studies done through a MEDLINE search by the WHO [33].

In 2004, an analysis was conducted for the WHO Comparative Risk Assessment project on data that related undernutrition and mortality from diarrhea, pneumonia, measles, and malaria [37]. Two cohort studies that were relevant to malaria were identified by a search of existing literature. The pooled relative risk for malaria among children having weight-for-age < 2 SDs was increased but statistically nonsignificant (RR 1.31, 95% confidence interval [95% CI] 0.92–1.88). The pooled relative risk estimate for malarial mortality among children having weight-for-age < 3 SDs was 9.5. From the pooled estimates, the investigators estimated that 549,200 malarial deaths were secondary to undernutrition [14]. Kang et al. used a combination of Mendelian randomization with the sickle cell trait and matched control subjects for confounders in determining the influence of stunting on malaria [81]. This study noted that before controlling for confounding variables, for every malarial episode, the risk of stunting increased by only 0.02 (weak association), whereas after controlling for confounding variables, the risk increased to 0.32 (p = .004, 95% CI 0.09–1), indicating a strong association between stunting and malaria. Not accounting for the effect of the sickle cell trait and other confounders may have influenced other investigators in their inability to detect the association between stunting and malaria [71,72]. Overall, reappraisal of old data together with a review of recent literature indicates that, in many instances, undernutrition increases host susceptibility to malarial infection and increases mortality.

IMPACT OF MALARIA ON PEM

Malaria affects the host nutritional status adversely. Malarial symptoms, namely fever, vomiting, and anorexia characteristic of malaria, lead to decreased food intake. A hypercatabolic state is created by the infection resulting in negative nitrogen balance. A study compared nutritional parameters in malaria-infected patients with healthy volunteers who had a history of malaria in the Amazon region of South America. The study showed that *P. falciparum*-infected patients had a markedly worse nutritional status and decreased serum total protein, albumin, and transferrin [82]. Randomized controlled trials conducted in Gambia and Kenya showed that by controlling malarial transmission by using insecticide (permethrin)-treated bed nets, nutritional status was improved not only in malnourished but also in nonmalnourished children [83,84].

Multiple studies done recently have looked at the impact of malaria in pregnancy and fetal growth. A study done on pregnant mothers showed that *P. falciparum* parasitemia in primigravida before 20 weeks' gestation increases the risk of intrauterine fetal growth restriction by 4-fold when compared with multigravida without early pregnancy malaria parasitemia [85]. Several other studies looking at pregnancy-associated malaria drew similar conclusions [86–89]. Overall, the evidence clearly indicates a negative influence of malaria on the nutritional status of the host.

MALARIA, NUTRITION, AND IMMUNITY

Malnutrition per se affects all arms of the immune system, resulting in increased susceptibility to infection (Figure 9.3). The mechanisms involved include impairment of cell-mediated immunity, humoral immunity, complement system and phagocyte function, and alteration of anatomical barriers and intestinal flora [27]. Human studies report impaired capacity of malnourished children to mount an immune response when exposed to pathogens. Micronutrient deficiencies such as zinc deficiency accompanying PEM have been shown to alter functioning of B and T cells, thus resulting in impaired immune function [90].

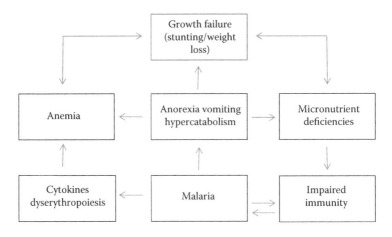

FIGURE 9.3 Interrelation between malnutrition, malaria, and immunity.

Malarial infection affects both cell-mediated immunity and humoral immunity. Thymic atrophy, which results in impaired T-lymphocyte production, is implicated in the pathogenesis of malarial infection [91]. Humoral immune responses, which play a vital role in naturally acquired immunity to malaria, has also been shown to be altered by direct interaction of the parasite with B cells [92]. A study done on peripheral blood mononuclear cells (PBMCs) of children showed that prior malarial infection suppresses the Th2 (regulatory) responses to the disease. In this study, micronutrient deficiencies, such as zinc and iron, have been shown to be associated with a hyperinflammatory state characterized by elevated proinflammatory cytokines [93]. It is well known that cerebral malaria is associated with a proinflammatory state. There is abundant evidence that malnutrition decreases the resistance to infection and malaria impairs immune function, which in turn increases the susceptibility to other infections. However, the mechanisms behind this effect are yet to be well characterized. A simplified view of the interaction between malaria, malnutrition, and immunity is shown in Figure 9.3.

MICRONUTRIENTS AND MALARIA

PEM is associated with multiple micronutrient deficiencies. Table 9.2 depicts the consequences of common micronutrient deficiencies with respect to malarial illness.

IMPACT OF NUTRIENT-BASED INTERVENTIONS ON MALARIA

Nutrient-based interventions have focused predominantly on four micronutrients thus far. A brief overview of the studies conducted on micronutrient supplementation is shown in Table 9.3.

TABLE 9.2
Influence of Micronutrient Deficiency on Malarial Illness

Deficiency	Potential Mechanism	Malarial Morbidity	References
Zinc	Impairs cellular and humoral immunity	Increased	[94]
Vitamin A	Depresses phagocytosis, lack of inhibition of proinflammatory cytokine response	Increased	[95,96]
Iron	Deprives iron, an essential nutrient for the parasite, impairs immune response	May decrease	[97,98]
Folate	Unclear. Increases susceptibility to malaria	Increased	[99]
Thiamin	Metabolic acidosis that could worsen the severity of malaria	Increased	[100,101]
Riboflavin	Accentuates oxidative state, which likely results in destruction of the parasite	Decreased	[102]
Vitamin E	Unbalanced oxidative state results in destruction of the parasite	Decreased	[103,104]

TABLE 9.3

Micronutrient Supplementation Trials in Malarial Endemic Regions

Supplementation	Study	Subjects	Effect of Supplementation	References
Zinc	RCT	Children	~30% reduction in health center visits for malaria in two of three studies. No difference in one study	[43,105,106]
Vitamin A	RCT	Children	Decrease in symptomatic malarial episodes, less splenomegaly, lower parasite density	[107,108]
Iron	PCT	Children, adults	Increased malarial episodes	[109,110]
	Review		Review of 13 studies: No worse outcomes with substantial reduction in anemia with mild worsening of malariometric indices and clinical malaria	[111]
Folate	RCT	Children, pregnant mothers	High-dose folic acid (2.5–5 mg) when given with sulfadoxine–pyrimethamine resulted in malarial treatment failure. No adverse effect at low doses. Standard folic acid supplements unlikely to affect malaria cure.	[112–114]

Note: PCT, placebo-controlled trials; RCT, randomized double-blind placebo-controlled trials.

PARASITIC INFECTIONS OTHER THAN MALARIA AND HUMAN NUTRITION

Parasitic infections are frequent worldwide, and it is estimated that nearly 48% of the world's population is infected with one of the intestinal nematodes [115]. *Ascaris lumbricoides*, *Trichuris trichiura*, and the hookworms cause the most impact on the population especially in children [116]. In 1968, the WHO published a monograph to define changes in the severity of infections in the nutritionally deprived host [117]. Interestingly, while in most of the studies reviewed (325) malnutrition was found to increase the severity of disease, in 93 studies the opposite was true, and in 66 studies there was no apparent difference in the severity of disease as related to nutritional deficiency. The authors concluded that interactions may be synergistic (preexisting malnutrition lowered resistance to infection, thereby worsening severity) or antagonistic. A systematic review on the impact of nematode infections in children concluded that treatment of infected children leads to better growth and development [118]. However, the improvement in growth may also depend on local epidemiology and supplementation of deficient macronutrients and micronutrients. We will focus our chapter on the important nematodes mentioned previously and on giardiasis, amoebiasis, and leishmaniasis. We intend to discuss the nutritional effects of the above parasitic infections on the host and vice versa.

NEMATODES

Of these, three soil-transmitted helminthes (*A. lumbricoides*, *T. trichiura*, and the hookworms [e.g., *Necator americanus* and *Ancylostoma duodenale*]) are the most prevalent nematode infections.

Hookworm

Patients with hookworm infection are usually asymptomatic; however, chronic infection may lead to hypochromic microcytic anemia, while heavy infection may cause hypoproteinemia and edema [24]. Chronic intestinal blood loss resulting from the feeding habits of hookworms has long been recognized as a major contributing factor to the IDA seen in these patients. Many of the world's cases of IDA occur in countries where hookworms are endemic [25]. Current estimates indicate that from 30 to 44 million pregnant women may harbor hookworms [119]. Sixteen percent to 20% of maternal deaths are complicated by IDA in the developing world, including India [120]. The incidence of premature deliveries in severely anemic women can be three times that in nonanemic women. Low birth weight (<2 kg) is frequently observed in babies of anemic mothers [119].

Hookworm infections are known to impair host immune responses by (i) reducing mitogen-mediated lymphocyte proliferation, (ii) impairing antigen-presenting pathways, and (iii) reducing CD4$^+$ T cells in the spleen and mesenteric lymph nodes. Animal studies reveal a 3-fold higher mean intestinal worm burden and more severe anemia in CD4-depleted hosts. The CD4 cell depletion, in turn, impairs humoral (serum and mucosal) immune responses to hookworm antigens [17,121].

Ascariasis

Recent data suggest that >1.2 billion people are infected globally [18,20]. While acute symptoms are typically due to the larval form and tend to involve the lungs, the chronic disease (by the adult worm) causes abdominal distension, pain, nausea, and diarrhea. Rarely, entangled adult worms lead to mechanical intestinal obstruction (0.005–2 per 1000 infections per year). There has been much debate about the improvement in growth parameters in patients treated with antihelminthic drugs. The results of 10 longitudinal studies comparing the growth of children infected with *A. lumbricoides* treated with antihelminthic drugs were reviewed and found to have significant improvements in weight and height in most cases [18]. Another meta-analysis of around 30 randomized controlled trials showed positive albeit inconsistent results [122]. Jejunal biopsies of *Ascaris*-infected children revealed abnormalities including shortened villi, elongated crypts, a decrease in the villus/crypt ratio, and cellular infiltration of the lamina propria [123]. Preschool children with *Ascaris* infection produce significantly more breath hydrogen after a lactose load than uninfected children, and the lactose tolerance returned to normal about 3 weeks after treatment [124]. Several clinical studies have shown that absorption of an oral dose of vitamin A was lower in *Ascaris*-infected children compared with uninfected controls. Impaired vitamin A absorption may be related to the effects of infection on fat absorption [125].

Trichuriasis

The prevalence of *T. trichiura* in children is particularly high (up to 95%) in parts of the world where PEM and anemia are prevalent and access to medical care is limited. The *Trichuris* dysentery syndrome is characterized by chronic dysentery, anemia, and poor growth, and, in many cases, severe stunting and cognitive deficits. The severe stunting is likely to be a reaction partly due to a chronic inflammatory response and concomitant decreases in plasma insulin-like growth factor-1, increases in tumor necrosis factor-α (TNF-α) in the lamina propria of the colonic mucosa and peripheral blood (which likely decrease appetite and intake of all nutrients), and a decrease in collagen synthesis [22].

GIARDIASIS

In addition to being a significant cause of diarrheal disease worldwide, giardiasis can also lead to malnutrition and cognitive deficits in children in developing countries [126]. A cross-sectional study conducted in primary-school children in Malaysia revealed a statistically significant association of giardiasis with low serum retinol levels (odds ratio [OR] 2.7, 95% CI 1.3–5.5) [7]. A cross-sectional study in northwest Mexico conducted in schoolchildren with similar z-scores for nutritional indices and similar mean daily vitamin A intake found that *Giardia*-infected children were more likely to be vitamin A deficient than *Giardia*-free children (OR 3.2, 95% CI 1.2–8.5) [127]. Another study found that giardiasis may be a risk factor for zinc deficiency in schoolchildren in northwestern Mexico [9].

AMOEBIASIS

A large prospective observational study of amoebiasis conducted in an urban slum in Dhaka, Bangladesh, found a decrease of interferon-γ (IFN-γ) accompanied by an increase in IL-5 production in PBMCs in malnourished children. They found that *Entamoeba histolytica* was negatively associated with growth in the 3-year observational period. They suggested that malnutrition may in fact have predisposed the children to amoebiasis by suppressing the normally protective cell-mediated response. This study revealed a positive correlation of PBMC production of IFN-γ and height-associated z-scores and weight-associated z-scores [6].

LEISHMANIASIS

A murine model revealed that malnourished mice that were fed protein-, iron-, and zinc-deficient diets and inoculated with *Leishmania chagasi* had lower liver and spleen weights, higher parasite loads, and lower serum glucose and protein concentrations. These data suggest that malnutrition alters the immune response to *L. chagasi* infection in this model [128].

MALNUTRITION, PARASITIC INFECTIONS, AND IMMUNITY

The immune system is an intricate, highly complex system of cell–cell interactions, feedback pathways, control signals, and memory properties. In addition to its humoral and cell-mediated arms, it relies on a number of additional factors such as complement, lymphokines, cytokines, phagocytic cells, and hormones. The syntheses of these molecules require DNA replication, RNA expression, protein synthesis, and secretion. These pathways require additional energy and a constant supply of building blocks that would be provided by an optimum nutritional status. It would be safe to say that the nutritional status of the host determines outcomes of infection. The immune impairment in the face of macronutrient and micronutrient deficiency is shown in Tables 9.4 and 9.5, respectively.

TABLE 9.4
Immune Impairment in Macronutrient Deficiency

Form of Malnutrition	Mechanism of Immune Impairment
Acute PEM	Phagocytosis, RNI, ROI, antigen presentation, T-cell activation, T-cell memory, antibody titers (IgG, IgA), cytokine secretion, leptin levels, macrophage activation
Chronic PEM	Thymic development, T-cell differentiation, T-cell expansion, T-cell memory, IgA, IgG, complement, leptin levels decreased, macrophage activation
Overnutrition	Permanent preactivation of leukocytes, increased TNF-α/IFN-γ, suppressed NK cell and T-cell activation, reduced phagocytosis, increased leptin concentrations with relative leptin resistance

Source: Schaible, U.E. and S.H. Kaufmann, *PLoS Med*, 4, p. e115, 2007.
Note: RNI, reactive nitrogen intermediate; ROI, reactive oxygen intermediate.

TABLE 9.5
Immune Impairment in Micronutrient Deficiency

Micronutrient	Immune Impairment from Deficiency
Vitamin A	Deficit of retinol for acute phase reactants
Vitamin C	Impaired T-lymphocyte response, delayed cutaneous hypersensitivity, impaired complement function, reduced phagocytic function
Vitamin E	Impaired T-cell response, impaired B-cell function and humoral response, impaired cytokine function, reduced phagocytic function, delayed cutaneous hypersensitivity
Copper	Possible involvement of acute phase response to infection
Iron	Impaired T-cell response, impaired B-cell function and humoral response, impaired cytokine function, reduced phagocytic function, delayed cutaneous hypersensitivity
Selenium	Impairment of both cellular and humoral immune responses
Zinc	Impaired T-cell response, impaired B-cell function and humoral response, impaired cytokine function, reduced phagocytic function, delayed cutaneous hypersensitivity

Malnourished hosts may have reduced lymphocyte counts in Peyer's patches and reduced immunoglobulin A (IgA) secretion that facilitate parasitic infestations [129]. IL-4 production, expansion of eosinophils, and IgE secretion are some of the Th2-type protective T-cell responses against helminth infections. However, malnourished children are deficient for protective IgE antibodies against *A. lumbricoides* [130,131]. While the concentrations of total IgE in malnourished children with helminth infections are high, the antibodies are neither worm specific nor protective. Moreover, their memory T cells do not recognize helminth antigens [132].

EFFECTS OF MACRONUTRIENT AND MICRONUTRIENT DEFICIENCIES ON PARASITIC INFECTIONS

PROTEIN–ENERGY MALNUTRITION

PEM is the most common cause of human secondary immunodeficiency ("nutritional immunodeficiency") [133,134]. Diarrheal diseases in malnourished individuals, especially children, further exacerbate the problem by decreasing nutrient uptake. Severe protein malnutrition in children has been shown to be associated with atrophy of the thymus and poorly developed peripheral lymphoid organs (lymph nodes and spleen). This may lead to leukopenia, decreased CD4/CD8 ratio, decreased functional T-cell numbers, and the appearance of immature T cells in the circulation. As the structure and function of this organ are diminished, so is the memory T-cell response to antigens [135]. PEM is a major determinant of both progression and severity of visceral leishmaniasis and greatly increases the case-fatality rate [15,16,136,137]. In a study to assess the influence of nutrition on the outcome of *Leishmania* infection, a decrease in body mass index and mid-upper arm circumference by age z-scores for children with the disease was observed [138]. PEM in individuals with visceral leishmaniasis has been associated with increased risk of in-hospital morbidity, mortality, increased length of hospital stay, increased cost, and use of health-care resources [17].

MICRONUTRIENTS

Several trace elements (iron, zinc, and selenium) serve to modulate immune function, thereby influencing host susceptibility to infection.

Zinc Deficiency and Parasitic Infections

Studies conducted in a zinc-deficient, nematode-infected mouse model revealed that parasites are better able to survive in zinc-deficient hosts than in well-nourished hosts. A decrease in the splenic production of IL-4, decrease in levels of IgE, IgG_1, and eosinophils, and impaired T-cell and antigen-presenting cell function were noted in zinc-deficient hosts. Prolonged parasite infection results in suppressed local gut mucosa and systemic immune systems due to a combination of zinc deficiency and energy restriction [139]. Both Th1 and Th2 responses were impaired in zinc-deficient mice infected with nematodes [139]. Other studies have shown that *Trypanosoma cruzi* and zinc deficiency interact synergistically to increase mortality (80% vs. 10%) and overwhelmingly increase parasitemia in zinc-deficient mice as compared with control mice [134].

Selenium Deficiency and Parasitic Infections

Significant amounts of selenium are found in the liver, spleen, and lymph nodes, and its deficiency can lead to the impairment of both cellular and humoral immune responses [140]. Moreover, selenium has immune-stimulant properties that include enhanced clonal expansion and natural killer cell activity to antigen stimulation [141]. Beneficial effects of selenium supplementation have been reported in murine models, and increasing severity of *T. cruzi* has been associated with chronic inflammatory myopathy in the selenium-deficient state [142].

VAD and Parasitic Infections

The available evidence indicates a beneficial effect of vitamin A supplementation on intestinal integrity in children with severe infections or undernutrition. This might explain the decreased risk of mortality and morbidity from some forms of diarrhea in vitamin A-supplemented preschool children [143]. T-cell immunocompetence can be affected by VAD at various levels, including lymphopoiesis, distribution, expression of surface molecules, and cytokine production [143]. Maciel et al. demonstrated lower levels of vitamin A (serum retinol) in children with active visceral leishmaniasis [138].

NUTRITIONAL INTERVENTIONAL PROGRAMS AND PARASITIC INFECTIONS

An intervention study conducted in western India, aimed at school-going, 8–12-year-old children, evaluated the effect of deworming alone vs. deworming and weekly iron–folic acid (IFA) supplementation on growth, hemoglobin level, and physical work capacity of their subjects. As compared with only deworming medication, deworming + IFA supplementation was more effective in increasing the hemoglobin levels of the children, with 65% of the children converting to a nonanemic status after IFA + deworming supplementation [144]. Another study examining the relation of intestinal parasite treatment and oral supplementation for iodine deficiency revealed that intestinal parasites interfered with absorption, thereby reducing the efficacy of oral iodine supplementation [145].

The most recent Cochrane database review examining the effects of deworming drugs for soil-transmitted intestinal worms on nutritional indicators, hemoglobin, and school performance in children showed marked variability in results [146]. While treating only infected children with a single dose of deworming medication may have increased weight and hemoglobin, cognitive function appeared unchanged. The Cochrane review concluded that there was a lack of good-quality data to determine the effect of deworming on cognitive function. In a recent review, Bundy et al. eloquently assessed some of the challenges in interpreting studies incorporating the impact of deworming on nutritional status within the context of a Cochrane review and makes the case for sources of evidence other than traditional medical trials that document the benefits of deworming [147].

A 12-month longitudinal study conducted with 2–5-year-old Bangladeshi children showed that while treatment with mebendazole reduced the prevalence of *A. lumbricoides*, *T. trichiura*, and hookworm infections, no significant difference in growth or intestinal permeability or plasma albumin were observed after deworming [8]. In fact, significant decreases in total protein (p < .001) and α1-antichymotrypsin (p < .001) were observed in the treatment group, indicating possible reductions in inflammation and immunoglobulin concentration after deworming.

A double-blind placebo-controlled trial to evaluate the effect of vitamin A and zinc supplementation on gastrointestinal infections and growth among 584 infants aged 5–15 months was conducted in Mexico City. Infants aged 5–15 months were assigned to receive either a vitamin A supplement every 2 months (20,000 IU of retinol for infants ≤ 1 year or 45,000 IU for infants > 1 year), a daily supplement of 20 mg of zinc, a combined vitamin A–zinc supplement, or a placebo, and were followed for 1 year. Vitamin A- and zinc-supplemented children infected with any parasite and zinc-supplemented children infected with either *A. lumbricoides* or *Giarda duodenalis* had significantly lower growth than did noninfected children. It was concluded that gastrointestinal parasite infections may modify the effect that zinc or vitamin A supplementation has on childhood growth [10].

CONCLUSIONS

Parasitic infections, including malaria and soil-transmitted helminthic infections, significantly impair the nutritional status of the infected population. Parasitic infections impair growth and cognitive function, and deworming programs improve growth and possibly cognitive function. Interventions to prevent parasitic infections, such as deworming, are feasible, have a favorable cost–benefit ratio, and are paramount in improving the health of the community as a whole. Coupled with targeted nutritional supplemental programs, a great deal can be achieved in terms of productivity and health of the population in endemic areas. Nutrition plays a seminal role in modulating the morbidity and mortality resulting from malarial and parasitic infections. Despite the complex interrelation between nutrition and parasitic infestations, overall the evidence emphasizes that malnutrition and specific micronutrient deficiencies exacerbate malaria and other parasitic infections and vice versa. The limited clinical trials done on micronutrient supplementation, especially vitamin A and zinc, suggest that improving specific nutrition deficiencies by nutrition intervention programs is highly warranted. Nutritional programs should be coupled with general preventative strategies, such as provision of clean drinking water, sanitary facilities, better housing, mosquito nets, and measures to eliminate poverty to combat these debilitating diseases. It is paramount that the impact of these interventions is assessed periodically and systematically.

REFERENCES

1. WHO, Neglected tropical diseases: PCT databank. Geneva: World Health Organization, 2010. Available from: http://www.who.int/neglected_diseases/preventive_chemotherapy/databank/en/.
2. Pullan, R. and S. Brooker, The health impact of polyparasitism in humans: Are we under-estimating the burden of parasitic diseases? *Parasitology*, 2008. 135(7): 783–94.

3. Balci, Y.I. et al., The distribution of intestinal parasites among children in Denizli. *Turkiye Parazitol Derg*, 2009. 33(4): 298–300.
4. Koroma, J.B. et al., Geographical distribution of intestinal schistosomiasis and soil-transmitted helminthiasis and preventive chemotherapy strategies in Sierra Leone. *PLoS Negl Trop Dis*, 2010. 4(11): e891.
5. Pezzani, B.C. et al., Community participation in the control of intestinal parasitoses at a rural site in Argentina. *Rev Panam Salud Pub*, 2009. 26(6): 471–7.
6. Petri, W.A., Jr. et al., Association of malnutrition with amoebiasis. *Nutr Rev*, 2009. 67 Suppl 2: S207–15.
7. Al-Mekhlafi, H.M. et al., Giardiasis and poor vitamin A status among aboriginal school children in rural Malaysia. *Am J Trop Med Hyg*, 2010. 83(3): 523–7.
8. Northrop-Clewes, C.A. et al., Anthelmintic treatment of rural Bangladeshi children: Effect on host physiology, growth, and biochemical status. *Am J Clin Nutr*, 2001. 73(1): 53–60.
9. Quihui, L. et al., Could giardiasis be a risk factor for low zinc status in schoolchildren from northwestern Mexico? A cross-sectional study with longitudinal follow-up. *BMC Public Health*, 2010. 10(1): 85.
10. Rosado, J.L. et al., Interaction of zinc or vitamin A supplementation and specific parasite infections on Mexican infants' growth: A randomized clinical trial. *Eur J Clin Nutr*, 2009. 63(10): 1176–84.
11. World Health Organization, World Malaria Report 2011. Geneva: World Health Organization, 2011.
12. Global Malaria Programme: Information for travellers, 2011. Available from: http://www.who.int/malaria/travellers/en/.
13. Arinaitwe, E. et al., The association between malnutrition and the incidence of malaria among young HIV-infected and -uninfected Ugandan children: A prospective study. *Malar J*, 2012. 11: 90.
14. Caulfield, L.E. et al., Undernutrition as an underlying cause of child deaths associated with diarrhea, pneumonia, malaria, and measles. *Am J Clin Nutr*, 2004. 80(1): 193–8.
15. Anstead, G.M. et al., Malnutrition alters the innate immune response and increases early visceralization following *Leishmania donovani* infection. *Infect Immun*, 2001. 69(8): 4709–18.
16. Cerf, B.J. et al., Malnutrition as a risk factor for severe visceral leishmaniasis. *J Infect Dis*, 1987. 156(6): 1030–3.
17. Malafaia, G., Protein–energy malnutrition as a risk factor for visceral leishmaniasis: A review. *Parasite Immunol*, 2009. 31(10): 587–96.
18. O'Lorcain, P. and C.V. Holland, The public health importance of *Ascaris lumbricoides*. *Parasitology*, 2000. 121 Suppl: S51–71.
19. Hlaing, T., Ascariasis and childhood malnutrition. *Parasitology*, 1993. 107 Suppl: S125–36.
20. Dold, C. and C.V. Holland, *Ascaris* and ascariasis. *Microbes Infect*, 2011. 13(7): 632–7.
21. Bundy, D.A. and E.S. Cooper, *Trichuris* and trichuriasis in humans. *Adv Parasitol*, 1989. 28: 107–73.
22. Stephenson, L.S., C.V. Holland, and E.S. Cooper, The public health significance of *Trichuris trichiura*. *Parasitology*, 2000. 121 Suppl: S73–95.
23. Hotez, P.J. et al., Helminth infections: The great neglected tropical diseases. *J Clin Invest*, 2008. 118(4): 1311–21.
24. AAP, Hookworm Infections, in *2012 Report of the Committee on Infectious Diseases*, L.K. Pickering et al., Editors. Elk Grove Village, IL: American Academy of Pediatrics, 2012. 411–3.
25. Pawlowski, Z.S. et al., *Hookworm Infection and Anaemia: Approaches to Prevention and Control*. Geneva: World Health Organization, 1991, 96.

26. Schaible, U.E. and S.H. Kaufmann, Malnutrition and infection: Complex mechanisms and global impacts. *PLoS Med*, 2007. 4(5): e115.
27. WHO, Nutrition: Challenges. Geneva: World Health Organization, 2013.
28. Scrimshaw, N.S. and J.P. SanGiovanni, Synergism of nutrition, infection, and immunity: An overview. *Am J Clin Nutr*, 1997. 66(2): 464S–77S.
29. Ambrus, J.L., Sr. and J.L. Ambrus, Jr., Nutrition and infectious diseases in developing countries and problems of acquired immunodeficiency syndrome. *Exp Biol Med (Maywood)*, 2004. 229(6): 464–72.
30. Stephenson, L.S., M.C. Latham, and E.A. Ottesen, Global malnutrition. *Parasitology*, 2000. 121 Suppl: S5–22.
31. World Health Organization, ICCIDD, UNICEF, Assessment of iodine deficiency disorders and monitoring their elimination, in *A Guide for Program Managers*. 2nd ed. Geneva, Switzerland: World Health Organization, 2001, 17.
32. Pelletier, D.L., E.A. Frongillo, Jr., and J.P. Habicht, Epidemiologic evidence for a potentiating effect of malnutrition on child mortality. *Am J Public Health*, 1993. 83(8): 1130–3.
33. Rice, A.L. et al., Malnutrition as an underlying cause of childhood deaths associated with infectious diseases in developing countries. *Bull World Health Organ*, 2000. 78(10): 1207–21.
34. Victora, C.G. et al., Risk factors for pneumonia among children in a Brazilian metropolitan area. *Pediatrics*, 1994. 93(6 Pt 1): 977–85.
35. Man W.D. et al., Nutritional status of children admitted to hospital with different diseases and its relationship to outcome in The Gambia, West Africa. *Trop Med Int Health*, 1998. 3(8): 678–86.
36. Gore, F.M. et al., Global burden of disease in young people aged 10–24 years: A systematic analysis. *Lancet*, 2011. 377(9783): 2093–102.
37. Fishman, S., Caulfield, L, De Onis, M., Blossner, M., Hyder, A., Mullany, L., Black, R., Childhood and maternal underweight, in Comparative Quantification of Health Risks: Global and Regional Burden of Disease Attribution to Selected Major Risk Factors, Vol. 1. Geneva, Switzerland: World Health Organization, 2004.
38. Hendrickse, R.G. et al., Malaria in early childhood. An investigation of five hundred seriously ill children in whom a "clinical" diagnosis of malaria was made on admission to the children's emergency room at University College Hospital, Ibadan. *Ann Trop Med Parasitol*, 1971. 65(1): 1–20.
39. Murray, M.J. et al., Refeeding—Malaria and hyperferraemia. *Lancet*, 1975. 1(7908): 653–4.
40. Murray, M.J. et al., The adverse effect of iron repletion on the course of certain infections. *Br Med J*, 1978. 2(6145): 1113–5.
41. Murray, M.J. et al., Diet and cerebral malaria: The effect of famine and refeeding. *Am J Clin Nutr*, 1978. 31(1): 57–61.
42. Richard, S.A. et al., Zinc and iron supplementation and malaria, diarrhea, and respiratory infections in children in the Peruvian Amazon. *Am J Trop Med Hyg*, 2006. 75(1): 126–32.
43. Shankar, A.H. et al., The influence of zinc supplementation on morbidity due to *Plasmodium falciparum*: A randomized trial in preschool children in Papua New Guinea. *Am J Trop Med Hyg*, 2000. 62(6): 663–9.
44. Shankar, A.H. et al., Effect of vitamin A supplementation on morbidity due to *Plasmodium falciparum* in young children in Papua New Guinea: A randomised trial. *Lancet*, 1999. 354(9174): 203–9.
45. Cusick, S.E. et al., Short-term effects of vitamin A and antimalarial treatment on erythropoiesis in severely anemic Zanzibari preschool children. *Am J Clin Nutr*, 2005. 82(2): 406–12.

46. Saaka, M., J. Oosthuizen, and S. Beatty, Effect of joint iron and zinc supplementation on malarial infection and anaemia. *East Afr J Public Health*, 2009. 6(1): 55–62.

47. Smith, T., J.A. Schellenberg, and R. Hayes, Attributable fraction estimates and case definitions for malaria in endemic areas. *Stat Med*, 1994. 13(22): 2345–58.

48. McGuinness, D. et al., Clinical case definitions for malaria: Clinical malaria associated with very low parasite densities in African infants. *Trans R Soc Trop Med Hyg*, 1998. 92(5): 527–31.

49. Bloland, P.B. et al., Longitudinal cohort study of the epidemiology of malaria infections in an area of intense malaria transmission II. Descriptive epidemiology of malaria infection and disease among children. *Am J Trop Med Hyg*, 1999. 60(4): 641–8.

50. Kau, A.L. et al., Human nutrition, the gut microbiome and the immune system. *Nature*, 2011. 474(7351): 327–36.

51. Arroyave, G. et al., Epidemiology and prevention of severe protein malnutrition (kwashiorkor) in Central America. *Am J Public Health Nations Health*, 1957. 47(1): 53–62.

52. Scrimshaw, N.S. and F.E. Viteri, INCAP studies of kwashiorkor and marasmus. *Food Nutr Bull*, 2010. 31(1): 34–41.

53. Gordon, J.E. and N.S. Scrimshaw, Infectious disease in the malnourished. *Med Clin North Am*, 1970. 54(6): 1495–508.

54. Tatke, M. and G. Bazaz-Malik, Brain histomorphology in protein deprived rhesus monkeys with fatal malarial infection. *Indian J Med Res*, 1989. 89: 404–10.

55. Ray, A.P., Haematological studies in simian malaria. II. Blood picture in monkeys during acute and chronic stages of *P. knowlesi* infection. *Indian J Malariol*, 1957. 11(4): 369–88.

56. Ramakrishnan, S.P., Studies on *Plasmodium berghei* N. sp. Vincke and Lips, 1948. VIII. The course of blood-induced infection in starved albino rats. *Indian J Malariol*, 1953. 7(1): 53–60.

57. Etkin, N. and J. Eaton, *Erythrocyte, Structure, and Function. Malaria Induced Erythrocyte Oxidant Sensitivity*, G. Brewer (Ed.). New York: Alan R. Liss, 1975, 219–32.

58. Eckman, J.R. et al., Role of vitamin E in regulating malaria expression. *Trans Assoc Am Physicians*, 1976. 89: 105–15.

59. Taylor, D.W. et al., Vitamin E-deficient diets enriched with fish oil suppress lethal *Plasmodium yoelii* infections in athymic and scid/bg mice. *Infect Immun*, 1997. 65(1): 197–202.

60. Herbas, M.S. et al., Alpha-tocopherol transfer protein disruption confers resistance to malarial infection in mice. *Malar J*, 2010. 9: 101.

61. Edirisinghe, J.S., E.B. Fern, and G.A. Targett, Resistance to superinfection with *Plasmodium berghei* in rats fed a protein-free diet. *Trans R Soc Trop Med Hyg*, 1982. 76(3): 382–6.

62. Bhatia, A. et al., Interactions of protein calorie malnutrition, malaria infection and immune responses. *Aust J Exp Biol Med Sci*, 1983. 61(Pt 5): 589–97.

63. Cornet, S. et al., Impact of host nutritional status on infection dynamics and parasite virulence in a bird-malaria system. *J Anim Ecol*, 2014, 83(1): 256–65.

64. Edington, G.M., Cerebral malaria in the Gold Coast African: Four autopsy reports. *Ann Trop Med Parasitol*, 1954. 48(3): 300–6.

65. Shankar, A.H., Nutritional modulation of malaria morbidity and mortality. *J Infect Dis*, 2000. 182 Suppl 1: S37–53.

66. Murray, M.J. et al., Somali food shelters in the Ogaden famine and their impact on health. *Lancet*, 1976. 1(7972): 1283–5.

67. Olumese, P.E. et al., Protein energy malnutrition and cerebral malaria in Nigerian children. *J Trop Pediatr*, 1997. 43(4): 217–9.

68. Renaudin, P., Evaluation of the nutritional status of children less than 5 years of age in Moundou, Chad: Correlations with morbidity and hospital mortality. *Med Trop (Mars)*, 1997. 57(1): 49–54.

69. Faye, O. et al., Malaria lethality in Dakar pediatric environment: Study of risk factors. *Med Trop (Mars)*, 1998. 58(4): 361–4.
70. Tshikuka, J.G. et al., Relationship of childhood protein–energy malnutrition and parasite infections in an urban African setting. *Trop Med Int Health*, 1997. 2(4): 374–82.
71. Crookston, B.T. et al., Exploring the relationship between chronic undernutrition and asymptomatic malaria in Ghanaian children. *Malar J*, 2010. 9: 39.
72. Deribew, A. et al., Malaria and under-nutrition: A community based study among under-five children at risk of malaria, south-west Ethiopia. *PLoS One*, 2010. 5(5): e10775.
73. Mitangala, P.N. et al., Malaria infection and nutritional status: Results from a cohort survey of children from 6–59 months old in the Kivu province, Democratic Republic of the Congo. *Rev Epidemiol Sante Publique*, 2013. 61(2): 111–20.
74. Genton, B. et al., Relation of anthropometry to malaria morbidity and immunity in Papua New Guinean children. *Am J Clin Nutr*, 1998. 68(3): 734–41.
75. Ehrhardt, S. et al., Malaria, anemia, and malnutrition in African children—Defining intervention priorities. *J Infect Dis*, 2006. 194(1): 108–14.
76. Deen, J.L., G.E. Walraven, and L. von Seidlein, Increased risk for malaria in chronically malnourished children under 5 years of age in rural Gambia. *J Trop Pediatr*, 2002. 48(2): 78–83.
77. Muller, O. et al., The association between protein–energy malnutrition, malaria morbidity and all-cause mortality in West African children. *Trop Med Int Health*, 2003. 8(6): 507–11.
78. Razanamparany, M.S. et al., The malaria epidemic in Antananarivo from 1983 to 1994 as seen through the Pediatric Service A in the Befelatanana General Hospital. *Sante*, 1995. 5(6): 382–5.
79. Schellenberg, D. et al., African children with malaria in an area of intense *Plasmodium falciparum* transmission: Features on admission to the hospital and risk factors for death. *Am J Trop Med Hyg*, 1999. 61(3): 431–8.
80. Mockenhaupt, F.P. et al., Manifestation and outcome of severe malaria in children in northern Ghana. *Am J Trop Med Hyg*, 2004. 71(2): 167–72.
81. Kang, H. et al., The causal effect of malaria on stunting: A Mendelian randomization and matching approach. *Int J Epidemiol*, 2013. 42(5): 1390–8.
82. Fillol, F. et al., Impact of child malnutrition on the specific anti-*Plasmodium falciparum* antibody response. *Malar J*, 2009. 8: 116.
83. D'Alessandro, U. et al., Mortality and morbidity from malaria in Gambian children after introduction of an impregnated bednet programme. *Lancet*, 1995. 345(8948): 479–83.
84. ter Kuile, F.O. et al., Impact of permethrin-treated bed nets on malaria and all-cause morbidity in young children in an area of intense perennial malaria transmission in western Kenya: Cross-sectional survey. *Am J Trop Med Hyg*, 2003. 68(4 Suppl): 100–7.
85. Griffin, J.B. et al., *Plasmodium falciparum* parasitaemia in the first half of pregnancy, uterine and umbilical artery blood flow, and foetal growth: A longitudinal Doppler ultrasound study. *Malar J*, 2012. 11: 319.
86. Schmiegelow, C. et al., Malaria and fetal growth alterations in the 3(rd) trimester of pregnancy: A longitudinal ultrasound study. *PLoS One*, 2013. 8(1): e53794.
87. Huynh, B.T. et al., Influence of the timing of malaria infection during pregnancy on birth weight and on maternal anemia in Benin. *Am J Trop Med Hyg*, 2011. 85(2): 214–20.
88. Rijken, M.J. et al., Effect of malaria on placental volume measured using three-dimensional ultrasound: A pilot study. *Malar J*, 2012. 11: 5.
89. Rijken, M.J. et al., Ultrasound evidence of early fetal growth restriction after maternal malaria infection. *PLoS One*, 2012. 7(2): e31411.
90. Gruber, K. et al., Zinc deficiency adversely influences interleukin-4 and interleukin-6 signaling. *J Biol Regul Homeost Agents*, 2013. 27(3): 661–71.
91. Caulfield, L.E. et al., Undernutrition as an underlying cause of child deaths associated with diarrhea, pneumonia, malaria, and measles. *Am J Clin Nutr*, 2004. 80: 55–63.

92. Scholzen, A. and R.W. Sauerwein, How malaria modulates memory: Activation and dysregulation of B cells in *Plasmodium* infection. *Trends Parasitol*, 2013. 29(5): 252–62.

93. Mbugi, E.V. et al., Effect of nutrient deficiencies on *in vitro* Th1 and Th2 cytokine response of peripheral blood mononuclear cells to *Plasmodium falciparum* infection. *Malar J*, 2010. 9: 162.

94. Shankar, A.H. and A.S. Prasad, Zinc and immune function: The biological basis of altered resistance to infection. *Am J Clin Nutr*, 1998. 68(2 Suppl): 447S–63S.

95. Serghides, L. and K.C. Kain, Peroxisome proliferator-activated receptor gamma-retinoid X receptor agonists increase CD36-dependent phagocytosis of *Plasmodium falciparum*-parasitized erythrocytes and decrease malaria-induced TNF-alpha secretion by monocytes/macrophages. *J Immunol*, 2001. 166(11): 6742–8.

96. Hautvast, J.L. et al., Malaria is associated with reduced serum retinol levels in rural Zambian children. *Int J Vitam Nutr Res*, 1998. 68(6): 384–8.

97. Harvey, P.W., R.G. Bell, and M.C. Nesheim, Iron deficiency protects inbred mice against infection with *Plasmodium chabaudi*. *Infect Immun*, 1985. 50(3): 932–4.

98. Oppenheimer, S.J., Iron and its relation to immunity and infectious disease. *J Nutr*, 2001. 131(2S–2): 616S–33S; discussion 633S–5S.

99. Fleming, A.F. and B. Werblinska, Anaemia in childhood in the guinea savanna of Nigeria. *Ann Trop Paediatr*, 1982. 2(4): 161–73.

100. Mayxay, M. et al., Thiamin deficiency and uncomplicated falciparum malaria in Laos. *Trop Med Int Health*, 2007. 12(3): 363–9.

101. Krishna, S. et al., Thiamine deficiency and malaria in adults from southeast Asia. *Lancet*, 1999. 353(9152): 546–9.

102. Thurnham, D.I., S.J. Oppenheimer, and R. Bull, Riboflavin status and malaria in infants in Papua New Guinea. *Trans R Soc Trop Med Hyg*, 1983. 77(3): 423–4.

103. Levander, O.A. et al., Qinghaosu, dietary vitamin E, selenium, and cod-liver oil: Effect on the susceptibility of mice to the malarial parasite *Plasmodium yoelii*. *Am J Clin Nutr*, 1989. 50(2): 346–52.

104. Levander, O.A. et al., Menhaden-fish oil in a vitamin E-deficient diet: Protection against chloroquine-resistant malaria in mice. *Am J Clin Nutr*, 1989. 50(6): 1237–9.

105. Bates, C.J. et al., A trial of zinc supplementation in young rural Gambian children. *Br J Nutr*, 1993. 69(1): 243–55.

106. Muller, O. et al., Effect of zinc supplementation on malaria and other causes of morbidity in west African children: Randomised double blind placebo controlled trial. *BMJ*, 2001. 322(7302): 1567.

107. Binka, F.N. et al., Vitamin A supplementation and childhood malaria in northern Ghana. *Am J Clin Nutr*, 1995. 61(4): 853–9.

108. Fawzi, W.W. et al., A randomized trial of vitamin A supplements in relation to mortality among human immunodeficiency virus-infected and uninfected children in Tanzania. *Pediatr Infect Dis J*, 1999. 18(2): 127–33.

109. Oppenheimer, S.J. et al., Iron supplementation increases prevalence and effects of malaria: Report on clinical studies in Papua New Guinea. *Trans R Soc Trop Med Hyg*, 1986. 80(4): 603–12.

110. Sazawal, S. et al., Effects of routine prophylactic supplementation with iron and folic acid on admission to hospital and mortality in preschool children in a high malaria transmission setting: Community-based, randomised, placebo-controlled trial. *Lancet*, 2006. 367(9505): 133–43.

111. International Nutritional Anemia Consultative Group, Safety of iron supplementation programs in malaria-endemic regions. *Acta Trop* 2002. 82: 321–7.

112. van Hensbroek, M.B. et al., Iron, but not folic acid, combined with effective antimalarial therapy promotes haematological recovery in African children after acute falciparum malaria. *Trans R Soc Trop Med Hyg*, 1995. 89(6): 672–6.

113. Ouma, P. et al., A randomized controlled trial of folate supplementation when treating malaria in pregnancy with sulfadoxine–pyrimethamine. *PLoS Clin Trials*, 2006. 1(6): e28.

114. Carter, J.Y. et al., Reduction of the efficacy of antifolate antimalarial therapy by folic acid supplementation. *Am J Trop Med Hyg*, 2005. 73(1): 166–70.

115. de Silva, N.R. et al., Soil-transmitted helminth infections: Updating the global picture. *Trends Parasitol*, 2003. 19(12): 547–51.

116. Hall, A. et al., A review and meta-analysis of the impact of intestinal worms on child growth and nutrition. *Matern Child Nutr*, 2008. 4 Suppl 1: 118–236.

117. Scrimshaw, N.S., C.E. Taylor, and J.E. Gordon, Interactions of nutrition and infection. *Monogr Ser World Health Organ*, 1968. 57: 3–329.

118. Wiersma, P. et al., Catheter-related polymicrobial bloodstream infections among pediatric bone marrow transplant outpatients—Atlanta, Georgia, 2007. *Infect Control Hosp Epidemiol*, 31(5): 522–7.

119. Crompton, D.W. and M.C. Nesheim, Nutritional impact of intestinal helminthiasis during the human life cycle. *Annu Rev Nutr*, 2002. 22: 35–59.

120. Seshadri, S., Nutritional anaemia in South Asia, in *Malnutrition in South Asia: A Regional Profile*, S. Gillespie, Editor. ROSA Publication Kathmandu, Nepal: UNICEF Regional Office for South Asia, 1997. 75–124.

121. Dondji, B. et al., CD4 T cells mediate mucosal and systemic immune responses to experimental hookworm infection. *Parasite Immunol*, 2010. 32(6): 406–13.

122. Dickson, R. et al., Effects of treatment for intestinal helminth infection on growth and cognitive performance in children: Systematic review of randomised trials. *BMJ*, 2000. 320(7251): 1697–701.

123. Tripathy, K. et al., Malabsorption syndrome in ascariasis. *Am J Clin Nutr*, 1972. 25(11): 1276–81.

124. Taren, D.L. et al., Contributions of ascariasis to poor nutritional status in children from Chiriqui Province, Republic of Panama. *Parasitology*, 1987. 95(Pt 3): 603–13.

125. Reddy, V., K. Vijayaraghavan, and K.K. Mathur, Effect of deworming and vitamin A administration on serum vitamin A levels in preschool children. *J Trop Pediatr*, 1986. 32(4): 196–9.

126. Laishram, S., G. Kang, and S.S. Ajjampur, Giardiasis: A review on assemblage distribution and epidemiology in India. *Indian J Gastroenterol*, 2012. 31(1): 3–12.

127. Quihui-Cota, L. et al., Impact of *Giardia intestinalis* on vitamin A status in schoolchildren from northwest Mexico. *Int J Vitam Nutr Res*, 2008. 78(2): 51–6.

128. Serafim, T.D. et al., Immune response to *Leishmania* (*Leishmania*) *chagasi* infection is reduced in malnourished BALB/c mice. *Mem Inst Oswaldo Cruz*, 2010. 105(6): 811–7.

129. Beisel, W.R., Nutrition in pediatric HIV infection: Setting the research agenda. Nutrition and immune function: Overview. *J Nutr*, 1996. 126(10 Suppl): 2611S–5S.

130. Hagel, I. et al., Nutritional status and the IgE response against *Ascaris lumbricoides* in children from a tropical slum. *Trans R Soc Trop Med Hyg*, 1995. 89(5): 562–5.

131. Hagel, I. et al., Defective regulation of the protective IgE response against intestinal helminth *Ascaris lumbricoides* in malnourished children. *J Trop Pediatr*, 2003. 49(3): 136–42.

132. Ing, R. et al., Suppressed T helper 2 immunity and prolonged survival of a nematode parasite in protein-malnourished mice. *Proc Natl Acad Sci U S A*, 2000. 97(13): 7078–83.

133. Katona, P. and J. Katona-Apte, The interaction between nutrition and infection. *Clin Infect Dis*, 2008. 46(10): 1582–8.

134. Fraker, P.J., R. Caruso, and F. Kierszenbaum, Alteration of the immune and nutritional status of mice by synergy between zinc deficiency and infection with *Trypanosoma cruzi*. *J Nutr*, 1982. 112(6): 1224–9.

135. Savino, W. et al., The thymus gland: A target organ for growth hormone. *Scand J Immunol*, 2002. 55(5): 442–52.
136. Badaro, R. et al., A prospective study of visceral leishmaniasis in an endemic area of Brazil. *J Infect Dis*, 1986. 154(4): 639–49.
137. Collin, S. et al., Conflict and kala-azar: Determinants of adverse outcomes of kala-azar among patients in southern Sudan. *Clin Infect Dis*, 2004. 38(5): 612–9.
138. Maciel, B.L. et al., Association of nutritional status with the response to infection with *Leishmania chagasi. Am J Trop Med Hyg*, 2008. 79(4): 591–8.
139. Scott, M.E. and K.G. Koski, Zinc deficiency impairs immune responses against parasitic nematode infections at intestinal and systemic sites. *J Nutr*, 2000. 130(5S Suppl): 1412S–20S.
140. Spallholz, J.E., L.M. Boylan, and H.S. Larsen, Advances in understanding selenium's role in the immune system. *Ann N Y Acad Sci*, 1990. 587: 123–39.
141. Kiremidjian-Schumacher, L. et al., Supplementation with selenium and human immune cell functions. II. Effect on cytotoxic lymphocytes and natural killer cells. *Biol Trace Elem Res*, 1994. 41(1–2): 115–27.
142. Davis, C.D. et al., Beneficial effect of selenium supplementation during murine infection with Trypanosoma cruzi. *J Parasitol*, 1998. 84(6): 1274–7.
143. Villamor, E. and W.W. Fawzi, Effects of vitamin a supplementation on immune responses and correlation with clinical outcomes. *Clin Microbiol Rev*, 2005. 18(3): 446–64.
144. Bhoite, R.M. and U.M. Iyer, Effect of deworming vs iron–folic acid supplementation plus deworming on growth, hemoglobin level, and physical work capacity of schoolchildren. *Indian Pediatr*, 2012. 49(8): 659–61.
145. Furnee, C.A. et al., Effect of intestinal parasite treatment on the efficacy of oral iodized oil for correcting iodine deficiency in schoolchildren. *Am J Clin Nutr*, 1997. 66(6): 1422–7.
146. Taylor-Robinson, D.C. et al., Deworming drugs for soil-transmitted intestinal worms in children: Effects on nutritional indicators, haemoglobin and school performance. *Cochrane Database Syst Rev*, 2012. 11: CD000371.
147. Bundy, D.A., J.L. Walson, and K.L. Watkins, Worms, wisdom, and wealth: Why deworming can make economic sense. *Trends Parasitol*, 2013. 29(3): 142–8.

10 Gut Microbiome in the Nutrition– Infection Interaction

A Focus on Malnourished Children

Dorottya Nagy-Szakal, Richard Kellermayer, and Sanjiv Harpavat

CONTENTS

Introduction 247
Malnourished Children Have Altered Microbiomes 248
Which Comes First, Infection/Altered Microbiome or Malnutrition? 249
Breaking the Cycle: Antibiotics 251
Breaking the Cycle: Changing the Microbiome 252
Conclusions 253
References 253

INTRODUCTION

In the last decade, the gut microbiome has emerged as a metabolic powerhouse influencing a wide variety of physiological processes. Gut microorganisms account for 10 times as many cells in the human body, coding for 150 times more genes than our genome (Gill et al., 2006). They may play pivotal roles in the pathogenesis of all the major diseases of our time, including cancer, heart disease, autoimmune disease, and metabolic diseases. Furthermore, their regulation and manipulation may be the foundation for powerful therapies in the future. Given their diverse roles, perhaps it is not surprising that gut microorganisms seem to also play a critical role in the human nutrition–infection interaction, as best demonstrated by studies in malnourished children.

Malnourished children worldwide are caught in a vicious cycle between infection and poor nutrition. They experience various gastrointestinal infections, which damage intestinal tissue and hamper absorption of nutrients. Without nutrients, they lack the building blocks to repair mucosa and mount an effective immune response. As a result, they remain vulnerable to more infections, which lead to further malnutrition, which perpetuates tragic loops that continue through the most critical years of physical and mental growth. The cycle's consequences are far-reaching, resulting in stunted and cognitively impaired children, thereby permanently crippling the most productive future members of many societies.

This chapter discusses the gut microbiome's role in malnourished children and the infection-poor nutrition cycle. We first discuss recent studies establishing that healthy and malnourished children have distinctly different gut microbiomes. We next consider how manipulating the microbiome through antibiotics has proven successful in halting the infection-poor nutrition cycle in some cases. Finally, we end by considering an alternative approach—adding "good" microbes, rather than eliminating "bad" ones with antibiotics—which may prove an attractive option in the future. Such an approach is in its infancy for many other diseases, and deserves special consideration in malnourished children.

MALNOURISHED CHILDREN HAVE ALTERED MICROBIOMES

New, powerful techniques are allowing us to better determine the microorganisms harbored by malnourished children. Previously, physicians would culture stool from malnourished children, in order to identify individual pathogens responsible for diarrhea and malabsorption. Now, scientists undertaking the Human Microbiome Project have refined culture-independent, sequencing techniques that sample bacterial DNA from a patient's feces and then compare those sequences to known sequences from bacterial species (Human Microbiome Project Consortium, 2012; Turnbaugh et al., 2007). In this way, a bacterial catalogue of all the stool species can be created and compared between patients, to determine differences between disease and physiological states. These techniques are less biased because they do not require culturing; however, they are limited in that they infer the bacterial composition of the intestines by relying on bacteria passed in stools. They are also limited by our inability to separately culture about 80% of intestinal bacteria, so genome libraries for many organisms do not exist. As a result, many sequences generated lack an exact species match.

Such techniques are now being applied to malnourished children. For example, in one of the first such studies, Gupta et al. (2011) analyzed stool from two 16-month-old females from Kolkata, one apparently healthy and one malnourished. Neither received antibiotics for at least 3 months before stool collection. Stool from the malnourished child had more sequences of human DNA, suggesting that the malnourished child had epithelial cell exfoliation. Furthermore, stool from the malnourished child was enriched in organisms from the pathogenic bacterial families Campylobacteraceae and Helicobacteraceae (order Campylobacterales). The authors argue that their findings confirm what is already suspected in the malnourished child: gut infection causes mucosal damage and exfoliation, leading to malabsorption and susceptibility to pathogenic microorganisms.

Perhaps less obvious is that the authors also found global changes in the microbiome between patients, i.e., a change in the entire microbiome rather than a difference of a few pathogenic organisms. As mentioned, malnourished children may have excessive numbers of species belonging to families Campylobacteraceae and Helicobacteraceae. Excessive amounts of species from families Bacteroidaceae (whose phylum is associated with thinner individuals) and Porphyromonadaceae (which the authors note is also enriched in Crohn's disease) were also noted. In contrast, the healthy patient had a more diverse stool profile, rich with organisms from a variety of families including Streptococcaceae, Enterobacteriaceae, Methanosarcinaceae, Thermotogaceae, Shewanellaceae, and Eubacteriaceae. These findings, although limited by comparing only two subjects, hint at systemic microbiome differences in healthy versus malnourished children.

WHICH COMES FIRST, INFECTION/ALTERED MICROBIOME OR MALNUTRITION?

One important challenge in breaking the malnutrition cycle is understanding the cause-and-effect relation between nutrition and the microbiome. On the one hand, the diet shapes the microbiome. The microbiome feeds on undigested or unabsorbed nutrients, and organisms most fit to metabolize these nutrients are the most likely to survive. In fact, some have categorized the human microbiome into three bacterial "enterotypes" determined by the food humans consume (Table 10.1) (Arumugam et al., 2011). Those who eat modern diets rich in animal protein and saturated fat have the *Bacteroides* enterotype, whereas those who consume high amounts of carbohydrates similar to ancient rural communities have the *Prevotella* enterotype. Those that consume high levels of polyunsaturated fat and alcohol have the *Ruminococcus*-dominated enterotype. While these enterotype designations are useful conceptually, recent data suggest that gut microbiome composition may be more complicated with overlap among the different enterotypes (Yatsunenko et al., 2012).

Supporting the central role of diet in shaping the microbiome, dietary changes have been shown to alter the microbiome. For example, those switching from the Western diet to a vegetarian lifestyle had decreased amounts of *Bacteroides* and the related genus *Escherichia* and increased amounts of *Prevotella* (Zimmer et al., 2012). As a result, these subjects have less exposure to inflammation-inducing endotoxin

---

TABLE 10.1
Nutrition-Associated Modifications of the Microbiota Composition

Dietary Habits	Microbiota Alteration
"Western" diet (animal protein, saturated fat)	*Bacteroides* enterotype
High-carbohydrate diet	*Prevotella* enterotype
Ancient rural communities (high carbohydrates, plants)	↑*Bacteroidetes* (*Prevotella*)
Polyunsaturated fat and alcohol	*Ruminococcus* enterotype
Vegetarian lifestyle	↓*Bacteroides, Escherichia*
High fiber	↑*Bacteroidetes, Actinobacteria*
	↓*Firmicutes, Proteobacteria*
High fat	↑*Firmicutes, Proteobacteria*
	↓*Bacteroidetes*
High carbohydrate	↑*Firmicutes*
	↓*Bacteroidetes*

from *Bacteroides* and *Escherichia*, as well as faster transit times and more intestinal trophic factors associated with *Prevotella*. However, while significant short-term dietary changes can induce detectable microbiome changes within 24 h, such effects level out and do not lead to major enterotype changes over a short period (Wu et al., 2011). Rather, the intestinal microbiome has been recently observed to be surprisingly stable during a few years in adults whose body mass index does not change significantly (Faith et al., 2013). Hence, these findings suggest it is likely for only long-term (months or years) and large diet changes (i.e., from mixed to vegetarian diet) to lead to more global microbiome switches among the three enterotypes.

The hypothesis that malnourishment also alters the microbiome is supported by a recent study on children in the developing world. Smith et al. (2013) report the microbiome composition of 9 Malawian healthy twins and 13 Malawian twins discordant for nutrition (one with kwashiorkor, a form of severe acute malnutrition characterized by edema, skin changes, and fatty liver). By studying twins, the authors controlled for genetic and age differences that may affect the microbiome. The authors found that the microbiome composition of the healthy twins was similar and changed to a mature configuration with time. In contrast, in twins discordant for kwashiorkor, the undernourished twin's microbiome composition differed from the healthy sibling and did not mature with time, even when both twins were fed ready-to-use therapeutic (RUTF) food for 4 weeks. These results hint at the possibility that malnourishment may have generated an altered microbiome, resistant to short-term improvements in nutrition.

Just as malnutrition may help determine an impaired microbiome, the opposite is also true: an impaired microbiome may cause malnutrition. A less diverse microbiome, as seen in patients with kwashiorkor, for example, allows for the colonization of pathogenic species. For example, in the Gupta et al. (2011) report, the malnourished child had a microbiome with limited diversity, allowing for overcolonization with organisms from the order Campylobacterales at the expense of others. The authors speculate that *Helicobacter* species belonging to the order Campylobacterales may be present in higher quantities, reducing stomach acid secretion and predisposing infants to infections from opportunistic pathogens such as *Vibrio cholerae*. *Vibrio cholerae*, in turn, generates a watery diarrhea, which hinders the child's ability to renourish and grow.

In addition to preventing colonization of pathogenic bacteria, an impaired microbiome will also be unable to generate important nutrients for the growing child. For example, Yatsunenko et al. (2012) showed that the microbiome diversifies with time in humans from varied geographies. The maturing microbiome codes for a number of enzymes that provide nutrition for the host. Microorganisms making vitamin B_{12} (cobalamin) increase with age, as do those making vitamin B_7 and B_1 (Nicholson et al., 2012; Saulnier et al., 2011). Bacteria also provide balanced homeostasis of bone and vascular health by producing vitamin K_1 (phylloquinone), vitamin K_2 (menaquinone), and choline (Conly et al., 1994; Wang et al., 2011). Without proper representation from these microorganisms, the malnourished child would be missing essential gut-generated vitamins required for proper growth and development.

In addition to vitamins, gut bacteria also produce a number of other important nutrients. Perhaps the best studied are short-chain fatty acids (SCFAs), which are produced when bacteria ferment undigested/unabsorbed sugars (Wong et al., 2006). SCFAs, including butyrate, acetate, and propionate, are the main energy source for colonic epithelial cells. Butyrate has also been shown to influence cell growth and differentiation, and may have an antiproliferative effect on adenoma growth and colon cancer. Acetate influences lipogenesis, serving as the starting substrate for endogenous fatty-acid production in cells, and has anti-inflammatory effects in the mammalian colon (Maslowski et al., 2009). Propionate serves as a substrate for gluconeogenesis but can also inhibit glucose synthesis through its metabolites (succinyl CoA and methymalonyl CoA). Hence, an impaired microbiome that cannot produce proper amounts of SCFAs would negatively influence its host's normal metabolic pathways.

BREAKING THE CYCLE: ANTIBIOTICS

One way to limit the malnutrition–infection cycle is through antibiotics. Antibiotics could have two theoretical beneficial effects. First, they could eliminate offending pathogens, clearing the child of gut infection and allowing the mucosa to repair and return to its normal absorptive functions. Second, antibiotics could "reset" the impaired microbiome in the malnourished child. This may give a chance for more diverse bacteria to colonize the gut and restore normal functions, such as generating vitamins and providing trophic support to epithelial cells. Antibiotics also pose potential risk, including promoting antibiotic-resistant pathogens and clearing normal flora, which normally inhibits overgrowth of pathogenic bacterial strains.

A recent clinical study by Trehan et al. (2013) tested whether antibiotics improve nutrition in malnourished children. The authors randomized 2767 malnourished infants to placebo, amoxicillin, or cefdinir for 7 days at the time of diagnosis. In addition, all children received RUTF composed of peanut paste, sugar, vegetable oil, and milk fortified with vitamin and minerals. The authors found a significant improvement in recovery and decrease in mortality with antibiotics, no matter which antibiotics were used. Furthermore, those receiving antibiotics had a more rapid weight gain. These studies show that the benefits of antibiotics likely outweigh the risks and suggest that manipulating the microbiome composition through antibiotics can help treat malnutrition. This conclusion could be further supported with studies characterizing the gut microbiome of the subjects, as well as screening for infectious agents before treatment.

How antibiotics exert this effect remains unknown, although a recent study by Cho et al. (2012) argues that antibiotics select for a microbiome that promotes adiposity. The authors' objective was to understand why farm animals gain weight when fed antibiotics. They used a mouse model, in which pups were fed a 7-week antibiotic cocktail at weaning. The antibiotic-treated mice had normal weights but significantly more adiposity compared with their untreated counterparts. The authors showed that chronic antibiotics do not alter the number of bacterial species in the feces and cecum but rather changed their composition. Antibiotic-fed mice had an increased ratio of Firmicutes to Bacteroidetes, which had also been observed in other mouse models of obesity. Furthermore, the authors noted an increase in the SCFAs butyrate and acetate in the cecum of antibiotic-treated mice. They speculate that one way the microbiome in antibiotic-treated animals could promote adiposity is by supplying more energy to colonocytes.

BREAKING THE CYCLE: CHANGING THE MICROBIOME

Given the close relation between malnutrition and the gut microbiome, another approach would be to modify the microbiome rather than disrupt them with antibiotics. One option is to use a healthy diet to promote a particular microbiome. Smith et al. (2013) studied this in the laboratory, first by creating mice with "malnourished" and "healthy" microbiomes. To do this, the authors used germ-free mice and implanted the microbiomes from discordant Malawain twins, resulting in mouse lines with defined different microbial compositions. These "xenobiotic" mouse models are advantageous in that they allow scientists to determine the effects of introducing particular bacterial strains. They are limited, however, because the mice lack the normal host–bacteria interactions that occur during normal development that would affect how they respond to the newly introduced bacteria.

The authors then fed the xenobiotic mice a typical Malawian diet. Mice receiving bacteria from the kwashiorkor twin lost weight compared with mice receiving bacteria from the healthy twin. However, when the mice were then placed on an RUTF diet, the mice with the kwashiorkor microbiome rapidly regained weight. Concurrently, their microbiome changed dramatically, including an increase in bacteria known to modulate the immune system (*Lactobacillus* and *Ruminococcus*), hinting that RUTFs changed the microbiome, which then improved weight gain. These results argue that certain diets (i.e., the Malawian diet) perpetuate a certain microbiome, whereas a more nutritious diet (i.e., RUTFs) can therapeutically improve the microbiome composition into a richer, healthier one.

While RUTFs in this case may be a form of "prebiotics," or nondigestible food ingredients that promote growth of beneficial microorganisms in the intestines, an analogous treatment would be to give live bacteria that simply replace the microbiome. "Probiotic" treatment may be one possibility. Probiotic therapy requires predicting which individual bacterial species are beneficial and then providing them in oral preparation. Probiotics in otherwise healthy human infants do reduce the length of rotavirus illness by modest amounts (Huang et al., 2013). Whether probiotics actually improve malnutrition has yet to be seen, and some groups have developed mouse models to examine this question in more depth (Preidis et al., 2012a,b).

As the extreme spectrum of probiotic use is the modulation of the entire microbiome with a "healthy" one, through fecal microbiome transplantation (FMT). FMT has proved incredibly successful for diseases caused by altered microbiomes, such as life-threatening intestinal *Clostridium difficile* infections (CDI). In the first randomized trial, patients with recurrent CDI recalcitrant to standard antibiotics received one of three treatments: (1) vancomycin, (2) vancomycin followed by bowel lavage, or (3) vancomycin followed by nasogastric infusion of fecal samples from healthy donors (van Nood et al., 2013). Eighty-one percent (13 of 16) of patients in group 3 had resolution of CDI. In contrast, only 30.8% (4 of 13) of group 1 and 23% (3 of 13) of group 2 patients benefitted. In addition, as expected, group 3 patients demonstrated improved diversity in their microbiome, including increase in species of Bacteroidetes and Firmicutes (*Clostridium* clusters IV and XIVa) phyla and a decrease of Proteobacteria.

How FMT achieves such dramatic success remains a matter of controversy. Some argue that donor microbiota engrafts into the colon of recipients (Hamilton et al., 2013).

However, microbiome changes in FMT do not seem to be permanent. For example, in another study, patients with CDI were given a bacterial preparation of 33 species after failing antibiotic therapy (Petrof et al., 2013). When their microbiome was tracked over time, there was a steady decline in the transplanted strains. By 6 months, only about 25–30% of the species received remained in the recipient. Hence, another possibility is that healthy donor bacterial communities "shock" the recipient microbiome and help restructure it acutely. A few bacterial species may engraft to provide long-term support; however, the acute value lies in the sudden change, which capitalizes on the dynamic nature of the microbiome and encourages it to "reset" to a healthier, more diverse state.

FMT as a treatment for malnourished children is only a theoretical idea at this point, with many issues that need to be resolved. For example, FMT risks transferring pathogenic bacteria as well as beneficial bacteria, which could have devastating consequences in malnourished children who are already vulnerable to infection. FMT as a concept also is not fully accepted, in large part because most cultural traditions do not accept transferring stools among individuals. Still, FMT is affordable and universally available. It has also been used successfully in a number of conditions, including inflammatory bowel diseases (Anderson et al., 2012), irritable bowel syndrome (Borody et al., 1989), metabolic syndrome (Vrieze et al., 2012), and even in isolated cases of neurological diseases (Borody and Campbell, 2012). An FMT workgroup now exists to establish guidelines for donor screening and recipient selection (Bakken et al., 2011). The establishment and adherence to stringent guidelines and methods should aid the safety and future utilization of this unconventional treatment option for various human diseases.

CONCLUSIONS

The malnourished child provides a case study for the gut microbiome's role in the human nutrition–infection interaction. As shown in recent studies, poor nutrition may select for an altered microbiome. The altered microbiome, in turn, may exacerbate the malnutrition in two ways: (i) allowing pathogenic organisms to colonize and (ii) producing fewer nutrients for the host. As a result, a cycle ensues that any successful treatment must break. Antibiotics are one such theoretical treatment, which may reset the microbiome and allow healthier, more diverse organisms to colonize. In contrast to antibiotics, promoting an improved microbiome through food (prebiotics) or bacterial replacement (prebiotics, FMT) may be safe and affordable therapies that are easy to implement. As our understanding of the microbiome in the malnourished child deepens, we will be able to test these therapies and hopefully provide long-standing relief to many of the world's malnourished children.

REFERENCES

Anderson, J. L., R. J. Edney, and K. Whelan. 2012. Systematic review: Faecal microbiota transplantation in the management of inflammatory bowel disease. *Aliment Pharmacol Ther* 36 (6):503–16.

Arumugam, M., J. Raes, E. Pelletier, D. Le Paslier, T. Yamada, D. R. Mende, G. R. Fernandes et al. 2011. Enterotypes of the human gut microbiome. *Nature* 473 (7346):174–80.

Bakken, J. S., T. Borody, L. J. Brandt, J. V. Brill, D. C. Demarco, M. A. Franzos, C. Kelly et al. 2011. Treating *Clostridium difficile* infection with fecal microbiota transplantation. *Clin Gastroenterol Hepatol* 9 (12):1044–9.

Borody, T. J., and J. Campbell. 2012. Fecal microbiota transplantation: Techniques, applications, and issues. *Gastroenterol Clin North Am* 41 (4):781–803.

Borody, T. J., L. George, P. Andrews, S. Brandl, S. Noonan, P. Cole, L. Hyland, A. Morgan, J. Maysey, and D. Moore-Jones. 1989. Bowel-flora alteration: A potential cure for inflammatory bowel disease and irritable bowel syndrome? *Med J Aust* 150 (10):604.

Cho, I., S. Yamanishi, L. Cox, B. A. Methe, J. Zavadil, K. Li, Z. Gao et al. 2012. Antibiotics in early life alter the murine colonic microbiome and adiposity. *Nature* 488 (7413):621–6.

Conly, J. M., K. Stein, L. Worobetz, and S. Rutledge-Harding. 1994. The contribution of vitamin K2 (menaquinones) produced by the intestinal microflora to human nutritional requirements for vitamin K. *Am J Gastroenterol* 89 (6):915–23.

Faith, J. J., J. L. Guruge, M. Charbonneau, S. Subramanian, H. Seedorf, A. L. Goodman, J. C. Clemente et al. 2013. The long-term stability of the human gut microbiota. *Science* 341 (6141):1237439.

Gill, S. R., M. Pop, R. T. Deboy, P. B. Eckburg, P. J. Turnbaugh, B. S. Samuel, J. I. Gordon, D. A. Relman, C. M. Fraser-Liggett, and K. E. Nelson. 2006. Metagenomic analysis of the human distal gut microbiome. *Science* 312 (5778):1355–9.

Gupta, S. S., M. H. Mohammed, T. S. Ghosh, S. Kanungo, G. B. Nair, and S. S. Mande. 2011. Metagenome of the gut of a malnourished child. *Gut Pathog* 3:7.

Hamilton, M. J., A. R. Weingarden, T. Unno, A. Khoruts, and M. J. Sadowsky. 2013. High-throughput DNA sequence analysis reveals stable engraftment of gut microbiota following transplantation of previously frozen fecal bacteria. *Gut Microbes* 4 (2):125–35.

Huang, Y. F., P. Y. Liu, Y. Y. Chen, B. R. Nong, I. F. Huang, K. S. Hsieh, and K. T. Chen. 2013. Three-combination probiotics therapy in children with salmonella and rotavirus gastroenteritis. *J Clin Gastroenterol* 48 (1):37–42.

Human Microbiome Project Consortium. 2012. Structure, function and diversity of the healthy human microbiome. *Nature* 486 (7402):207–14.

Maslowski, K. M., A. T. Vieira, A. Ng, J. Kranich, F. Sierro, D. Yu, H. C. Schilter et al. 2009. Regulation of inflammatory responses by gut microbiota and chemoattractant receptor GPR43. *Nature* 461 (7268):1282–6.

Nicholson, J. K., E. Holmes, J. Kinross, R. Burcelin, G. Gibson, W. Jia, and S. Pettersson. 2012. Host–gut microbiota metabolic interactions. *Science* 336 (6086):1262–7.

Petrof, E. O., G. B. Gloor, S. J. Vanner, S. J. Weese, D. Carter, M. C. Daigneault, E. M. Brown, K. Schroeter, and E. Allen-Vercoe. 2013. Stool substitute transplant therapy for the eradication of *Clostridium difficile* infection: 'RePOOPulating' the gut. *Microbiome* 1 (1):3. http://www.microbiomejournal.com/content/1/1/3.

Preidis, G. A., D. M. Saulnier, S. E. Blutt, T. A. Mistretta, K. P. Riehle, A. M. Major, S. F. Venable et al. 2012a. Host response to probiotics determined by nutritional status of rotavirus-infected neonatal mice. *J Pediatr Gastroenterol Nutr* 55 (3):299–307.

Preidis, G. A., D. M. Saulnier, S. E. Blutt, T. A. Mistretta, K. P. Riehle, A. M. Major, S. F. Venable, M. J. Finegold, J. F. Petrosino, M. E. Conner, and J. Versalovic. 2012b. Probiotics stimulate enterocyte migration and microbial diversity in the neonatal mouse intestine. *FASEB J* 26 (5):1960–9.

Saulnier, D. M., F. Santos, S. Roos, T. A. Mistretta, J. K. Spinler, D. Molenaar, B. Teusink, and J. Versalovic. 2011. Exploring metabolic pathway reconstruction and genome-wide expression profiling in *Lactobacillus reuteri* to define functional probiotic features. *PLoS One* 6 (4):e18783.

Smith, M. I., T. Yatsunenko, M. J. Manary, I. Trehan, R. Mkakosya, J. Cheng, A. L. Kau et al. 2013. Gut microbiomes of Malawian twin pairs discordant for kwashiorkor. *Science* 339 (6119):548–54.

Trehan, I., H. S. Goldbach, L. N. LaGrone, G. J. Meuli, R. J. Wang, K. M. Maleta, and M. J. Manary. 2013. Antibiotics as part of the management of severe acute malnutrition. *N Engl J Med* 368 (5):425–35.

Turnbaugh, P. J., R. E. Ley, M. Hamady, C. M. Fraser-Liggett, R. Knight, and J. I. Gordon. 2007. The human microbiome project. *Nature* 449 (7164):804–10.

van Nood, E., A. Vrieze, M. Nieuwdorp, S. Fuentes, E. G. Zoetendal, W. M. de Vos, C. E. Visser et al. 2013. Duodenal infusion of donor feces for recurrent *Clostridium difficile*. *N Engl J Med* 368 (5):407–15.

Vrieze, A., E. Van Nood, F. Holleman, J. Salojarvi, R. S. Kootte, J. F. Bartelsman, G. M. Dallinga-Thie et al. 2012. Transfer of intestinal microbiota from lean donors increases insulin sensitivity in individuals with metabolic syndrome. *Gastroenterology* 143 (4):913–6.e7.

Wang, Z., E. Klipfell, B. J. Bennett, R. Koeth, B. S. Levison, B. Dugar, A. E. Feldstein et al. 2011. Gut flora metabolism of phosphatidylcholine promotes cardiovascular disease. *Nature* 472 (7341):57–63.

Wong, J. M., R. de Souza, C. W. Kendall, A. Emam, and D. J. Jenkins. 2006. Colonic health: Fermentation and short chain fatty acids. *J Clin Gastroenterol* 40 (3):235–43.

Wu, G. D., J. Chen, C. Hoffmann, K. Bittinger, Y. Y. Chen, S. A. Keilbaugh, M. Bewtra et al. 2011. Linking long-term dietary patterns with gut microbial enterotypes. *Science* 334 (6052):105–8.

Yatsunenko, T., F. E. Rey, M. J. Manary, I. Trehan, M. G. Dominguez-Bello, M. Contreras, M. Magris et al. 2012. Human gut microbiome viewed across age and geography. *Nature* 486 (7402):222–7.

Zimmer, J., B. Lange, J. S. Frick, H. Sauer, K. Zimmermann, A. Schwiertz, K. Rusch, S. Klosterhalfen, and P. Enck. 2012. A vegan or vegetarian diet substantially alters the human colonic faecal microbiota. *Eur J Clin Nutr* 66 (1):53–60.

Enteric Syndromes
Leading to Malnutrition
and Infections

Vi Lier Goh and Praveen S. Goday

CONTENTS

Celiac Disease 257
Tropical Sprue 262
Autoimmune Enteropathy (AIE) and IPEX Syndrome 263
    IPEX Syndrome (AIE Type 1) 263
    AIE Type 2 (IPEX-Like without Mutations in the *FOXP3* Gene) 265
    AIE Type 3 (without or with Extraintestinal Manifestations) 266
    Treatment 266
Intestinal Lymphangiectasia 267
Inflammatory Bowel Disease 269
Intestinal Failure 272
Acrodermatitis Enteropathica and Zinc Deficiency 274
References 275

Malnutrition is an important risk factor contributing to the high mortality rate of childhood diarrhea in developing countries. In case-control studies, malnutrition, infections, and prolonged duration of diarrhea[1,2] are associated with fatal outcomes in children. As malnutrition in these children is also associated with other infections such as pneumonia, urinary tract infections, and sepsis. Persistent diarrhea is a key determinant of prolonged illness. Absorption of nutrients may also be impaired as a consequence of altered mucosal structure of the small intestine in the malnourished host. It is frequently difficult to distinguish what comes first, the persistent diarrhea or the malnutrition. While prolonged childhood diarrheal illnesses are common in the developing world, there are a host of enteric syndromes that also are associated with malnutrition. In this chapter, we will discuss the common gastrointestinal syndromes that cause nutritional deficiencies and also predispose patients to infections.

CELIAC DISEASE

Celiac disease (CD) is a T-cell-mediated, chronic systemic inflammatory disorder, elicited by the ingestion of wheat gliadin and related prolamins. CD affects individuals with a strong genetic predisposition that is associated with human leukocyte antigen

HLA-DQ2 and HLA-DQ8, and characterized by the presence of CD-specific anti-bodies and/or gluten-dependent manifestations, including enteropathy.[3] CD-specific antibodies include autoantibodies against tissue transglutaminase (tTG), including endomysial antibodies (EMA), and antibodies against deaminated forms of gliadin antibodies (DGP). Glutens are present in wheat, rye, barley, and, to a lesser extent, oats.[3] The disease prevalence among the first-degree relatives of a proband varies from 1% to 18%, with an average prevalence of about 10%.[4]

The three prominent features of CD are the following: (i) it is induced solely by an environmental trigger, namely ingested gluten, and disease remission is highly dependent on a strict gluten-free diet; (ii) it requires a unique genetic background—HLA class II molecules DQ2 or DQ8; and (iii) the ingested gluten mediates both intestinal adaptive and innate immune responses, where TG-2, the autoantigen, is also targeted by specific autoantibodies.[4–7]

Characteristically, CD manifests before school age. In the classic form of childhood CD, signs and symptoms of malabsorption become evident within several months of starting a gluten-containing diet. The child presents with chronic diarrhea, vomiting, and abdominal distention. Typically, the child presents with a malabsorption syndrome with prolonged diarrhea, hypotonia, and may have other symptoms of severe enteropathies, such as dehydration, hypoproteinemia, hypokalemia, hypoprothrombinemia, and hypocalcemia. Rickets may be a presenting symptom in one-fourth of the children with CD.[8] In older children, the presenting signs of malabsorption may include short stature, failure to thrive, delayed puberty, iron deficiency anemia, and osteoporosis.[9,10] During the early 1980s, it was reported that the prevalence of childhood CD was decreasing[11]; however, this seemed not to be the case. Rather, clinicians were seeing a changing pattern of disease presentation with milder symptomatology and an increase in the age at diagnosis. Today, it is clear that CD with typical gastrointestinal symptoms represents only the tip of the iceberg.[12] CD is associated with a number of other diseases and syndromes (Table 11.1) and it can also present with extraintestinal symptoms (Table 11.2).[3,13]

CD can be diagnosed by elevated IgA-tTG and/or EMA, and the presence of HLA-DQ2/DQ8. The gold standard for clinical diagnosis is the presence of histological changes in the small intestine manifested as increased density of intraepithelial lymphocytes, villous atrophy, and crypt hyperplasia[14,15] (Figure 11.1). However,

TABLE 11.1
Diseases and Syndromes Associated with Celiac Disease

Insulin-dependent diabetes mellitus
Autoimmune endocrinopathies
IgA deficiency
Down syndrome
Turner syndrome
Connective tissue disorders

TABLE 11.2

Extraintestinal Manifestation of
Celiac Disease

Unexplained anemia	Aphthous stomatitis
Arthritis or arthralgia	Osteoporosis
Ataxia or polyneuropathy	Alopecia
Enamel hypoplasia	Infertility
Elevation of hepatic transaminases	Intractable seizures

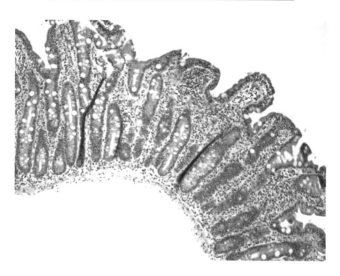

FIGURE 11.1 **(See color insert.)** Histological findings of celiac disease with increased density of intraepithelial lymphocytes, villous atrophy, and crypt hyperplasia. (Picture courtesy of Dr. Michael O'Brien, MD MPH, Boston Medical Center.)

the most recent European Society of Pediatric Gastroenterology, Hepatology, and Nutrition guidelines recommend that histological assessment may be omitted in symptomatic patients who have high IgA-tTG levels (10 times above upper limit of normal), verified by EMA positivity, and are HLA-DQ2 and/or HLA-DQ8 heterodimer positive.[16] This has been verified in a population in Spain[17] but is not yet considered the standard of care in North America.

CD is a common cause of hematological disorders, the most common being anemia. It is also frequently implicated in the etiology of other hematological disease states, including thrombocytopenia, thrombocytosis, thromboembolism, leukopenia, coagulopathy, splenic hypofunction, and intestinal lymphomas.[18,19] The anemia of CD is usually due to malabsorption of micronutrients such as iron, folic acid, and vitamin B12. Iron is absorbed in the proximal small intestine and its absorption is dependent on an intact mucosal surface and intestinal acidity.[20] Iron deficiency anemia has been reported in 46% of cases of subclinical CD, with a higher prevalence in adults than in children.[19] Iron deficiency anemia manifests as microcytic, hypochromic anemia, and patients characteristically have low serum iron levels, elevated total iron-binding capacity, and low ferritin levels.[21]

Folic acid is an essential element of amino acid and nucleic acid metabolism and metabolic regulation.[22] Adequate folic acid is required for normal hematopoiesis and development of the nervous system. Folic acid is primarily absorbed in the jejunum.[22,23] Deficiency in folic acid usually presents as macrocytic and megaloblastic anemia but abnormalities in other cell lines are common. Concomitant iron deficiency, as can be seen in CD, can result in atypical findings on blood smear. Severe folic acid deficiency can result in a decrease in both leukocytes and platelets and even manifest as severe pancytopenia. The diagnosis is made by measuring red blood cell folate. Previous studies have shown that many untreated patients with CD are folate deficient.[24–26]

Vitamin B12 is an essential cofactor and coenzyme in multiple biochemical pathways, including the pathways of DNA and methionine synthesis. While the main site of vitamin B12 absorption is the distal ileum, where it is absorbed bound to an intrinsic factor, a small proportion is also absorbed passively along the entire small bowel.[27] The cause of vitamin B12 deficiency in CD is not known but may include decreased gastric acid, bacterial overgrowth, autoimmune gastritis, decreased efficiency of mixing with transfer factors in the intestine, or perhaps subtle dysfunction of the distal small intestine.[28,29] Studies have shown that 8%–41% of untreated patients with CD are deficient in vitamin B12.[30,31] Vitamin B12 deficiency should be considered in all CD patients with hematologic and/or neurologic abnormalities. Measurement of vitamin B12 levels can be misleading and difficult to interpret, especially when the results fall within the lower range of normal or if there is a coexisting deficiency of folate.[32] Elevated levels of serum methylmalonic acid may enhance the diagnostic accuracy under these circumstances.[33] Patients with vitamin B12 deficiency should receive therapy with parenteral vitamin B12. Although studies have suggested that large doses of oral vitamin B12 may be as effective as parenteral vitamin B12,[34] studies have not been performed in patients with vitamin B12 deficiency secondary to CD.

The anemia seen in CD can also result from malabsorption of various micronutrients necessary for normal hematopoiesis. Copper deficiency has been described in adults and children with CD and may result in anemia and thrombocytopenia.[35,36] Abnormally low white blood cell counts have been reported in a few children with CD.[37] These findings appear to be rare, and deficiencies in folate and copper have been implicated as a possible etiology of leukopenia.[38] The data on treatment of these patients are extremely limited.

Venous thrombosis has been reported in CD. Hyperhomocysteinemia is a frequent finding in CD and may be related to an increased tendency to form clots.[39] Increased levels of thrombin-activatable fibrinolysis inhibitor (TAFI) recently have been reported in patients with inflammatory bowel disease (IBD) and CD.[40,41] Elevated levels of TAFI have been shown to be a risk factor for venous thromboembolism.[41] A decreased level of vitamin K–dependent anticoagulant proteins, protein C and S, has been suggested as a cause for thrombosis associated with CD.[42] This can result in prolongation of coagulation assays such as the prothrombin time, international normalized ratio, and the activated partial thromboplastin time.[43,44] Patients with CD can present with hemorrhagic diathesis. The resulting hemorrhage can be minimal to severe.[45,46] Therapy is in the form of parenteral vitamin K; however, occasionally, plasma products may be needed in bleeding patients.

Splenic atrophy associated with malabsorption and CD has been described.[47,48] Splenic dysfunction can be demonstrated using scintigraphy and measurement of the clearance of labeled heat-damaged red blood cells.[47] A commonly used method of assessing splenic function in patients with CD is to count "pitted" erythrocytes by interference contrast microscopy.[49] A pitted erythrocyte count of > 2% to 4% is indicative of hyposplenism.[49] The prevalence of hyposplenism in patients with CD ranges from 21% to 60%.[19] The risks associated with hyposplenism in patients with CD are unknown. Infectious complications appear to be rare, given the high frequency of hyposplenism. However, several case reports of severe and even fatal bacterial infections in such patients have been published.[50–52] These are mostly associated with *Streptococcus pneumoniae* infection. Cavitating lesions in mesenteric lymph nodes and the lungs have also been reported in patients with CD and hyposplenism, and can be associated with significant mortality, presumably due to overwhelming infections.[53–55] The etiology of these cavitating lesions is unknown; however, it has been suggested that immune complexes result in endothelial damage leading to intranodal hemorrhagic necrosis.[55] It is recommended that patients with hyposplenism be treated as patients who are asplenic secondary to other reasons. Immunizations against the encapsulated bacteria *Streptococcus pneumoniae*, *Haemophilius influenzae* type b, and *Neisseria meningitidis* are recommended.[56,57] One small study suggested that the antibody response to the polyvalent pneumococcal vaccine is intact in patients with CD.[58] Younger patients should be considered for prophylactic therapy with antibiotics, and all patients should receive education on the infectious complications associated with hyposplenism.[56]

CD and IgA deficiency are commonly associated. Patients with IgA deficiency have a 10-fold higher risk of developing CD, and the prevalence of IgA deficiency among CD patients is 10- to 16-fold higher than expected in the general population.[59,60] IgA-deficient individuals are prone to enteric conditions such as IBD and chronic parasite infections, especially giardiasis, which can mimic CD. A recent study showed that patients with CD have lower seroconversion to hepatitis B and A vaccine compared with controls.[61]

In CD, a lifelong gluten-free diet is the only effective treatment. Wheat-, rye-, and barley-based products should be avoided. Oats do not contain gluten but are frequently contaminated by being processed together with gluten-containing products. A strict gluten-free diet often restricts social activities, limits nutritional variety, is expensive, and is difficult to maintain in many countries. Alternative or adjunctive treatments are desired but presently are unavailable. Therapeutic strategies are being tested as alternative therapy for CD. These include genetic modifications of wheat, oral enzyme therapy, neutralizing gluten antibodies, inhibition of intestinal permeability, transglutaminase inhibitors, and mesenchymal stem cell therapy.[62]

TROPICAL SPRUE

Tropical sprue (TS), although endemic to certain tropical regions of the world, is rarely seen in North America and Europe. It is an acquired intestinal malabsorption syndrome of unknown etiology that affects residents and tourists of tropical regions, including West Africa, Central America, South America, the Caribbean islands, Puerto Rico, Southeast Asia, and the Indian subcontinent.[63,64] It still accounts for almost 40% of malabsorption in adults and children in South Asia.[65,66] Interestingly, TS is becoming rare in expatriates living in endemic countries, presumably owing to wider use of antibiotics in acute diarrheal illnesses and better sanitation practices.[67]

The etiology of TS remains elusive. The fact that the disease occurs in epidemics is more prevalent in poorly sanitized environments, and response to antibiotic treatment strongly suggests an infectious etiology.[68] Contamination of the small bowel by aerobic enteric bacteria has been reported in TS patients, but no specific causal agent has been identified.[69,70] It is also postulated that bacterial colonization is secondary to slowing of small-bowel transit induced by the ileal brake responding to unabsorbed fat.[70] HLA of the Aw-19 series has been associated with TS in Puerto Ricans with the strongest association being with Aw-31 (relative risk 10.6).[70] It has also been suggested that TS is caused by fecal bacteria ingested in large quantities by young children living in conditions of poor sanitation and hygiene. The ingested high concentrations of fecal bacteria, which colonize the small intestine, presumably induces TS through a T-cell-mediated process. The hyperpermeable gut facilitates translocation of microbes, which trigger the metabolic changes associated with an immune response.[71] Growth falters when these changes coincide with reduced nutrient absorption by atrophied villi in addition to the marginal dietary intake and high growth demands of children living in developing countries.[72]

Typical symptoms of TS include chronic diarrhea, glossitis, bloating, prominent bowel sounds, and weight loss. The signs of nutritional deficiency include pallor due to anemia, angular stomatitis, cheilitis, and glossitis due to vitamin B12 deficiency, and peripheral edema and skin and hair changes secondary to hypoproteinemia.[66]

Histological findings in TS may be indistinguishable from those in CD. However, TS involves the entire length of the small bowel while CD typically spares the terminal ileum. Villous blunting is noted, but complete villous flattening seen in CD is rare in TS.[73] Typically, laboratory findings include macrocytic anemia, low folate and B12, hypoalbuminemia, steatorrhea, D-xylose malabsorption, and often abnormal vitamin B12 absorption (Schilling test). Small-bowel histological changes include variable degrees of villous atrophy, crypt hyperplasia, and inflammatory cell infiltrate. In the endemic areas of the tropics, it is important to rule out specific enteric infections by stool examination before a diagnosis of TS is made.[74]

Nutrient malabsorption arises from involvement of both the proximal and distal small intestine. Ultrastructural studies show degenerating cells in the crypts of the small intestine, suggesting stem cell damage.[75] Reduction in the total absorptive surface area as a consequence of villous atrophy and loss of epithelial cell microvilli results in reduced D-xylose absorption and malabsorption of fat and fat-soluble vitamins. Folate and iron deficiency represent proximal small-bowel involvement, whereas B12 malabsorption reflects terminal ileal involvement. Folate may be depleted both by damage to the host epithelium and by bacterial uptake.[69] Bile acid malabsorption occurs as a result of terminal ileal involvement and may contribute to diarrhea. Colonic malabsorption of water and electrolytes contributes considerably to diarrhea in patients with TS, and may result from the action of unabsorbed bile acids and free unsaturated fatty acids.[76,77] Lymphocytic infiltration of the colonic mucosa is also seen.[78] Rarely, vitamin A deficiency, which is caused by fat-soluble vitamin malabsorption, may manifest with night blindness and corneal xerosis, while vitamin B12 deficiency can lead to subacute combined degeneration of the spinal cord.[79]

Restoration of fluid and electrolyte balance is necessary in dehydrated patients, and deficiencies of magnesium and potassium need to be corrected in those with long-standing illness. Specific deficiencies of vitamins A, D, and B complex vitamins may be treated with either parenteral or oral supplements. Parenteral vitamin B12, oral folate, and iron replacement result in prompt resolution of symptoms of anemia, glossitis, and anorexia, and may result in weight gain before improvement in intestinal absorption.[80] Folate supplementation improves macrocytic anemia and also villous atrophy.[81] Antimicrobial agents are widely used for treatment; oral tetracycline, 250 mg four times daily for 3 to 6 months, is the antibiotic of choice but cannot be used in young children. Restriction of long-chain fatty acids in the diet helps reduce diarrhea, which is one of the major symptoms. Medium-chain triglycerides (MCTs) may be substituted for long-chain fatty acids.[66] In endemic sprue, relapses are common, occurring in 50% of affected people.

AUTOIMMUNE ENTEROPATHY (AIE) AND IPEX SYNDROME

The hallmark of the different forms of autoimmune enteropathy (AIE) is the occurrence of profuse diarrhea—most often in the form of massive protein-losing enteropathy—along with villous atrophy and a massive mononuclear inflammatory infiltrate of the lamina propria on duodenal/jejunal histology as well as the occurrence of anti-enterocyte antibodies. AIE is typically a T-cell-mediated disorder, which has to be distinguished from classic immune deficiencies.[82]

IPEX Syndrome (AIE Type 1)

Immune dysregulation, polyendocrinopathy, enteropathy X-linked (IPEX) syndrome is a rare monogenic primary immunodeficiency characterized by multiorgan autoimmunity. It is caused by mutations in the transcription factor *Forkhead box P3 (FOXP3)*, the master gene of T-regulatory (Treg) cells. The disease shows an X-linked hereditary pattern: only males are affected, whereas the carrier mothers are healthy.

Most IPEX patients are born normally at term after an uneventful pregnancy from unrelated parents. A careful family history may reveal the presence of male subjects in the maternal lineage with a similar clinical phenotype, early death, or multiple spontaneous abortions.[83] The onset of IPEX syndrome usually occurs within the first months of life; however, in some cases, symptoms begin after a few days or weeks and can be rapidly fatal if not diagnosed and treated. The main clinical characteristic of IPEX syndrome is a combination of early onset type 1 diabetes mellitus (T1DM), severe immune-mediated enteropathy,[84] X chromosome linkage, and eczema-like dermatitis.[82]

AIE is the hallmark of IPEX syndrome. Patients present with watery, and sometimes mucoid or bloody diarrhea. This acute severe enteropathy often begins in the first days of life or during breast-feeding. It can be worsened by switching from breast-feeding to regular formula. The onset of diarrhea is often within the first 3 months of life; however, later onset has been occasionally described.[85,86] Characteristically, diarrhea is secretory and persists despite bowel rest. Patients often develop a protein-losing enteropathy with a marked increase of α-1 antitrypsin in the stool and serum hypoalbuminemia.[82] Since it results in severe malabsorption and significant failure to thrive, parenteral nutrition (PN) is often required. In addition to diarrhea, other gastrointestinal manifestations such as vomiting, gastritis, ileus, and colitis can be present.[84,87–89] T1DM can precede or follow the development of enteritis. T1DM is present in the majority of patients, including newborns, and is usually difficult to control.[90,91] Imaging studies or histological examination at autopsy often reveal destruction of the pancreas and intense lymphocytic infiltrate, suggesting that immune-mediated tissue damage plays a role in the pathogenesis.[92,93] Cutaneous manifestations appear in the first months of life and can be the first signs of the disease. Dermatitis can be in the form of eczematiform, ichthyosiform, or psoriasiform rashes.[94–97] Skin involvement is severe and diffuse, characterized by erythematous exudative plaques that can evolve into more lichenified plaques.[98] Pruritis is a major complaint in these patients, and it is intense and difficult to control with antihistamines. Cutaneous lesions often are resistant to standard treatments such as topical steroids or tacrolimus and can be complicated by bacterial infections with the potential development of sepsis. Other manifestations include chelitis, onychodystrophy, and alopecia.[90,98] The clinical picture can be complicated by the presence of other autoimmune conditions such as thyroiditis, cytopenias (hemolytic anemia, thrombocytopenia, and neutropenia), and hepatitis with positive autoantibodies.[82,90,92,98] Renal disease can be related either to autoimmunity or to prolonged administration of nephrotoxic drugs and can present as tubulonephropathy or nephrotic syndrome.[89,90,93] Splenomegaly and lymphadenopathy may progress as a result of an ongoing autoimmune lymphoproliferation, as evidenced by the extensive lymphocytic infiltrates in secondary lymphoid organs found in several patients at autopsy.[94,99] The clinical spectrum is complicated by infections; however, a clear causative role of pathogens in the onset of autoimmunity has not been demonstrated and infections can often be the consequence of multiple immunosuppressive medications.

Laboratory tests can be normal at the onset. There are no specific diagnostic findings in IPEX syndrome, although laboratory abnormalities consistent with T1DM and severe enteropathy are common. Moreover, other alterations may suggest ongoing autoimmune manifestations in other target organs, such as hypothyroidism, cytopenias, hepatitis, or nephropathy. Patients in the acute phase of disease can have normal or elevated white blood cell counts. Leukocytosis, if present, is due to an increase in lymphocytes but the percentage of lymphocyte subpopulations (CD3, CD4, CD8, CD16, CD19) remains unchanged despite immune dysregulation. The CD4/CD8 ratio is usually normal.[82] The CD4$^+$ CD25$^+$ FOXP3$^+$ Treg cells are present; however, FOXP3 protein expression can be reduced if FOXP3 mutations are present or if the patient is exposed to immunosuppressive therapy.[90,100] T-cell proliferation assays (mitogens and antigens) are within the low–normal range or completely normal in the majority of patients. Humoral immunity is normal with normal vaccination titers and normal immunoglobulin levels (IgG, IgM, and IgA). In contrast, IgE levels are often dramatically elevated and can be considered a diagnostic criterion for IPEX.[82] In addition, persistent or periodic eosinophilia is frequent, reflecting an atopic–allergic background. In fact, skin prick tests for immediate hypersensitivity are usually consistent with heightened allergic response.[101,102] A variety of autoantibodies are detected in most patients, and their presence usually correlates with signs of pathology in target organs, but their production may also be a sign of immune dysregulation without obvious pathological linkage.[103] There is increasing evidence that anti-enterocyte antibodies are present in IPEX patients, although these are not seen in all patients.[86,104] The AIE-related 75-kDa antigen (AIE-75), predominantly expressed in the brush border of the small intestine and proximal tubules of the kidney, has been identified as a specific target of the autoantibodies present in IPEX patients.[105,106]

Upper and lower gastrointestinal endoscopy are indicated when AIE is suspected. The entire gastrointestinal tract can be involved. In most cases, there is a marked discrepancy between macroscopic endoscopic and histological findings. Macroscopically, the mucosa of the stomach, duodenum, jejunum, and ileum show only mild abnormalities with a variable degree of enhanced mucosal granularity along with erythema. Most often, no aphthae or ulcerations are observed. Colonic lesions can be more pronounced with loss of the normal vascular pattern due to edema, along with erythema, potentially involving the entire colonic mucosa. In addition, a marked granular aspect of the mucosa is regularly observed. These findings are most often homogenous along the entire colon.[82] Obligate histological findings in IPEX are the combination of villous atrophy and a massive mucosal mononuclear cell infiltration. This infiltrate consists predominantly of T lymphocytes and eosinophils, but is not specific for the disease.[107] In most cases, severe-to-total villous atrophy is associated with crypt hyperplasia. Total villous atrophy on duodenal biopsies can initially lead to a suspicion of CD. In some patients, villous atrophy is associated with epithelial cell death and crypt abscess formation. Recent studies indicate that enterocyte cell death occurs through apoptosis probably induced by activated cytotoxic lymphocytes. The number of goblet cells is also reduced, and in some cases, goblet cells are almost absent[107] (Figure 11.2). These changes are often observed in small-bowel mucosa, but can also be seen in other parts of the digestive tract, such as the stomach or colon.[108] Extensive digestive involvement is usually associated with a poor outcome.

AIE Type 2 (IPEX-Like without Mutations in the *FOXP3* Gene)

The observation of rare cases of AIE in girls and atypical IPEX presentation in boys without mutations or alterations of the regulation of the *FOXP3* gene suggests that there might be a different, non-X-linked mode of disease. In most cases, girls present with multiple extraintestinal autoimmune manifestations, such as thyroiditis or diabetes.[82] There is a defect in Treg cells, which might be FOXP3+ or FOXP3- Treg cells.

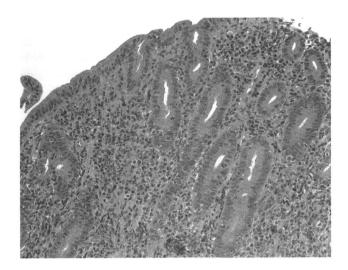

FIGURE 11.2   **(See color insert.)** Histological findings in AIE with villous atrophy, mucosal mononuclear cell infiltration, and decreased number of goblet cells. (Picture courtesy of Dr. Michael O'Brien, MD MPH, Boston Medical Center.)

AIE Type 3 (without or with Extraintestinal Manifestations)

Some patients present with symptoms exclusively limited to the gastrointestinal tract in the form of secretory diarrhea with positive-circulating anti-enterocyte or anti-colonocyte antibodies and positive anti-AIE-75 antibodies. In these patients, no extraintestinal manifestations are observed.[108] FOXP3 mutations are not a characteristic of these patients. Other mutations in regulatory genes controlling T-cell functions at the level of the intestinal mucosa are presumed to be the cause.[82] In general, endoscopic and histologic analyses are indistinguishable from IPEX syndrome, and a marked mononuclear cell infiltration of the intestinal lamina propria along with villous atrophy and epithelial cell apoptosis has been described. The diagnosis of AIE type 3 is established by the presence of anti-enterocyte and/or anti-colonocyte antibodies along with positive anti-AIE-75 antibodies.

Treatment

IPEX syndrome can be fatal in early infancy if not recognized. Therefore, a timely diagnosis is essential to initiate appropriate treatment. Owing to the limited number of cases reported in the literature, it has been difficult to compare different therapeutic strategies and relative outcomes. The current treatments available for IPEX syndrome include supportive therapy, immunosuppressive therapy, and hematopoietic stem cell transplantation. Nutritional support and immunosuppressive therapy should be started promptly to counteract the initial acute manifestations. A wasting syndrome can acutely affect the outcome of patients. At onset, patients are hospitalized and receive supportive care such as fluids, antibiotics, and albumin. All patients are initially dependent on PN. Management by PN can be additionally complicated in patients presenting with diabetes. Immunosuppressive medications and bone marrow transplantation have been shown to be effective in the treatment of IPEX.[83,104,109–111] Monotherapy or combination immunosuppression has been partially effective in controlling the autoimmune manifestations.[104,110,111] However, multiple immunosuppressive therapies are often required to control symptoms.[90]

Over the years, some experience has been gained in treating AIE patients with steroids alone or in combination with azathioprine, cyclosporine A, or tacrolimus.[87,112–114] Chronic immunosuppression can be effective in some patients but ineffective in others. Remission can most often be induced by the combination of methylprednisolone and tacrolimus.[82] The ultimate goal of immunosuppressive therapy is to stop secretory diarrhea, allowing the child to be weaned from PN and start oral or enteral nutrition. Chronic immunosuppression increases the risk of viral, bacterial, or fungal infections. *Pneumocystis jiroveci* pneumonia is not uncommon so patients are routinely placed on trimethoprim/sulfamethoxazole prophylaxis. In patients who survive the first years of life, immunosuppression may stabilize the existing symptoms; however, flares of the disease may occur and new symptoms may develop despite therapy.

Allogenic hematopoietic stem cell transplantation is considered the treatment of choice for IPEX syndrome. Early stem cell transplantation leads to the best outcome when the organs are yet to be damaged from autoimmunity and/or the adverse effects of therapy. Therefore, early diagnosis is fundamental. Among 15 cases of transplanted IPEX patients, an 80% survival rate has been reported.[83]

INTESTINAL LYMPHANGIECTASIA

Intestinal lymphangiectasia is a rare protein-losing gastroenteropathy caused by congenital malformation or obstruction of the intestinal lymphatic drainage resulting in lymph leakage into the small-bowel lumen. This loss of lymph is responsible for a protein-losing enteropathy leading to lymphopenia, hypoalbuminemia, and hypogammaglobulinemia.[115] Any factor causing an elevation of pressure against which the lymph has to drain from the intestinal wall leads to dilatation and even rupture of the lymphatic vessels, which, in turn, results in the leakage of lymphatic fluid.[116] As lymphatic fluid contains large amounts of fat, protein, and lymphocytes, leakage causes hypoproteinemia, lymphopenia, and decreased serum levels of immunoglobulin. Depending on the cause, it can be classified into primary or secondary intestinal lymphangiectasia. In 53% of cases, the age of onset of primary lymphangiectasia (PIL) was <2 years.[117] Peripheral edema of variable degree, usually symmetrical, from moderate (lower limb edema) to severe, including the face and external genitalia, is the main clinical feature, which accounts for 95% of the clinical manifestations of PIL.[115] Moderate serous effusions (pleural effusion, pericardial effusion, and chylous ascites) are common, and life-threatening anasarca may occur rarely throughout the course of the disease. The edema is pitting because the oncotic pressure is low due to hypoalbuminemia resulting from exudative enteropathy. Other common signs include diarrhea and ascites.[117] PIL may be suspected at birth or during pregnancy based on ultrasound images, which can detect fetal ascites or lower limb lymphedema.[118] PIL may be complicated by fatigue, abdominal pain, nausea, vomiting, and failure to thrive. Malabsorption may cause fat-soluble vitamin deficiencies and hypocalcaemia leading to convulsions.[115]

Several genes, such as *vascular endothelial growth factor receptor 3 (VEGFR3), prospero-related homeobox-transcription factor (PROC1), forkhead box C2 (FOXC2),* and *SOX18* have been implicated in the development of the lymphatic system. In a recent report, Hokari et al. reported inconsistent changes in the expression of regulatory molecules for lymphangiogenesis in the duodenal mucosa of PIL patients.[119] Diagnosis is confirmed by the presence of intestinal lymphangiectasia based on endoscopic findings with the corresponding histology of intestinal biopsies. Macroscopic abnormalities are usually obvious with the creamy yellow of jejunal villi corresponding to marked dilatation of the lymphatics within the intestinal mucosa. Histological examination of duodenal, jejunal, and ileal biopsies confirms the presence of lacteal juice, dilated mucosal and submucosal lymphatic vessels with polyclonal normal plasma cells. Intestinal lesions can be segmental or localized. Video capsule endoscopy has been used to diagnose PIL.[120] A high-fat diet before endoscopic examination leads to more prominent abnormal lymphatics and facilitates the endoscopic and histological diagnosis of intestinal lymphangiectasia.[116] Indirect biological abnormalities are suggestive of PIL and include hypoproteinemia; hypoalbuminemia; hypogammaglobulinemia with low IgG, IgA, and IgM levels; or lymphocytopenia. Elevated IgE levels without underlying allergic diathesis or disease has also been reported.[117] Exudative enteropathy is confirmed by high stool α-1-antitrypsin levels due to enteric protein loss.

PIL patients also have immunological abnormalities involving both B-cell and T-cell lineages of the immune system. The B-cell defects are characterized by low immunoglobulin levels (IgA, IgG, IgM) and poor antibody responses.[121] The T-cell defects are characterized by lymphocytopenia, prolonged skin–allograft rejection, and impaired *in vitro* proliferative responses to various stimulants (anti-CD3, anti-CD28).[122] Peripheral blood samples may contain extremely low counts of CD4+ T cells, especially naïve CD45RA+ CD62L+, while CD45RO+ memory cells are only moderately below normal. CD45RA+ and CD45RO+CD8+ T cells also are moderately below normal.[122]

Although PIL patients have moderate-to-severe hypogammaglobulinemia and lymphopenia, their risk of pyogenic bacterial infection and opportunistic infections has not been well described. However, severe and recurrent infections have been reported in case reports and case series.[123–125] In patients with very low CD4+ counts and immunoglobulin G levels, recurrent and opportunistic infections have been reported and contribute to higher morbidity and mortality.[125] Prophylactic antimicrobial therapy may be considered in these patients.

The first-line treatment of PIL is a low-fat diet with supplementary MCTs. The absence of long-chain triglyceride in the diet may decrease the engorgement of the intestinal lymphatics with chyle, thereby preventing their rupture with ensuing protein and T-cell loss. Since MCTs are directly absorbed into the portal venous circulation, they provide nutrients while avoiding lacteal engorgement. After a few weeks, this treatment may lead to reversal of clinical and laboratory measures such as hypoalbuminemia and lymphocytopenia.[126] In patients not responding to low-fat diet, enteral nutritional therapy (elemental, semielemental, and polymeric diets) may be required. In very severe cases, PN may be warranted.[127] The need for dietary control is permanent, as clinical and biochemical abnormalities reappear after a low-fat diet has been withdrawn. In cases with segmental lesions, local bowel resection has been successful.[117,128] Other treatments that have been proposed and usually used after or in combination with a low-fat diet (with MCT supplementation) include antiplasmin, octreotide, corticosteroids, and albumin infusions.[129–132] However, their efficacies are variable and have not been adequately evaluated.

INFLAMMATORY BOWEL DISEASE

IBD is a chronic inflammatory disorder that involves the colon in ulcerative colitis (UC) and may involve any part of the gastrointestinal tract in Crohn's disease. The disruption of the gastrointestinal tract by inflammation and the associated symptoms of pain, nausea, and diarrhea lead to reduced food intake, reduced nutrient use, and ultimately to impaired nutrition status in these patients (Figure 11.3). Decreased food intake, increased nutritional requirements, malabsorption and maldigestion, increased intestinal losses, disease activity, surgical resections, and medications are all potential factors in the etiology of malnutrition in IBD.[133–135]

Malnutrition is common in patients with IBD, especially in active Crohn's disease. Several studies have documented weight loss in 70%–80% of hospitalized patients and 20%–40% of outpatients with Crohn's disease. The prevalence of malnutrition is lower in patients with UC, but nutritional deficiencies can develop quickly in these patients during periods of active disease.[136–138] Growth failure is seen in approximately 30% of children with Crohn's disease (9 years of age to adolescence) and in 5%–10% of children with UC.[139,140] The cause of growth failure is multifactorial, given that patients with IBD face many nutritional obstacles. During active disease,

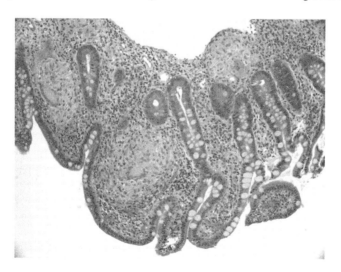

FIGURE 11.3 **(See color insert.)** Granuloma seen in the terminal ileum in a patient with Crohn's disease. (Picture courtesy of Dr. Michael O'Brien, MD MPH, Boston Medical Center.)

patients often experience anorexia, early satiety, and pain associated with eating. These symptoms limit oral intake and therefore overall caloric intake. Active disease within the small bowel can also lead to both macronutrient and micronutrient malabsorption. Although nutrition intervention can ameliorate adverse effects on growth failure, permanent growth impairment can still occur in 19%–35% of children with Crohn's disease.[141–143] However, permanent growth failure is rare in children with UC.[141,143]

Deficiencies of specific vitamins and minerals are not uncommon in IBD.[138,144,145] However, the clinical significance of these micronutrient deficiencies is not always apparent. Bone deficits have been well documented in children and adults with IBD.[146–148] Pediatric IBD is associated with multiple risk factors for impaired bone development, including growth failure, delayed maturation, malnutrition, malabsorption, micronutrient deficiencies, alterations in growth hormone axis, decreased muscle mass and weight-bearing activity, effects of cumulative corticosteroid therapy, and increased circulating inflammatory cytokines.[148,149] Avoidance of specific foods such as dairy products, which patients often undertake in an attempt to improve symptoms, can also lead to deficiencies in micronutrients such as calcium and vitamin D.[150] The prevalence of vitamin D deficiency ranges from 16% to 35% in pediatric patients with IBD.[151,152] Risk factors for low vitamin D status were wintertime measurement, African American race, upper gastrointestinal tract disease, and increased lifetime corticosteroid use.[151] These effects combined with decreased calcium and vitamin D intake may contribute to the high prevalence of osteopenia and osteoporosis in patients with IBD. Increased rates of fractures have also been demonstrated.[153–155] In addition to potential implications for immediate fracture risk, failure of bone mass accrual in childhood IBD may compromise adult bone health and result in skeletal fragility later in life. Dual-energy x-ray absorptiometry is widely accepted as a quantitative measurement technique for assessing skeletal status at all ages. Children should be assessed relative to age or body size and sex, with bone mineral density expressed as z-scores. Vitamin D supplementation and higher serum 25-hydroxyvitamin D levels have also been shown to be associated with quiescent disease activity.[156]

Other fat-soluble vitamin deficiencies have been reported in IBD. In a study of 97 children with IBD, 14% were deficient in vitamin A and 6% were deficient in vitamin E. Hypovitaminosis of either vitamin A or E was associated with increased disease activity; was present in 26% and 43% of those with moderately to severe active Crohn's disease and UC, respectively; and was rare in those with inactive disease.[157] These data may indicate that vitamin A and E status are more related to disease severity than nutritional status, although the clinical significance is unclear. Vitamin K has also been reported to be lower in adults with CD.[158] Low levels of vitamin K have been shown to be an independent risk factor for osteoporosis as vitamin K is a cofactor in the carboxylation of osteocalcin, a protein essential for calcium binding to bone.[159] Pediatric data on vitamin K are lacking.

Iron deficiency is the most common micronutrient deficiency to cause anemia in IBD. The prevalence of iron deficiency anemia in adults with IBD is reported to be between 6% and 73% of patients depending on disease type as well as laboratory definitions.[160] The prevalence of iron deficiency in pediatric patients with IBD is reported to be 17%.[161] Treating iron deficiency anemia can include nutrition counseling to increase dietary iron sources, addition of oral or parenteral iron supplements, and treatment of the underlying disease.[162,163] Iron dosing for the treatment of anemia in children ranges from 2 to 6 mg/kg per day of elemental iron for younger children. In most adult studies, between 100 and 200 mg of ferrous salts were used. Ferric iron has been used as well with reportedly reduced side effects and good efficacy.[164]

Vitamin B12 deficiency causing anemia should be considered when inflammation or surgery compromises normal function of the ileum, if macrocytic anemia is present, or if anemia does not respond to iron supplementation.[160] Plasma total homocysteine levels are higher in children with IBD and are linked to low plasma folate levels.[165] The concern for folic acid deficiency in IBD patients, especially in patients being treated with medications that interfere with folate metabolism (i.e., methotrexate or sulfasalazine), has led to the empiric folate supplementation in IBD patients. Although a dose of 1 mg of folic acid is commonly used in pediatrics, the folic acid requirement of children with Crohn's disease has not been determined.[145]

Nutrition therapy has been used in pediatric IBD with two main goals: (i) to correct nutrient deficiencies and (ii) to provide dietary therapy to improve disease activity and symptoms. It is essential to identify caloric deficiencies that are usually manifested by decreased body mass index and/or height for age as well as specific nutrient deficiencies in children and adolescents with IBD. Stunting is usually seen in patients with long-standing uncontrolled disease or delayed diagnosis. Undernourished children with CD who are provided long-term supplemental feedings can achieve catch-up growth, with average height and weight gain of 7–9 cm/year and 7 kg/year, respectively, with daily dietary energy intakes approximating 133% of recommended values for ideal body weight[166] or 60–75 kcal/kg actual body weight.[167] Patients at risk of or with identified micronutrient deficiencies will require appropriate vitamin and mineral supplementation based on the degree of deficiency and clinical considerations. Well-nourished patients should try to achieve recommended caloric intakes and recommended daily allowances of vitamins and micronutrients.

A number of randomized-controlled trials suggest that primary exclusive enteral nutrition (EEN) therapy not only achieves remission rates comparable to corticosteroids in children but also improves growth compared with patients receiving corticosteroids. EEN requires that the patient stop eating regular food and receive all dietary intake as an elemental or polymeric formula. Effective also in maintaining remission in pediatric IBD.[168–172] For adults with IBD, EEN has yielded conflicting results. A more recent systematic review confirmed higher rates of remission in corticosteroid-treated patients.[173,174] On the basis of methodological quality, the best adult study cited had an impressive nutrition-induced remission rate of 80%.[175]

Immunomodulators and biological therapy have become the standard of care in the medical management of moderate-to-severe IBD because of demonstrated efficacy. However, clinical studies, registries, and case reports warn of the increased risk of infections, particularly tuberculosis and fungal infections.[176] A randomized, multicenter, open-labeled study to evaluate safety and efficacy of maintenance therapy demonstrated that infliximab given every 8 weeks was more efficacious than when given every 12 weeks. The incidence of infections, however, increased in patients given infliximab more frequently. Infections occurred in 73.6% of children treated every 8 weeks compared with 38.0% of children treated every 12 weeks. During the 36-month follow-up, the most prevalent adverse events were respiratory infections. Ten percent of 60 patients at follow-up had severe respiratory infection.[177] A recent review of children who received adalimumab identified two deaths, both related to sepsis. In both cases, the children were receiving other immunosuppressive treatments and had central venous catheters (CVCs) in place.[178] In IBD, antibiotic prophylaxis is generally not recommended but can be used in special situations such as surgery.[179] Cotrimoxazole prophylaxis for *Pneumocystis jiroveci* is advised in children who are receiving three different immunosuppressive agents, in malnourished children with dual immunosuppressive therapy including infliximab or calcineurin inhibitors, and in children younger than 6 years with severe manifestations of IBD, in whom a primary immunodeficiency disorder is likely or cannot be excluded.[179]

There is also epidemiologic evidence that in patients with IBD, *Clostridium difficile* infection occurs more frequently than in the general population and these rates have been increasing over the past several decades.[180,181] Advances in our understanding of the epidemiology, immunology, and pathogenesis of *C. difficile* infection have not altered the increasing incidence.[182] Compounding this issue is the fact that asymptomatic colonization by *C. difficile* has been reported more frequently in the IBD population compared with the general population.[183] Clinically, there is a variable host response to *C. difficile* infection in patients with IBD ranging from asymptomatic carrier state to severe life-threatening colitis requiring colectomy and death.

INTESTINAL FAILURE

Intestinal failure (IF), a relatively new term, has superseded the traditional term "short-bowel syndrome." A clinically measurable definition of IF is the dependence on PN for >90 days. Functionally, IF encompasses all states wherein the absorptive capacity of the intestine is inadequate to meet nutrition, hydration, electrolyte, and growth requirements of the patient. The estimated incidence of IF is <1 to 10 per million.[184]

IF states are most commonly divided into three categories: (i) traditional short-bowel syndrome, resulting from significant loss of intestinal length; (ii) malabsorptive states such as microvillus inclusion disease, tufting enteropathy; and (iii) motility disorders, such as intestinal pseudoobstruction. IF in children is usually due to perinatal and congenital diseases. Intestinal atresia, gastroschisis, intestinal aganglionosis, volvulus, and necrotizing enterocolitis are the most common causes.[184] Among adults, the most common causes are intestinal infarction, radiation enteritis, and IBD.[184]

The major nutritional consequences of IF result from the loss of functional absorptive surface, which may be physical or functional, resulting in malabsorption of macronutrients and micronutrients, electrolytes, and water. The immediate manifestations are voluminous diarrhea, hypovolemia, hyponatremia, and hypokalemia. As the absorption of some nutrients is restricted to certain areas of the small intestine, the manifestations of IF caused by shortened bowel length may vary according to the specific areas that are involved. Iron, phosphorus, and water-soluble vitamins are predominantly absorbed in the proximal intestine. As most patients with short-bowel syndrome have an intact duodenum and proximal jejunum, deficiencies of these entities are rare but patients tend to develop calcium and magnesium deficiencies. Loss of part or whole of the ileum can result in vitamin B12 and bile salt malabsorption. Gastrointestinal hormones, such as gastrin, cholecystokinin, secretin, gastric inhibitory polypeptide, and motilin, are produced by endocrine cells in the proximal intestinal tract. These hormones usually remain intact. Glucagon-like peptide 1 and 2, neurotensin, and peptide YY are produced in the ileum and proximal colon, which may be deficient in short-bowel syndrome, and this may lead to rapid gastric emptying, shortened intestinal transit, and hypergastrinemia.[185,186] The presence of the ileocecal junction was previously thought to be an important variable for achieving enteral independence attributed to the barrier function and transit prolonging property of ileocecal valve.[187] As more is learned about the process of intestinal adaptation and the relative importance of ileum in this process, this advantage may actually be related to the specialized property of the terminal ileum itself.[188] In IF, deficiencies of specific micronutrients should be looked for and supplemented if needed. H2-receptor antagonists, proton pump inhibitors, antidiarrheal agents, cholestyramine, and octreotide have all been used to control the diarrhea.

Studies that have analyzed the natural history of IF in children report an overall survival rate of ~90% during a follow-up period of 1 to 5 years.[189–192] In children, the most common causes of death are bacterial infection and cholestatic liver disease.[190] Adequate homeostasis and growth are the goal of nutrition therapy in IF. The mainstay of this therapy in the initial phase of management of IF is PN. Long-term treatment with PN at home has become an established treatment option for adult and pediatric patients with severe IF. Home PN requires the presence of a CVC for safe and effective venous access. A common complication in patients with IF and indwelling CVC access is catheter-related blood stream infection (CRBSI), which may lead to sepsis and, potentially, death. Therefore, any patient with IF and an indwelling CVC that presents with fever, lethargy, and ileus must be presumed to have a CRBSI until proven otherwise. The gold standard for diagnosing a CRBSI is to collect blood cultures through all lumens of the CVC, as well as peripheral blood cultures. The standard practice has been to treat empirically with broad-spectrum intravenous antibiotics through the CVC until the blood cultures remain negative for 48 h or an infection is proven and the antibiotics can be tailored to the pathogen's susceptibilities. In certain cases, removal of the CVC will be necessary. Clearly, prevention of CRBSI is the main goal. Multiple studies have looked at methods including protocols centered on checklists for the placement of CVCs and specific protocols for changing the dressings.[193,194] Other methods evaluated include the use of chlorhexidine-based cleansing solutions and chlorhexidine-impregnated dressings, the use of antimicrobial-impregnated CVCs, and the use of antibiotic locks.[195] The most recent promising method is the use of 70% ethanol locks. This intervention is associated with a decrease in the rate of CRBSI in IF patients from 9.9 per 1000 catheter-days to 2.1 per 1000 catheter-days with no demonstrated adverse effects.[196]

ACRODERMATITIS ENTEROPATHICA AND ZINC DEFICIENCY

Acrodermatitis enteropathica (AE) is a rare autosomal recessive disorder of zinc deficiency. Individuals with AE have severe zinc deficiency derived from a defect of zinc absorption in the duodenum and jejunum. The genetic defect in AE has been mapped to 8q24 and the defective gene identified as *SLC39A4*, which encodes the zinc transporter Zip4. Inherited zinc deficiency, AE, occurs worldwide with an estimated incidence of 1 per 500,000 children. It has no predilection for race or sex.[197] In contrast to the United States, dietary zinc deficiency is a major factor contributing to the burden of disease in children in developing countries. Inadequate zinc intake affects a third of some populations in Southeast Asia and sub-Saharan Africa, where children are most severely affected. In these countries, zinc-related growth stunting affects 40% of preschool children and zinc supplementation has been shown to dramatically reduce common infant morbidities and mortalities.[198] In developed countries, groups at risk of dietary zinc deficiency include vegetarians, alcoholics, malnourished patients, and premature infants.[199]

Given the diverse physiologic functions of zinc, it is not surprising that there are multiple signs and symptoms of AE. AE usually presents in infancy–within days if an infant is bottled-fed, and days to weeks after weaning in breast-fed infants. The clinical presentation of AE is similar to the deficiency dermatitis caused by low dietary zinc. AE presents with eczematous pink scaly plaques, which can become vesicular, bullous, pustular, or desquamative. The lesions develop over the extremities, and anogenital and periorificial areas. Angular cheilitis is a common early manifestation followed by paronychia. Without treatment, skin lesions slowly evolve into erosions and patients develop generalized alopecia and diarrhea. The triad of total alopecia, skin lesions with localization around the body orifices and on the extremities, and diarrhea or other obscure gastrointestinal dysfunction was once thought to be essential in making the diagnosis of AE. Patients with advanced disease will also experience growth delay, mental slowing, poor wound healing, anemia, photophobia, hypogeusia, anorexia, delayed puberty, and hypogonadism in boys and men. Skin lesions can be secondarily infected with bacteria and *Candida albicans*.[199]

Establishing a diagnosis of zinc deficiency may be complicated by the fact that zinc levels may decrease during states of inflammation. Thus, the presence of a depressed serum or plasma zinc level does not always indicate zinc deficiency. In addition, the zinc level may be within normal limits in a deficiency dermatitis that nevertheless responds to zinc replacement therapy.[199]

Zinc replacement therapy should be started at 3 mg/kg per day of elemental zinc. Serum or plasma zinc levels and zinc-dependent enzyme levels should be monitored every 3 to 6 months and the dose of zinc should be adjusted appropriately. Typically, clinical improvement is seen very rapidly, within days to weeks, before a significant change in serum zinc levels. In deficiency dermatitis caused by low dietary zinc, replacement therapy should be initiated at 0.5 to 1 mg/kg per day of elemental zinc. Importantly, in patients who are malnourished, a multinutrient replacement approach is warranted.[199]

REFERENCES

1. Shahid NS, Sack DA, Rahman M, Alam AN, Rahman N. Risk factors for persistent diarrhoea. *BMJ*. Oct 22, 1988;297(6655):1036–1038.
2. Sibal A, Patwari AK, Anand VK, Chhabra AK, Chandra D. Associated infections in persistent diarrhoea—Another perspective. *Journal of Tropical Pediatrics*. Apr 1996;42(2):64–67.
3. Maki M. Celiac disease. In Kleinman R, Goulet O, Mieli-Vergani G, Sanderson I, eds. *Walker's Pediatric Gastrointestinal Disease*, Vol. 1, 5th ed. Hamilton, Ontario: BC Decker, 2008.
4. Koning F, Schuppan D, Cerf-Bensussan N, Sollid LM. Pathomechanisms in celiac disease. *Best Practice & Research. Clinical Gastroenterology*. Jun 2005;19(3):373–387.
5. Dieterich W, Ehnis T, Bauer M et al. Identification of tissue transglutaminase as the autoantigen of celiac disease. *Nature Medicine*. Jul 1997;3(7):797–801.
6. Jabri B, Sollid LM. Mechanisms of disease: Immunopathogenesis of celiac disease. Nature clinical practice. *Gastroenterology & Hepatology*. Sep 2006;3(9):516–525.
7. Kagnoff MF. Celiac disease: Pathogenesis of a model immunogenetic disease. *The Journal of Clinical Investigation*. Jan 2007;117(1):41–49.
8. Rawashdeh MO, Khalil B, Raweily E. Celiac disease in Arabs. *Journal of Pediatric Gastroenterology and Nutrition*. Nov 1996;23(4):415–418.
9. Verkasalo M, Kuitunen P, Leisti S, Perheentupa J. Growth failure from symptomless celiac disease. A study of 14 patients. *Helvetica Paediatrica Acta*. Dec 1978;33(6): 489–495.
10. Bonamico M, Scire G, Mariani P et al. Short stature as the primary manifestation of monosymptomatic celiac disease. *Journal of Pediatric Gastroenterology and Nutrition*. Jan 1992;14(1):12–16.
11. Dossetor JF, Gibson AA, McNeish AS. Childhood coeliac disease is disappearing. *Lancet*. Feb 7, 1981;1(8215):322–323.
12. Catassi C, Ratsch IM, Fabiani E et al. Coeliac disease in the year 2000: Exploring the iceberg. *Lancet*. Jan 22, 1994;343(8891):200–203.
13. Maki M, Hallstrom O, Verronen P et al. Reticulin antibody, arthritis, and coeliac disease in children. *Lancet*. Feb 27, 1988;1(8583):479–480.
14. Oberhuber G, Granditsch G, Vogelsang H. The histopathology of coeliac disease: Time for a standardized report scheme for pathologists. *European Journal of Gastroenterology & Hepatology*. Oct 1999;11(10):1185–1194.
15. Marsh MN. Grains of truth: Evolutionary changes in small intestinal mucosa in response to environmental antigen challenge. *Gut*. Jan 1990;31(1):111–114.
16. Husby S, Koletzko S, Korponay-Szabo IR et al. European Society for Pediatric Gastroenterology, Hepatology, and Nutrition guidelines for the diagnosis of coeliac disease. *Journal of Pediatric Gastroenterology and Nutrition*. Jan 2012;54(1):136–160.
17. Klapp G, Masip E, Bolonio M et al. Celiac disease: The new proposed ESPGHAN diagnostic criteria do work well in a selected population. *Journal of Pediatric Gastroenterology and Nutrition*. Mar 2013;56(3):251–256.
18. Brousse N, Meijer JW. Malignant complications of coeliac disease. *Best Practice & Research. Clinical Gastroenterology*. Jun 2005;19(3):401–412.
19. Halfdanarson TR, Litzow MR, Murray JA. Hematologic manifestations of celiac disease. *Blood*. Jan 15, 2007;109(2):412–421.

20. Goodnough LT, Nemeth E. Iron deficiency and related disorder. In Arber DA, Glader B, List AF, eds. *Wintrobe's Clinical Hematology*, Vol. 1, 13th ed. Philadelphia: Lippincott Williams and Wilkins, 2013.

21. Cook JD. Diagnosis and management of iron-deficiency anaemia. *Best Practice & Research. Clinical Haematology*. Jun 2005;18(2):319–332.

22. Gregory JF 3rd, Quinlivan EP. *In vivo* kinetics of folate metabolism. *Annual Review of Nutrition*. 2002;22:199–220.

23. Pawson R, Mehta A. Review article: The diagnosis and treatment of haematinic deficiency in gastrointestinal disease. *Alimentary Pharmacology & Therapeutics*. Aug 1998;12(8):687–698.

24. Pittschieler K. Folic acid concentration in the serum and erythrocytes of patients with celiac disease. *Padiatrie und Padologie*. 1986;21(4):363–366.

25. Howard MR, Turnbull AJ, Morley P, Hollier P, Webb R, Clarke A. A prospective study of the prevalence of undiagnosed coeliac disease in laboratory defined iron and folate deficiency. *Journal of Clinical Pathology*. Oct 2002;55(10):754–757.

26. Haapalahti M, Kulmala P, Karttunen TJ et al. Nutritional status in adolescents and young adults with screen-detected celiac disease. *Journal of Pediatric Gastroenterology and Nutrition*. May 2005;40(5):566–570.

27. Kuzminski AM, Del Giacco EJ, Allen RH, Stabler SP, Lindenbaum J. Effective treatment of cobalamin deficiency with oral cobalamin. *Blood*. Aug 15, 1998;92(4):1191–1198.

28. Gillberg R, Kastrup W, Mobacken H, Stockbrugger R, Ahren C. Gastric morphology and function in dermatitis herpetiformis and in coeliac disease. *Scandinavian Journal of Gastroenterology*. Mar 1985;20(2):133–140.

29. Dickey W, Hughes DF. Histology of the terminal ileum in coeliac disease. *Scandinavian Journal of Gastroenterology*. Jul 2004;39(7):665–667.

30. Dahele A, Ghosh S. Vitamin B12 deficiency in untreated celiac disease. *The American Journal of Gastroenterology*. Mar 2001;96(3):745–750.

31. Dickey W. Low serum vitamin B12 is common in coeliac disease and is not due to autoimmune gastritis. *European Journal of Gastroenterology & Hepatology*. Apr 2002;14(4):425–427.

32. Ward PC. Modern approaches to the investigation of vitamin B12 deficiency. *Clinics in Laboratory Medicine*. Jun 2002;22(2):435–445.

33. Klee GG. Cobalamin and folate evaluation: Measurement of methylmalonic acid and homocysteine vs vitamin B(12) and folate. *Clinical Chemistry*. Aug 2000;46(8 Pt 2):1277–1283.

34. Vidal-Alaball J, Butler CC, Cannings-John R et al. Oral vitamin B12 versus intramuscular vitamin B12 for vitamin B12 deficiency. *Cochrane Database of Systematic Reviews*. 2005(3):CD004655.

35. Goyens P, Brasseur D, Cadranel S. Copper deficiency in infants with active celiac disease. *Journal of Pediatric Gastroenterology and Nutrition*. Aug 1985;4(4):677–680.

36. Jameson S, Hellsing K, Magnusson S. Copper malabsorption in coeliac disease. *The Science of the Total Environment*. Mar 15, 1985;42(1–2):29–36.

37. Fisgin T, Yarali N, Duru F, Usta B, Kara A. Hematologic manifestation of childhood celiac disease. *Acta Haematologica*. 2004;111(4):211–214.

38. Pittschieler K. Neutropenia, granulocytic hypersegmentation and coeliac disease. *Acta Paediatrica*. Jun 1995;84(6):705–706.

39. Saibeni S, Lecchi A, Meucci G et al. Prevalence of hyperhomocysteinemia in adult gluten-sensitive enteropathy at diagnosis: Role of B12, folate, and genetics. *Clinical Gastroenterology and Hepatology: The Official Clinical Practice Journal of the American Gastroenterological Association*. Jun 2005;3(6):574–580.

40. Saibeni S, Bottasso B, Spina L et al. Assessment of thrombin-activatable fibrinolysis inhibitor (TAFI) plasma levels in inflammatory bowel diseases. *The American Journal of Gastroenterology*. Oct 2004;99(10):1966–1970.

41. van Tilburg NH, Rosendaal FR, Bertina RM. Thrombin activatable fibrinolysis inhibitor and the risk for deep vein thrombosis. *Blood*. May 1, 2000;95(9):2855–2859.
42. Thorburn D, Stanley AJ, Foulis A, Campbell Tait R. Coeliac disease presenting as variceal haemorrhage. *Gut*. May 2003;52(5):758.
43. Krasinski SD, Russell RM, Furie BC, Kruger SF, Jacques PF, Furie B. The prevalence of vitamin K deficiency in chronic gastrointestinal disorders. *The American Journal of Clinical Nutrition*. Mar 1985;41(3):639–643.
44. Jacobs P, Wood L. Macronutrients. *Disease-a-Month: DM*. Feb 2004;50(2):46–115.
45. Granel B, Rossi P, Frances Y, Henry JF. Bilateral massive adrenal haemorrhage revealing coeliac disease. *QJM: Monthly Journal of the Association of Physicians*. Jan 2005;98(1):70–71.
46. Lubel JS, Burrell LM, Levidiotis V. An unexpected cause of macroscopic haematuria. *The Medical Journal of Australia*. Sep 19, 2005;183(6):321–323.
47. Marsh GW, Stewart JS. Splenic function in adult coeliac disease. *British Journal of Haematology*. Oct 1970;19(4):445–457.
48. Ferguson A, Hutton MM, Maxwell JD, Murray D. Adult coeliac disease in hyposplenic patients. *Lancet*. Jan 24, 1970;1(7639):163–164.
49. Corazza GR, Bullen AW, Hall R, Robinson PJ, Losowsky MS. Simple method of assessing splenic function in coeliac disease. *Clinical Science (London)*. Jan 1981;60(1):109–113.
50. Johnston SD, Robinson J. Fatal pneumococcal septicaemia in a coeliac patient. *European Journal of Gastroenterology & Hepatology*. Apr 1998;10(4):353–354.
51. O'Donoghue DJ. Fatal pneumococcal septicaemia in coeliac disease. *Postgraduate Medical Journal*. Mar 1986;62(725):229–230.
52. Parnell N, Thomas P. Fatal pneumococcal septicaemia in a coeliac patient. *European Journal of Gastroenterology & Hepatology*. Oct 1998;10(10):899–900.
53. Stevens FM, Connolly CE, Murray JP, McCarthy CF. Lung cavities in patients with coeliac disease. *Digestion*. 1990;46(2):72–80.
54. Howat AJ, McPhie JL, Smith DA et al. Cavitation of mesenteric lymph nodes: A rare complication of coeliac disease, associated with a poor outcome. *Histopathology*. Oct 1995;27(4):349–354.
55. Schmitz F, Herzig KH, Stuber E et al. On the pathogenesis and clinical course of mesenteric lymph node cavitation and hyposplenism in coeliac disease. *International Journal of Colorectal Disease*. May 2002;17(3):192–198.
56. Melles DC, de Marie S. Prevention of infections in hyposplenic and asplenic patients: An update. *The Netherlands Journal of Medicine*. Feb 2004;62(2):45–52.
57. Pediatrics. AAo. Immunization in special clinical circumstances: Immunocompromised children. In Pickering LK, ed. *Red Book*, 27th ed. Elk Grove Village, IL: American Academy of Pediatrics, 2006.
58. McKinley M, Leibowitz S, Bronzo R, Zanzi I, Weissman G, Schiffman G. Appropriate response to pneumococcal vaccine in celiac sprue. *Journal of Clinical Gastroenterology*. Mar 1995;20(2):113–116.
59. Cataldo F, Marino V, Ventura A, Bottaro G, Corazza GR. Prevalence and clinical features of selective immunoglobulin A deficiency in coeliac disease: An Italian multicentre study. Italian Society of Paediatric Gastroenterology and Hepatology (SIGEP) and "Club del Tenue" Working Groups on Coeliac Disease. *Gut*. Mar 1998;42(3):362–365.
60. Meini A, Pillan NM, Villanacci V, Monafo V, Ugazio AG, Plebani A. Prevalence and diagnosis of celiac disease in IgA-deficient children. *Annals of Allergy, Asthma & Immunology: Official Publication of the American College of Allergy, Asthma, & Immunology*. Oct 1996;77(4):333–336.
61. Kalyoncu D, Urganci N. Response to hepatitis A and B vaccination in patients with chronic hepatitis C: 8-year follow-up. *Paediatrics and International Child Health*. Aug 2012;32(3):136–139.

62. Schuppan D, Junker Y, Barisani D. Celiac disease: From pathogenesis to novel therapies. *Gastroenterology.* Dec 2009;137(6):1912–1933.
63. Cook GC. Aetiology and pathogenesis of postinfective tropical malabsorption (tropical sprue). *Lancet.* Mar 31, 1984;1(8379):721–723.
64. Booth C. Tropical sprue. *Lancet.* May 5, 1984;1(8384):1018.
65. Khokhar N, Gill ML. Tropical sprue: Revisited. *JPMA. The Journal of the Pakistan Medical Association.* Mar 2004;54(3):133–134.
66. Ramakrishna BS, Venkataraman S, Mukhopadhya A. Tropical malabsorption. *Postgraduate Medical Journal.* Dec 2006;82(974):779–787.
67. Klipstein FA. Tropical sprue in travelers and expatriates living abroad. *Gastroenterology.* Mar 1981;80(3):590–600.
68. Tomkins A. Tropical malabsorption: Recent concepts in pathogenesis and nutritional significance. *Clinical Science (London).* Feb 1981;60(2):131–137.
69. Walker MM. What is tropical sprue? *Journal of Gastroenterology and Hepatology.* Aug 2003;18(8):887–890.
70. Ghoshal UC, Ghoshal U, Ayyagari A et al. Tropical sprue is associated with contamination of small bowel with aerobic bacteria and reversible prolongation of orocecal transit time. *Journal of Gastroenterology and Hepatology.* May 2003;18(5):540–547.
71. Haghighi P, Wolf PL. Tropical sprue and subclinical enteropathy: A vision for the nineties. *Critical Reviews in Clinical Laboratory Sciences.* 1997;34(4):313–341.
72. Humphrey JH. Child undernutrition, tropical enteropathy, toilets, and handwashing. *Lancet.* Sep 19, 2009;374(9694):1032–1035.
73. Owens SR, Greenson JK. The pathology of malabsorption: Current concepts. *Histopathology.* Jan 2007;50(1):64–82.
74. Westergaard H. Tropical sprue. *Current Treatment Options in Gastroenterology.* Feb 2004;7(1):7–11.
75. Mathan M, Mathan VI, Baker SJ. An electron-microscopic study of jejunal mucosal morphology in control subjects and in patients with tropical sprue in southern India. *Gastroenterology.* Jan 1975;68(1):17–32.
76. Ramakrishna BS, Mathan VI. Water and electrolyte absorption by the colon in tropical sprue. *Gut.* Oct 1982;23(10):843–846.
77. Ramakrishna BS, Mathan VI. Role of bacterial toxins, bile acids, and free fatty acids in colonic water malabsorption in tropical sprue. *Digestive Diseases and Sciences.* May 1987;32(5):500–505.
78. Puri AS, Khan EM, Kumar M, Pandey R, Choudhuri G. Association of lymphocytic (microscopic) colitis with tropical sprue. *Journal of Gastroenterology and Hepatology.* Jan–Feb 1994;9(1):105–107.
79. Iyer GV, Taori GM, Kapadia CR, Mathan VI, Baker SJ. Neurologic manifestations in tropical sprue. A clinical and electrodiagnostic study. *Neurology.* Sep 1973;23(9): 959–966.
80. Tomkins AM, Smith T, Wright SG. Assessment of early and delayed responses in vitamin B12 absorption during antibiotic therapy in tropical malabsorption. *Clinical Science and Molecular Medicine. Supplement.* Dec 1978;55(6):533–539.
81. Sheehy TW, Baggs B, Perez-Santiago E, Floch MH. Prognosis of tropical sprue. A study of the effect of folic acid on the intestinal aspects of acute and chronic sprue. *Annals of Internal Medicine.* Dec 1962;57:892–908.
82. Ruemmele FM, Brousse N, Goulet O. Autoimmune enteropathy and IPEX syndrome. *Walker's Pediatric Gastrointestinal Disease,* Vol. 1, 5th ed. Hamilton, Ontario: BC Decker Inc., 2008.
83. Barzaghi F, Passerini L, Bacchetta R. Immune dysregulation, polyendocrinopathy, enteropathy, x-linked syndrome: A paradigm of immunodeficiency with autoimmunity. *Frontiers in Immunology.* 2012;3:211.

84. Scaillon M, Van Biervliet S, Bontems P et al. Severe gastritis in an insulin-dependent child with an IPEX syndrome. *Journal of Pediatric Gastroenterology and Nutrition*. Sep 2009;49(3):368–370.
85. Goulet OJ, Brousse N, Canioni D, Walker-Smith JA, Schmitz J, Phillips AD. Syndrome of intractable diarrhoea with persistent villous atrophy in early childhood: A clinico-pathological survey of 47 cases. *Journal of Pediatric Gastroenterology and Nutrition*. Feb 1998;26(2):151–161.
86. Russo PA, Brochu P, Seidman EG, Roy CC. Autoimmune enteropathy. *Pediatric and Developmental Pathology: The Official Journal of the Society for Pediatric Pathology and the Paediatric Pathology Society*. Jan–Feb 1999;2(1):65–71.
87. Ferguson PJ, Blanton SH, Saulsbury FT et al. Manifestations and linkage analysis in X-linked autoimmunity-immunodeficiency syndrome. *American Journal of Medical Genetics*. Feb 28, 2000;90(5):390–397.
88. Levy-Lahad E, Wildin RS. Neonatal diabetes mellitus, enteropathy, thrombocytopenia, and endocrinopathy: Further evidence for an X-linked lethal syndrome. *The Journal of Pediatrics*. Apr 2001;138(4):577–580.
89. Otsubo K, Kanegane H, Kamachi Y et al. Identification of FOXP3-negative regulatory T-like (CD4(+)CD25(+)CD127(low)) cells in patients with immune dysregulation, polyendocrinopathy, enteropathy, X-linked syndrome. *Clinical Immunology*. Oct 2011;141(1):111–120.
90. Gambineri E, Perroni L, Passerini L et al. Clinical and molecular profile of a new series of patients with immune dysregulation, polyendocrinopathy, enteropathy, X-linked syndrome: Inconsistent correlation between forkhead box protein 3 expression and disease severity. *The Journal of Allergy and Clinical Immunology*. Dec 2008;122(6):1105–1112.e1101.
91. Baud O, Goulet O, Canioni D et al. Treatment of the immune dysregulation, polyendocrinopathy, enteropathy, X-linked syndrome (IPEX) by allogeneic bone marrow transplantation. *The New England Journal of Medicine*. Jun 7, 2001;344(23):1758–1762.
92. Wildin RS, Ramsdell F, Peake J et al. X-linked neonatal diabetes mellitus, enteropathy and endocrinopathy syndrome is the human equivalent of mouse scurfy. *Nature Genetics*. Jan 2001;27(1):18–20.
93. Rubio-Cabezas O, Klupa T, Malecki MT. Permanent neonatal diabetes mellitus—The importance of diabetes differential diagnosis in neonates and infants. *European Journal of Clinical Investigation*. Mar 2011;41(3):323–333.
94. Wildin RS, Smyk-Pearson S, Filipovich AH. Clinical and molecular features of the immunodysregulation, polyendocrinopathy, enteropathy, X linked (IPEX) syndrome. *Journal of Medical Genetics*. Aug 2002;39(8):537–545.
95. Ruemmele FM, Moes N, de Serre NP, Rieux-Laucat F, Goulet O. Clinical and molecular aspects of autoimmune enteropathy and immune dysregulation, polyendocrinopathy autoimmune enteropathy X-linked syndrome. *Current Opinion in Gastroenterology*. Nov 2008;24(6):742–748.
96. Rao A, Kamani N, Filipovich A et al. Successful bone marrow transplantation for IPEX syndrome after reduced-intensity conditioning. *Blood*. Jan 1, 2007;109(1):383–385.
97. De Benedetti F, Insalaco A, Diamanti A et al. Mechanistic associations of a mild phenotype of immunodysregulation, polyendocrinopathy, enteropathy, x-linked syndrome. *Clinical Gastroenterology and Hepatology: The Official Clinical Practice Journal of the American Gastroenterological Association*. May 2006;4(5):653–659.
98. Halabi-Tawil M, Ruemmele FM, Fraitag S et al. Cutaneous manifestations of immune dysregulation, polyendocrinopathy, enteropathy, X-linked (IPEX) syndrome. *The British Journal of Dermatology*. Mar 2009;160(3):645–651.
99. Ochs HD, Torgerson TR. Immune dysregulation, polyendocrinopathy, enteropathy, X-linked inheritance: Model for autoaggression. *Advances in Experimental Medicine and Biology*. 2007;601:27–36.

100. Bacchetta R, Gambineri E, Roncarolo MG. Role of regulatory T cells and FOXP3 in human diseases. *The Journal of Allergy and Clinical Immunology.* Aug 2007;120(2):227–235; quiz 236–237.

101. Bennett CL, Yoshioka R, Kiyosawa H et al. X-linked syndrome of polyendocrinopathy, immune dysfunction, and diarrhea maps to Xp11.23-Xq13.3. *American Journal of Human Genetics.* Feb 2000;66(2):461–468.

102. Cuenod B, Brousse N, Goulet O et al. Classification of intractable diarrhea in infancy using clinical and immunohistological criteria. *Gastroenterology.* Oct 1990;99(4):1037–1043.

103. Tsuda M, Torgerson TR, Selmi C et al. The spectrum of autoantibodies in IPEX syndrome is broad and includes anti-mitochondrial autoantibodies. *Journal of Autoimmunity.* Nov 2010;35(3):265–268.

104. Jonas MM, Bell MD, Eidson MS, Koutouby R, Hensley GT. Congenital diabetes mellitus and fatal secretory diarrhea in two infants. *Journal of Pediatric Gastroenterology and Nutrition.* Nov 1991;13(4):415–425.

105. Moes N, Rieux-Laucat F, Begue B et al. Reduced expression of FOXP3 and regulatory T-cell function in severe forms of early-onset autoimmune enteropathy. *Gastroenterology.* Sep 2010;139(3):770–778.

106. Gambineri E, Torgerson TR, Ochs HD. Immune dysregulation, polyendocrinopathy, enteropathy, and X-linked inheritance (IPEX), a syndrome of systemic autoimmunity caused by mutations of FOXP3, a critical regulator of T-cell homeostasis. *Current Opinion in Rheumatology.* Jul 2003;15(4):430–435.

107. Patey-Mariaud de Serre N, Canioni D, Ganousse S et al. Digestive histopathological presentation of IPEX syndrome. *Modern Pathology: An Official Journal of the United States and Canadian Academy of Pathology, Inc.* Jan 2009;22(1):95–102.

108. Hill SM, Milla PJ, Bottazzo GF, Mirakian R. Autoimmune enteropathy and colitis: Is there a generalised autoimmune gut disorder? *Gut.* Jan 1991;32(1):36–42.

109. Seidman EG, Lacaille F, Russo P, Galeano N, Murphy G, Roy CC. Successful treatment of autoimmune enteropathy with cyclosporine. *The Journal of Pediatrics.* Dec 1990;117(6):929–932.

110. Walker-Smith JA, Unsworth DJ, Hutchins P, Phillips AD, Holborow EJ. Autoantibodies against gut epithelium in child with small-intestinal enteropathy. *Lancet.* Mar 6, 1982;1(8271):566–567.

111. Unsworth J, Hutchins P, Mitchell J et al. Flat small intestinal mucosa and autoantibodies against the gut epithelium. *Journal of Pediatric Gastroenterology and Nutrition.* 1982;1(4):503–513.

112. Satake N, Nakanishi M, Okano M et al. A Japanese family of X-linked auto-immune enteropathy with haemolytic anaemia and polyendocrinopathy. *European Journal of Pediatrics.* Apr 1993;152(4):313–315.

113. Torgerson TR, Linane A, Moes N et al. Severe food allergy as a variant of IPEX syndrome caused by a deletion in a noncoding region of the FOXP3 gene. *Gastroenterology.* May 2007;132(5):1705–1717.

114. Kobayashi I, Kawamura N, Okano M. A long-term survivor with the immune dysregulation, polyendocrinopathy, enteropathy, X-linked syndrome. *The New England Journal of Medicine.* Sep 27, 2001;345(13):999–1000.

115. Vignes S, Bellanger J. Primary intestinal lymphangiectasia (Waldmann's disease). *Orphanet Journal of Rare Diseases.* 2008;3:5.

116. Lee J, Kong MS. Primary intestinal lymphangiectasia diagnosed by endoscopy following the intake of a high-fat meal. *European Journal of Pediatrics.* Feb 2008;167(2):237–239.

117. Wen J, Tang Q, Wu J, Wang Y, Cai W. Primary intestinal lymphangiectasia: Four case reports and a review of the literature. *Digestive Diseases and Sciences.* Dec 2010;55(12):3466–3472.

118. Schmider A, Henrich W, Reles A, Vogel M, Dudenhausen JW. Isolated fetal ascites caused by primary lymphangiectasia: A case report. *American Journal of Obstetrics and Gynecology.* Jan 2001;184(2):227–228.

119. Hokari R, Kitagawa N, Watanabe C et al. Changes in regulatory molecules for lymphangiogenesis in intestinal lymphangiectasia with enteric protein loss. *Journal of Gastroenterology and Hepatology.* Jul 2008;23(7 Pt 2):e88–e95.

120. Rivet C, Lapalus MG, Dumortier J et al. Use of capsule endoscopy in children with primary intestinal lymphangiectasia. *Gastrointestinal Endoscopy.* Oct 2006;64(4):649–650.

121. Heresbach D, Raoul JL, Genetet N et al. Immunological study in primary intestinal lymphangiectasia. *Digestion.* 1994;55(1):59–64.

122. Fuss IJ, Strober W, Cuccherini BA et al. Intestinal lymphangiectasia, a disease characterized by selective loss of naive CD45RA+ lymphocytes into the gastrointestinal tract. *European Journal of Immunology.* Dec 1998;28(12):4275–4285.

123. Hallevy C, Sperber AD, Almog Y. Group G streptococcal empyema complicating primary intestinal lymphangiectasia. *Journal of Clinical Gastroenterology.* Sep 2003; 37(3):270.

124. Cole SL, Ledford DK, Lockey RF, Daas A, Kooper J. Primary gastrointestinal lymphangiectasia presenting as cryptococcal meningitis. *Annals of Allergy, Asthma & Immunology: Official Publication of the American College of Allergy, Asthma, & Immunology.* May 2007;98(5):490–492.

125. Dierselhuis MP, Boelens JJ, Versteegh FG, Weemaes C, Wulffraat NM. Recurrent and opportunistic infections in children with primary intestinal lymphangiectasia. *Journal of Pediatric Gastroenterology and Nutrition.* Mar 2007;44(3):382–385.

126. Alfano V, Tritto G, Alfonsi L, Cella A, Pasanisi F, Contaldo F. Stable reversal of pathologic signs of primitive intestinal lymphangiectasia with a hypolipidic, MCT-enriched diet. *Nutrition.* Apr 2000;16(4):303–304.

127. Aoyagi K, Iida M, Matsumoto T, Sakisaka S. Enteral nutrition as a primary therapy for intestinal lymphangiectasia: Value of elemental diet and polymeric diet compared with total parenteral nutrition. *Digestive Diseases and Sciences.* Aug 2005;50(8): 1467–1470.

128. Chen CP, Chao Y, Li CP et al. Surgical resection of duodenal lymphangiectasia: A case report. *World Journal of Gastroenterology: WJG.* Dec 2003;9(12):2880–2882.

129. Mine K, Matsubayashi S, Nakai Y, Nakagawa T. Intestinal lymphangiectasia markedly improved with antiplasmin therapy. *Gastroenterology.* Jun 1989;96(6):1596–1599.

130. MacLean JE, Cohen E, Weinstein M. Primary intestinal and thoracic lymphangiectasia: A response to antiplasmin therapy. *Pediatrics.* Jun 2002;109(6):1177–1180.

131. Klingenberg RD, Homann N, Ludwig D. Type I intestinal lymphangiectasia treated successfully with slow-release octreotide. *Digestive Diseases and Sciences.* Aug 2003;48(8):1506–1509.

132. Fleisher TA, Strober W, Muchmore AV, Broder S, Krawitt EL, Waldmann TA. Corticosteroid-responsive intestinal lymphangiectasia secondary to an inflammatory process. *The New England Journal of Medicine.* Mar 15, 1979;300(11):605–606.

133. Han PD, Burke A, Baldassano RN, Rombeau JL, Lichtenstein GR. Nutrition and inflammatory bowel disease. *Gastroenterology Clinics of North America.* Jun 1999;28(2): 423–443, ix.

134. Dieleman LA, Heizer WD. Nutritional issues in inflammatory bowel disease. *Gastroenterology Clinics of North America.* Jun 1998;27(2):435–451.

135. Stokes MA. Crohn's disease and nutrition. *The British Journal of Surgery.* May 1992;79(5):391–394.

136. Lanfranchi GA, Brignola C, Campieri M et al. Assessment of nutritional status in Crohn's disease in remission or low activity. *Hepato-gastroenterology.* Jun 1984;31(3): 129–132.

137. Rocha R, Santana GO, Almeida N, Lyra AC. Analysis of fat and muscle mass in patients with inflammatory bowel disease during remission and active phase. *The British Journal of Nutrition*. Mar 2009;101(5):676–679.
138. Hartman C, Eliakim R, Shamir R. Nutritional status and nutritional therapy in inflammatory bowel diseases. *World Journal of Gastroenterology: WJG*. Jun 7, 2009;15(21): 2570–2578.
139. Rosenthal SR, Snyder JD, Hendricks KM, Walker WA. Growth failure and inflammatory bowel disease: Approach to treatment of a complicated adolescent problem. *Pediatrics*. Oct 1983;72(4):481–490.
140. Motil KJ, Grand RJ, Davis-Kraft L, Ferlic LL, Smith EO. Growth failure in children with inflammatory bowel disease: A prospective study. *Gastroenterology*. Sep 1993;105(3):681–691.
141. Markowitz J, Grancher K, Rosa J, Aiges H, Daum F. Growth failure in pediatric inflammatory bowel disease. *Journal of Pediatric Gastroenterology and Nutrition*. May 1993;16(4):373–380.
142. Sentongo TA, Semeao EJ, Piccoli DA, Stallings VA, Zemel BS. Growth, body composition, and nutritional status in children and adolescents with Crohn's disease. *Journal of Pediatric Gastroenterology and Nutrition*. Jul 2000;31(1):33–40.
143. Hildebrand H, Karlberg J, Kristiansson B. Longitudinal growth in children and adolescents with inflammatory bowel disease. *Journal of Pediatric Gastroenterology and Nutrition*. Feb 1994;18(2):165–173.
144. Oliva MM, Lake AM. Nutritional considerations and management of the child with inflammatory bowel disease. *Nutrition*. Mar 1996;12(3):151–158.
145. Kleinman RE, Baldassano RN, Caplan A et al. Nutrition support for pediatric patients with inflammatory bowel disease: A clinical report of the North American Society for Pediatric Gastroenterology, Hepatology and Nutrition. *Journal of Pediatric Gastroenterology and Nutrition*. Jul 2004;39(1):15–27.
146. Burnham JM, Shults J, Semeao E et al. Whole body BMC in pediatric Crohn disease: Independent effects of altered growth, maturation, and body composition. *Journal of Bone and Mineral Research: The Official Journal of the American Society for Bone and Mineral Research*. Dec 2004;19(12):1961–1968.
147. Bischoff SC, Herrmann A, Goke M, Manns MP, von zur Muhlen A, Brabant G. Altered bone metabolism in inflammatory bowel disease. *The American Journal of Gastroenterology*. Jul 1997;92(7):1157–1163.
148. Mascarenhas MR, Thayu M. Pediatric inflammatory bowel disease and bone health. *Nutrition in Clinical Practice: Official Publication of the American Society for Parenteral and Enteral Nutrition*. Aug 2010;25(4):347–352.
149. Gokhale R, Favus MJ, Karrison T, Sutton MM, Rich B, Kirschner BS. Bone mineral density assessment in children with inflammatory bowel disease. *Gastroenterology*. May 1998;114(5):902–911.
150. Mishkin S. Dairy sensitivity, lactose malabsorption, and elimination diets in inflammatory bowel disease. *The American Journal of Clinical Nutrition*. Feb 1997;65(2):564–567.
151. Sentongo TA, Semaeo EJ, Stettler N, Piccoli DA, Stallings VA, Zemel BS. Vitamin D status in children, adolescents, and young adults with Crohn disease. *The American Journal of Clinical Nutrition*. Nov 2002;76(5):1077–1081.
152. Pappa HM, Grand RJ, Gordon CM. Report on the vitamin D status of adult and pediatric patients with inflammatory bowel disease and its significance for bone health and disease. *Inflammatory Bowel Diseases*. Dec 2006;12(12):1162–1174.
153. Semeao EJ, Stallings VA, Peck SN, Piccoli DA. Vertebral compression fractures in pediatric patients with Crohn's disease. *Gastroenterology*. May 1997;112(5):1710–1713.
154. van Staa TP, Cooper C, Brusse LS, Leufkens H, Javaid MK, Arden NK. Inflammatory bowel disease and the risk of fracture. *Gastroenterology*. Dec 2003;125(6):1591–1597.

155. Bernstein CN, Blanchard JF, Leslie W, Wajda A, Yu BN. The incidence of fracture among patients with inflammatory bowel disease. A population-based cohort study. *Annals of Internal Medicine.* Nov 21, 2000;133(10):795–799.

156. Samson CM, Morgan P, Williams E et al. Improved outcomes with quality improvement interventions in pediatric inflammatory bowel disease. *Journal of Pediatric Gastroenterology and Nutrition.* Dec 2012;55(6):679–688.

157. Bousvaros A, Zurakowski D, Duggan C et al. Vitamins A and E serum levels in children and young adults with inflammatory bowel disease: Effect of disease activity. *Journal of Pediatric Gastroenterology and Nutrition.* Feb 1998;26(2):129–135.

158. Schoon EJ, Muller MC, Vermeer C, Schurgers LJ, Brummer RJ, Stockbrugger RW. Low serum and bone vitamin K status in patients with longstanding Crohn's disease: Another pathogenetic factor of osteoporosis in Crohn's disease? *Gut.* Apr 2001;48(4):473–477.

159. Kuwabara A, Tanaka K, Tsugawa N et al. High prevalence of vitamin K and D deficiency and decreased BMD in inflammatory bowel disease. *Osteoporosis International: A Journal Established as Result of Cooperation between the European Foundation for Osteoporosis and the National Osteoporosis Foundation of the USA.* Jun 2009;20(6):935–942.

160. Kulnigg S, Gasche C. Systematic review: Managing anaemia in Crohn's disease. *Alimentary Pharmacology & Therapeutics.* Dec 2006;24(11–12):1507–1523.

161. Revel-Vilk S, Tamary H, Broide E et al. Serum transferrin receptor in children and adolescents with inflammatory bowel disease. *European Journal of Pediatrics.* Aug 2000;159(8):585–589.

162. Erichsen K, Ulvik RJ, Nysaeter G et al. Oral ferrous fumarate or intravenous iron sucrose for patients with inflammatory bowel disease. *Scandinavian Journal of Gastroenterology.* Sep 2005;40(9):1058–1065.

163. Schroder O, Mickisch O, Seidler U et al. Intravenous iron sucrose versus oral iron supplementation for the treatment of iron deficiency anemia in patients with inflammatory bowel disease—A randomized, controlled, open-label, multicenter study. *The American Journal of Gastroenterology.* Nov 2005;100(11):2503–2509.

164. Harvey RS, Reffitt DM, Doig LA et al. Ferric trimaltol corrects iron deficiency anaemia in patients intolerant of iron. *Alimentary Pharmacology & Therapeutics.* Sep 1998;12(9): 845–848.

165. Nakano E, Taylor CJ, Chada L, McGaw J, Powers HJ. Hyperhomocystinemia in children with inflammatory bowel disease. *Journal of Pediatric Gastroenterology and Nutrition.* Nov 2003;37(5):586–590.

166. Belli DC, Seidman E, Bouthillier L et al. Chronic intermittent elemental diet improves growth failure in children with Crohn's disease. *Gastroenterology.* Mar 1988;94(3): 603–610.

167. Polk DB, Hattner JA, Kerner JA, Jr. Improved growth and disease activity after intermittent administration of a defined formula diet in children with Crohn's disease. *JPEN. Journal of Parenteral and Enteral Nutrition.* Nov–Dec 1992;16(6):499–504.

168. Heuschkel RB, Menache CC, Megerian JT, Baird AE. Enteral nutrition and corticosteroids in the treatment of acute Crohn's disease in children. *Journal of Pediatric Gastroenterology and Nutrition.* Jul 2000;31(1):8–15.

169. Day AS, Whitten KE, Lemberg DA et al. Exclusive enteral feeding as primary therapy for Crohn's disease in Australian children and adolescents: A feasible and effective approach. *Journal of Gastroenterology and Hepatology.* Oct 2006;21(10):1609–1614.

170. Hartman C, Berkowitz D, Weiss B et al. Nutritional supplementation with polymeric diet enriched with transforming growth factor-beta 2 for children with Crohn's disease. *The Israel Medical Association Journal: IMAJ.* Jul 2008;10(7):503–507.

171. Dziechciarz P, Horvath A, Shamir R, Szajewska H. Meta-analysis: Enteral nutrition in active Crohn's disease in children. *Alimentary Pharmacology & Therapeutics.* Sep 15, 2007;26(6):795–806.

172. Fernandez-Banares F, Cabre E, Esteve-Comas M, Gassull MA. How effective is enteral nutrition in inducing clinical remission in active Crohn's disease? A meta-analysis of the randomized clinical trials. *JPEN. Journal of Parenteral and Enteral Nutrition.* Sep–Oct 1995;19(5):356–364.

173. Griffiths AM, Ohlsson A, Sherman PM, Sutherland LR. Meta-analysis of enteral nutrition as a primary treatment of active Crohn's disease. *Gastroenterology.* Apr 1995;108(4):1056–1067.

174. Zachos M, Tondeur M, Griffiths AM. Enteral nutritional therapy for induction of remission in Crohn's disease. *Cochrane Database of Systematic Reviews.* 2007(1):CD000542.

175. Gonzalez-Huix F, de Leon R, Fernandez-Banares F et al. Polymeric enteral diets as primary treatment of active Crohn's disease: A prospective steroid controlled trial. *Gut.* Jun 1993;34(6):778–782.

176. Veereman-Wauters G, de Ridder L, Veres G et al. Risk of infection and prevention in pediatric patients with IBD: ESPGHAN IBDPorto Group commentary. *Journal of Pediatric Gastroenterology and Nutrition.* 2012 Jun;54(6):830–837.

177. Hyams J, Walters TD, Crandall W et al. Safety and efficacy of maintenance infliximab therapy for moderate-to-severe Crohn's disease in children: REACH open-label extension. *Current Medical Research and Opinion.* Mar 2011;27(3):651–662.

178. Russell RK, Wilson ML, Loganathan S et al. A British Society of Paediatric Gastroenterology, Hepatology and Nutrition survey of the effectiveness and safety of adalimumab in children with inflammatory bowel disease. *Alimentary Pharmacology & Therapeutics.* Apr 2011;33(8):946–953.

179. Veereman-Wauters G, de Ridder L, Veres G et al. ESPGHAN IBD Porto Group commentary on risk of infection and prevention in pediatric IBD patients. *Journal of Pediatric Gastroenterology and Nutrition.* June 2012;54(6):830–837.

180. Bossuyt P, Verhaegen J, Van Assche G, Rutgeerts P, Vermeire S. Increasing incidence of *Clostridium difficile*–associated diarrhea in inflammatory bowel disease. *Journal of Crohn's & Colitis.* Feb 2009;3(1):4–7.

181. Issa M, Vijayapal A, Graham MB et al. Impact of *Clostridium difficile* on inflammatory bowel disease. *Clinical Gastroenterology and Hepatology: The Official Clinical Practice Journal of the American Gastroenterological Association.* Mar 2007;5(3):345–351.

182. Berg AM, Kelly CP, Farraye FA. *Clostridium difficile* infection in the inflammatory bowel disease patient. *Inflammatory Bowel Diseases.* Jan 2013;19(1):194–204.

183. Clayton EM, Rea MC, Shanahan F et al. The vexed relationship between *Clostridium difficile* and inflammatory bowel disease: An assessment of carriage in an outpatient setting among patients in remission. *The American Journal of Gastroenterology.* May 2009;104(5):1162–1169.

184. Koffeman GI, van Gemert WG, George EK, Veenendaal RA. Classification, epidemiology and aetiology. *Best Practice & Research. Clinical Gastroenterology.* Dec 2003;17(6):879–893.

185. Williams NS, Evans P, King RF. Gastric acid secretion and gastrin production in the short bowel syndrome. *Gut.* Sep 1985;26(9):914–919.

186. Nightingale JM, Kamm MA, van der Sijp JR et al. Disturbed gastric emptying in the short bowel syndrome. Evidence for a 'colonic brake.' *Gut.* Sep 1993;34(9):1171–1176.

187. Wilmore DW. Factors correlating with a successful outcome following extensive intestinal resection in newborn infants. *The Journal of Pediatrics.* Jan 1972;80(1):88–95.

188. Gutierrez IM, Kang KH, Jaksic T. Neonatal short bowel syndrome. *Seminars in Fetal & Neonatal Medicine.* Jun 2011;16(3):157–163.

189. Quiros-Tejeira RE, Ament ME, Reyen L et al. Long-term parenteral nutritional support and intestinal adaptation in children with short bowel syndrome: A 25-year experience. *The Journal of Pediatrics.* Aug 2004;145(2):157–163.

190. Wales PW, de Silva N, Kim JH, Lecce L, Sandhu A, Moore AM. Neonatal short bowel syndrome: A cohort study. *Journal of Pediatric Surgery.* May 2005;40(5):755–762.
191. Vantini I, Benini L, Bonfante F et al. Survival rate and prognostic factors in patients with intestinal failure. *Digestive and Liver Disease: Official Journal of the Italian Society of Gastroenterology and the Italian Association for the Study of the Liver.* Jan 2004;36(1):46–55.
192. Diamond IR, de Silva N, Pencharz PB, Kim JH, Wales PW. Neonatal short bowel syndrome outcomes after the establishment of the first Canadian multidisciplinary intestinal rehabilitation program: Preliminary experience. *Journal of Pediatric Surgery.* May 2007;42(5):806–811.
193. Lee OK, Johnston L. A systematic review for effective management of central venous catheters and catheter sites in acute care paediatric patients. *Worldviews on Evidence-Based Nursing/Sigma Theta Tau International, Honor Society of Nursing.* 2005;2(1):4–13.
194. Wheeler DS, Giaccone MJ, Hutchinson N et al. A hospital-wide quality-improvement collaborative to reduce catheter-associated bloodstream infections. *Pediatrics.* Oct 2011;128(4):e995–e1004.
195. Huang EY, Chen C, Abdullah F et al. Strategies for the prevention of central venous catheter infections: An American Pediatric Surgical Association Outcomes and Clinical Trials Committee systematic review. *Journal of Pediatric Surgery.* Oct 2011;46(10):2000–2011.
196. Jones BA, Hull MA, Richardson DS et al. Efficacy of ethanol locks in reducing central venous catheter infections in pediatric patients with intestinal failure. *Journal of Pediatric Surgery.* Jun 2010;45(6):1287–1293.
197. Van Wouwe JP. Clinical and laboratory assessment of zinc deficiency in Dutch children. A review. *Biological Trace Element Research.* Aug–Sep 1995;49(2–3):211–225.
198. Shrimpton R, Gross R, Darnton-Hill I, Young M. Zinc deficiency: What are the most appropriate interventions? *BMJ.* Feb 12, 2005;330(7487):347–349.
199. Maverakis E, Fung MA, Lynch PJ et al. Acrodermatitis enteropathica and an overview of zinc metabolism. *Journal of the American Academy of Dermatology.* Jan 2007;56(1):116–124.

12 Relationship of Probiotics, Prebiotics, Synbiotics to Infections, Immunity, and Nutrition

Diomel de la Cruz and Josef Neu

CONTENTS

Introduction 287
Intestinal Environment 288
Functions of the Intestinal Environment and Associations with Disease 288
Probiotics 293
    Immunomodulation 293
    Safety of Probiotics 294
    Drug Interactions..296
    Metabolic Activities 296
    Other Effects 296
Prebiotics and Synbiotics..297
Future Perspectives 298
Conclusions and Recommendations 298
References...299

INTRODUCTION

With the development of new technologies, there has been a rapid growth in our knowledge of the intestinal microbiota in terms of taxonomy, function, early development, and impact on lifelong health. The recent emergence of non-culture-based techniques to evaluate microbial DNA through the Human Genome Project is providing new insights into the relation that exists between microbes and their mammalian hosts. Microbial organisms found in the gastrointestinal tract play a significant role in innate and adaptive immunity, intestinal growth, metabolism, and nutrition. They also influence the balance of mucosal inflammatory and anti-inflammatory processes, which play a significant role in overall illness and health.

INTESTINAL ENVIRONMENT

A complex ecosystem composed of eukaryotes, bacteria, and other organisms reside within the human body. These organisms inhabit the human body in large numbers, from the nasal and oral cavities down to the rectum. The gastrointestinal tract represents the body's most colonized organ. The colon alone contains >70% of all the microbes in the human body. The human gut is dominated by several bacterial taxa that are composed of 10–100 trillion microorganisms. This number suggests that the human "superorganism" is made up of only 10% human cells (Kunz, Kuntz, and Rudloff 2009; Neish 2009; Morelli 2008).

The fetal gastrointestinal tract was previously thought to be sterile. However, with the knowledge that amniotic fluid is frequently not sterile (DiGiulio et al. 2010), it is likely that the gastrointestinal tract of the fetus is exposed to microbes through swallowing of amniotic fluid. In fact, microbial DNA has been found in the meconium (Mshvildadze, Neu, and Mai 2008; Jiménez et al. 2008), indicating that the microbiota found in the meconium has an intrauterine origin. Organisms from the mother and the environment begin to further inhabit the gastrointestinal tract of the infant, ultimately leading to a dense and diverse bacterial population (Dominguez-Bello et al. 2011; Palmer et al. 2007). It is not surprising that the intestinal microbiota has a profound effect on intestinal physiology, the development and functions of the intestinal epithelium, and the regulation of inflammation. Studies suggest that an interaction of the gut microflora with intestinal epithelial cells as well as other mucosal cell types contributes to the development of mucosal and systemic immunity and plays a role in several disease states, including rheumatoid arthritis, inflammatory bowel diseases, periodontal disease, allergy, multiorgan failure, and colon carcinoma.

Preterm infants are at risk for abnormal colonization or "dysbiosis" for a multitude of reasons, including antibiotic use, delayed initiation of feeds, and immature gut mucosa. The administration of substances, such as antibiotics, probiotics, prebiotics, or synbiotics, may alter colonization and provide beneficial effects through different mechanisms such as anti-inflammatory properties, immunomodulation, and nutritional and metabolic activities. However, questions remain whether introduction of these substances may promote inappropriate colonization that may also have adverse effects on the health of the individual.

FUNCTIONS OF THE INTESTINAL ENVIRONMENT AND ASSOCIATIONS WITH DISEASE

The functions of the intestinal microbiota can be split into two major categories, and several subcategories that are interactive: the metabolic role and the immunologic role (see Figure 12.1).

The metabolic role of the intestinal microbiota involves fermentation and metabolism of nondigestible substrates, which leads to the production of short-chain fatty acids and contributes to microbial growth. These short-chain fatty acids have been shown to have a protective effect on the intestinal epithelium by their immunomodulatory capabilities (Wong et al. 2006; Tedelind et al. 2007). Salminen et al. (1998) has shown that butyrate, a four-carbon short-chain fatty acid, has an effect

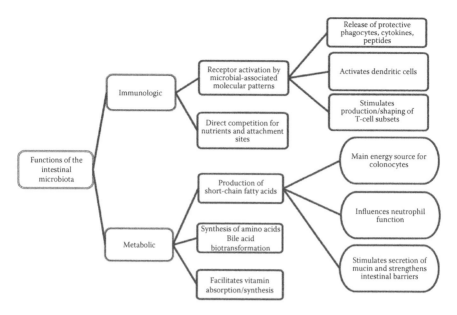

FIGURE 12.1 Selected functions of intestinal microbiota.

on the regulation of cell growth and differentiation. Evidence indicates that butyrate generates the secretion of factors such as mucin and antibacterial peptides that, in turn, strengthens the intestinal mucosal barrier by establishing an impediment to proinflammatory compounds and a hindrance to antigens (Hamer et al. 2008). The discovery of GPR43, a G-protein-coupled receptor, has been implicated in the anti-inflammatory action of the short-chain fatty acids such as butyrate, acetate, and propionate. GPR43 is expressed by neutrophils, eosinophils, and monocytes (Le Poul et al. 2003). The interactions between short-chain fatty acids and GPR43 influence neutrophil function. Neutrophils lacking GPR43 and mice deficient in GPR43, with limited interaction with short-chain fatty acids, have higher sensitivity to inflammatory processes.

It is widely recognized that metabolic activities, such as digestion and production of biologically active substances, are influenced by the action of gut microbes. The microbiota of the colon use butyrate as a lone source of energy, while acetate serves as a substrate for the synthesis of cholesterol. Gut microbes are also implicated in the synthesis of amino acids, biotransformation of bile, and the production of various vitamins. In turn, bile acid biotransformation has a crucial role in the metabolism of glucose and cholesterol (Lefebvre et al. 2009). Bile acids contribute to the absorption of dietary fats and lipid-soluble vitamins, and maintain intestinal barrier function (Groh, Schade, and Hörhold-Schubert 1993; Ridlon, Kang, and Hylemon 2006). Turnbaugh et al. (2006) provided data suggesting that the gastrointestinal microbiota is an important factor in the development of obesity and type 2 diabetes mellitus (DM). The study proposed that an altered bacterial colonization promotes an increasing energy harvest from food, which ultimately promotes insulin resistance and generation of increased adipocytes. Moreover, Cani and Delzenne (2009) have implicated gut microbiota as a contributing factor in the development of these metabolic disorders. Obese individuals have been found to have a greater number of Firmicutes as compared with Bacteroidetes (De Filippo et al. 2010; Ley et al. 2005). Vael and colleagues (2011) performed a prospective trial that suggests that a microbiota with an elevated concentration of *Bacteroides fragilis* and low *Staphylococcus* concentrations placed a person at a higher risk of obesity during preschool age. Other studies that dealt with microbial composition identified trends of decreased bifidobacteria and its association with obesity (Kalliomaki et al. 2008; Luoto et al. 2011). A similar finding has been reported in children with type 2 DM as compared with nondiabetics (Wu et al. 2010). Apart from its function in terms of energy recovery and digestion, the gut microbiota has a role in the synthesis of vitamin K, B-group vitamins, and other water-soluble vitamins (LeBlanc et al. 2013). There is evidence that *Lactobacillus reuteri* produces a cobalamin-like compound (Taranto et al. 2003; Santos et al. 2007). Further studies are warranted to have a thorough understanding on the role of the microbiota on the development of obesity and other metabolic disorders.

The microbiota also plays a substantial function in the development of cells of the immune system. Bacterial sensing by Toll-like receptors activates inherent immune responses and intestinal pathways. These Toll-like receptors are transmembrane proteins found on the surface of cells. Toll-like receptors attach to specific microbial macromolecules such as lipopolysaccharides, flagellin, peptidoglycan, and *N*-formylated peptides. The activation of these Toll-like receptors leads to the production and release of protective phagocytes, cytokines, and peptides. Subsequently, this can produce inflammatory responses to pathogens, or otherwise protective mechanisms to commensal organisms. The development of intestinal villi is also dependent on indigenous microbes. Commensal organisms may produce antimicrobial compounds and also serve as competition for nutrients and attachment sites preventing overgrowth of pathogenic strains (Tlaskalová-Hogenová et al. 2011). The development of the immune system is also influenced by the signals from the intestinal bacteria that stimulate production of T cells. Certain microbes control T-cell differentiation in the lamina propria, where CD4+ T-cell subsets are numerous (Mazmanian et al. 2005; Ivanov et al. 2009; Atarashi et al. 2011). It is important to note that Th17 cells in the gut of germ-free mice are drastically reduced, further supporting the theory that T-cell differentiation is modulated by gut microbes. Clarke et al. (2010) have reported that the peptidoglycan component of the bacterial cell membrane influences neutrophil priming. Peptidoglycans bind to a pattern recognition receptor called nucleotide-binding oligomerization domain-containing protein-1 (Nod-1). Nods are cytoplasmic proteins expressed in host defense cells. Nod-1 is specific to peptidoglycans from gram-negative organisms. Impaired killing of pathogenic *Staphylococcus pneumoniae* and *Staphylococcus aureus* has been exhibited by neutrophils without Nod-1. Therefore, gram-negative bacteria are able to enhance immune response through peptidoglycans (Clarke et al. 2010). Furthermore, *Bacteroides fragilis*, an anaerobic organism found in great number in the human gut, produces polysaccharide A, which, in turn, induces different T-cell responses (Könönen, Jousimies-Somer, and Asikainen 1992). Germ-free mice monocolonized with *B. fragilis* were able to correct abnormal splenic structure, restore previously low levels of CD4+

T-cell numbers in the spleen, and remedy increased levels of interleukin (IL)-4 cytokine production (Krinos et al. 2001; Mazmanian et al. 2005).

There is strong evidence pointing to a link between the gut microbiota and the development of immune-related disorders, especially atopic disease (Wang et al. 2008; Kirjavainen et al. 2002; Gore et al. 2008; Forno et al. 2008). Higher amounts of fecal *Clostridium difficile* and *Escherichia coli* in the gut microbiota of infants were linked to a higher risk of atopic dermatitis, allergies, and eczema (Penders et al. 2007). Remarkably, Björkstén et al. (2001) revealed that a reduced number of bifidobacteria and lactobacilli were found in the gut of children who developed atopy. The diversity of gut microbiota has also been found to be reduced in those children with atopic disease and may actually be more relevant than the prevalence of specific species (Wang et al. 2008; Abrahamsson et al. 2012). Clearly, a variability in the microbiota of children with atopic disease compared with those who do not develop them shows a link between gut microbes to these immunologic diseases.

Aside from the immunomodulatory and metabolic action of the microbiota, the enteric nervous system plays a role in gastrointestinal motility, function, and vice versa. Interactions between the brain and intestine are known to have an effect on the regulation of intestinal function. The brain influences gastrointestinal motility and secretion, intestinal permeability, and, by releasing molecules to the gut lumen (neurons, enterochromaffin cells, immune cells), may effect changes to the microbiota. Communication is facilitated by receptor-mediated signaling through epithelial cells and also through direct stimulation of host cells in the lamina propria. Enterochromaffin cells serve a fundamental responsibility of regulating transmissions between the gut and brain. The disturbance of this two-way pathway between the nervous system and the gut microbiota may be implicated in the pathophysiology of some gastrointestinal disorders, such as inflammatory bowel disease and functional abdominal pain (Rhee, Pothoulakis, and Mayer 2009).

Beneficial organisms inhabiting the gastrointestinal tract contribute to the maintenance and development of gut motor and sensory functions. Commensal bacteria regulate gut function by the release of bacterial cell components, fermentation products, and neuroendocrine factors (Rondeau 2003; Cherbut 2003). Short-chain fatty acids and products of enteric fermentation participate in the modulation of gut motor activity. Intestinal motility requires an interaction between interstitial cells of Cajal, smooth muscle cells, and enteric motor neurons. This functional coordination acts by way of neuroimmune peptide receptor effects on immune cells and receptors expressed on enteric nerves. In conjunction with this, intestinal propulsion represents a major factor in the regulation of gut microflora through the removal of excess bacteria from the lumen. The enteric nervous system affects gut motility related to contractions and also by its indirect influence on gut immunity and epithelial cells. This communication relies on the interplay of Toll-like receptor activation by bacterial components that, in turn, trigger innate immune responses (Indrio and Neu 2011). Studies in germ-free animals and exposure to specific organisms have provided insight into this bidirectional interaction between the gut and the brain (Forsythe and Kunze 2012). Both Heijtz et al. (2011) and Neufeld et al. (2011) demonstrated that complete absence of gut bacteria resulted in a decreased state of anxiety compared with conventional animals. Heijtz et al. (2011) strikingly revealed that there is a correction of germ-free behavioral patterns of the hypothalamic–pituitary–adrenal (HPA) axis set points that persisted into adulthood only when these animals are colonized early, rather than late in life. Brain-derived neurotrophic factor (BDNF) expression was found to be lower in the study of Heijtz et al. (2011) but elevated in the study by Neufeld et al. (2011) in germ-free mice that exhibited this decreased state of anxiety. This window of vulnerability has been suggested wherein gut microbiota influences developmental programming that may have lifelong physiologic consequences (Sudo et al. 2004; Lucas 1991).

A number of studies exhibited that BDNF levels are influenced by gut bacteria (Heijtz et al. 2011; Neufeld et al. 2011; Sudo et al. 2004; Bercik et al. 2010). BDNF has been known to have an influence on the regulation of behavior, and is also involved in neuronal growth and survival (Nguyen et al. 2009; Deng, Zhong, and Zhou 2000; Garraway, Petruska, and Mendell 2003). Interestingly, BDNF was decreased significantly in patients who were clinically depressed, and in hippocampal tissue of depressed suicide patients (Karege et al. 2002, 2005; Shimizu, Hashimoto, and Iyo 2004). Moreover, several studies also suggest an association between the gut microflora and changes in the HPA axis. The gut microbiota, as a response to stress, affect the HPA axis and thus may influence behavior (Neufeld et al. 2011; Sudo et al. 2004; Desbonnet et al. 2010).

The gastrointestinal tract provides a steady environment for commensal bacteria, which then supports its integrity. Changes in natural gastrointestinal physiology can

TABLE 12.1
Summary of Associations between Different Disease Conditions with Accompanying Microbial Perturbation

Pathologic Condition	Microbial Pertubation That Results in Dysbiosis	Reference
Obesity	Elevated Firmicutes and reduced bifidobacteria	(Ley et al. 2005)
Necrotizing enterocolitis	Increased Gammaproteobacteria decrease in Firmicutes, low diversity	(Wang et al. 2010)
Diabetes type 2	Reduced Firmicutes abundance of Proteobacteria	(Larsen et al. 2010)
Diabetes type 1	Increased *Bacteroides*, decreased *Bifidobacterium*, Firmicutes	(Roesch et al. 2010; Brugman et al. 2006)
Eczema	Decreased *Bacteroides* and proteobacterium, low diversity	(Abrahamsson et al. 2012)
Inflammatory bowel disease	Increased vs. decreased Bacteroidetes, decreased Firmicutes and Enterobacteriae	(Takaishi et al. 2008; Walker et al. 2011)
Irritable bowel syndrome	Prevalance of *Lactobacillus*, *Streptococcus*, *Ruminococcus*, *Veillonella*	(Malinen et al. 2005)

destabilize the environment, which results in differences in its microbial constitution. On the other hand, disturbances in the microbial composition, antibiotic use, inflammation, or infection may have severe consequences on gastrointestinal function and physiology and overall health (Rhee, Pothoulakis, and Mayer 2009) (see Table 12.1). It is therefore imperative to establish homeostasis when this ecosystem is disturbed. As we learn more about the intestine–microbiota interactions and their effects on human physiology and the occurrence of disease, new treatments, such as the use of prebiotics, probiotics, and a combination of both (synbiotics), have been proposed.

PROBIOTICS

Probiotics are live microorganisms that, when administered, confer a health benefit to the host. It has been proposed that probiotics not only have effects on intestinal diseases but also may have beneficial roles in allergic disorders and other systemic diseases (Ouwehand 2007; Gratz, Mykkanen, and El-Nezami 2010). Moreover, probiotic strains should be nontoxic and nonpathogenic, and resistant to the host. Since there have been multiple studies of species, strains, genera, and even doses of probiotics, the practice of combining the information from these studies provide us with only limited conclusions about specific interventions.

IMMUNOMODULATION

Probiotics are thought to enhance the protective barrier against pathogenic organisms by competing for nutrient binding sites. Probiotics may also strengthen the immunological properties of the gut by increasing mucus production, modulation of inflammatory responses, and nitric oxide production. Additionally, probiotics may be linked to improved intestinal motility (Indrio et al. 2009). They also appear to simulate commensal microbes; in this way, they alter gut intestinal community without necessarily becoming permanent residents of the lumen (Murguía-Peniche et al. 2013).

There is evidence suggesting that probiotics are protective for the host from diseases with inflammatory activity in the bowel. Immunomodulation may be effected by intestinal barrier reinforcement, whereby there is a reduction of bacterial translocation across the gut epithelium. VSL#3, a mixture of different species of *Bifidobacterium*, *Lactobacillus*, and *Streptococcus*, was found to prevent *Salmonella*-induced transepithelial reduction in epithelial resistance, while strengthening the barriers by increasing mucin production and stabilizing tight junctions (Otte and Podolsky 2004). *Bacillus subtilis* secreted a molecule that stimulated the production of heat shock proteins that help protect the intestinal lumen from oxidant-induced injury (Fujiya et al. 2007). Furthermore, probiotics stimulate the immune system through a process involving dendritic cells (Macpherson and Uhr 2004). Dendritic cells incorporate commensal organisms and transport them to lymphatic tissue, where they induce an immune response that activates B cells to produce IgA (Macpherson and Uhr 2004). Probiotic mixtures containing three *Bifidobacterium* species, four *Lactobacillus* species, and *Streptococcus thermophilus* have been studied to induce IL-10 production by these dendritic cells (Hart et al. 2004). Moreover, Von Der Weid, Bulliard, and Schiffrin (2001) report that regulatory T-cell production was regulated by *Lactobacillus paracasei*. This is also supported by recent studies that reveal that regulatory T cells are stimulated by dendritic cell maturation induced by bacteria (Baba et al. 2008).

Probiotic organisms with Toll receptor agonists can decrease nuclear factor-κB (NF-κB) activation to preserve the inhibitor (Petrof et al. 2004). *Bacteroides thetaiotaomicron* promotes the clearance of NF-κB by nuclear peroxisome proliferator activated receptor-γ (Kelly et al. 2004). *Lactobacillus plantarum* and *Bacillus subtilis* stimulated the production of proliferation-inducing ligands that mediates class-switching recombinations of B cells to IgA2 (He et al. 2007). Gut-associated lymphoid tissue found mostly in the small intestine mediates an immune response with intestinal microbes. Within the large intestine, short-chain fatty acids are produced through fermentation processes mediated by probiotics (Neish 2009). Probiotics have also been shown to demonstrate cytoprotective effects and antiviral activity (Mikhaĭlova et al. 2010).

In neonatal intensive care, one of the most devastating diseases is necrotizing enterocolitis (NEC) (Neu and Walker 2011). Interestingly, high NF-κB activity has been found in infants who developed NEC (Chung et al. 2001). A meta-analysis of 13 randomized controlled trials reported on the association of probiotics with sepsis or NEC incidence, although the quality of these studies varies. There is no convincing evidence showing that probiotics have a significant effect on the incidence of sepsis. On the other hand, some of the available studies using meta-analysis suggest that probiotics decrease the incidence of NEC (Deshpande et al. 2010). However, Rojas et al. (2012) studied 750 babies, all <2000 g, and did not show any significant differences in mortality and nosocomial infections between control and those given *L. reuteri*. They did reveal a nonsignificant 40% decrease in NEC in the probiotic group, but this might be explained by the lack of power of the study. That being said, most of the studies on probiotics used various strains of bacteria, with different doses. Treatment duration also varied among studies. Large, multicenter trials are central in the determination of a specific product for routine use in neonates. Available trials do not indicate an optimal strain, dose, and method of delivery nor protocol. Further studies with similar strains, dose, delivery, and treatment protocols are needed to truly establish long-term effects of probiotics in children.

SAFETY OF PROBIOTICS

In healthy individuals, probiotics are thought to be safe. Conversely, probiotic therapy has been found to have correlation with sepsis, endocarditis, or bacteremia in patients who were immunocompromised or in premature infants (Petrof et al. 2004; Mackay et al. 1999; Rautio et al. 1999; Bayer et al. 1978). Reports of *Saccharomyces cerevisiae*, *Bifidobacterium breve*, *Lactobacillus bacteremia*, and *Saccharomyces boulardii* fungemia in children with risk factors such as immune deficiency, complex cardiac diseases, or short gut syndrome have also been documented (Perapoch et al.

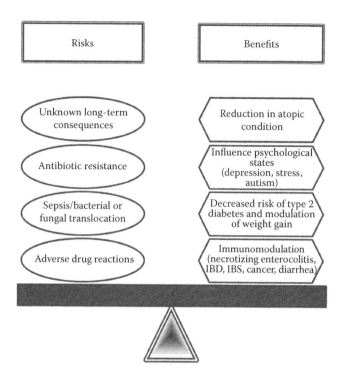

FIGURE 12.2 Presumed risks and benefits of probiotics, prebiotics, and synbiotics.

2000; Ohishi et al. 2010; Land et al. 2005; De Groote et al. 2005). It is hypothesized that bacterial or fungal translocation may explain this phenomenon, mostly probably due to any gut injury to the epithelial barrier. Risk factors for probiotic sepsis, such as immune compromise, catheter in place, impaired intestinal barrier, prematurity, gastric acid bypass, administration of broad spectrum antibiotics, probiotics of high mucosal adhesion, and cardiac valvular disease, are all mentioned by Boyle, Robins-Browne, and Tang (2006) (see Figure 12.2).

A potential risk of antimicrobial resistance from probiotic to pathogenic strains of bacteria is present. The National Institutes of Health has published an assessment on probiotic safety and has come to the conclusion that better documentation of adverse events and interventions are necessitated (Hempel et al. 2011). In the United States, probiotics are not highly regulated since they are considered food additives. The Food and Drug Administration merely consider them GRAS (Generally Recognized as Safe) (Caplan and Frost 2011). Thus, they are not regulated to the same quality control standards as pharmacologic agents. Manipulations of the gut flora in neonates have significant immunomodulatory effects. The very premature infant differs in a multitude of ways from term infants (Claud 2012). They have very primitive host defense systems, altered intestinal flora, and exaggerated inflammatory responses. Therefore, further investigation is needed on their long-term effects, how they work on whole bacterial communities, and their specific mechanisms of action, before being standard of care (Martin 2013; Claud 2012; Caplan and Frost 2011).

Drug Interactions

Probiotics have been studied to have varied interactions with certain drugs. Studies have shown that the administration of antibiotics could kill a large amount of the live microorganisms contained in probiotics and reduce their efficacy. Furthermore, antifungal medications have been found to reduce the usefulness of certain probiotics such as *S. boulardii*. It is also hypothesized that probiotics may affect the sensitivity of a subject to warfarin and coumadin, and vitamin K uptake (Vyas and Ranganathan 2012). Since probiotics contain live microorganisms, caution is necessary in patients taking immunosuppression medications.

Metabolic Activities

The gut microbiota play an integral role in many metabolic activities. Compared with mice not exposed to any microbes, those that were exposed grew fatter, although the ability of probiotics to promote weight gain is controversial at this time (Bäckhed et al. 2004). Mugambi et al. (2012) revealed that there is no significant difference in weight gain when infant formula was supplemented with prebiotics, probiotics, or synbiotics. It is possible that only specific microbes with certain immunomodulatory activities may be beneficial. More studies need to be done to determine which specific strains of probiotics are truly helpful. Studies have shown that adults with obesity and type 2 DM have different gut microbial flora compared with controls. Administration of *Lactobacillus acidophilus* and *Lactobacillus gasseri* demonstrated a decreased risk of insulin resistance and type 2 DM in obese individuals (Kadooka et al. 2010; Andreasen et al. 2010). Several studies on inulin-type fructans have revealed encouraging results on the obese and diabetic populations (Parnell and Reimer 2009; Luo et al. 2000; Daubioul et al. 2005). Garcia et al. (2006) also demonstrate positive results with the use of arabinoxylan fiber consumption in diabetics.

Other Effects

Several studies have evaluated the effects of probiotics on atopic diseases in children. *Lactobacillus fermentum* improved symptomatology of eczema, while supplementation with a combination of *Bifidobacterium bifidum* and *Bifidobacterium lactis* and *Lactococcus lactis* had positive effects on infants with eczema (Niers et al. 2009; Weston et al. 2005). In terms of cancer prevention, bifidobacteria and lactobacilli have been studied to reduce the number of precancerous lesions in the colon and bladder (Bolognani et al. 2001; Pool-Zobel et al. 2002). Multiple recent studies have also shown significant effects of the gut–brain axis on behavior. Volunteers who were treated for a month with *Lactobacillus helveticus* R0052 and *Bifidobacterium longum* R0173 in a randomized controlled trial showed a reduction in psychological distress (Messaoudi et al. 2011). This was also shown to reduce anxiety-induced behavior in rats (Messaoudi et al. 2011). Rats fed with *Lactobacillus rhamnosus* and *L. helveticus* showed a reduction in stress response and visceral pain (Zareie et al. 2006). Several meta-analyses of randomized controlled trials have been done on the effects of probiotics on common gastrointestinal diseases. Johnston et al. (2011) and D'Souza et al. (2002) both have shown that *Lactobacillus* spp., combined with other probiotics, reduced the risk of antibiotic-associated diarrhea. A multicenter study by Guandalini et al. (2010) performed on children with irritable bowel syndrome reveals that a VSL#3 probiotic combination provided symptomatic relief compared with controls.

PREBIOTICS AND SYNBIOTICS

Prebiotics are nondigestible dietary products that, when administered, result in specific changes in the gastrointestinal microbiota that result in beneficial effects to the host. They are typically oligosaccharides that are used by beneficial bacteria. Prebiotics, in combination with probiotics, theoretically enhances survival and function of probiotics.

Human milk contains extensive amounts of a variety of different oligosaccharides—human milk oligosaccharides (HMO). HMOs are very complex glycans that are abundant in human breast milk, and comparatively, found in only trace amounts in bovine milk products. Most oligosaccharides resist digestion in the small intestine and undergo fermentation in the colon. Oligosaccharides (inulin, galactose, fructose, acidic oligosaccharides, and/or lactulose) are implicated in maintaining normal gut flora and inhibiting growth of pathogenic bacteria. The products of the fermentation of these HMOs, short-chain fatty acids, are involved in the provision of nutrition and energy for colonocytes, and anti-infection roles in the respiratory, intestinal, and urinary systems (Murguía-Peniche et al. 2013). Long-chain polyunsaturated fatty acids (LC-PUFAs) from human milk are involved in inflammatory modulation. Interestingly, the incidence of NEC in rats was reduced when fed with formula supplemented with LC-PUFAs (Lu et al. 2009). Beyond these prebiotic effects, HMOs have been shown to have immunomodulation properties such as anti-adhesive effects and the mimicking or alteration of the attachment sites of pathogenic strains (Bode 2009).

Synbiotics refer to nutritional supplements that contain both probiotics and prebiotics. They selectively stimulate the growth of live microbial supplements by metabolizing a number of health-promoting bacteria. There have been several relevant studies that show the effects of prebiotics and synbiotics. Kukkonen et al. (2007) reveal that there is a reduction on antibiotic prescription and respiratory infections in children with allergic disorders who are given a four-species probiotic mixture. *Bifidobacterium lactis* combined with oligofructose and acacia gum reduced the number of days of diarrhea by 20% in children in day-care centers (Binns et al. 2007). A randomized control trial on the administration of *B. longum* combined with inulin–oligofructose significantly reduced mucosal inflammatory markers (Furrie et al. 2005). Supplementation of preterm infant formula with prebiotics has not been shown to change the characteristics of their stool. Modi et al. (2010) also suggest that prebiotics improve feeding tolerance in preterm infants, but the evidence is not conclusive. There are conflicting reports concerning whether prebiotics significantly increase the number of bifidobacteria or decrease the pathogenic strains in the stool.

Current research has hypothesized that routine use of prebiotics reduces the incidence of hospital-acquired infections, necrotizing enterocolitis, and improves long-term development. There is also a suggestion that prebiotics affect gastrointestinal motility and have a positive effect on overall immune function. However, no convincing outcome on NEC and sepsis has been generated in randomized control trials. No studies have been sufficiently powered to generate a conclusion about their effect on neonatal health (Salminen et al. 1998). Prebiotics and synbiotics, therefore, cannot be routinely recommended for these indications.

FUTURE PERSPECTIVES

With the advent of the Human Microbiome Project in 2008, the understanding of the human microbiota increases exponentially with the development of new technologies. We are also learning that the gut microbiota is also affected by changes in our ecosystem. Overall hygiene, clean water, smaller family sizes, and increased number of caesarian sections can have a profound effect on the microbial community of a human being. Initial research on the effects of the gut microbiota and behavioral pathologies such as autism are already under way. An emerging sector comes from research on the potentially beneficial effects of lactobacilli on cardiovascular disease and hypercholesterolemia (Oxman et al. 2001; De Roos and Katan 2000; Lam et al. 2012).

The field of microbial ecosystem therapeutics (MET) also comes into the fray when dealing with the human microbiota and its believed functions on normal homeostasis. MET deals with the replacement of a damaged ecosystem with a fully developed, bacterial community derived directly from the gastrointestinal tract, which differs from the probiotic approach (Petrof et al. 2012). This new paradigm leads to novel approaches in the management of human disease. Fecal transplantation and fecal bacteriotherapy are emerging fields in the treatment of *C. difficile* infections (Gough, Shaikh, and Manges 2011). Furthermore, the natural progression from fecal bacteriotherapy would be the creation of synthetic stool substitutes. Petrof et al. (2013) revealed that the formulation of cultures mixed with saline was curative when administered through colonoscopy on two patients with *C. difficile* infections.

CONCLUSIONS AND RECOMMENDATIONS

The gastrointestinal microbiota has multiple mechanisms of actions to influence a host's growth and development. Disturbances in this complex environment may result in a wide array of diseases. There is encouraging preliminary information that indicates the safety and efficacy of probiotics in the prevention of NEC. However, these studies need to be performed in larger randomized control studies. Data showing benefits from a specific probiotic does not apply to another probiotic. The safety and efficacy of each strain should be tested individually. Furthermore, there has been no agreement among all studies about the optimal dosing regimen, probiotic strain, or mode of delivery. Future areas of research are promising in the realms of oncology, renal diseases, and metabolic diseases such as diabetes and obesity. It remains to be seen whether the administration of probiotics, prebiotics, or synbiotics would have any effect on individuals with behavioral and neurological conditions. Large, multicenter, well-designed randomized control trials in infants are needed to confirm their efficacy and safety. Certainly, the amount of knowledge accrued over the past decade points to an exciting future in the field of microbial therapeutics.

REFERENCES

Abrahamsson, T R, H E Jakobsson, A F Andersson, B Björkstén, L Engstrand, and M C Jenmalm. 2012. "Low Diversity of the Gut Microbiota in Infants with Atopic Eczema." *The Journal of Allergy and Clinical Immunology* 129 (2): 434–440, 440.e1–2. doi:10.1016/j. jaci.2011.10.025. http://www.ncbi.nlm.nih.gov/pubmed/22153774.

Andreasen, A S, N Larsen, T Pedersen-Skovsgaard, R M G Berg, K Møller, K D Svendsen, M Jakobsen, and B K Pedersen. 2010. "Effects of *Lactobacillus acidophilus* NCFM on Insulin Sensitivity and the Systemic Inflammatory Response in Human Subjects." *The British Journal of Nutrition* 104 (12): 1831–1838. http://www.ncbi.nlm.nih.gov/pubmed/20815975.

Atarashi, K, T Tanoue, T Shima, A Imaoka, T Kuwahara, Y Momose, G Cheng et al. 2011. "Induction of Colonic Regulatory T Cells by Indigenous *Clostridium* Species." *Science (New York, N.Y.)* 331 (6015): 337–341. doi:10.1126/science.1198469. http://www.ncbi. nlm.nih.gov/pubmed/21205640.

Baba, N, S Samson, R Bourdet-Sicard, M Rubio, and M Sarfati. 2008. "Commensal Bacteria Trigger a Full Dendritic Cell Maturation Program That Promotes the Expansion of Non-Tr1 Suppressor T Cells." *Journal of Leukocyte Biology* 84 (2): 468–476. http:// www.ncbi.nlm.nih.gov/pubmed/18511576.

Bäckhed, F, H Ding, T Wang, L V Hooper, G Y Koh, A Nagy, C F Semenkovich, and J I Gordon. 2004. "The Gut Microbiota as an Environmental Factor That Regulates Fat Storage." *Proceedings of the National Academy of Sciences of the United States of America* 101 (44): 15718–15723. http://www.pubmedcentral.nih.gov/articlerender.fcgi? artid=524219&tool=pmcentrez&rendertype=abstract.

Bayer, A S, A W Chow, D Betts, and L B Guze. 1978. "Lactobacillemia—Report of Nine Cases. Important Clinical and Therapeutic Considerations." *The American Journal of Medicine* 64 (5): 808–813. http://www.ncbi.nlm.nih.gov/pubmed/645745.

Bercik, P, E F Verdu, J A Foster, J Macri, M Potter, X Huang, P Malinowski et al. 2010. "Chronic Gastrointestinal Inflammation Induces Anxiety-Like Behavior and Alters Central Nervous System Biochemistry in Mice." *Gastroenterology* 139 (6): 2102–2112.e1. http://www.ncbi.nlm.nih.gov/pubmed/20600016.

Binns, C W, A H Lee, H Harding, M Gracey, and D V Barclay. 2007. "The CUPDAY Study: Prebiotic–Probiotic Milk Product in 1–3-year-old Children Attending Childcare Centres." *Acta Paediatrica* 96 (11): 1646–1650. http://www.ncbi.nlm.nih.gov/entrez/query.fcgi?cmd= Retrieve&db=PubMed&dopt=Citation&list_uids=17937689.

Björkstén, B, E Sepp, K Julge, T Voor, and M Mikelsaar. 2001. "Allergy Development and the Intestinal Microflora during the First Year of Life." *The Journal of Allergy and Clinical Immunology* 108 (4): 516–520. http://www.ncbi.nlm.nih.gov/pubmed/11590374.

Bode, L. 2009. "Human Milk Oligosaccharides: Prebiotics and Beyond." *Nutrition Reviews* 67 Suppl 2: S183–S191. doi:10.1111/j.1753-4887.2009.00239.x. http://www.ncbi.nlm. nih.gov/pubmed/19906222.

Bolognani, F, C J Rumney, B L Pool-Zobel, and I R Rowland. 2001. "Effect of Lactobacilli, Bifidobacteria and Inulin on the Formation of Aberrant Crypt Foci in Rats." *European Journal of Nutrition* 40 (6): 293–300. http://www.ncbi.nlm.nih.gov/pubmed/11876494.

Boyle, R J, R M Robins-Browne, and M L K Tang. 2006. "Probiotic Use in Clinical Practice: What Are the Risks?" *The American Journal of Clinical Nutrition* 83 (6): 1256–1264; quiz 1446–1447. http://www.ncbi.nlm.nih.gov/pubmed/16762934.

Brugman, S, F A Klatter, J T J Visser, A C M Wildeboer-Veloo, H J M Harmsen, J Rozing, and N A Bos. 2006. "Antibiotic Treatment Partially Protects against Type 1 Diabetes in the Bio-Breeding Diabetes-Prone Rat. Is the Gut Flora Involved in the Development of Type 1 Diabetes?" *Diabetologia* 49 (9): 2105–2108. doi:10.1007/s00125-006-0334-0. http://www.ncbi.nlm.nih.gov/pubmed/16816951.

Cani, P D, and N M Delzenne. 2009. "The Role of the Gut Microbiota in Energy Metabolism and Metabolic Disease." *Current Pharmaceutical Design* 15 (13): 1546–1558. http://www.ncbi.nlm.nih.gov/pubmed/19442172.

Caplan, M, and B Frost. 2011. "Seminars in Fetal & Neonatal Medicine Myth: Necrotizing Enterocolitis: Probiotics Will End the Disease, and Surgical Intervention Improves the Outcome." *Seminars in Fetal and Neonatal Medicine* 16 (5): 264–268. doi:10.1016/j.siny.2011.03.004. http://dx.doi.org/10.1016/j.siny.2011.03.004.

Cherbut, C. 2003. "Motor Effects of Short-Chain Fatty Acids and Lactate in the Gastrointestinal Tract." *The Proceedings of the Nutrition Society* 62 (1): 95–99.

Chung, D H, R T Ethridge, S Kim, S Owens-Stovall, A Hernandez, D R Kelly, and B M Evers. 2001. "Molecular Mechanisms Contributing to Necrotizing Enterocolitis." *Annals of Surgery* 233 (6): 835–842. http://www.pubmedcentral.nih.gov/articlerender.fcgi?artid=1421327&tool=pmcentrez&rendertype=abstract.

Clarke, T B, K M Davis, E S Lysenko, A Y Zhou, Y Yu, and J N Weiser. 2010. "Recognition of Peptidoglycan from the Microbiota by Nod1 Enhances Systemic Innate Immunity." *Nature Medicine* 16 (2): 228–231. http://www.ncbi.nlm.nih.gov/pubmed/20081863.

Claud, E C. 2012. "First Do No Harm." *Journal of Pediatric Pharmacology and Therapeutics* 17 (4): 298–301.

D'Souza, A L, C Rajkumar, J Cooke, and C J Bulpitt. 2002. "Probiotics in Prevention of Antibiotic Associated Diarrhoea: Meta-analysis." *BMJ British Medical Journal* 324 (7350): 1361. http://www.pubmedcentral.nih.gov/articlerender.fcgi?artid=115209&tool=pmcentrez&rendertype=abstract.

Daubioul, C A, Y Horsmans, P Lambert, E Danse, and N M Delzenne. 2005. "Effects of Oligofructose on Glucose and Lipid Metabolism in Patients with Nonalcoholic Steatohepatitis: Results of a Pilot Study." *European Journal of Clinical Nutrition* 59: 723–726.

Deng, Y S, J H Zhong, and X F Zhou. 2000. "Effects of Endogenous Neurotrophins on Sympathetic Sprouting in the Dorsal Root Ganglia and Allodynia following Spinal Nerve Injury." *Experimental Neurology* 164 (2): 344–350. http://www.ncbi.nlm.nih.gov/pubmed/10915573.

Desbonnet, L, L Garrett, G Clarke, B Kiely, J F Cryan, and T G Dinan. 2010. "Effects of the Probiotic *Bifidobacterium infantis* in the Maternal Separation Model of Depression." *Neuroscience* 170 (4): 1179–1188. http://www.ncbi.nlm.nih.gov/pubmed/20696216.

Deshpande, G, S Rao, S Patole, and M Bulsara. 2010. "Updated Meta-analysis of Probiotics for Preventing Necrotizing Enterocolitis in Preterm Neonates." *Pediatrics* 125 (5): 921–930. doi:10.1542/peds.2009-1301. http://www.ncbi.nlm.nih.gov/pubmed/20403939.

De Filippo, C, D Cavalieri, M Di Paola, M Ramazzotti, J B Poullet, S Massart, S Collini, G Pieraccini, and P Lionetti. 2010. "Impact of Diet in Shaping Gut Microbiota Revealed by a Comparative Study in Children from Europe and Rural Africa." *Proceedings of the National Academy of Sciences of the United States of America* 107 (33): 14691–14696. http://www.pubmedcentral.nih.gov/articlerender.fcgi?artid=2930426&tool=pmcentrez&rendertype=abstract.

De Groote, M A, D N Frank, E Dowell, M P Glode, and N R Pace. 2005. "*Lactobacillus rhamnosus* GG Bacteremia Associated with Probiotic Use in a Child with Short Gut Syndrome." *The Pediatric Infectious Disease Journal* 24 (3): 278–280. http://www.ncbi.nlm.nih.gov/pubmed/15750472.

De Roos, N M, and M B Katan. 2000. "Effects of Probiotic Bacteria on Diarrhea, Lipid Metabolism, and Carcinogenesis: A Review of Papers Published between 1988 and 1998." *The American Journal of Clinical Nutrition* 71 (2): 405–411. http://www.ncbi. nlm.nih.gov/pubmed/10648252.

DiGiulio, D B, R Romero, J P Kusanovic, R Gómez, C J Kim, K S Seok, F Gotsch et al. 2010. "Prevalence and Diversity of Microbes in the Amniotic Fluid, the Fetal Inflammatory Response, and Pregnancy Outcome in Women with Preterm Pre-labor Rupture of Membranes." *American Journal of Reproductive Immunology (New York: 1989)* 64 (1): 38–57. doi:10.1111/ j.1600-0897.2010.00830.x. http://www.pubmedcentral.nih.gov/articlerender.fcgi?artid=2907 911&tool=pmcentrez&rendertype=abstract.

Dominguez-Bello, M G, M J Blaser, R E Ley, and R Knight. 2011. "Development of the Human Gastrointestinal Microbiota and Insights from High-Throughput Sequencing." *Gastroenterology* 140 (6): 1713–1719. doi:10.1053/j.gastro.2011.02.011. http://www.ncbi. nlm.nih.gov/pubmed/21530737.

Forno, E, A B Onderdonk, J McCracken, A A Litonjua, D Laskey, M L Delaney, A M DuBois et al. 2008. "Diversity of the Gut Microbiota and Eczema in Early Life." *Clinical and Molecular Allergy CMA* 6: 11. http://www.pubmedcentral.nih.gov/articlerender.fcgi?art id=2562383&tool=pmcentrez&rendertype=abstract.

Forsythe, P, and W A Kunze. 2012. "Voices from Within: Gut Microbes and the CNS." *Cellular and Molecular Life Sciences CMLS* 70 (1): 55–69. doi:10.1007/s00018-012-1028-z. http://www.ncbi.nlm.nih.gov/pubmed/22638926.

Fujiya, M, M W Musch, Y Nakagawa, S Hu, J Alverdy, Y Kohgo, O Schneewind, B Jabri, and E B Chang. 2007. "The *Bacillus subtilis* Quorum-Sensing Molecule CSF Contributes to Intestinal Homeostasis via OCTN2, a Host Cell Membrane Transporter." *Cell Host Microbe* 1 (4): 299–308. http://www.ncbi.nlm.nih.gov/pubmed/18005709.

Furrie, E, S Macfarlane, A Kennedy, J Cummings, S Walsh, D A O'Neil, and G Macfarlane. 2005. "Synbiotic Therapy (*Bifidobacterium longum*/Synergy 1) Initiates Resolution of Inflammation in Patients with Active Ulcerative Colitis: A Randomised Controlled Pilot Trial." *Gut* 54 (2): 242–249. http://dx.doi.org/10.1136/gut.2004.044834.

Garcia, A L, J Steiniger, S C Reich, M O Weickert, I Harsch, A Machowetz, M Mohlig et al. 2006. "Arabinoxylan Fibre Consumption Improved Glucose Metabolism, But Did Not Affect Serum Adipokines in Subjects with Impaired Glucose Tolerance." *Hormone and Metabolic Research Hormon und Stoffwechselforschung Hormones Et Metabolisme* 38 (11): 761–766. http://eprints.gla.ac.uk/22764/.

Garraway, S M, J C Petruska, and L M Mendell. 2003. "BDNF Sensitizes the Response of Lamina II Neurons to High Threshold Primary Afferent Inputs." *European Journal of Neuroscience* 18 (9): 2467–2476. http://doi.wiley.com/10.1046/j.1460-9568.2003.02982.x.

Gore, C, K Munro, C Lay, R Bibiloni, J Morris, A Woodcock, A Custovic, and G W Tannock. 2008. "*Bifidobacterium pseudocatenulatum* Is Associated with Atopic Eczema: A Nested Case–Control Study Investigating the Fecal Microbiota of Infants." *The Journal of Allergy and Clinical Immunology* 121 (1): 135–140. http://www.ncbi.nlm.nih.gov/pubmed/17900682.

Gough, E, H Shaikh, and A R Manges. 2011. "Systematic Review of Intestinal Microbiota Transplantation (Fecal Bacteriotherapy) for Recurrent *Clostridium difficile* Infection." *Clinical Infectious Diseases* 53 (10): 994–1002. doi:10.1093/cid/cir632. http://www. ncbi.nlm.nih.gov/pubmed/22002980.

Gratz, S W, H Mykkanen, and H S El-Nezami. 2010. "Probiotics and Gut Health: A Special Focus on Liver Diseases." *World Journal of Gastroenterology: WJG* 16 (4): 403–410. http://www.pubmedcentral.nih.gov/articlerender.fcgi?artid=2811790&tool=pmcentrez& rendertype=abstract.

Groh, H, K Schade, and C Hörhold-Schubert. 1993. "Steroid Metabolism with Intestinal Microorganisms." *Journal of Basic Microbiology* 33 (1): 59–72. http://dx.doi.org/10.1002/ jobm.3620330115.

Guandalini, S, G Magazzù, A Chiaro, V La Balestra, G Di Nardo, S Gopalan, A Sibal et al. 2010. "VSL#3 Improves Symptoms in Children with Irritable Bowel Syndrome: A Multicenter, Randomized, Placebo-Controlled, Double-Blind, Crossover Study." *Journal of Pediatric Gastroenterology and Nutrition* 51 (1): 24–30. doi:10.1097/MPG.0b013e3181ca4d95. http://www.ncbi.nlm.nih.gov/pubmed/20453678.

Hamer, H M, D Jonkers, K Venema, S Vanhoutvin, F J Troost, and R-J Brummer. 2008. "Review Article: The Role of Butyrate on Colonic Function." *Alimentary Pharmacology & Therapeutics* 27 (2): 104–119. doi:10.1111/j.1365-2036.2007.03562.x. http://www.ncbi.nlm.nih.gov/pubmed/17973645.

Hart, A L, K Lammers, P Brigidi, B Vitali, F Rizzello, P Gionchetti, M Campieri, M A Kamm, S C Knight, and A J Stagg. 2004. "Modulation of Human Dendritic Cell Phenotype and Function by Probiotic Bacteria." *Gut* 53 (11): 1602–1609. http://www.pubmedcentral.nih.gov/articlerender.fcgi?artid=1774301&tool=pmcentrez&rendertype=abstract.

He, B, W Xu, P A Santini, A D Polydorides, A Chiu, J Estrella, M Shan et al. 2007. "Intestinal Bacteria Trigger T Cell–Independent Immunoglobulin A(2) Class Switching by Inducing Epithelial-Cell Secretion of the Cytokine APRIL." *Immunity* 26 (6): 812–826. http://www.ncbi.nlm.nih.gov/pubmed/17570691.

Heijtz, R D, S Wang, F Anuar, Y Qian, B Björkholm, A Samuelsson, M L Hibberd, H Forssberg, and S Pettersson. 2011. "Normal Gut Microbiota Modulates Brain Development and Behavior." *Proceedings of the National Academy of Sciences of the United States of America* 108 (7): 3047–3052. http://www.pubmedcentral.nih.gov/articlerender.fcgi?artid=3041077&tool=pmcentrez&rendertype=abstract.

Hempel, S, S Newberry, A Ruelaz, Z Wang, J N V Miles, M J Suttorp, B Johnsen et al. 2011. "Safety of Probiotics Used to Reduce Risk and Prevent or Treat Disease." *Evidence Report/Technology Assessment* (200): 1–645. http://www.ncbi.nlm.nih.gov/pubmed/23126627.

Indrio, F, G Riezzo, F Raimondi, M Bisceglia, L Cavallo, and R Francavilla. 2009. "Effects of Probiotic and Prebiotic on Gastrointestinal Motility in Newborns." *Journal of Physiology and Pharmacology: An Official Journal of the Polish Physiological Society* 60 Suppl 6: 27–31. http://www.ncbi.nlm.nih.gov/pubmed/20224148.

Indrio, F, and J Neu. 2011. "The Intestinal Microbiome of Infants and the Use of Probiotics." *Current Opinion in Pediatrics* 23 (2): 145–150. doi:10.1097/MOP.0b013e3283444ccb. http://www.pubmedcentral.nih.gov/articlerender.fcgi?artid=3155417&tool=pmcentrez&rendertype=abstract.

Ivanov, I I, K Atarashi, N Manel, E L Brodie, T Shima, U Karaoz, D Wei et al. 2009. "Induction of Intestinal Th17 Cells by Segmented Filamentous Bacteria." *Cell* 139 (3): 485–498. doi:10.1016/j.cell.2009.09.033. http://www.pubmedcentral.nih.gov/articlerender.fcgi?artid=2796826&tool=pmcentrez&rendertype=abstract.

Jiménez, E, M L Marín, R Martín, J M Odriozola, M Olivares, J Xaus, L Fernández, and J M Rodríguez. 2008. "Is Meconium from Healthy Newborns Actually Sterile?" *Research in Microbiology* 159 (3): 187–193. doi:10.1016/j.resmic.2007.12.007. http://www.ncbi.nlm.nih.gov/pubmed/18281199.

Johnston, B C, J Z Goldenberg, P O Vandvik, X Sun, and G H Guyatt. 2011. "Probiotics for the Prevention of Pediatric Antibiotic-Associated Diarrhea." *Cochrane Database of Systematic Reviews Online* 42 Suppl 2 (11): CD004827. doi:10.1002/14651858.CD004827.pub3. http://www.ncbi.nlm.nih.gov/pubmed/22071814.

Kadooka, Y, M Sato, K Imaizumi, A Ogawa, K Ikuyama, Y Akai, M Okano, M Kagoshima, and T Tsuchida. 2010. "Regulation of Abdominal Adiposity by Probiotics (*Lactobacillus gasseri* SBT2055) in Adults with Obese Tendencies in a Randomized Controlled Trial." *European Journal of Clinical Nutrition* 64 (6): 636–643. doi:10.1038/ejcn.2010.19. http://www.ncbi.nlm.nih.gov/pubmed/20216555.

Kalliomaki, M, M C Collado, S Saliminen, and E Isolauri. 2008. "Early Differences in Fecal Microbiota Composition in Children May." *American Journal of Clinical Nutrition* 87 (1): 534–538. http://www.ajcn.org/cgi/reprint/87/3/534.

Karege, F, G Perret, G Bondolfi, M Schwald, G Bertschy, and J-M Aubry. 2002. "Decreased Serum Brain-derived Neurotrophic Factor Levels in Major Depressed Patients." *Psychiatry Research* 109 (2): 143–148. http://www.ncbi.nlm.nih.gov/pubmed/11927139.

Karege, F, G Vaudan, M Schwald, N Perroud, and R La Harpe. 2005. "Neurotrophin Levels in Postmortem Brains of Suicide Victims and the Effects of Antemortem Diagnosis and Psychotropic Drugs." *Brain Research Molecular Brain Research* 136 (1–2): 29–37. http://www.ncbi.nlm.nih.gov/pubmed/15893584.

Kelly, D, J I Campbell, T P King, G Grant, E A Jansson, A G P Coutts, S Pettersson, and S Conway. 2004. "Commensal Anaerobic Gut Bacteria Attenuate Inflammation by Regulating Nuclear–Cytoplasmic Shuttling of PPAR-Gamma and RelA." *Nature Immunology* 5 (1): 104–112. http://www.ncbi.nlm.nih.gov/pubmed/14691478.

Kirjavainen, P V, T Arvola, S J Salminen, and E Isolauri. 2002. "Aberrant Composition of Gut Microbiota of Allergic Infants: A Target of Bifidobacterial Therapy at Weaning?" *Gut* 51 (1): 51–55. http://www.pubmedcentral.nih.gov/articlerender.fcgi?artid=1773282&tool =pmcentrez&rendertype=abstract.

Könönen, E, H Jousimies-Somer, and S Asikainen. 1992. "Relationship between Oral Gram-Negative Anaerobic Bacteria in Saliva of the Mother and the Colonization of Her Edentulous Infant." *Oral Microbiology and Immunology* 7 (5): 273–276.

Krinos, C M, M J Coyne, K G Weinacht, A O Tzianabos, D L Kasper, and L E Comstock. 2001. "Extensive Surface Diversity of a Commensal Microorganism by Multiple DNA Inversions." *Nature* 414 (6863): 555–558. http://www.ncbi.nlm.nih.gov/pubmed/11734857.

Kukkonen, K, E Savilahti, T Haahtela, K Juntunen-Backman, R Korpela, T Poussa, T Tuure, and M Kuitunen. 2007. "Probiotics and Prebiotic Galacto-Oligosaccharides in the Prevention of Allergic Diseases: A Randomized, Double-Blind, Placebo-Controlled Trial." *The Journal of Allergy and Clinical Immunology* 119 (1): 192–198. http://www.ncbi.nlm.nih.gov/pubmed/17208601.

Kunz, C, S Kuntz, and S Rudloff. 2009. "Intestinal Flora." *Annales De Gastroenterologie et Dhepatologie* 639 (4): 67–79.

Lam, V, J Su, S Koprowski, A Hsu, J S Tweddell, P Rafiee, G J Gross, N H Salzman, and J E Baker. 2012. "Intestinal Microbiota Determine Severity of Myocardial Infarction in Rats." *The FASEB Journal Official Publication of the Federation of American Societies for Experimental Biology* 26 (4): 1727–1735. doi:10.1096/fj.11-197921. http://www.ncbi.nlm.nih.gov/pubmed/22247331.

Land, M H, K Rouster-Stevens, C R Woods, M L Cannon, J Cnota, and A K Shetty. 2005. "*Lactobacillus* Sepsis Associated with Probiotic Therapy." *Pediatrics* 115 (1): 178–181. doi:10.1542/peds.2004-2137. http://www.ncbi.nlm.nih.gov/pubmed/15629999.

Larsen N, Vogensen F K, van den Berg F W J, Nielsen D S, Andreasen A S et al. 2010. "Gut Microbiota in Human Adults with Type 2 Diabetes Differs from Non-Diabetic Adults." *PLoS ONE* 5(2): e9085. doi:10.1371/journal.pone.0009085.

LeBlanc, J G, C Milani, G S de Giori, F Sesma, D van Sinderen, and M Ventura. 2013. "Bacteria as Vitamin Suppliers to Their Host: A Gut Microbiota Perspective." *Current Opinion in Biotechnology* 24 (2): 160–168. doi:10.1016/j.copbio.2012.08.005. http://www.ncbi.nlm.nih.gov/pubmed/22940212.

Lefebvre, P, B Cariou, F Lien, F Kuipers, and B Staels. 2009. "Role of Bile Acids and Bile Acid Receptors in Metabolic Regulation." *Physiological Reviews* 89 (1): 147–191. doi:10.1152/physrev.00010.2008. http://www.ncbi.nlm.nih.gov/pubmed/19126757.

Le Poul, E, C Loison, S Struyf, J-Y Springael, V Lannoy, M-E Decobecq, S Brezillon et al. 2003. "Functional Characterization of Human Receptors for Short Chain Fatty Acids and Their Role in Polymorphonuclear Cell Activation." *The Journal of Biological Chemistry* 278 (28): 25481–25489. doi:10.1074/jbc.M301403200. http://www.ncbi.nlm.nih.gov/pubmed/12711604.

Ley, R E, F Bäckhed, P Turnbaugh, C A Lozupone, R D Knight, and J I Gordon. 2005. "Obesity Alters Gut Microbial Ecology." *Proceedings of the National Academy of Sciences of the United States of America* 102 (31): 11070–11075. http://www.pubmedcentral.nih.gov/articlerender.fcgi?artid=1176910&tool=pmcentrez&rendertype=abstract.

Lu, J, T Jilling, D A N Li, M S Caplan, and E Northwestern. 2009. "NIH Public Access" 61 (4): 427–432. doi:10.1203/pdr.0b013e3180332ca5.Polyunsaturated.

Lucas, A. 1991. "Programming by Early Nutrition in Man." Ed. G R Bock and J Whelan. *Ciba Foundation Symposium* 156 (38): 38–50; discussion 50–55. http://ovidsp.ovid.com/ovidweb.cgi?T=JS&CSC=Y&NEWS=N&PAGE=fulltext&D=med3&AN=1855415.

Luo, J, M Van Yperselle, S W Rizkalla, F Rossi, F R Bornet, and G Slama. 2000. "Chronic Consumption of Short-Chain Fructooligosaccharides Does Not Affect Basal Hepatic Glucose Production or Insulin Resistance in Type 2 Diabetics." *The Journal of Nutrition* 130. AMER INST NUTRITION, 1572–1577.

Luoto, R, M Kalliomäki, K Laitinen, N M Delzenne, P D Cani, S Salminen, and E Isolauri. 2011. "Initial Dietary and Microbiological Environments Deviate in Normal-weight Compared to Overweight Children at 10 Years of Age." *Journal of Pediatric Gastroenterology and Nutrition* 52 (1): 90–95. http://www.ncbi.nlm.nih.gov/pubmed/21150648.

Mackay, A D, M B Taylor, C Kibbler, and J M T Hamilton-Miller. 1999. "*Lactobacillus endocarditis* Caused by a Probiotic Organism." *Clinical Microbiology and Infection: The Official Publication of the European Society of Clinical Microbiology and Infectious Diseases* 5 (5): 290–292. http://www.ncbi.nlm.nih.gov/pubmed/11856270.

Macpherson, A J, and T Uhr. 2004. "Induction of Protective IgA by Intestinal Dendritic Cells Carrying Commensal Bacteria." *Science* 303 (5664): 1662–1665. doi:10.1126/science.1091334. http://www.ncbi.nlm.nih.gov/pubmed/15016999.

Malinen, E, T Rinttilä, K Kajander, J Mättö, A Kassinen, L Krogius, M Saarela, R Korpela, and A Palva. 2005. "Analysis of the Fecal Microbiota of Irritable Bowel Syndrome Patients and Healthy Controls with Real-time PCR." *The American Journal of Gastroenterology* 100 (2): 373–382. doi:10.1111/j.1572-0241.2005.40312.x. http://www.ncbi.nlm.nih.gov/pubmed/15667495.

Martin, C R. 2013. "Probiotics for the Prevention of Necrotizing Enterocolitis: Not Just Which Ones, But Why?" *Journal of Pediatric Gastroenterology and Nutrition* 57 (1): 3. doi:10.1097/MPG.0b013e31829291d2. http://www.ncbi.nlm.nih.gov/pubmed/23535765.

Mazmanian, S K, C H Liu, A O Tzianabos, and D L Kasper. 2005. "An Immunomodulatory Molecule of Symbiotic Bacteria Directs Maturation of the Host Immune System." *Cell* 122 (1): 107–118. doi:10.1016/j.cell.2005.05.007. http://www.ncbi.nlm.nih.gov/pubmed/16009137.

Messaoudi, M, R Lalonde, N Violle, H Javelot, D Desor, A Nejdi, J-F Bisson et al. 2011. "Assessment of Psychotropic-like Properties of a Probiotic Formulation (*Lactobacillus helveticus* R0052 and *Bifidobacterium longum* R0175) in Rats and Human Subjects." *The British Journal of Nutrition* 105 (5): 755–764. http://www.ncbi.nlm.nih.gov/pubmed/20974015.

Mikhaĭlova, N A, F G Nagieva, O M Grin'ko, and V V Zverev. 2010. "Experimental Study of Antiviral Activity of Spore-Forming Bacterium *Bacillus pumilus* 'Pashkov'." *Zhurnal Mikrobiologii, Epidemiologii, i Immunobiologii* (2): 69–74. http://www.ncbi.nlm.nih.gov/pubmed/20465005.

Modi, N, S Uthaya, J Fell, and E Kulinskaya. 2010. "A Randomized, Double-Blind, Controlled Trial of the Effect of Prebiotic Oligosaccharides on Enteral Tolerance in Preterm Infants (ISRCTN77444690)." *Pediatric Research* 68 (5): 440–445. http://www.ncbi.nlm.nih.gov/pubmed/20639792.

Morelli, L. 2008. "Postnatal Development of Intestinal Microflora as Influenced by Infant Nutrition." *The Journal of Nutrition* 138 (9): 1791S–1795S. http://www.ncbi.nlm.nih. gov/pubmed/18716188.

Mshvildadze, M, J Neu, and V Mai. 2008. "Intestinal Microbiota Development in the Premature Neonate: Establishment of a Lasting Commensal Relationship?" *Nutrition Reviews* 66 (11): 658–663. http://www.ncbi.nlm.nih.gov/pubmed/19019028.

Mugambi, M N, A Musekiwa, M Lombard, T Young, and R Blaauw. 2012. "Probiotics, Prebiotics Infant Formula Use in Preterm or Low Birth Weight Infants: A Systematic Review." *Nutrition Journal* 11:58. doi:10.1186/1475-2891-11-58. http://www.pubmed central.nih.gov/articlerender.fcgi?artid=3487753&tool=pmcentrez&rendertype= abstract.

Murguía-Peniche, T, W A Mihatsch, J Zegarra, S Supapannachart, Z-Y Ding, and J Neu. 2013. "Intestinal Mucosal Defense System, Part 2. Probiotics and Prebiotics." *The Journal of Pediatrics* 162 (3): S64–S71. doi:10.1016/j.jpeds.2012.11.055. http://linkinghub. elsevier.com/retrieve/pii/S0022347612013893.

Neish, A S. 2009. "Microbes in Gastrointestinal Health and Disease." *Gastroenterology* 136 (1): 65–80. doi:10.1053/j.gastro.2008.10.080. http://www.pubmedcentral.nih.gov/articlerender. fcgi?artid=2892787&tool=pmcentrez&rendertype=abstract.

Neu, J, and W A Walker. 2011. "Necrotizing Enterocolitis." *The New England Journal of Medicine* 364 (3): 255–264. doi:10.1056/NEJMra1005408. http://www.pubmedcentral. nih.gov/articlerender.fcgi?artid=3628622&tool=pmcentrez&rendertype=abstract.

Neufeld, K M, N Kang, J Bienenstock, and J A Foster. 2011. "Reduced Anxiety-Like Behavior and Central Neurochemical Change in Germ-Free Mice." *Neurogastroenterology and Motility* 23 (3): 255–264, e119. doi:10.1111/j.1365-2982.2010.01620.x. http://www. ncbi.nlm.nih.gov/pubmed/21054680.

Nguyen, N, S B Lee, Y S Lee, K-H Lee, and J-Y Ahn. 2009. "Neuroprotection by NGF and BDNF against Neurotoxin-Exerted Apoptotic Death in Neural Stem Cells Are Mediated through Trk Receptors, Activating PI3-Kinase and MAPK Pathways." *Neurochemical Research* 34 (5): 942–951. http://www.ncbi.nlm.nih.gov/pubmed/18846424.

Niers, L, R Martín, G Rijkers, F Sengers, H Timmerman, N Van Uden, H Smidt, J Kimpen, and M Hoekstra. 2009. "The Effects of Selected Probiotic Strains on the Development of Eczema (the PandA Study)." *Allergy* 64 (9): 1349–1358. http://www.ncbi.nlm.nih. gov/pubmed/19392993.

Ohishi, A, S Takahashi, Y Ito, Y Ohishi, K Tsukamoto, Y Nanba, N Ito et al. 2010. "*Bifidobacterium* Septicemia Associated with Postoperative Probiotic Therapy in a Neonate with Omphalocele." *The Journal of Pediatrics* 156 (4): 679–681. doi:10.1016/j. jpeds.2009.11.041. http://www.ncbi.nlm.nih.gov/pubmed/20303445.

Otte, J-M, and D K Podolsky. 2004. "Functional Modulation of Enterocytes by Gram-Positive and Gram-Negative Microorganisms." *American Journal of Physiology Gastrointestinal and Liver Physiology* 286 (4): G613–G626. http://www.ncbi.nlm.nih. gov/pubmed/15010363.

Ouwehand, A C. 2007. "Antiallergic Effects of Probiotics." *The Journal of Nutrition* 137 (3 Suppl 2): 794S–797S. http://www.ncbi.nlm.nih.gov/pubmed/17311977.

Oxman, T, M Shapira, R Klein, N Avazov, and B Rabinowitz. 2001. "Oral Administration of *Lactobacillus* Induces Cardioprotection." *Journal of Alternative and Complementary Medicine* 7 (4): 345–354. http://www.ncbi.nlm.nih.gov/pubmed/11558777.

Palmer, C, E M Bik, D B DiGiulio, D A Relman, and P O Brown. 2007. "Development of the Human Infant Intestinal Microbiota." *PLoS Biology* 5 (7): e177. doi:10.1371/journal. pbio.0050177. http://www.pubmedcentral.nih.gov/articlerender.fcgi?artid=1896187& tool=pmcentrez&rendertype=abstract.

Parnell, J A, and R A Reimer. 2009. "Weight Loss During Oligofructose Supplementation Is Associated with Decreased Ghrelin and Increased Peptide YY in Overweight and Obese

Adults." *The American Journal of Clinical Nutrition* 89 (6): 1751–1759. http://www.scopus.com/inward/record.url?eid=2-s2.0-66849129539&partnerID=40&md5=bbfa25 3c38f246e72bbd61bb9f3b88c3.

Penders, J, E E Stobberingh, P A Van Den Brandt, and C Thijs. 2007. "The Role of the Intestinal Microbiota in the Development of Atopic Disorders." *Allergy* 62 (11): 1223–1236. http://www.ncbi.nlm.nih.gov/pubmed/17711557.

Perapoch, J, A M Planes, A Querol, V López, I Martínez-Bendayán, R Tormo, F Fernández, G Peguero, and S Salcedo. 2000. "Fungemia with *Saccharomyces cerevisiae* in Two Newborns, Only One of Whom Had Been Treated with Ultra-Levura." *European Journal of Clinical Microbiology & Infectious Diseases: Official Publication of the European Society of Clinical Microbiology* 19 (6): 468–470. http://www.ncbi.nlm.nih.gov/pubmed/10947224.

Petrof, E O, K Kojima, M J Ropeleski, M W Musch, Y Tao, C De Simone, and E B Chang. 2004. "Probiotics Inhibit Nuclear Factor-KappaB and Induce Heat Shock Proteins in Colonic Epithelial Cells through Proteasome Inhibition." *Gastroenterology* 127 (5): 1474–1487. http://www.ncbi.nlm.nih.gov/pubmed/15521016.

Petrof, E O, E C Claud, G B Gloor, and E Allen-Vercoe. 2013. "Microbial Ecosystems Therapeutics: A New Paradigm in Medicine?" *Beneficial Microbes* 4 (1): 53–65. doi:10.3920/BM2012.0039. http://www.ncbi.nlm.nih.gov/pubmed/23257018.

Pool-Zobel, B, J Van Loo, I Rowland, and M B Roberfroid. 2002. "Experimental Evidences on the Potential of Prebiotic Fructans to Reduce the Risk of Colon Cancer." *The British Journal of Nutrition* 87 Suppl 2: S273–S281. http://www.journals.cambridge.org/abstract_S000711450200106X.

Rautio, M, H Jousimies-Somer, H Kauma, I Pietarinen, M Saxelin, S Tynkkynen, and M Koskela. 1999. "Liver Abscess due to a *Lactobacillus rhamnosus* Strain Indistinguishable from *L. rhamnosus* Strain GG." *Clinical Infectious Diseases: An Official Publication of the Infectious Diseases Society of America* 28 (5): 1159–1160. doi:10.1086/514766. http://www.ncbi.nlm.nih.gov/pubmed/10452653.

Rhee, S H, C Pothoulakis, and E A Mayer. 2009. "Principles and Clinical Implications of the Brain–Gut–Enteric Microbiota Axis." *Nature Reviews. Gastroenterology & Hepatology* 6 (5): 306–314. doi:10.1038/nrgastro.2009.35. http://www.ncbi.nlm.nih.gov/pubmed/19404271.

Ridlon, J M, D-J Kang, and P B Hylemon. 2006. "Bile Salt Biotransformations by Human Intestinal Bacteria." *Journal of Lipid Research* 47 (2): 241–259. http://www.ncbi.nlm.nih.gov/pubmed/16299351.

Roesch, L F W, G L Lorca, G Casella, A Giongo, A Naranjo, A M Pionzio, N Li et al. 2010. "The Onset of Diabetes in a Rat Model." *The ISME Journal* 3 (5): 536–548. doi:10.1038/ismej.2009.5.Culture-independent.

Rojas, M A, J M Lozano, M X Rojas, V A Rodriguez, M A Rondon, J A Bastidas, L A Perez et al. 2012. "Prophylactic Probiotics to Prevent Death and Nosocomial Infection in Preterm Infants." *Pediatrics* 130 (5): e1113–e1120. doi:10.1542/peds.2011-3584. http://www.ncbi.nlm.nih.gov/pubmed/23071204.

Rondeau, M. 2003. "Short Chain Fatty Acids Stimulate Feline Colonic Smooth Muscle Contraction." *Journal of Feline Medicine Surgery* 5 (3): 167–173. doi:10.1016/S1098-612X(03)00002-0. http://linkinghub.elsevier.com/retrieve/pii/S1098612X03000020.

Salminen, S, C Bouley, M C Boutron-Ruault, J H Cummings, A Franck, G R Gibson, E Isolauri, M C Moreau, M Roberfroid, and I Rowland. 1998. "Functional Food Science and Gastrointestinal Physiology and Function." *The British Journal of Nutrition* 80 Suppl 1: S147–S171. http://www.ncbi.nlm.nih.gov/pubmed/9849357.

Santos, F, J L Vera, P Lamosa, G F de Valdez, W M de Vos, H Santos, F Sesma, and J Hugenholtz. 2007. "Pseudovitamin B(12) Is the Corrinoid Produced by *Lactobacillus reuteri* CRL1098 Under Anaerobic Conditions." *FEBS Letters* 581 (25): 4865–4870. doi:10.1016/j.febslet.2007.09.012. http://www.ncbi.nlm.nih.gov/pubmed/17888910.

Shimizu, E, K Hashimoto, and M Iyo. 2004. "Major Depressive Disorders and BDNF (Brain-Derived Neurotrophic Factor)." *Nihon Shinkei Seishin Yakurigaku Zasshi Japanese Journal of Psychopharmacology* 24 (3): 147–150. http://www.ncbi.nlm.nih.gov/pubmed/22407616.

Sudo, N, Y Chida, Y Aiba, J Sonoda, N Oyama, X-N Yu, C Kubo, and Y Koga. 2004. "Postnatal Microbial Colonization Programs the Hypothalamic–Pituitary–Adrenal System for Stress Response in Mice." *The Journal of Physiology* 558 (Pt 1): 263–275. http://discovery.ucl.ac.uk/176047/.

Takaishi, H, T Matsuki, A Nakazawa, T Takada, S Kado, T Asahara, N Kamada et al. 2008. "Imbalance in Intestinal Microflora Constitution Could Be Involved in the Pathogenesis of Inflammatory Bowel Disease." *International Journal of Medical Microbiology: IJMM* 298 (5–6): 463–472. doi:10.1016/j.ijmm.2007.07.016. http://www.ncbi.nlm.nih.gov/pubmed/17897884.

Taranto, M P, L Vera, J Hugenholtz, G F De Valdez, and F Sesma. 2003. "*Lactobacillus reuteri* CRL1098 Produces Cobalamin" *Journal of Bacteriology* 185 (18): 5643–5647. doi:10.1128/JB.185.18.5643.

Tedelind, S, F Westberg, M Kjerrulf, and A Vidal. 2007. "Anti-inflammatory Properties of the Short-Chain Fatty Acids Acetate and Propionate: A Study with Relevance to Inflammatory Bowel Disease." *World Journal of Gastroenterology* 13 (20): 2826–2832. http://www.ncbi.nlm.nih.gov/pubmed/17569118.

Tlaskalová-Hogenová, H, R Štěpánková, H Kozáková, T Hudcovic, L Vannucci, L Tučková, P Rossmann et al. 2011. "The Role of Gut Microbiota (Commensal Bacteria) and the Mucosal Barrier in the Pathogenesis of Inflammatory and Autoimmune Diseases and Cancer: Contribution of Germ-Free and Gnotobiotic Animal Models of Human Diseases." *Cellular & Molecular Immunology* 8 (2): 110–120. doi:10.1038/cmi.2010.67. http://www.ncbi.nlm.nih.gov/pubmed/21278760.

Turnbaugh, P J, R E Ley, M A Mahowald, V Magrini, E R Mardis, and J I Gordon. 2006. "An Obesity-Associated Gut Microbiome with Increased Capacity for Energy Harvest." *Nature* 444 (7122): 1027–1031. doi:10.1038/nature05414. http://www.ncbi.nlm.nih.gov/pubmed/17183312.

Vael, C, S L Verhulst, V Nelen, H Goossens, and K N Desager. 2011. "Intestinal Microflora and Body Mass Index during the First Three Years of Life: An Observational Study." *Gut Pathogens* 3 (1): 8. http://www.pubmedcentral.nih.gov/articlerender.fcgi?artid=3118227&tool=pmcentrez&rendertype=abstract.

Von Der Weid, T, C Bulliard, and E J Schiffrin. 2001. "Induction by a Lactic Acid Bacterium of a Population of CD4(+) T Cells with Low Proliferative Capacity That Produce Transforming Growth Factor Beta and Interleukin-10." *Clinical and Diagnostic Laboratory Immunology* 8 (4): 695–701. http://www.ncbi.nlm.nih.gov/pubmed/11427413.

Vyas, U, and N Ranganathan. 2012. "Probiotics, Prebiotics, and Synbiotics: Gut and Beyond." *Gastroenterology Research and Practice* 2012: 872716. doi:10.1155/2012/872716. http://www.pubmedcentral.nih.gov/articlerender.fcgi?artid=3459241&tool=pmcentrez&rendertype=abstract.

Walker, A W, J D Sanderson, C Churcher, G C Parkes, B N Hudspith, N Rayment, J Brostoff, J Parkhill, G Dougan, and L Petrovska. 2011. "High-throughput Clone Library Analysis of the Mucosa-Associated Microbiota Reveals Dysbiosis and Differences between Inflamed and Non-inflamed Regions of the Intestine in Inflammatory Bowel Disease." *BMC Microbiology* 11 (1): 7. doi:10.1186/1471-2180-11-7. http://www.pubmedcentral.nih.gov/articlerender.fcgi?artid=3032643&tool=pmcentrez&rendertype=abstract.

Wang, M, C Karlsson, C Olsson, I Adlerberth, A E Wold, D P Strachan, P M Martricardi et al. 2008. "Reduced Diversity in the Early Fecal Microbiota of Infants with Atopic Eczema." *The Journal of Allergy and Clinical Immunology* 121 (1): 129–134. http://www.ncbi.nlm.nih.gov/pubmed/18028995.

Weston, S, A Halbert, P Richmond, and S L Prescott. 2005. "Effects of Probiotics on Atopic Dermatitis: A Randomised Controlled Trial." *Archives of Disease in Childhood* 90 (9): 892–897. http://www.pubmedcentral.nih.gov/articlerender.fcgi?artid=1720555&tool=pmcentrez&rendertype=abstract.

Wong, J M W, R de Souza, C W C Kendall, A Emam, and D J A Jenkins. 2006. "Colonic Health: Fermentation and Short Chain Fatty Acids." *Journal of Clinical Gastroenterology* 40 (3): 235–243. http://www.ncbi.nlm.nih.gov/pubmed/16633129.

Wu, X, C Ma, L Han, M Nawaz, F Gao, X Zhang, P Yu et al. 2010. "Molecular Characterisation of the Faecal Microbiota in Patients with Type II Diabetes." *Current Microbiology* 61 (1): 69–78. http://www.ncbi.nlm.nih.gov/pubmed/20087741.

Zareie, M, K Johnson-Henry, J Jury, P-C Yang, B-Y Ngan, D M McKay, J D Soderholm, M H Perdue, and P M Sherman. 2006. "Probiotics Prevent Bacterial Translocation and Improve Intestinal Barrier Function in Rats following Chronic Psychological Stress." *Gut* 55 (11): 1553–1560. http://www.pubmedcentral.nih.gov/articlerender.fcgi?artid=1860130&tool=pmcentrez&rendertype=abstract.

13 Immunonutrients and Evidence for Their Use in Hospitalized Adults Receiving Artificial Nutrition

Philip C. Calder

CONTENTS

Introduction 309
Concept of Immunonutrition 310
Scientific Rationale for the Specific Nutrients Included in Immune-
Modulating Artificial Nutrition (aka Immunonutrition) 311
    Glutamine 312
    Arginine 316
    N-Acetyl Cysteine 317
    Omega-3 Fatty Acids from Fish Oil 317
        Omega-3 Fatty Acids in Parenteral Nutrition 317
        Omega-3 Fatty Acids in Enteral Nutrition 319
    Antioxidant Micronutrients and Trace Elements 321
    Mixtures of Immunonutrients Used Enterally 322
Conclusion 324
References 325

INTRODUCTION

Systemic inflammatory response syndrome (SIRS) is the name given to the uncontrolled inflammatory response to an insult (e.g., surgery, trauma, burns) and involving excessive production of inflammatory cytokines, particularly tumor necrosis factor (TNF)-α, interleukin (IL)-1β, IL-6, and IL-8 (Bone et al., 1997). Sepsis is the presence of SIRS in response to, or in combination with, an infection (Bone et al., 1997). The mortality risk of sepsis is about 20%, and it predisposes to organ failure, which carries an even greater mortality risk. Septic shock is the occurrence of multiple organ failures, metabolic acidosis, and hypotension, and it carries a mortality risk of 40%–80% (Bone et al., 1997). Together with SIRS, sepsis and septic shock are termed "septic syndromes." Septic syndromes are the leading cause of death in critically ill patients in Western countries (Angus et al., 2001). This chapter is based on, and updated from, an earlier publication on this topic (Calder, 2007).

Animal studies show a central role for inflammatory cytokines in the septic response (see Sadeghi et al., 1999 for references), and patients with sepsis show markedly elevated circulating concentrations of TNF-α, TNF-receptor 1, IL-1β, IL-6, and IL-8, with those patients having the highest concentrations being more likely to die (Girardin et al., 1998; Hatherill et al., 2000; Arnalich et al., 2000). In addition, circulating white cells from septic patients have high levels of activated nuclear factor κB (NF-κB), a transcription factor that promotes the expression of numerous genes associated with inflammation (Arnalich et al., 2000). Furthermore, the levels of activated NF-κB were reported to be higher in those patients who went on to die (Arnalich et al., 2000). Mediators other than inflammatory cytokines are involved in the pathological processes that accompany critical illness. For example, prostaglandin E_2 is implicated in sepsis, burns, and critical illness (Grbic et al., 1991; Ertel et al., 1992), while leukotriene B_4 and oxidants released by neutrophils are involved in acute respiratory distress syndrome (Kollef and Schuster, 1995).

In addition to hyperinflammation, patients with sepsis, burns, and trauma can display immunosuppression, characterized by decreased monocyte expression of the human leukocyte antigens (HLA) involved in antigen presentation, impaired ability of monocytes to stimulate T cells (i.e., impaired antigen presentation activity), impaired T-cell proliferation, and low production of the T-helper (Th) 1-type cytokines (e.g., interferon [IFN]-γ) associated with host defense against bacteria and viruses but high levels of the Th2- and regulatory T-cell (Treg)-type cytokines (IL-4, IL-10) associated with inhibition of host defense against bacteria and viruses (see Calder, 2004 for references). It is believed that the immunosuppressed phase of sepsis lags behind the hyperinflammatory phase; that is, initially sepsis is characterized by increased generation of inflammatory mediators but, as it persists, there is a shift toward an anti-inflammatory, immunosuppressed state sometimes called the compensatory anti-inflammatory response syndrome, or CARS, although the precise timing of the two phases and the factors that influence their relative magnitudes are not entirely clear (Heidecke et al., 1999; Weighardt et al., 2000; Tschaikowsky et al., 2002).

CONCEPT OF IMMUNONUTRITION

The ability of nutrients to influence the activities of cells of the immune system has been termed "immunonutrition," although this term has most frequently been associated with the use of specific nutrients or combinations of nutrients in surgical, trauma, burned, or critically ill patients (Calder, 2003a). These patients will often receive artificial nutrition, either intravenously (referred to as parenteral nutrition) or directly into the stomach or small intestine through a tube (referred to as tube feeding or enteral nutrition). Although the specific immunonutrients provided through these approaches will contribute to the patient's nutrient supply, the underlying rationale for immunonutrition is that certain nutrients can improve cell-mediated immune responses in a way that is clinically meaningful. In the context of patients

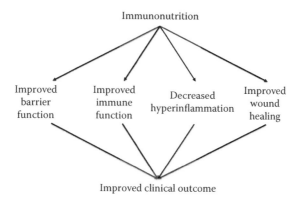

FIGURE 13.1 Concept of immunonutrition in the context of surgical or critically ill patients. (Reproduced from Calder, P. C., *British Journal of Nutrition* 98, S133, 2007.)

requiring artificial nutrition, this concept is extended to include modification of hyperinflammatory processes (including oxidative stress) and improvement in gut barrier function, thus preventing bacterial translocation (Figure 13.1).

SCIENTIFIC RATIONALE FOR THE SPECIFIC NUTRIENTS INCLUDED IN IMMUNE-MODULATING ARTIFICIAL NUTRITION (AKA IMMUNONUTRITION)

Nutrients considered for inclusion in immune-modulating (sometimes called immune-enhancing) artificial nutrition (i.e., immunonutrients) are generally those that have been shown to act in relevant animal models to improve immune function, regulate inflammation, maintain or improve gut barrier function, or improve antioxidant defenses, and which have been shown to be safe and efficacious (assessed according to the defined study outcome, which has not always been a clinical endpoint) in clinical trials in the relevant patient groups. In addition, theoretical considerations, experimental data from *in vitro* studies and healthy volunteer studies, and clinical findings in other patient groups have played a role in influencing the precise composition of immune-modulating artificial nutrition. It is important to appreciate that artificial nutrition itself provides macronutrients and micronutrients, including carbohydrate, lipid, protein, and/or peptides, and the full range of vitamins and minerals; immune-modulating artificial nutrition contains additional nutrients or increased amounts of nutrients normally present. Nutrients that have been identified as potentially important as components of immune-modulating artificial nutrition include

- Glutamine (sometimes provided as a dipeptide with either glycine or alanine)
- Arginine
- *N*-acetyl cysteine (as a cysteine precursor)
- Branched-chain amino acids
- Nucleotides

- Omega-3 fatty acids from fish oil
- Antioxidant vitamins
- Trace elements
- Taurine

The scientific rationale for the inclusion of these nutrients is summarized in Table 13.1. Mechanisms of action and preclinical evidence will not be discussed here, but may be found in the references listed in Table 13.1. The evidence of clinical efficacy of these nutrients, either alone or in combination, in hospitalized patients will be described below.

GLUTAMINE

Enteral glutamine increased the ratio of CD4[+] to CD8[+] cells in the blood of intensive care patients (Jensen et al., 1996), while parenteral administration of glutamine in patients having undergone colorectal cancer resection surgery increased mitogen-stimulated proliferation of blood lymphocytes (O'Riordain et al., 1994). Another study in postoperative patients who received parenteral glutamine showed increased blood lymphocyte numbers (Morlion et al., 1998) and, more recently, parenteral glutamine for 48 h after major abdominal surgery was shown to result in better maintenance of HLA-DR expression on blood monocytes (Spittler et al., 2001). Patients with esophageal cancer being treated with radiochemotherapy also had higher blood lymphocyte counts and better lymphocyte proliferative responses if they consumed glutamine for 28 days (Yoshida et al., 1998). In addition to a direct immunological effect, glutamine, even given parenterally, appears to improve gut barrier function in patients at risk of infection (van der Hulst et al., 1993), an effect that is likely to decrease translocation of bacteria from the gut and hence eliminate a key source of infection.

The improvements in immune function with glutamine administration have been suggested to result in clinical benefit. Parenteral glutamine after bone marrow transplantation reduced infections and length of hospital stay (Ziegler et al., 1992), with a later report showing that glutamine resulted in higher total blood lymphocyte, T-lymphocyte, and CD4[+] lymphocyte numbers after patients' discharge (Ziegler et al., 1998). In a study of patients in intensive care, glutamine decreased mortality compared with standard parenteral nutrition and changed the pattern of mortality (Griffiths et al., 1997). In another study in which patients received enteral glutamine or a standard enteral feed from within 48 h of the initiation of trauma, there was a significant reduction in the 15-day incidence of pneumonia, bacteremia, and severe sepsis in the glutamine group, although this was not associated with reduced mortality (Houdijk et al., 1998). This improved clinical outcome in patients receiving glutamine was associated with increased monocyte expression of HLA-DR (Boelens et al., 2002) and increased *ex vivo* IFN-γ production by T cells (Boelens et al., 2004). Enteral glutamine was found to decrease infection rate, *Pseudomonas aeruginosa* bacteremia, and mortality in adult burns patients (Garrel et al., 2003).

A number of systematic reviews and meta-analyses of the clinical efficacy of glutamine when used as a component of artificial nutrition have been conducted during the past 10 years or so. One of the earliest was by Novak et al. (2002), who conducted a meta-analysis of 14 studies of parenteral or enteral glutamine in surgical or critically ill patients excluding studies in bone marrow transplantation and in premature infants. The analysis included eight studies in ill postsurgical patients, all using parenteral glutamine, and six studies in critically ill patients (intensive care unit [ICU], trauma, or burns patients), three using parenteral glutamine and three using enteral glutamine. Overall, glutamine use was associated with significant decreases in infectious complications (7 studies; risk reduced by 20%) and in length of hospital stay (10 studies; 2.6 days shorter) and with a trend toward lower mortality (risk reduced by 22%). In surgical patients, glutamine decreased infections (risk reduced by 54%) and length of hospital stay (3.5 days shorter) but did not affect mortality. Mortality benefits were seen in the critically ill (risk reduced by 23%). Overall, the impact of glutamine was greater in surgical patients and was greater when used parenterally or at high dose. Murray and Pindoria (2002) conducted a meta-analysis of studies of parenteral glutamine in bone marrow transplantation and showed decreased length of hospital stay (three studies; 6.6 days shorter) and reduced development of positive blood cultures (two studies; risk reduced by 77%). They concluded that bone marrow transplant patients with gastrointestinal failure should receive parenteral glutamine. An updated meta-analysis including an additional study tempered this strong conclusion (Murray and Pindoria, 2009). Glutamine provision remained associated with reduced development of positive blood cultures (three studies; risk reduced by 54%) but the earlier identified effect on length of hospital stay was lost. It was still concluded that routine use of parenteral glutamine for bone marrow transplantation patients could be considered, but that benefits are not certain. Avenell (2009) reported a meta-analysis of parenteral and enteral glutamine in surgical and critically ill patients. The analysis evaluated a total of 27 studies, 11 in surgical (mainly gastrointestinal) patients, 15 in critically ill patients (mixed ICU, trauma, pancreatitis, surgical complications), and 1 in mixed surgical and critically ill patients. Of these studies, 19 were included in the meta-analysis of infection and 16 in the meta-analysis of mortality. No significant effect on mortality of either parenteral or enteral glutamine was seen in either surgical or critically ill patients, although when all studies were aggregated there was a strong trend to a reduction in mortality (risk reduced by 24%). Critically ill patients receiving enteral glutamine and surgical patients receiving parenteral glutamine were less likely to become infected (risk reduced by 24% and 55%, respectively). There was also a strong trend to reduced infections in critically ill patients receiving parenteral glutamine (risk reduced by 29%). When all studies were aggregated, there was a significant reduction in infections with glutamine (risk reduced by 24%). Parenteral, but not enteral, glutamine also lowered multiorgan failure (risk reduced by 33%). A meta-analysis of parenteral glutamine in abdominal surgery patients identified significant reductions in infections (four studies; risk reduced by 76%) and length of hospital stay (six studies; 3.5 days shorter) (Zheng et al., 2006). Another meta-analysis of parenteral glutamine in abdominal surgery patients identified significant reductions in infections (10 studies; risk reduced by 31%) and length of hospital stay (13 studies; 3.8 days shorter for alanyl-glutamine and 5.4 days shorter for glycyl-glutamine) (Wang et al., 2010). A meta-analysis of four studies of enteral glutamine in burn patients was recently published (Lin et al., 2013). Enteral glutamine reduced hospital mortality (two studies; risk reduced by 87%) but not the length of hospital stay.

TABLE 13.1
Scientific Rationale for Inclusion of Nutrients in Immune-Modulating Artificial Nutrition

Nutrient	Rationale	References
Glutamine	The most abundant amino acid in the blood and in free amino acid pool; an important fuel for cells of the immune system; intramuscular and plasma glutamine concentrations decrease postsurgery, in sepsis, cancer cachexia, and after burns. In animal experiments, glutamine improved T-cell function and enhanced resistance to infectious pathogens. In animal experiments, glutamine improved gut-associated immune tissue weight and cellularity and maintained intestinal integrity (infections, endotoxemia).	Calder and Yaqoob, 1999, 2004
Arginine	Involved in protein, urea, and nucleotide synthesis and ATP generation; precursor of nitric oxide, a potent immunoregulatory and blood flow mediator, which is cytotoxic to tumor cells and some microorganisms; precursor for synthesis of polyamines, which have a key role in DNA replication, regulation of the cell cycle, and cell division. In animal experiments, arginine decreased thymus involution associated with trauma, promoted thymus cellularity, lymphocyte proliferation, natural killer cell activity, and macrophage cytotoxicity, and improved delayed-type hypersensitivity, resistance to bacterial infections, survival to sepsis and burns, and wound healing. In healthy human subjects, arginine supplementation increased blood lymphocyte proliferation in response to mitogens and promoted wound healing.	Calder and Yaqoob, 2004; Popovic et al., 2007
N-acetyl cysteine	Cysteine is a component of the antioxidant glutathione. Glutathione concentrations in the liver, lung, small intestine, and immune cells fall in response to inflammation, and this fall can be prevented in some organs by provision of cysteine. Glutathione enhances the activity of T cells, improves cell-mediated immune function, and decreases the production of inflammatory cytokines.	Calder and Yaqoob, 2004
Branched-chain amino acids	Glutamine precursor; some (limited) evidence of improved immune function and increased resistance to infection from animal studies.	Calder, 2006a
Nucleotides	Involved in DNA and RNA structure, energy metabolism, signal transduction, biosynthesis of phospholipids, and regulation of enzyme activity. Activation of lymphocytes causes a rapid increase in demands for nucleotides to cover an early increase in energy requirements and a later need to synthesize RNA for protein production and DNA for cell division. In animal experiments, nucleotides improve T-cell functions, antibody responses, delayed-type hypersensitivity, and resistance to pathogens.	Carver et al., 1991; Gil, 2002

(continued)

TABLE 13.1 (Continued)
Scientific Rationale for Inclusion of Nutrients in Immune-Modulating Artificial Nutrition

Nutrient	Rationale	References
Omega-3 fatty acids from fish oil	Excessive arachidonic acid (long-chain n-6 fatty acid) may promote inflammatory processes and suppress cell-mediated immunity; arachidonic acid–derived eicosanoids associated with trauma, burns, and acute respiratory distress syndrome. Long-chain n-3 fatty acids oppose the action of arachidonic acid. *In vitro*, animal, and healthy volunteer experiments show that they are anti-inflammatory (decreased production of inflammatory eicosanoids and cytokines; increased production of anti-inflammatory resolvins); in animal experiments, increased resistance to endotoxin; generally associated with human health.	Calder, 2004
Antioxidant vitamins	Maintenance of antioxidant defenses; prevention of oxidative stress and lipid peroxidation (oxidative stress induces inflammation and lipid hydroperoxides are immunosuppressive). Vitamin E has been shown to improve T-cell responses and cell-mediated immunity.	Meydani et al., 2005
Trace elements	Zinc, copper, and selenium are components of the major antioxidant enzymes; maintenance of antioxidant protective mechanisms; postsurgical and critically ill patients lose trace elements; large losses in burns patients. Deficiencies in zinc, copper, or selenium are associated with immune impairments and increased susceptibility to infections, while zinc, copper, and selenium have all been shown to improve immune function in individuals with a low status.	Berger and Chiolero, 2003
Taurine	Taurine is present in high concentrations in most tissues and particularly in cells of the immune system. It contributes 50% of the free amino acid pool within lymphocytes, and is the most abundant free nitrogenous compound therein. Animal studies show that taurine prevents the decline in T-cell number seen with ageing and enhances the proliferative responses of T lymphocytes. In neutrophils, taurine maintains phagocytic capacity and microbicidal action through interaction with myeloperoxidase. In humans, plasma taurine concentrations are decreased by trauma and sepsis.	Calder and Yaqoob, 2004

Source: Modified from Calder, P. C., *British Journal of Nutrition* 98, S133, 2007.

Thus, a number of individual clinical trials published between the mid-1990s and 2011 report clinical benefits when glutamine is included in either parenteral or enteral nutrition given to postsurgical or critically ill patients, and these benefits are supported by several meta-analyses published between 1999 and 2013. This large dataset provides substantial evidence for the clinical efficacy of glutamine in these patient groups. However, two recent large studies of glutamine have questioned the robust-ness of this evidence base as far as critically ill patients are concerned. In the SIGNET trial, Andrews et al. (2011) conducted a randomized controlled trial of parenteral glu-tamine (20.2 g/day) and selenium (500 µg/day) either alone or together in 502 patients in intensive care. Glutamine did not affect antibiotic use, infections, length of hospital stay, or 6-month mortality. In the REDOXS trial, Heyland et al. (2013) randomized 1233 critically ill patients to glutamine or antioxidants including selenium or both. The immunonutrients were provided both parenterally and enterally, and very high doses of glutamine were administered. Glutamine did not reduce mortality (in fact, there was a strong trend toward increased mortality with glutamine), in-hospital mor-tality, 6-month mortality, ICU or hospital length of stay, or organ failure. It is difficult to understand why these two recent trials have been neutral (Andrews et al., 2011) and negative (Heyland et al., 2013) given the large number of positive earlier studies. However, the differences might be due to other advances in treatment negating the effects of glutamine, the specific characteristics of the patients studied, or, in the case of the REDOXS trial, the very high dose of glutamine used.

One meta-analysis of parenteral glutamine in surgical and critically ill patients has been published including the SIGNET trial (Bollhalder et al., 2013). This analysis identi-fied no significant effect on short-term mortality across all studies (15 studies); however, when the findings of the SIGNET trial were removed, glutamine had a significant effect (risk reduced by 28%). Glutamine reduced infections overall (27 studies; risk reduced by 17% [this became a 20% reduction when the SIGNET trial was removed]) and in sur-gical patients (risk reduced by 39%) (Bollhalder et al., 2013). There was a reduction in length of hospital stay overall (30 studies; 2.4 days shorter with glutamine) and in surgi-cal patients (15 studies; 2.9 days shorter with glutamine) but not in critically ill patients.

Meta-analyses are consistent in demonstrating that in postsurgical patients, gluta-mine, usually given parenterally, reduces risk of infections and shortens hospital stay (Novak et al., 2002; Zheng et al., 2006; Avenell, 2009; Wang et al., 2010; Bollhalder et al., 2013). Beneficial findings in critically ill patients are less consistently sup-ported through meta-analysis (Novak et al., 2002; Avenell, 2009; Lin et al., 2013; Bollhalder et al., 2013) and are questioned by the failure of two recent large studies to show a benefit of glutamine (Andrews et al., 2011; Heyland et al., 2013). There may be subgroups of critically ill patients who will benefit from glutamine given either parenterally or enterally, and it will be important to identify the characteristics of such subgroups and the most appropriate dose of glutamine to use.

ARGININE

Oral arginine supplementation for 7 days postsurgery was associated with an increased number of circulating CD4[+] cells and an enhanced response of peripheral blood lym-phocytes to mitogens by day 7 (Daly et al., 1988). Although the arginine-supplemented group achieved a positive nitrogen balance (by day 6), there was no difference in clini-cal outcome compared with the placebo group. Intravenous or enteral arginine has been given in various conditions, including in surgical and ICU patients, although these usually did not evaluate immune outcomes (see Zhou and Martindale, 2007 for references). Arginine is included in several immunonutrition formulas, including

IMPACT®, which are described in the later section "Mixtures of Immunonutrients Used Enterally." Marik and Zaloga conducted meta-analyses of immunonutrition in high-risk surgical patients (2010) and in critically ill patients (2008), and they included studies that used arginine alone as the immunonutrient (Mendez et al., 1997; Tsuei et al., 2005; de Luis et al., 2005; Wibbenmeyer et al., 2006; Casas-Rodera et al., 2008). In surgical patients, enteral arginine (two studies) had no effect on infection risk or length of hospital stay (Marik and Zaloga, 2010). Use of enteral arginine in burn patients (one study) or in trauma patients (two studies) was without effect on mortality (Marik and Zaloga, 2008). Thus, on the basis of clinical outcomes, evidence to support the use of arginine as the sole immunonutrient in postsurgical or critically ill patients is weak.

N-ACETYL CYSTEINE

Parenteral administration of *N*-acetyl cysteine in patients with sepsis increased blood glutathione concentration, decreased plasma concentrations of IL-8 and soluble TNF receptors, and improved respiratory function with a decreased number of days in intensive care (Bernard et al., 1997; Spapen et al., 1998). While not affecting mortality rates, *N*-acetyl cysteine also shortened hospital length of stay.

OMEGA-3 FATTY ACIDS FROM FISH OIL

Omega-3 Fatty Acids in Parenteral Nutrition

In the 1960s and 1970s, soybean oil became established as the lipid component of parenteral nutrition (Edgren and Wretlind, 1963; Hallberg et al., 1966; Wretlind, 1972), and mixtures of soybean oil and so-called "medium-chain triglycerides" (a derivative of coconut oil or palm kernel oil) were introduced in the mid-1980s (Sailer and Muller, 1981; Ulrich et al., 1996). Globally, soybean oil and mixtures of soybean oil and medium-chain triglycerides remain the major lipids used in parenteral nutrition. Soybean oil is rich in the omega-6 fatty acid linoleic acid, which comprises about 50% of the fatty acids present. A study in patients after a major gastrointestinal surgery identified that the amount of omega-6 fatty acid (i.e., linoleic acid) infused was one of two positive predictors of the length of hospital stay (increased by 1.6 days/100 g of n-6 fatty acid infused), the other being the delay in the onset of initiating nutritional support (Koch and Heller, 2005). However, clinical trials with soybean oil–based lipid emulsions, mainly in undernourished patients undergoing major gastrointestinal surgery, provide conflicting evidence, some showing selective immunosuppressive effects (Monson et al., 1988; Battistella et al., 1997; Furukawa et al., 2002), in some cases linked to poorer patient outcomes (Battistella et al., 1997), and others not showing effects on the immune system (Dionigi et al., 1985; Gogos et al., 1990; Sedmen et al., 1991) or on clinical outcomes (Lenssen et al., 1998). These studies have been described and discussed previously (Calder, 2006b, 2009). Despite the inconsistencies of the outcomes of studies with soybean-based lipid emulsions, a view has developed that the use of lipid emulsions based solely on soybean oil may not be optimal or may even be harmful, the concern being that n-6 fatty acids might be "proinflammatory, immunosuppressive, and procoagulatory." It is important to note, however, that despite these concerns, soybean oil remains widely used as the sole lipid provided in parenteral nutrition regimens.

One approach to decreasing the linoleic acid content in intravenous lipid emulsions is partial replacement of soybean oil with omega-3 fatty acid–rich fish oil. This not only decreases the omega-6 fatty acid content but also increases provision of biologically active omega-3 fatty acids. Several studies with fish oil containing lipid emulsions have been conducted in postsurgery patients, demonstrating decreased production of some inflammatory mediators (leukotriene B_4, TNF-α, IL-6) (Morlion et al., 1996; Wachtler et al., 1997; Koller et al., 2003; Grimm et al., 2006) and better preservation of some immune functions (e.g., monocyte expression of HLA-DR, IFN-γ production) (Schauder et al., 2002; Weiss et al., 2002). Some studies have also reported shorter postoperative stays in hospital (Grimm et al., 2006; Wichmann et al., 2007; Liang et al., 2008) with parenteral fish oil; however, most report no differences in infection rates or mortality. One study reported that perioperative fish oil decreased the need for mechanical ventilation, readmission to intensive care, mortality, and length of hospital stay (Tsekos et al., 2004), and similar findings were seen in the 230 postsurgical patients within a large study of >650 heterogeneous patients receiving intravenous fish oil (Heller et al., 2006).

Fish oil containing parenteral nutrition has also been examined experimentally in critically ill patients (Calder, 2006b, 2010, 2013). Reduced inflammation has been reported in some studies (Mayer et al., 2003a,b; Barbosa et al., 2010), as has improved gas exchange (Wang et al., 2008; Barbosa et al., 2010) and shorter length of hospital stay (Barbosa et al., 2010). However, not all studies show such benefits (Friesecke et al., 2008), although the small sample size of some of these studies may be a limitation. Heller et al. (2006) included patients with abdominal sepsis, multiple trauma, and severe head injury in an uncontrolled study of intravenous fish oil. They found a significantly lower rate of infection and shorter lengths of ICU and hospital stay in those patients receiving >0.05 g fish oil/kg per day than in those receiving less than this. Mortality was significantly decreased in those patients who received >0.1 g fish oil/kg per day. The survival advantage was greater in some patient groups than others (severe head injury > multiple trauma > abdominal sepsis > non-abdominal sepsis > postsurgery); however, the small numbers of patients in some groups make the interpretation of these data difficult. Nevertheless, the data are strongly suggestive of a genuine clinical benefit from the inclusion of fish oil in parenteral nutrition regimens given to critically ill patients.

Studies of intravenous fish oil in hospitalized adults have been subject to several meta-analyses during the last few years (Wei et al., 2010; Chen et al., 2010; Pradelli et al., 2012; Palmer et al., 2013; Manzanares et al., 2014). Wei et al. (2010) and Chen et al. (2010) both included studies of surgical patients, those undergoing surgery for gastrointestinal cancer removal, and both combined studies where patients were transferred into an ICU unit with those who were not. Despite the relatively small overlap, which were mainly in the included studies, these two meta-analyses produced very similar findings: including fish oil in parenteral nutrition reduced infections by about 50%, length of ICU stay by about 2 days, and length of hospital stay by about 3 days. There was no effect on mortality, but rate of mortality was typically very low in these studies anyway. The recent meta-analysis of Pradelli et al. (2012) included a combination of surgical patients who were not admitted to the ICU and patients in the ICU, irrespective of their origin (i.e., surgical, sepsis, critical illness);

they also conducted analyses in these two groups separately. Across all studies combined, Pradelli et al. (2012) identified that inclusion of fish oil reduced infections by about 40%, length of ICU stay by about 2 days, and length of hospital stay by about 3 days. Among the non-ICU patients (all gastrointestinal cancer surgery patients), fish oil reduced infections by about 50% and length of hospital stay by about 2 days, consistent with the two earlier meta-analyses in this patient group (Wei et al., 2010; Chen et al., 2010). The 30% reduction in infections in ICU patients was not significant, but fish oil shortened hospital stay by about 5 days in this group. Recently, Palmer et al. (2013) published the first meta-analysis of studies with parenteral fish oil restricted to critically ill patients. Eight studies were included, three of which had been published in abstract form only. The reductions in infections of about 20% and of ICU stay by about half a day seen with fish oil were not significant; however, there was a significantly shorter length of hospital stay by about 9 days with parenteral fish oil. More recently, Manzanares et al. (2014) also published a meta-analysis of studies with parenteral fish oil restricted to critically ill patients. Six studies were included, one of which had been published in abstract form only. Aggregation of these studies showed a strong trend toward reduced mortality (five studies; risk reduced by 29%); however, there was no effect on infections (three studies) or duration of ICU stay (five studies). Length of hospital stay was not evaluated in this meta-analysis.

Thus, meta-analyses suggest a benefit of intravenous fish oil in surgical patients with fewer complications and shorter hospital stay. If these patients happen to be admitted to an ICU, they stay for a shorter time. Two recent meta-analyses restricted to critically ill patients indicate that there may be clinical benefits, although small sample size and the lack of studies limit the conclusions that can be made. There is a need for larger studies of intravenous fish oil in critically ill patients either as a supplement to standard enteral nutrition or in those intolerant of enteral nutrition.

Omega-3 Fatty Acids in Enteral Nutrition

Fish oil omega-3 fatty acids are included in the enteral immunonutrition formula IMPACT, which also includes arginine and nucleotides. Studies with IMPACT are described below in the section "Mixtures of Immunonutrients Used Enterally." Here, the use of enteral formulas providing a high dose of omega-3 fatty acids and some other potential immunonutrients, but neither arginine nor glutamine, is discussed. The first such study compared a high-fat (55% energy from fat) control enteral formula that used corn oil as the fat source with a novel enteral formula (OxEPA®) providing fish oil (20% of fat), medium-chain triglycerides (25%), canola oil (32%), and borage oil (20%) along with additional antioxidants (vitamins C and E) and β-carotene, taurine, and carnitine in critically ill patients with acute respiratory distress syndrome (Gadek et al., 1999; Pacht et al., 2003). By 4 days of treatment, the numbers of total leukocytes and of neutrophils in the alveolar fluid declined significantly in the omega-3 fatty acid group and were lower than in controls (Gadek et al., 1999). Alveolar fluid IL-8 was lower in the experimental group compared with controls, and leukotriene B_4 and TNF-α tended to be lower (Pacht et al., 2003). Arterial oxygenation and gas exchange were also improved, and the treated patients had a decreased requirement for supplemental oxygen, decreased time on ventilation support, and a shorter length of stay in intensive care (5 days shorter) (Gadek et al., 1999). The total length of hospital stay tended to be shorter in the experimental group (by 5 days), and fewer patients developed new organ failure (8% vs. 28%) (Gadek et al., 1999). Mortality was 12% in the experimental group and 19% in the control group, but this difference was not statistically significant (Gadek et al., 1999). A second study made the same comparison in patients with acute lung injury during 14 days (Singer et al., 2006). By days 4 and 7, patients receiving the experimental formula showed improved oxygenation and a reduction in length of ventilation; however, there was no difference between the groups in mortality. It is not clear whether the effects reported in these two studies are due to omega-3 fatty acids since the experimental formula contained fewer omega-6 fatty acids and more medium-chain triglycerides, β-carotene, taurine, carnitine, vitamin C, and vitamin E than the control formula. This was partly addressed by a study (Pontes-Arruda et al., 2006) that compared OxEPA with a control formula that included a mix of lipids with a lower omega-6 fatty acid content (56% fat as canola oil, 14% as corn oil, 20% as medium-chain triglycerides, and 7% as high-oleic sunflower oil) as well as β-carotene (same as in OxEPA), taurine (50% of the amount on OxEPA), and carnitine (33% more than in OxEPA) in patients with severe sepsis and septic shock. Patients receiving the experimental formula showed lower 28-day mortality (risk reduced by 37%), improved oxygenation, more ventilator-free days, more ICU-free days, and reduced development of new organ failures. The findings suggest a benefit of omega-3 fatty acids and/or the γ-linolenic acid found in borage oil. These three studies were subjected to a meta-analysis (Pontes-Arruda et al., 2008), which identified that an experimental high-fat enteral formula providing omega-3 fatty acids and γ-linolenic acid reduced ventilation requirement (by 45%), reduced ICU stay (by 50%), reduced new organ failures (by 83%), and lowered 28-day mortality (by 60%). A more recent study in patients with sepsis compared OxEPA with a control formula providing less fat (29% of energy); more carbohydrate; a mixture of high-oleic sunflower oil (50% of fat), canola oil (30%), and medium-chain triglycerides (30%); and additional β-carotene, taurine, and carnitine (Pontes-Arruda et al., 2011). Patients receiving OxEPA were less likely to develop severe sepsis and septic shock and to develop cardiovascular and respiratory failures, had less need for mechanical ventilation, had more ICU-free days, and had shorter stays in the ICU and in hospital; there was no effect on mortality.

Thus, a number of individual clinical trials published between the late 1990s and 2010 report clinical benefits of a high-fat enteral formula containing fish oil omega-3 fatty acids and borage oil in critically ill patients, and these benefits are supported by a meta-analysis based on three of those trials. This dataset provides good evidence for the clinical efficacy of this formula in these patients. However, two recent large studies of enteral fish oil have questioned the robustness of this evidence base. Stapleton et al. (2011) reported a study in patients with acute lung injury who all received a standard low-fat enteral formula plus either saline or fish oil given as a bolus daily for 14 days. There was no difference between groups in lung lavage neutrophils, leukotriene B_4, IL-6, IL-8, or monocyte chemoattractant protein (MCP)-1; plasma IL-6, IL-8, or MCP-1; gas exchange; ventilation-free days; ICU-free days; organ dysfunction; hospital length of stay; hospital mortality; or 60-day mortality.

Rice et al. (2011) also reported a study in patients with acute lung injury who all received a standard low-fat enteral formula; the treatment group received a mix of fish oil, borage oil, and antioxidants as a bolus twice daily for 21 days. There was no difference between groups in plasma IL-6, IL-8, or leukotriene E_4; gas exchange; or the development of new infections. The treatment group had fewer ventilator-free days, fewer ICU-free days, and a near-significant higher 60-day mortality. The trial was stopped early. There are a number of possible explanations for why the studies of Stapleton et al. (2011) and Rice et al. (2011) show findings that are very different from the consistent earlier studies. Clearly, the designs of the two recent studies were rather different from the earlier studies, and this may be the reason for the different findings. The earlier studies used high-fat formulas with a high-omega-6 fatty acid content in the control group, and it is possible that either high-fat or high-omega-6 fatty acid is proinflammatory in the control group, allowing fish oil to appear anti-inflammatory and clinically beneficial in comparison. The nutrient mix was different in the recent studies compared with the earlier studies, and it may be that a key component was omitted from the formulas used in the recent studies. Also, the more recent studies used more protein than was used in the earlier studies. In the earlier studies, the fish oil was included within the enteral feed, whereas in the two recent studies it was given as a supplement. Furthermore, when included within the feed, the fish oil was given continuously compared with being given as a once- or twice-daily bolus in the recent studies. The earlier studies excluded patients who did not meet a particular feeding rate but later studies did not, meaning that they included a number of underfed patients. Finally, it is possible that there have been other improvements in patient care that have had an influence that negates the benefit of fish oil seen in earlier studies. It will be important that these discrepancies in formulation and study design be investigated in order to better evaluate the role of enteral fish oil, perhaps in combination with borage oil, in critically ill patients.

ANTIOXIDANT MICRONUTRIENTS AND TRACE ELEMENTS

Several studies investigating parenteral and/or enteral (mainly parenteral) anti-oxidant micronutrients and trace elements in postsurgery, burned, or critically ill patients have been conducted, and 21 studies in critical illness were included in a meta-analysis looking at clinical outcomes (Manzanares et al., 2012). The nutrients studied were zinc, copper, selenium, vitamin E, and vitamin C, alone or in various combinations. Most studies did not evaluate immune markers, although some did. One study showed that parenteral zinc, copper, and selenium did not influence blood lymphocyte subsets, neutrophil chemotaxis, or T-lymphocyte proliferation in burned patients in the ICU, although there was a decrease in blood IL-6 levels (Berger et al., 1998). Several studies show improved clinical outcome with antioxidant micronutri-ents, including fewer infections in burned patients (Berger et al., 1998; Porter et al., 1999) and fewer infections and organ failures in trauma patients (Tanaka et al., 2000). The meta-analysis (Manzanares et al., 2012) showed reduced mortality (20 studies; risk reduced by 18%), a trend toward fewer infectious complications (10 studies; risk reduced by 12%), and fewer days of artificial ventilation (four studies; reduced by 0.7 days), but no effect on ICU or hospital length of stay. Fifteen studies provided antioxidants parenterally and four provided them enterally. Mortality was reduced by enteral antioxidants (risk reduced by 32%) and tended to be lower with parenteral antioxidants (risk reduced by 11%). Parenteral antioxidants also tended to reduce infection rates (risk reduced by 11%). Sixteen studies evaluated selenium either alone or in combination with other antioxidants. There was a reduction in mortality whether selenium was present (risk reduced by 11%) or not (risk reduced by 44%). Studies using selenium tended to show reduced infections (risk reduced by 13%) but studies that did not include selenium did not. Parenteral selenium and use of selenium alone were superior to enteral selenium and use of selenium within a cocktail of antioxidants, respectively. Doses of selenium >500 µg/day were required for benefit to be seen.

Thus, a number of individual clinical trials report clinical benefits when antioxidant nutrients are provided parenterally or enterally to critically ill or burn patients, and these benefits, especially of high-dose parenteral selenium, are supported by a recent meta-analysis (Manzanares et al., 2012). This dataset provides some evidence for the clinical efficacy of antioxidants, especially selenium, in these patient groups. Two recent large trials described in the earlier section on glutamine (SIGNET and REDOXS) also studied the impact of antioxidants in ill patients receiving artificial nutrition. Andrews et al. (2011) conducted a randomized controlled trial of parenteral glutamine (20.2 g/day) and selenium (500 µg/day), either alone or together in 502 patients in intensive care. Selenium did not affect antibiotic use, length of hospital stay, or 6-month mortality. Selenium did not affect infection rate unless it was given for >5 days, in which case infections were reduced by an average of 43%. In the REDOXS trial, Heyland et al. (2013) randomized 1233 critically ill patients to glutamine and a mix of antioxidants including selenium, either alone or together. The immunonutrients including the antioxidants were provided both parenterally and enterally. Antioxidants did not affect mortality, in-hospital mortality, 6-month mortality, ICU or hospital length of stay, or organ failure. Once again, it is difficult to reconcile the neutral findings of these two recent large studies with the more positive findings of several earlier smaller trials, but there may still be a role for antioxidants in general, and selenium in particular, in artificial immunonutrition.

MIXTURES OF IMMUNONUTRIENTS USED ENTERALLY

Several enteral formulas using a combination of nutrients have been developed. The majority of trials in surgical and critically ill patients have used the commercially available product IMPACT, which is rich in arginine, nucleotides, and fish oil omega-3 fatty acids, and a number of these studies reported immune and/or inflammatory outcomes (see Calder, 2003b for references). Most studies reporting circulating lymphocyte numbers and subsets, and circulating immunoglobulin concentrations showed little difference between IMPACT-treated patients and controls, although some studies reported benefits on phagocytosis, respiratory burst, lymphocyte proliferation, HLA-DR expression on monocytes, and cytokine production (see Calder, 2003b). These effects could be due to any single specified nutrient (i.e., arginine, nucleotides, omega-3 fatty acids) or to the combination of these nutrients.

Trials of so-called immune-enhancing enteral formulas report a variety of clinical outcomes, most often infections, ventilation requirement, length of hospital stay, and mortality. These studies have been subject to a number of meta-analyses that have identified significant reductions in infections and length of hospital stay, with these effects being more evident in surgical rather than critically ill patients (Beale et al., 1999; Heys et al., 1999; Heyland et al., 2001; Montejo et al., 2003; Waitzberg et al., 2006); none of the meta-analyses shows a significant effect on mortality. Perhaps the most well known of these meta-analyses is that of Heyland et al. (2001). This analysis included 22 studies involving 2419 patients; there were 9 studies in surgical patients and 13 in critically ill, including trauma and burn, patients. All studies in surgical patients used IMPACT, while IMPACT was used by seven studies in the critically ill. The other studies in critical illness used Immunaid® (provides additional glutamine and arginine; two studies) or an "experimental formula" providing arginine and n-3 fatty acids (four studies). Mortality was reported in 22 studies, infections in 18, and length of hospital stay in 17. There was no effect of enteral immunonutrition on mortality overall or in either surgical or critically ill patients. Immunonutrition lowered the risk of new infections by 34% overall and by 47% in surgical patients, with no effect in critical illness. Immunonutrition shortened the length of hospital stay by 3.3 days overall and by 3.4 days in surgical patients and 3.3 days in critically ill patients. The meta-analysis indicated that beneficial effects were favored by having a high arginine content in the formula. Despite evidence and clear statements to the contrary in the earlier meta-analyses (Beale et al., 1999; Heys et al., 1999; Heyland et al., 2001), concern has been raised that these formulas may actually be detrimental in the seriously ill (Suchner et al., 2002; Heyland et al., 2003; Heyland and Samis, 2003). This is because a small number of studies of immunonutrition formulas in critically ill patients reported increased mortality (Beale et al., 1999; Heys et al., 1999; Heyland et al., 2001). The source of the concern is the high arginine content, which is thought to drive excessive production of nitric oxide (Suchner et al., 2002; Zhou and Martindale, 2007), although this is disputed.

More recently, Marik and Zaloga conducted meta-analyses of immunonutrition in high-risk surgical patients (2010) and in critically ill patients (2008). The meta-analysis of studies in surgical patients included 21 trials involving 1918 patients; of these, 16 trials used IMPACT, 2 used another formula (Stresson®, which provides glutamine, arginine, and omega-3 fatty acids), 2 used arginine, and 1 used fish oil. In 16 trials, patients had undergone surgery for gastrointestinal cancer. One other trial involved gastrointestinal surgery but not for cancer removal, three surgeries for head and neck cancer, and one cardiac surgery. One study administered the immunonutrition preoperatively, 15 postoperatively, and 5 perioperatively. Formulas providing arginine plus fish oil reduced the infection rate (reduced by 80% if provided preoperatively [but only 1 study], by 48% if provided postoperatively [12 studies], and by 58% if provided perioperatively [5 studies]). Such formulas reduced wound complications by 40% (11 studies). With regard to length of hospital stay, this was shorter by 3 days if the immunonutrition was provided preoperatively (1 study), by 3.5 days if provided postoperatively (10 studies), and by 2.2 days if provided perioperatively (3 studies). Mortality in these studies was low (about 1%) and was not different between groups. The meta-analysis of studies in critically ill patients (Marik and Zaloga, 2008) included 24 trials involving 3013 patients; of these, 7 trials used IMPACT, 2 used Stresson, 3 used OxEPA (these are the three trials included in the meta-analysis conducted by Pontes-Arruda et al. [2008], referred to in the section on omega-3 fatty acids), 1 used Immunaid, 3 used additional arginine, 6 used additional glutamine, and 2 used an "experimental" formula. Twelve studies were conducted in ICU patients, 5 in burns patients, and 7 in trauma patients. Mortality was reported in 23 studies, infections in 21, and length of hospital stay in 13. There was no effect of enteral immunonutrition on mortality overall or in any of the patient subgroups. Immunonutrition lowered the risk of new infections by 37% overall and by 31% in ICU patients and 51% in burns patients with no effect in trauma patients. Immunonutrition shortened the length of hospital stay by 5.1 days in ICU patients without an effect in burns or trauma patients. The meta-analysis suggests that the ingredient responsible for the benefits of immunonutrition is omega-3 fatty acids.

Results from meta-analyses are consistent with regard to the benefit of enteral immunonutrition in postsurgical patients, with clear benefits on infection risk and length of hospital stay (Beale et al., 1999; Heys et al., 1999; Heyland et al., 2001; Marik and Zaloga, 2010). Conclusions from meta-analyses of the studies in critically ill patients seem less clear; however, the most recent analysis by Marik and Zaloga (2008) demonstrates clinical benefits in ICU and burns patients but not in trauma patients. The compositions of the commonly used immunonutrition formulas such as IMPACT were established some years ago, and it is worth considering whether these might be refined in the context of better basic science understanding and greater clinical (and clinical trial) experience of using the formulas. Indeed, the original formulation of IMPACT did not include glutamine and a modified formulation, IMPACT Glutamine, has been recently launched.

CONCLUSION

Surgery, trauma, burns, and injury are insults that can induce an excessive inflammatory response that may be associated with a later immunosuppressed state. Hyperinflammation can lead to organ damage and failure, while immunosuppression increases susceptibility to infection. The resulting septic syndromes are associated with significant morbidity and mortality. A range of nutrients are able to modulate inflammation and its partner oxidative stress, and to maintain or improve immune function and the intestinal barrier. These include several amino acids (arginine and glutamine are the most studied), antioxidant vitamins and minerals, and omega-3 fatty acids. Experimental studies support a potential role for each of these nutrients in surgical, injured, or critically ill patients. There is good evidence that parenteral or enteral glutamine influences immune function in such patients, and that this is associated with clinical improvement, a conclusion that has been supported by meta-analyses. However, two recent studies failed to show a benefit of glutamine in critically ill patients. Evidence is also mounting for the use of intravenous omega-3 fatty acids in surgical and septic patients, again supported by recent meta-analyses; however, more evidence of efficacy is required in these groups. Enteral feeds that include fish oil and borage oil seem to benefit critically ill patients, although once again two recent studies have failed to demonstrate benefit. This may be due to the different study design of these recent studies. Mixtures of antioxidant vitamins and minerals are also clinically effective, especially if they include high doses of selenium. Their action appears not to involve improved immune function, although an anti-inflammatory mode of action has not been ruled out. Enteral immunonutrient mixtures, usually including arginine, nucleotides, and long-chain omega-3 fatty acids, have been used widely in surgical and critically ill patients. Evidence of efficacy is good in surgical patients; this conclusion is supported by meta-analyses. However, whether these same mixtures are beneficial, or should even be used, in a critically ill patient remains controversial. While some studies show decreased mortality with such mixtures, some show increased mortality. There is a view that this is due to a high arginine content driving nitric oxide production, although this is disputed. It is interesting that these mixtures often do not typically include glutamine, which may have a benefit. It seems likely that novel immunonutrient mixtures will be developed in the future. Clearly, more research using larger, better-designed trials will be needed to see whether these benefit immune function, with an improved clinical benefit in vulnerable patients.

REFERENCES

Andrews, P. J., A. Avenell, D. W. Noble, M. K. Campbell, B. L. Croal, W. G. Simpson, L. D. Vale, C. G. Battison, D. J. Jenkinson, J. A. Cook and the Scottish Intensive care Glutamine or seleNium Evaluative Trial Trials Group. 2011. Randomised trial of glutamine, selenium, or both, to supplement parenteral nutrition for critically ill patients. *British Medical Journal* 342:d1542.

Angus, D. C., W. T. Linde-Zwirble, J. Lidicker, G. Clermont, J. Carcillo and M. R. Pinsky. 2001. Epidemiology of severe sepsis in the United States: Analysis of incidence, outcome, and associated costs of care. *Critical Care Medicine* 29:1303–10.

Arnalich, F., E. Garcia-Palomero, J. Lopez, M. Jimenez, R. Madero, J. Renart, J. J. Vazquez and C. Montiel. 2000. Predictive value of nuclear factor κB activity and plasma cytokine levels in patients with sepsis. *Infection and Immunity* 68:1942–5.

Avenell, A. 2009. Current evidence and ongoing trials on the use of glutamine in critically-ill patients and patients undergoing surgery. *Proceedings of the Nutrition Society* 68:261–8.

Barbosa, V. M., E. A. Miles, C. Calhau, E. Lafuente and P. C. Calder. 2010. Effects of a fish oil containing lipid emulsion on plasma phospholipid fatty acids, inflammatory markers, and clinical outcomes in septic patients: A randomized, controlled clinical trial. *Critical Care* 14:R5.

Battistella, F. D., J. T. Widergren, J. T. Anderson, J. K. Siepler, J. C. Weber and K. MacColl. 1997. A prospective, randomized trial of intravenous fat emulsion administration in trauma victims requiring total parenteral nutrition. *Journal of Trauma* 43:52–8.

Beale, R. J., D. J. Bryg and D. J. Bihari. 1999. Immunonutrition in the critically ill: A systematic review of clinical outcome. *Critical Care Medicine* 27:2799–805.

Berger, M. M. and R. L. Chiolero. 2003. Key vitamins and trace elements in the critically ill. In *Nutrition and Critical Care*, eds. L. Cynober and F. A. Moore, 99–117. Vevey/Basel: Nestle/Karger.

Berger, M. M., F. Spertini, A. Shenkin, C. Wardle, L. Wiesner, C. Schindler and R. L. Chiolero. 1998. Trace element supplementation modulates pulmonary infection rates after major burns: A double-blind, placebo-controlled trial. *American Journal of Clinical Nutrition* 68:365–71.

Bernard, G. R., A. P. Wheeler, M. M. Arons, P. E. Morris, H. L. Paz, J. A. Russell and P. E. Wright. 1997. A trial of antioxidants *N*-acetylcysteine and procysteine in ARDS. *Chest* 112:164–72.

Boelens, P. G., A. P. Houdijk, J. C. Fonk, R. J. Nijveldt, C. C. Ferwerda, B. M. Von Blomberg-Van Der Flier, L. G. Thijs, H. J. Haarman, J. C. Puyana and P. A. Van Leeuwen. 2002. Glutamine-enriched enteral nutrition increases HLA-DR expression on monocytes of trauma patients. *Journal of Nutrition* 132:2580–6.

Boelens, P. G., A. P. Houdijk, J. C. Fonk, J. C. Puyana, H. J. Haarman, M. E. von Blomberg-van der Flier and P. A. van Leeuwen. 2004. Glutamine-enriched enteral nutrition increases *in vitro* interferon-gamma production but does not influence the *in vivo* specific antibody response to KLH after severe trauma. A prospective, double blind, randomized clinical study. *Clinical Nutrition* 23:391–400.

Bollhalder, L., A. M. Pfeil, Y. Tomonaga and M. Schwenkglenks. 2013. A systematic literature review and meta-analysis of randomized clinical trials of parenteral glutamine supplementation. *Clinical Nutrition* 32:213–23.

Bone, R. C., R. A. Balk, F. B. Cerra, R. P. Dellinger, A. M. Fein, W. A. Knaus, R. M. Schein and W. J. Sibbald. 1997. Definitions for sepsis and organ failure and guidelines for the use of innovative therapies in sepsis. *Chest* 101:1644–55.

Calder, P. C. 2003a. Immunonutrition. *British Medical Journal* 327:117–8.

Calder, P. C. 2003b. Long-chain n-3 fatty acids and inflammation: Potential application in surgical and trauma patients. *Brazilian Journal of Medical and Biological Research* 36:433–46.

Calder, P. C. 2004. N-3 fatty acids, inflammation and immunity—Relevance to postsurgical and critically ill patients. *Lipids* 39:1147–61.

Calder, P. C. 2006a. Branched-chain amino acids and immunity. *Journal of Nutrition* 136:288S–93S.

Calder, P. C. 2006b. Use of fish oil in parenteral nutrition: Rationale and reality. *Proceedings of the Nutrition Society* 65:264–77.

Calder, P. C. 2007. Immunonutrition in surgical and critically ill patients. *British Journal of Nutrition* 98:S133–9.

Calder, P. C. 2009. Rationale for using new lipid emulsions in parenteral nutrition and a review of the trials performed in adults. *Proceedings of the Nutrition Society* 68:252–60.

Calder, P. C. 2010. Rationale and use of n-3 fatty acids in artificial nutrition. *Proceedings of the Nutrition Society* 69:565–73.

Calder, P. C. 2013. Lipids for intravenous nutrition in hospitalised adult patients: A multiple choice of options. *Proceedings of the Nutrition Society* 72:263–76.

Calder, P. C. and P. Yaqoob. 1999. Glutamine and the immune system. *Amino Acids* 17:227–41.

Calder, P. C. and P. Yaqoob. 2004. Amino acids and immune function. In *Metabolic and Therapeutic Aspects of Amino Acids in Clinical Nutrition*, ed. L. Cynober, 305–20. Boca Raton: CRC Press.

Carver, J. D., B. Pimental, W. I. Cox and L. A. Barness. 1991. Dietary nucleotide effects upon immune function in infants. *Pediatrics* 88:359–63.

Casas-Rodera, P., C. Gómez-Candela, S. Benítez, R. Mateo, M. Armero, R. Castillo and J. M. Culebras. 2008. Immunoenhanced enteral nutrition formulas in head and neck cancer surgery: A prospective, randomized clinical trial. *Nutrición Hospitalaria* 23:105–10.

Chen, B., Y. Zhou, P. Yang, H.-W. Wan and X.-T. Wu. 2010. Safety and efficacy of fish oil-enriched parenteral nutrition regimen on postoperative patients undergoing major abdominal surgery: A meta-analysis of randomized controlled trials. *Journal of Parenteral and Enteral Nutrition* 34:387–94.

Daly, J. M., J. Reynolds, A. Thom, L. Kinsley, M. Dietrick-Gallagher, J. Shou and B. Ruggieri. 1988. Immune and metabolic effects of arginine in the surgical patient. *Annals of Surgery* 208:512–23.

de Luis, D. A., O. Izaola, R. Aller, L. Cuellar and M. C. Terroba. 2005. A randomized clinical trial with oral immunonutrition (omega 3-enhanced formula vs. arginine-enhanced formula) in ambulatory head and neck cancer patients. *Annals of Nutrition and Metabolism* 49:95–9.

Dionigi, P., R. Dionig, U. Prati, F. Pavesi, V. Jemos and S. Nazari. 1985. Effect of Intralipid® on some immunological parameters and leukocyte functions in patients with esophageal and gastric cancer. *Clinical Nutrition* 4:229–34.

Edgren, B. and A. Wretlind. 1963. The theoretical background of the intravenous nutrition with fat emulsions. *Nutritio et Dieta: European Review of Nutrition and Dietetics* 13:364–86.

Ertel, W., M. H. Morrison, D. R. Meldrum, A. Ayala and I. H. Chaudry. 1992. Ibuprofen restores cellular immunity and decreases susceptibility to sepsis following hemorrhage. *Journal of Surgical Research* 53:55–61.

Friesecke, S., C. Lotze, J. Köhler, A. Heinrich, S. B. Felix and P. Abel. 2008. Fish oil supplementation in the parenteral nutrition of critically ill medical patients: A randomised controlled trial. *Intensive Care Medicine* 34:1411–20.

Furukawa, K., H. Yamamori, K. Takagi, N. Hayashi, R. Suzuki, N. Nakajima and T. Tashiro. 2002. Influences of soybean oil emulsion on stress response and cell-mediated immune function in moderately or severely stressed patients. *Nutrition* 18:235–40.

Gadek, J. E., S. J. DeMichele, M. D. Karlstad, E. R. Pacht, M. Donahoe, T. E. Albertson, C. Van Hoozen, A. K. Wennberg, J. Nelson, M. Noursalehi and the Enteral Nutrition in ARDS Study Group. 1999. Effect of enteral feeding with eicosapentaenoic acid, γ-linolenic acid, and antioxidants in patients with acute respiratory distress syndrome. *Critical Care Medicine* 27:1409–20.

Garrel, D., J. Patenaude, B. Nedelec, L. Samson, J. Dorais, J. Champoux, M. 'Elia and J. Bernier. 2003. Decreased mortality and infectious morbidity in adult burn patients given enteral glutamine supplements: A prospective, controlled, randomized clinical trial. *Critical Care Medicine* 31:2444–9.

Gil, A. 2002. Modulation of the immune response mediated by dietary nucleotides. *European Journal of Clinical Nutrition* 56 Suppl 3:S1–4.

Girardin, E., G. E. Grau, J.-M. Dayer, P. Roux-Lombard, J5 Study Group and P. H. Lambert. 1998. Tumor necrosis factor and interleukin-1 in the serum of children with severe infectious purpura. *New England Journal of Medicine* 319:397–400.

Gogos, C. A., F. E. Kalfarentzos and N. C. Zoumbos. 1990. Effect of different types of total parenteral nutrition on T-lymphocyte subpopulations and NK cells. *American Journal of Clinical Nutrition* 51:119–22.

Grbic, J. T., J. A. Mannick, D. B. Gough and M. L. Rodrick. 1991. The role of prostaglandin E2 in immune suppression following injury. *Annals of Surgery* 214:253–63.

Griffiths, R. D., C. Jones and T. E. A. Palmer. 1997. Six-month outcome of critically ill patients given glutamine-supplemented parenteral nutrition. *Nutrition* 13:295–302.

Grimm, H., N. Mertes, C. Goeters, E. Schlotzer, K. Mayer, F. Gimminger and P. Furst. 2006. Improved fatty acid and leukotriene pattern with a novel lipid emulsion in surgical patients. *European Journal of Nutrition* 45:55–60.

Hallberg, D., O. Schuberth and A. Wretlind. 1966. Experimental and clinical studies with fat emulsion for intravenous nutrition. *Nutritio et Dieta: European Review of Nutrition and Dietetics* 8:245–81.

Hatherill, M., S. M. Tibby, C. Turner, N. Ratnavel and I. A. Murdoch. 2000. Procalcitonin and cytokine levels: Relationship to organ failure and mortality in pediatric septic shock. *Critical Care Medicine* 28:2591–4.

Heidecke, C. D., T. Hensler, H. Weighardt, N. Zantl, H. Wagner, J. R. Siewert and B. Holzmann. 1999. Selective defects of T lymphocyte function in patients with lethal intraabdominal infection. *American Journal of Surgery* 178:288–92.

Heller, A. R., S. Rössler, R. J. Litz, S. N. Stehr, S. C. Heller, R. Koch and T. Koch. 2006. Omega-3 fatty acids improve the diagnosis-related clinical outcome. *Critical Care Medicine* 34:972–9.

Heyland, D. K., R. Dhaliwal, J. W. Drover, L. Gramlich, P. Dodek and the Canadian Critical Care Clinical Practice Guidelines Committee. 2003. Canadian clinical practice guidelines for nutrition support in mechanically ventilated, critically ill adult patients. *Journal of Parenteral and Enteral Nutrition* 27:355–73.

Heyland, D., J. Muscedere, P. E. Wischmeyer, D. Cook, G. Jones, M. Albert, G. Elke, M. M. Berger and A. G. Day for the Canadian Critical Care Trials Group. 2013. A randomized trial of glutamine and antioxidants in critically ill patients. *New England Journal of Medicine* 368:1489–97.

Heyland, D. K., F. Novak, J. W. Drover, M. Jain, X. Su and U. Suchner. 2001. Should immuno-nutrition become routine in critically ill patients? A systematic review of the evidence. *Journal of the American Medical Association* 286:944–53.

Heyland, D. K. and A. Samis. 2003. Does immunonutrition in patients with sepsis do more harm than good? *Intensive Care Medicine* 29:669–71.

Heys, S. D., L. G. Walker, I. Smith and O. Eremin. 1999. Enteral nutritional supplementation with key nutrients in patients with critical illness and cancer—A meta-analysis of randomized controlled clinical trials. *Annals of Surgery* 229:467–77.

Houdijk, A. P., E. R. Rijnsburger, J. Jansen, R. I. Wesdorp, J. K. Weiss, M. A. McCamish, T. Teerlink, S. G. Meuwissen, H. J. Haarman, L. G. Thijs and P. A. van Leeuwen. 1998. Randomised trial of glutamine-enriched parenteral nutrition on infectious morbidity in patients with multiple trauma. *Lancet* 352:772–6.

Jensen, G. L., R. H. Miller, D. G. Talabiska, J. Fish and L. Gianferante. 1996. A double blind, prospective, randomized study of glutamine-enriched compared with standard peptide-based feeding in critically ill patients. *American Journal of Clinical Nutrition* 64:615–21.

Koch, T. and A. R. Heller. 2005. Auswirkungen einer parenteralen ernahrung mit n-3-fettsauren auf das therapieergebnis—Eine multizentrische analyse bei 661 patienten. *Akt Ernahrungstherapie* 30:15–22.

Kollef, M. H. and D. P. Schuster. 1995. The acute respiratory distress syndrome. *New England Journal of Medicine* 332:27–37.

Koller, M., M. Senkal, M. Kemen, W. Konig, V. Zumtobel and G. Muhr. 2003. Impact of omega-3 fatty acid enriched TPN on leukotriene synthesis by leukocytes after major surgery. *Clinical Nutrition* 22:59–64.

Lenssen, P., B. A. Bruemmer, R. A. Bowden, T. Gooley, S. N. Aker and D. Mattson. 1998. Intravenous lipid dose and incidence of bacteremia and fungemia in patients undergoing bone marrow transplantation. *American Journal of Clinical Nutrition* 67:927–33.

Liang, B., S. Wang, Y. J. Ye, X. D. Yang, Y. L. Wang, J. Qu, Q. W. Xie and M. J. Yin. 2008. Impact of postoperative omega-3 fatty acid-supplemented parenteral nutrition on clinical outcomes and immunomodulations in colorectal cancer patients. *World Journal of Gastroenterology* 14:2434–9.

Lin, J. J., X. J. Chung, C. Y. Yang and H. L. Lau. 2013. A meta-analysis of trials using the intention to treat principle for glutamine supplementation in critically ill patients with burn. *Burns* 39:565–70.

Manzanares, W., R. Dhaliwal, X. Jiang, L. Murch and D. K. Heyland. 2012. Antioxidant micronutrients in the critically ill: A systematic review and meta-analysis. *Critical Care* 16:R66.

Manzanares, W., R. Dhaliwal, B. Jurewitsch, R. D. Stapleton, K. N. Jeejeebhoy and D. K. Heyland. 2014. Parenteral fish oil lipid emulsions in the critically ill: A systematic review and meta-analysis. *Journal of Parenteral and Enteral Nutrition*, in press, 28:20–8.

Marik, P. E. and G. P. Zaloga. 2008. Immunonutrition in critically ill patients: A systematic review and analysis of the literature. *Intensive Care Medicine* 34:1980–90.

Marik, P. E. and G. P. Zaloga. 2010. Immunonutrition in high-risk surgical patients: A systematic review and analysis of the literature. *Journal of Parenteral and Enteral Nutrition* 34:378–86.

Mayer, K., C. Fegbeutel, K. Hattar, U. Sibelius, H. J. Kramer, K. U. Heuer, B. Temmesfeld-Wollbruck, S. Gokorsch, F. Grimminger and W. Seeger. 2003a. ω-3 vs. ω-6 Lipid emulsions exert differential influence on neutrophils in septic shock patients: Impact on plasma fatty acids and lipid mediator generation. *Intensive Care Medicine* 29:1472–81.

Mayer, K., S. Gokorsch, C. Fegbeutel, K. Hattar, S. Rosseau, D. Walmrath, W. Seeger and F. Grimminger. 2003b. Parenteral nutrition with fish oil modulates cytokine response in patients with sepsis. *American Journal of Respiratory and Critical Care Medicine* 167:1321–8.

Mendez, C., G. J. Jurkovich, I. Garcia, D. Davis, A. Parker and R. V. Maier. 1997. Effects of an immune-enhancing diet in critically injured patients. *Journal of Trauma* 42:933–40.

Meydani, S. N., S. N. Han and D. Wu. 2005. Vitamin E and immune response in the aged: Mechanisms and clinical implications. *Immunology Reviews* 205:269–84.

Monson, J. R. T., P. C. Sedman, C. W. Ramsden, T. G. Brennan and P. J. Guillou. 1988. Total parenteral nutrition adversely influences tumour-directed cellular cytotoxic responses in patients with gastrointestinal cancer. *European Journal of Surgical Oncology* 14:435–43.

Montejo, J. C., A. Zarazaga, J. López-Martínez, G. Urrútia, M. Roqué, A. L. Blesa, S. Celaya et al. 2003. Immunonutrition in the intensive care unit. A systematic review and consensus statement. *Clinical Nutrition* 22:221–33.

Morlion, B. J., P. Stehle, P. Wachtler, H. P. Siedhoff, M. Köller, W. König, P. Fürst and C. Puchstein. 1998. Total parenteral nutrition with glutamine dipeptide after major abdominal surgery—A randomized, double-blind, controlled study. *Annals of Surgery* 227:302–8.

Morlion, B. J., E. Torwesten, A. Lessire, G. Sturm, B. M. Peskar, P. Furst and C. Puchstein. 1996. The effect of parenteral fish oil on leukocyte membrane fatty acid composition and leukotriene-synthesizing capacity in postoperative trauma. *Metabolism* 45:1208–13.

Murray, S. M. and S. Pindoria. 2002. Nutrition support for bone marrow transplant patients. *Cochrane Database of Systematic Reviews* 2:CD002920.

Murray, S. M. and S. Pindoria. 2009. Nutrition support for bone marrow transplant patients. *Cochrane Database of Systematic Reviews* 1:CD002920.

Novak, F., D. K. Heyland, A. Avenell, J. W. Drover and X. Su. 2002. Glutamine supplementation in serious illness: A systematic review of the evidence. *Critical Care Medicine* 30:2022–9.

O'Riordain, M. G., K. C. Fearon, J. A. Ross, P. Rogers, J. S. Falconer, D. C. Bartolo, O. J. Garden and D. C. Carter. 1994. Glutamine supplemented parenteral nutrition enhances T-lymphocyte response in surgical patients undergoing colorectal resection. *Annals of Surgery* 220:212–21.

Pacht, E. R., S. J. DeMichele, J. L. Nelson, J. Hart, A. K. Wennberg and J. E. Gadek. 2003. Enteral nutrition with eicosapentaenoic acid, gamma-linolenic acid, and antioxidants reduces alveolar inflammatory mediators and protein influx in patients with acute respiratory distress syndrome. *Critical Care Medicine* 31:491–500.

Palmer, A. J., C. K. M. Ho, O. Ajibola and A. Avenell. 2013. The role of ω-3 fatty acid supplemented parenteral nutrition in critical illness in adults: A systematic review and meta-analysis. *Critical Care Medicine* 41:307–16.

Pontes-Arruda, A., A. M. Aragão and J. D. Albuquerque. 2006. Effects of enteral feeding with eicosapentaenoic acid, gamma-linolenic acid, and antioxidants in mechanically ventilated patients with severe sepsis and septic shock. *Critical Care Medicine* 34:2325–33.

Pontes-Arruda, A., S. Demichele, A. Seth and P. Singer. 2008. The use of an inflammation-modulating diet in patients with acute lung injury or acute respiratory distress syndrome: A meta-analysis of outcome data. *Journal of Parenteral and Enteral Nutrition* 32:596–605.

Pontes-Arruda, A., L. F. Martins, S. M. de Lima, A. M. Isola, D. Toledo, E. Rezende, M. Maia and G. B. Magnan for the Investigating Nutritional Therapy with EPA, GLA and Antioxidants Role in Sepsis Treatment (INTERSEPT) Study Group. 2011. Enteral nutrition with eicosapentaenoic acid, γ-linolenic acid and antioxidants in the early treatment of sepsis: Results from a multicenter, prospective, randomized, double-blinded, controlled study: The INTERSEPT study. *Critical Care* 15:R144.

Popovic, P. J., H. J. Zeh and J. B. Ochoa. 2007. Arginine and immunity. *Journal of Nutrition* 137:1681S–6S.

Porter, J. M., R. R. Ivatury, K. Azimuddin and R. Swami. 1999. Antioxidant therapy in the prevention of organ dysfunction syndrome and infectious complications after trauma: Early results of a prospective randomized study. *American Surgeon* 65:478–83.

Pradelli, L., K. Mayer, M. Muscaritoli and A. R. Heller. 2012. N-3 fatty acid-enriched parenteral nutrition regimens in elective surgical and ICU patients: A meta-analysis. *Critical Care* 216:R184.

Rice, T. W., A. P. Wheeler, B. T. Thompson, B. P. deBoisblanc, J. Steingrub and P. Rock for the NIH NHLBI Acute Respiratory Distress Syndrome Network of Investigators. 2011. Enteral omega-3 fatty acid, gamma-linolenic acid, and antioxidant supplementation in acute lung injury. *Journal of the American Medical Association* 306:1574–81.

Sadeghi, S., F. A. Wallace and P. C. Calder. 1999. Dietary lipids modify the cytokine response to bacterial lipopolysaccharide in mice. *Immunology* 96:404–10.

Sailer, D. and M. Muller. 1981. Medium chain triglycerides in parenteral nutrition. *Journal of Parenteral and Enteral Nutrition* 5:115–9.

Schauder, P., U. Rohn, G. Schafer, G. Korff and H.-D. Schenk. 2002. Impact of fish oil enriched total parenteral nutrition on DNA synthesis, cytokine release and receptor expression by lymphocytes in the postoperative period. *British Journal of Nutrition* 87:S103–10.

Sedman, P. C., S. S. Somers, C. W. Ramsden, T. G. Brennan and P. J. Guillou. 1991. Effects of different lipid emulsions on lymphocyte function during total parenteral nutrition. *British Journal of Surgery* 78:1396–9.

Singer, P., M. Theilla, H. Fisher, L. Gibstein, E. Grozovski and J. Cohen. 2006. Benefit of an enteral diet enriched with eicosapentaenoic acid and gamma-linolenic acid in ventilated patients with acute lung injury. *Critical Care Medicine* 34:1033–8.

Spapen, H., H. Zhang, C. Demanet, W. Vleminckx, J. L. Vincent and L. Huyghens. 1998. Does *N*-acetyl cysteine influence the cytokine response during early human septic shock? *Chest* 113:1616–24.

Spittler, A., T. Sautner, A. Gornikiewicz, N. Manhart, R. Oehler, M. Bergmann, R. Függer and E. Roth. 2001. Postoperative glycyl-glutamine infusion reduces immunosuppression: Partial prevention of the surgery induced decrease in HLA-DR expression on monocytes. *Clinical Nutrition* 20:37–42.

Stapleton, R. D., T. R. Martin, N. S. Weiss, J. J. Crowley, S. J. Gundel, A. B. Nathens, S. R. Akhtar et al. 2011. A phase II randomized placebo-controlled trial of omega-3 fatty acids for the treatment of acute lung injury. *Critical Care Medicine* 39:1655–62.

Suchner, U., D. K. Heyland and K. Peter. 2002. Immune-modulatory actions of arginine in the critically ill. *British Journal of Nutrition* 87:S121–32.

Tanaka, H., T. Matsuda, Y. Miyagantani, T. Yukioka, H. Matsuda and S. Shimazaki. 2000. Reduction of resuscitation fluid volumes in severely burned patients using ascorbic acid administration: A randomized, prospective study. *Archives of Surgery* 135:326–31.

Tschaikowsky, K., M. Hedwig-Geissing, A. Schiele, F. Bremer, M. Schywalsky and J. Schutter. 2002. Coincidence of pro- and anti-inflammatory responses in the early phase of severe sepsis: Longitudinal study of mononuclear histocompatibility leukocyte antigen-DR expression, procalcitonin, C-reactive protein, and changes in T-cell subsets in septic and postoperative patients. *Critical Care Medicine* 30:1015–23.

Tsekos, E., C. Reuter, P. Stehle and G. Boeden. 2004. Perioperative administration of parenteral fish oil supplements in a routine clinical setting improves patient outcome after major abdominal surgery. *Clinical Nutrition* 23:325–30.

Tsuei, B. J., A. C. Bernard, A. R. Barksdale, A. K. Rockich, C. F. Meier and P. A. Kearney. 2005. Supplemental enteral arginine is metabolized to ornithine in injured patients. *Journal of Surgical Research* 123:17–24.

Ulrich, H., S. McCarthy Pastores, D. P. Katz and V. Kvetan. 1996. Parenteral use of medium-chain triglycerides: A reappraisal. *Nutrition* 12:231–8.

van der Hulst, R. R., B. K. van Kreel, M. F. von Meyenfeldt, R. J. Brummer, J. W. Arends, N. E. Deutz and P. B. Soeters. 1993. Glutamine and the preservation of gut integrity. *Lancet* 341:1363–5.

Wachtler, P., W. Konig, M. Senkal, M. Kemen and M. Koller. 1997. Influence of a total parenteral nutrition enriched with ω-3 fatty acids on leukotriene synthesis of peripheral leukocytes and systemic cytokine levels in patients with major surgery. *Journal of Trauma* 42:191–8.

Waitzberg, D. L., H. Saito, L. D. Plank, G. G. Jamieson, P. Jagannath, T. L. Hwang, J. M. Mijares and D. Bihari. 2006. Postsurgical infections are reduced with specialized nutrition support. *World Journal of Surgery* 30:1592–604.

Wang, X., W. Li, N. Li and J. Li. 2008. Omega-3 fatty acids-supplemented parenteral nutrition decreases hyperinflammatory response and attenuates systemic disease sequelae in severe acute pancreatitis: A randomized and controlled study. *Journal of Parenteral and Enteral Nutrition* 32:236–41.

Wang, Y., Z. M. Jiang, M. T. Nolan, H. Jiang, H. R. Han, K. Yu, H. L. Li, B. Jie and X. K. Liang. 2010. The impact of glutamine dipeptide-supplemented parenteral nutrition on outcomes of surgical patients: A meta-analysis of randomized clinical trials. *Journal of Parenteral and Enteral Nutrition* 34:521–9.

Wei, C., J. Hua, C. Bin and K. Klassen. 2010. Impact of lipid emulsion containing fish oil on outcomes in surgical patients: Systematic review of randomized controlled trials from Europe and Asia. *Nutrition* 26:474–81.

Weighardt, H., C. D. Heidecke, K. Emmanuilidis, S. Maier, H. Bartels, J. W. Siewert and B. Holzmann. 2000. Sepsis after major visceral surgery is associated with sustained and interferon-γ-resistant defects of monocyte cytokine production. *Surgery* 127:309–15.

Weiss, G., F. Meyer, B. Matthies, M. Pross, W. Koenig and H. Lippert. 2002. Immunomodulation by perioperative administration of n-3 fatty acids. *British Journal of Nutrition* 87:S89–94.

Wibbenmeyer, L. A., M. A. Mitchell, I. M. Newel, L. D. Faucher, M. J. Amelon, T. O. Ruffin, R. D. Lewis 2nd, B. A. Latenser and P. G. Kealey. 2006. Effect of a fish oil and arginine-fortified diet in thermally injured patients. *Journal of Burn Care Research* 27:694–702.

Wichmann, M. W., P. Thul, H. D. Czarnetzki, B. J. Morlion, M. Kemen and K. W. Jauch. 2007. Evaluation of clinical safety and beneficial effects of a fish oil containing lipid emulsion (Lipoplus, MLF541): Data from a prospective, randomized, multicenter trial. *Critical Care Medicine* 35:700–6.

Wretlind, A. 1972. Complete intravenous nutrition. Theoretical and experimental background. *Nutrition and Metabolism* 14 Suppl:1–57.

Yoshida, S., M. Matsui, Y. Shirouzu, H. Fujita, H. Yamana and K. Shirouzu. 1998. Effects of glutamine supplements and radiochemotherapy on systemic immune and gut barrier function in patients with advanced esophageal cancer. *Annals of Surgery* 227:485–91.

Zheng, Y. M., F. Li, M. M. Zhang and X. T. Wu. 2006. Glutamine dipeptide for parenteral nutrition in abdominal surgery: A meta-analysis of randomized controlled trials. *World Journal of Gastroenterology* 12:7537–41.

Zhou, M. and R. G. Martindale. 2007. Arginine in the critical care setting. *Journal of Nutrition* 137:1687S–92S.

Ziegler, T. R., R. L. Bye, R. L. Persinger, L. S. Young, J. H. Antin and D. W. Wilmore. 1998. Effects of glutamine supplementation on circulating lymphocytes after bone marrow transplantation: A pilot study. *American Journal of Medical Science* 315:4–10.

Ziegler, T. R., L. S. Young, K. Benfell, M. Scheltinga, K. Hortos, R. Bye, F. D. Morrow, D. O. Jacobs, R. J. Smith, J. H. Antin and D. W. Wilmore. 1992. Clinical and metabolic efficacy of glutamine-supplemented parenteral nutrition following bone marrow transplantation: A double-blinded, randomized, controlled trial. *Annals of Internal Medicine* 116:821–8.

14 Impact of Infection– Nutrient Interactions in Infants, Children, and Adolescents

Renán A. Orellana and Jorge A. Coss-Bu

CONTENTS

Introduction..333
Effects of Acute and Chronic Infection on Growth and Development 335
    Ontogeny of the Circle of Malnutrition and Infection 336
        Fetal Period 336
        Newborn and Infant...337
        Children and Adolescents..338
        Failure to Thrive and Hindered Development 338
        Immune Weakness and Recurrence of Infections...339
    Cachexia, Chronic Diseases, and Immune Compromise 340
    Adaptive Mechanisms of Disease Tolerance and Alterations in the Microbiota... 342
        Pathogen/Disease Tolerance 342
        Alterations in the Microbiota 343
    Environmental Hostility, Undernutrition, and Infection 344
Effects of Acute and Chronic Infection on Nutrient Availability and Utilization ...345
    Effects on Appetite, Absorption, and Requirements 346
    Acquired Nutritional Deficiencies..346
    Nutrient Utilization 349
    Nutrient Distribution and Reprioritization 349
Conclusions..350
References..351

INTRODUCTION

The reciprocal effects of the interactions between nutrition and infection are being increasingly recognized in the past few decades, especially in children.[1] At present, it is understood that malnutrition and infection interact in a complex and synergistic way[1–3] (Figure 14.1). The complex interactions between nutrition and infection affect humans at genetic, molecular, microbiological, physiological, epidemiological, and

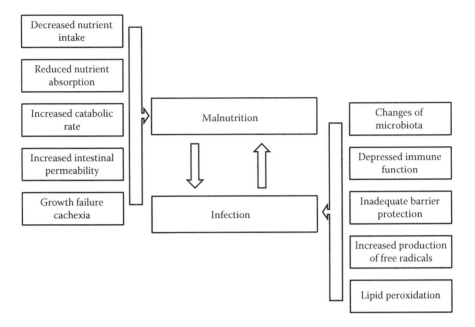

FIGURE 14.1 Relation between nutrition and infection.

ecologic levels.[2,4,5] Moreover, when such impact occurs during early development, the consequences may last throughout the life of the affected individual or even carried forward to future generations.[6–9]

Infectious diseases and malnutrition drive morbidity and mortality in vulnerable populations such as children and the elderly.[4,10] Individuals highly vulnerable to acquire infectious and communicable diseases, such as those with chronic debilitating diseases or those in extreme poverty, are generally malnourished and prone to experience recurrent infections. A periodic or constant infective state exacerbates the undernourished condition and perpetuates a vicious cycle. Infection promotes malnutrition by inducing anorexia, affecting the metabolic homeostasis, inducing consumption of nutrients to sustain the inflammatory response, impairing nutrient absorption, and causing microbial dysbiosis.[3,11] Healthy individuals may develop an acute malnutrition state when infected, even when nutrient intake is optimal.[2,12]

Nutrient–infection interactions weaken the host's ability to fight infections. Malnutrition impairs the activation and function of the humoral and cellular immune response to an infectious agent. Nutrition deficiency states also weaken the epithelial barrier integrity in the skin and in the intestinal and respiratory tracts, alter the symbiotic interaction with endogenous microbial flora, and induce oxidative stress.[4,13–15] These defects in the immune defense mechanisms are particularly critical during early growth and development,[16] leading to infant morbidity and mortality. Recurrences of infections or enhanced severity of infections in the pediatric host may lead to macronutrient and micronutrient deficiencies.

EFFECTS OF ACUTE AND CHRONIC INFECTION ON GROWTH AND DEVELOPMENT

Infants, children, and adolescents differ from adults in their need for a continuous supply of nutrients to maintain growth in addition for immunologic defense and tissue repair. They comprise a vulnerable population for whom the interaction between malnutrition and infection significantly affects clinical outcomes of morbidity and mortality. Pediatric patients are biologically immature and extremely dependent on their interactions with the caregiver and the environment. The smaller size of children accounts for lower protein and metabolic reserves. However, when compared with adults, infants, children, and adolescents have higher metabolic demands because of their need to use nutrients for growth. In addition, newborn infants and children have an immature immune system that makes them vulnerable to infections, which, in turn, exacerbates or perpetuates malnutrition.

In the pediatric population, besides recognizing the complex interactions between nutrient and infections at the individual level, it is important to recognize it at the level of the community and the country. Globally, most of the 10.8 million estimated deaths in children aged <5 years are caused by five infectious diseases: pneumonia, diarrhea, malaria, measles, and acquired immunodeficiency syndrome (AIDS). More than one-half of those deaths are associated with malnutrition,[2–4] and even mild malnutrition can substantially increase the risk of death due to these infections.[17] Epidemiological evidence suggests that malnutrition-associated infection is the leading cause of death in children <5 years old, worldwide.[18] Several investigators have suggested that one-third of the childhood deaths can be prevented by just correcting malnutrition.

The effect of malnutrition on mortality is not unique to children, as both malaria and influenza have mortality rates proportionate to the degree of malnutrition even in the general population.[2] Poverty and a hostile environment prolong the continuum of exposure of vulnerable children to respiratory and intestinal infections and parasitic infestations.[2] In developed countries, child mortality has declined below 10%, owing to high vaccination rates, adequate food availability and nutrition, healthy social and environmental conditions, and availability of high-quality medical care. In such countries, the causes for childhood mortality and morbidity are not directly related to infectious diseases resulting from malnutrition. However, malnutrition results from excess nutrient intake, resulting in obesity, or from other disorders such as genetic and metabolic disorders and malignancies. Large cohorts of these children with chronic medical conditions have increased medical instrumentation, frequent hospital admissions, frequent infections, immunosuppression,[19–21] and higher mortality.[22] Obesity has been associated with immune disequilibrium, involving low levels of persistent inflammation.[10] Close to 40%–50% of children with chronic medical conditions will have some degree of malnutrition,[23,24] and severe malnutrition is reported in nearly one-third of these patients.[19] Appropriate macronutrient and micronutrient supplementation in the critically ill child appears to decrease the incidence of infections, especially in children with nutrition-associated immune deficiencies.[19,20,25]

ONTOGENY OF THE CIRCLE OF MALNUTRITION AND INFECTION

The interaction between malnutrition and infection is prominent at the various developmental stages of humans. The fetus, newborn, infants, children, and adolescents present different anatomic and physiologic characteristics, which may increase their vulnerability to the effects of malnutrition. Nutrition is essential for adequate growth in children, and infection-induced metabolic impairment significantly affects body mass expansion and growth velocity.[4] Accretion of tissue protein and muscle mass in response to nutrients is a major component of growth, and this anabolic drive decreases with development.[26] Infection induces a catabolic state and blunts the anabolic drive associated with growth.[27,28] Because of this temporal association, it was previously considered that growth arrest induced by chronic malnutrition (stunting) does not occur before the age of 2 years and that any nutritional interventions to correct chronic malnutrition must occur before that age.[29] It is now recognized that a second critical window for interventions to correct growth deficits is during the second biological period of growth spurt in the adolescent years.[29] In addition to growth deficits, children who present with failure to thrive will also have cognitive deficits and intellectual delay that influence their developmental maturation.[30]

Fetal Period

The prenatal environment is a critical developmental window that can be affected by maternal (including the placenta) and/or fetal infections. The mother herself may be affected by the circle of malnutrition and infection. The prenatal environment can adjust the developmental program in the fetus to build up fitness/survival in later life, a process recognized as developmental plasticity.[8] The presence of malnutrition has been shown to modify gene expression during critical periods of development, in an effort to adapt growth to a hostile environment. Prenatal regulation of gene expression in response to environmental influences include those that regulate glucose homeostasis, metabolism, and blood pressure, and this can continue later in life. Limited availability of choline, methionine, and folate limits the disposition of the methyl group necessary to cause DNA and histone methylation to control gene expression, a process called epigenetic regulation.[7] Epigenetic changes can be sustained lifelong, affecting adult life and even can be transmitted to future generations.[7] Maternal nutritional deficits may be associated with fetal exposure to elevated stress hormones that undermines fetal growth and manifests as low birth weight (LBW)/intrauterine growth restriction (IUGR).[31] LBW/IUGR newborns have increased morbidity, mortality, faulty growth, developmental deficits, and adult-onset metabolic diseases.[31] Maternal undernutrition is also associated with diminished quality and quantity of maternal immune factors that are transferred to the fetus and the newborn through the placenta and breast milk. Immune competence of the newborn is highly dependent on the immunomodulatory functions of the maternally transferred factors, and deficient immune transference from the malnourished mother reduces immune protection of the infant and increases allergic tendencies in the infant.[16,32] LBW and IUGR infants have increased infant mortality and childhood and adolescent morbidity in underdeveloped societies.[32] It is plausible that nutritional interventions before conception and during pregnancy may improve the growth and development of the fetus and the newborn infant. However, attempts to supplement macronutrients or micronutrients in women before delivery has shown only limited effect on fetal and infant growth.[29] Antenatal supplementation of vitamin A, folic acid, and zinc has improved infant mortality and infectious morbidity.[32] A combined supplementation of proteins, calories, and multiple micronutrients, such as zinc and vitamins, to malnourished mothers has shown to improve the growth of the newborn.[31,32]

Newborn and Infant

The newborn and infantile periods are very vulnerable to the effects of malnutrition and infection interactions. The metabolic reserve of a developing organism includes not only endogenous macronutrient and macronutrient storage, but also the biochemical fitness and maturity of the metabolic processes to respond to fasting, feeding, and stress to maintain homeostasis and growth. High mortality in the newborn due to infections occurs owing to the immaturity of the immune response; however, immature metabolic stress responses also limit their ability to survive an acute infection.[27,33,34] Birth weight is the most important single predictor of early childhood mortality due to infectious diseases.[2,32] In developing countries, LBW infants are mostly small for gestational age, born malnourished, considered more immunocompromised, more prone to respiratory infections, and have a shorter duration of breast-feeding than infants with normal weight.[35] During their first months of life, infants rely on antibodies transferred from the mother through the placenta or through breast milk until they start to produce antibodies.[16,33] The sterile intrauterine environment limits pathogen challenge to the developing immune system of the fetus.[16,32]

The metabolic stress response of the rapidly growing infants is not fully mature,[27] although they are efficient at using their nutrients for growth.[26,28] Infants have a relatively smaller reserve of macronutrients compared with adults, low glycogen and protein reserves, immature gluconeogenic response, high protein and fat tissue turnover at baseline, and a high metabolic rate.[27,33,34] In addition, infants are dependent on the caregiver for provision of adequate nutrition to sustain their metabolic needs during the acute phase of the infection process.

Infections in children <2 years of age are the most common cause of morbidity and mortality in developing countries, and commonly coexist with malnutrition.[36] In this group of children, infants <6 months of age are the most vulnerable to have high morbidity and mortality from the synergy between infection and malnutrition. Nutritional interventions aimed at reducing malnutrition could prevent up to one-third of their deaths from infections.[35] In this group, breast-feeding is an important nutritional intervention that has been proven to reduce morbidity and mortality from infections.[16,35] Several studies have shown that malnutrition is linked to the incidence and risk of death from acute respiratory infections in children, and such incidence is higher in non-breast-fed children.[35] Breast-feeding has been shown to enhance the development of immune fitness in newborns and infants.[16] After 6 months of age, the addition of appropriate complementary foods to breast-feeding is recommended to meet the nutritional needs of the infant.[31] The period between 6 and 24 months of age is critical for childhood growth, and nutritional interventions during this time may help minimize malnutrition.

Children and Adolescents

Children and adolescents have a more mature metabolic reserve that may approach that of adults.[2] However, the presence of chronic, recurrent, or subacute infections may negatively influence the periods of rapid growth that occur during mid-infancy and early puberty. Although adolescents and older children with stunting respond to nutritional interventions with improvements in growth, they still retain maturational delay and a delayed completion of the growth period.[29]

Failure to Thrive and Hindered Development

In adults, infections produce a state of acute malnutrition characterized by an imbalance between energy, protein, and other nutrient requirements and intake.[37] As opposed to adults, children that face nonlethal chronic or recurrent infections will present with delayed growth and development. The nutritional status of the host is critical in determining the outcome of infection. Acutely, an infection triggers the loss of muscle and fat mass and leads to emaciation and micronutrient deficiencies.[3,20,38,39] A perennial inflammatory state devours the nutrients reserved for growth and building new tissue. If the infection becomes chronic, recurrent, or subacute, the child is unable to sustain both the metabolic response to infection and their growth results in the arrest of linear growth. In the presence of chronic malnutrition, chronic, recurrent, or subacute infections alter the protective epithelial barrier in the intestine, skin, and respiratory tract; impair the immune cellular response; alter the commensal flora; and further increase the susceptibility for infections.[4] Thus, impaired immune defense mechanisms after infections play a key role in the maintenance or perpetuation of the synergy between infection and malnutrition. Activation of the innate immune system by an infectious agent leads to inflammation, in which the presence of cytokines and other inflammatory mediators alter hunger, nutrient utilization, hormonal regulation of nutrients, and utilization of endogenous reserves.[14,39] In this vicious cycle, macronutrient and micronutrient deficiency further impairs the cellular immune response, perpetuating the infectious process and aggravating the nutritional deficit. Several of these alterations may be adaptive, involving activation of epigenetic mechanisms that allow survival of the host at the expense of loss of function or deficit tolerance.

Protein–energy malnutrition (PEM) can be classified according to severity (undernutrition, mild or severe, and obesity), chronicity (acute, chronic), or physiologic features (marasmus or wasting, stunting, kwashiorkor, cachexia).[13] Underweight PEM (low weight for age) and its more severe form, wasting (low weight for length/height), reflect an acute depletion of nutritional reserves as a result of acute illness or recurrent infections or famine.[40,41] Stunting (short height for age) includes linear growth retardation and has been more studied and associated with maternal malnutrition and infection, infant and child malnourishment, poverty, and recurrent infections.[40,41] Children will conserve weight for height at the expense of growth in length to adapt to a chronic deficit or insult. Important public health indicators that combine information about linear growth retardation and weight for length/height may predict mortality and the burden of infectious disease in children.[40,41] Stunting and wasting are associated with higher mortality than underweight PEM, and the mortality hazard ratio to die from respiratory tract infections and diarrhea is twice as high during wasting than stunting.[41]

Malnutrition has been shown to affect patient outcomes and represents a continuous spectrum ranging from marginal nutrient deficiency or excess status to severe metabolic and functional alterations, with different degrees of relative alterations of body weight and body composition.[42] Early studies on protein metabolism in the pregenomic era revealed human adaptation to chronic low protein intake with maintenance of appropriate health.[43] Currently, those concepts have been confirmed and widened by our understanding of metabolic adaptation and plasticity, nutrigenomics,[44] metabolomics, and epigenetics.[45] Recently, it has been shown that cells can sense amino acid (AA) deprivation during conditions of protein starvation, and regulate global protein synthesis by gene expression or translation to maintain metabolic homeostasis.[44]

Immune Weakness and Recurrence of Infections

The human responds to invasion of an infectious agent by eliciting biological defense responses aimed to contain and eliminate the infection. The immune responses can be innate, that is, nonspecific and independent of memory before exposure. This is the first and most immediate response that the host develops against an infection. A secondary immune response is adaptive, that is, antigen specific and dependent on memory built by prior exposure. Both innate and adaptive responses may cause collateral tissue injury in the host in the attempt to contain the infection. The systemic inflammation triggered by immune activation uses nutrients that otherwise would be used for homeostasis and growth, and would lead to undernutrition and malnutrition, either acutely or in a chronic state. In addition, immune paralysis has been shown to occur in severe infections that overwhelm the immune system, and it is associated with perpetuation of the infectious process.[21]

Epithelial layers in the skin and in mucosal surfaces of the respiratory and gastrointestinal tract interact with the colonizing bacteria and the immune system to contain infection and invasion by pathologic agents. The integrity of such barriers requires macronutrients and micronutrients to sustain their rapid turnover and the metabolic process necessary to perform their physiologic functions. Macronutrient and micronutrient deficiencies lead to loss of the epithelial integrity, higher risk of pathogenic invasion, and reduced healing of damaged tissue. As discussed below, alterations in epithelial commensal microbiota induced by infection may also influence metabolism in the host.

The innate immune system is modulated by activation of innate cell receptors that are not pathogen specific. The innate immune response is fundamental in restricting the infection until the adaptive immune response appears. Several components of this response are not fully developed at birth, as tissue macrophages, natural killer (NK) cells, complement, and NK cytolytic activity do not reach adult levels until later in childhood[32] and the cytokine response differs to that achieved with maturation.[16] Innate immunity is genetically predetermined by germline-encoded receptors that recognize pathogen-associated molecular patterns (PAMPs). PAMPs are highly conserved structures present in microorganisms, such as membrane lipopolysaccharides, peptidoglycan, bacterial DNA, double-stranded RNA, and others. Pattern-recognition receptors, such as human Toll-like receptors, recognize PAMPs leading to the production of cytokines, such as tumor necrosis factor-α (TNF-α), interleukins (ILs), and several other costimulatory molecules.

The adaptive immune system is a complex immune response that is antigen specific, uses immunologic memory, and requires exposure to the offending agent. Adaptive immune responses involve cellular programming of the B and the T lymphocytes to recognize and discriminate a pathogen. In the adaptive immune response, clonal expansion of lymphocytes in response to infection is absolutely critical, takes 3 to 5 days, and sufficient nutrient availability is necessary for clonal expansion to produce sufficient numbers of "effector" cells. While the innate immune system and most secondary lymphoid organs are qualitatively complete at birth, there are significant delays in the maturation of the adaptive immune response. Contact with offending pathogens during infancy and early childhood is critical for expansion and priming of adaptive lymphocyte cell populations. In severely malnourished patients, both innate host defense mechanisms and acquired immunity are diminished, thereby rendering them easy targets for infectious agents, and perpetuating the vicious cycle of infection–malnutrition[4] (Table 14.1).

The critical periods of development during fetal life, birth, and early infancy are highly vulnerable to insult and perturbations to the emerging immune system, particularly from nutritional imbalances. Maternal immune competence is relevant not only to the health of the mother but also for continued immune protection of the infant after birth. Maternal malnutrition may affect maternal immunological competency and its surrogate immunologic defense to the fetus and therefore decrease the immunocompetence in the newborn.[32] Both nutrient deficiency and excess may cause lifelong modifications to the response of the immune defenses;[32] in particular, lymphoid tissues in the intestine retain considerable plasticity to environmental stimuli throughout life.

CACHEXIA, CHRONIC DISEASES, AND IMMUNE COMPROMISE

It is important to recognize that infection can lead to malnutrition in the normal host, but that the continuum of infection–malnutrition as a chronic state may lead to cachexia or precachexia. Perhaps the major effect of infection–malnutrition interaction in increasing mortality is the development of cachectic syndrome.[12,38,39] Chronic, recurrent, or subacute infections will sustain a chronic state of inflammation and inadequate utilization of substrates and micronutrients, leading to malnutrition. In certain pediatric groups, malnutrition will develop as a consequence of chronic debilitating diseases (cancer, chronic pulmonary and cardiac disorders, chronic renal failure, and severe injuries), immune deficiencies, and in the elderly, sarcopenia. All cachectic patients are invariably malnourished, but not all malnourished patients are cachectic.[37] In the presence of cachexia and precachexia, malnutrition worsens even in the presence of adequate estimated feeds, leading to a cachectic syndrome.[37] Hallmarks of cachexia include inflammation and anorexia, with a resultant decreased intake and altered substrate metabolism, which makes a cachectic state resistant to feeding.[12,46] In contrast, malnutrition is a state of depleted endogenous substrate reserves and loss of body mass and function due to an imbalance between intake and requirements of energy, protein, and other nutrients; however, it can be resolved if the deficient macronutrient or micronutrient is supplemented.

TABLE 14.1
Influence of Nutritional State on Host Defense and Associated Infections

Condition	Physiologic Alteration during PEM	Immune Mechanisms Affected	Associated Infections	Metabolic Alterations and Deficiencies
Acute PEM	Underweight (low weight for age), wasting (more severe form: low weight for length/height)	Phagocytosis, RNIs, ROIs, antigen presentation, leukocyte migration, inflammation, T-cell activation, T-cell memory, antibodies (IgG, IgA), cytokine production, leptin levels, macrophage activation	Opportunistic, respiratory, and intestinal infections; helminthiasis; tuberculosis; measles; influenza; *P. jirovecii*	Frequent reinfections with high severity, low metabolic reserve in response to acute infections, low AA concentrations, diminished LBM
Chronic PEM	Stunting (short height for age), kwashiorkor, cachexia	Development of the thymus, T-cell differentiation, T-cell expansion, T-cell memory, IgA, IgG, decreased levels of complement and leptin, macrophage activation, decreased vaccine efficacy	Respiratory and intestinal infections, helminthiasis, BCG, malaria, AIDS, measles, influenza, skin infections, Noma, BCG anergy, active tuberculosis, encapsulated bacteria, measles	Changes in microbiota, zinc deficiency, diminished LBM
Obesity and overnutrition	Overweight, obese, metabolic syndrome	Permanent preactivation of leukocytes, increased levels of IFN-γ/TNF-α, suppressed NK and T-cell activation, reduced phagocytosis, increased plasma concentrations of leptin and leptin resistance	Opportunistic and fungal infections	Changes in microbiota, frequent cutaneous fungal infections and intertrigo, chronic inflammation, insulin resistance, hyperglycemia

Note: AA, amino acid; AIDS, acquired immunodeficiency syndrome; BCG, *Bacillus* Calmette–Guérin; IFN-γ, interferon γ; IgA, immunoglobulin A; IgG, immunoglobulin G; LBM, lean body mass; NK, natural killer; Noma, gangrenous stomatitis; PEM, protein–energy malnutrition; RNIs, reactive nitrogen intermediates; ROIs, reactive oxygen intermediates; TNFα, tumor necrosis factor α.

Cachexia is characterized by anorexia, inflammation, and >5% weight loss and loss of muscle mass. In children, failure to thrive is a hallmark of cachexia, usually presenting as a wasting syndrome.[12] The pathogenesis of cachexia is an imbalance between proinflammatory (e.g., TNF-α, IL-1, IL-6, interferon-γ [IFN-γ]) and anti-inflammatory (e.g., IL-4, IL-12, IL-15) cytokines and high C-reactive protein values, leading to anorexia, loss of weight, and lean body mass.[12,37,46] Such systemic inflammatory features are similar to those seen during malnutrition coexisting with many infectious diseases; however, in a precachectic or cachectic state, malnutrition does not respond to normal nourishment.[37]

Several infectious diseases that are prevalent in developing countries are associated with cachexia, e.g., tuberculosis, helminthiasis, NOMA (gangrenous stomatitis), brucellosis, chronic viral infections (i.e., hepatitis C), *Pneumocystis jiroveci* infection, and AIDS. Reversal of the infectious process improves the nutritional status in these patients. In other circumstances, where chronic debilitating diseases (i.e., cancer, chronic pulmonary and cardiac disorders, chronic renal failure, severe injuries, immune deficiencies) are the cause of the cachectic syndrome, malnutrition will be persistent and likely to coexist with frequent reinfections.[21,24]

ADAPTIVE MECHANISMS OF DISEASE TOLERANCE AND ALTERATIONS IN THE MICROBIOTA

Stunted children will conserve weight for height at the expense of growth in length to adapt to a chronic deficit or insult. Such alterations in the metabolic economy allow them to survive and keep metabolic and immune fitness in conditions of nutritional deficit, tolerating a decrease in their overall health. Similarly, two adaptive mechanisms have been described recently in the malnourished child that refocuses the metabolic and immunologic economy toward survival and adaptation rather than collateral damage and metabolic expense from fighting infection: pathogen/disease tolerance and alterations in the microbiota.

Pathogen/Disease Tolerance

The optimal immune response is determined by the balance between efficient pathogen clearance and an acceptable level of immunopathology. Immune recognition of a pathogen is followed by the production of effectors, which results in interactions between immune cells, often accompanied by collateral tissue damage and a metabolic cost to normal tissue function.[47] Immune activation against an infection agent is a defense mechanism aimed to fight and clear infection by attacking the pathogen, offering resistance against infection but also spending energy and substrate normally used for growth and homeostasis. Thus, it becomes partially detrimental to the host when frequent exposure and reinfection occurs. Adaptive tolerance mechanisms such as immune tolerance aim to restore homeostasis and normal tissue function, to reduce the fitness costs associated with fighting infections. The term "tolerance" used in this context is not to be confused with immunological tolerance, defined as unresponsiveness to self-antigens. Rather, it is an adaptive mechanism of host defense when immune resistance is exposed to constant infection and reinfection from evolutionary biology.[47,48] There is a tradeoff between these defense mechanisms, as increasing tolerance will decrease immunologic resistance to the pathogen.[47,49]

Infectious disease tolerance is a defense mechanism developed in evolutionary biology through epigenetic changes and alterations in molecular signaling responses that confer survival advantage against infection in simple organisms.[50] Several of those study models using cells and insects may suggest genetic regulatory links between the metabolic economy, tolerance to infection, and changes in microbiota.[50] In one example, in the *Drosophila melanogaster* fly, activation of insulin signaling conferred protection against death by wasting after *Mycobacterium marinum* infection without decreasing the infectious load.[49] In a second example, a methionine salvage enzyme signals the nutritional status of the host for sulfur-containing AAs and regulates cell death through pyroptosis.[50,51] Molecular adaptations mentioned above may be present in vertebrates and suggest that the development of immune tolerance mechanisms improve the metabolic economy of the host and confers survival benefit.

Alterations in the Microbiota

The development of immune tolerance allows bacteria to survive in the host while establishing a microbiota–host immune relation.[52] Recent biologic, molecular, and clinical data suggest that the gut microbiota is a metabolic organ that is needed for healthy postnatal development, and that the impact of the microbiota–host immune relation may have lifelong lasting modifications in the metabolic homeostasis of the host.[6] These bacterial commensals in the gastrointestinal tract have the potential to modulate human metabolism and systemic immunity.[9,53] The gut microbiota is now recognized as a biomarker and mediator of key metabolic functions needed to promote the nutritional health of mothers and the healthy growth of their offspring,[6] and can be altered by malnutrition, reshaping the immune and metabolic fitness of the host. Thus, the gut microbiome provides essential functions needed for healthy postnatal growth and development.

Interactions between the gut microbiota and the host immune system begin at birth with colonization of the intestinal surface by bacteria,[54] and changes as infant diet is initiated.[9] Diet and nutrients ingested through childhood, as well as infectious events, shape the configuration of host-associated microbial communities.[53] Although localized in the intestinal tract, the microbiota can trigger systemic inflammation in immunocompromised hosts[53] and that effect has been associated with systemic low-grade inflammation associated with lifelong risk of obesity, insulin resistance, metabolic syndrome, and autoimmune disorders,[55] even presenting with the onset in adulthood.[6]

The complex interactions between the host and microbiota include bacterial genomes that modulate metabolic reactions of the host–microbe, organizing metabolic signals comprising substrates generated by the microbiome and host genome, such as bile acids, choline, and short-chain fatty acids. The host–microbiota interaction is modulated by metabolite-sensing signals that facilitate communication of the microbiome with the host.[6] In the host, those metabolic signals are associated with low-grade chronic inflammation and activation of immune inflammatory axes that physiologically connect the gut, liver, muscle, and brain.[54]

Malnutrition and infection affects the assembly of metabolic functions encoded and expressed by the gut microbiome. The innate immune system defects associated with malnutrition can result in dysbiosis of the intestinal microbiota with downstream metabolic consequences for the host.[53] The interaction between chronic malnutrition and recurrent enteric infectious diseases produce environmental enteropathy (also known as tropical enteropathy).[6] This environmental enteropathy is characterized by damaged gut mucosal architecture and function, malabsorption, dysregulation of mucosal permeability, and inflammation.[55] It has been shown recently that disturbances in microbiome development and function caused by enteropathogenic infections increase the risk for kwashiorkor. In addition, malnutrition affects the gut microbiome functions involved in determining nutritional status, thus further worsening health status and perpetuating the interaction between malnutrition and infection.[18]

Perpetuation of the infection and malnutrition cycle is an immunopathological state linked to defects in gut microbiota maturation that leads to decreased nutrient availability, abnormal nutrient processing by the microbiota, aberrant nutrient and metabolite sensing by immune cells, the presence of enteropathogens, and epigenetic adaptation.[6,56] Our understanding of this immunopathological state may lead to effective clinical and public health interventions. As such, it has been shown that the metabolic capacity of the microbiota affects the development of kwashiorkor in children.[18] Moreover, antibiotic therapy together with ready-to-use therapeutic food (RUTF) improves recovery and reduces mortality in children with kwashiorkor, which was better than supplementing RUTF with placebo.[57] RUTF not only improves the symptoms of kwashiorkor but also has major effects on the gut microbiota.[57] The gut microbiome in healthy twins has been shown to be more differentiated than that in twins with kwashiorkor. Moreover, symptoms of malnutrition are transmissible into gnotobiotic mice by combining stool transplantation from children with kwashiorkor and region-specific diet.[6,58]

Environmental Hostility, Undernutrition, and Infection

Perpetuation of the interaction between malnutrition–infection is linked to the environment where individuals live. The malnutrition–infection binomia is highly prevalent in poor countries, where resources are limited, exposing the general population to food insecurity, frequent exposure to pathogens, vector proliferation, crowding, decreased access to sanitation, health care, and, for children, lack of an adequate and safe environment to thrive and achieve their maximal growth and intellectual potential. Such environmental hostility to the host enables infectious disease transmission risks and limited nutrition availability to satisfy needs and metabolic requirements. Chronic diseases resulting from overnutrition in industrial societies lead to a high prevalence of childhood obesity, and it is of equal concern.

The high prevalence of infectious disease in societies with limited resources and poverty worsens the prevalence of malnutrition, independently of food scarcity or agricultural insecurity[2,59] (Figure 14.2). Social ecosystems that limit the availability of food and waste disposal, and present inappropriate living conditions to children, create a hostile nonhygienic environment that perpetuates the interaction between malnutrition and infection. Poverty and such conditions promote vector and

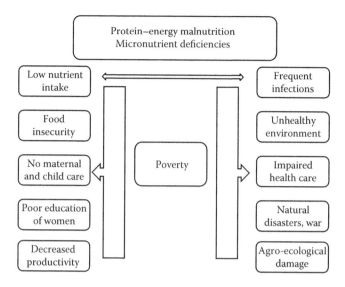

FIGURE 14.2 Social and ecosystem characteristics that perpetuate malnutrition and infection. Social ecosystems that limit the availability of food and waste disposal, and present inappropriate living conditions to children, create a hostile nonhygienic environment that perpetuates the interaction between malnutrition and infection.

infectious agent proliferation, leading to endemic prevalence and reinfection of many infectious diseases.[59] Frequent infections reduce social productivity, resources, and income, and worsen child malnourishment by affecting the sustainability of food production. Both ecosystems and climate also have an impact on the agricultural–food system by affecting the sustainability of food security. In addition, overexploitation and damage to the ecosystem health can affect human health by the presence of pollutants or toxins, the exposure of infectious agents and vectors, and the availability of clean water for human use. Thus, malnutrition and disease interact in an important feedback loop with the environment and with food and nutrition security.

The role of a hostile environment in the perpetuation of malnutrition–infection interaction has been modeled in a Pasteur's quadrant to delineate a global framework to understand bio-nutrition and the relation between basic science, eco-sociology, public health, and food technology designed to fight malnutrition and prevent the perpetual spiral of chronic malnutrition, infection, disease, and reduced economic productivity in poor societies.[4,5] Morbidity and mortality in children younger than 5 years due to the interaction between nutrition and infection in poor countries reflects the influence of an ecosystem that is hostile to the host and promotes malnutrition and infection–reinfection cycles.[4,59]

EFFECTS OF ACUTE AND CHRONIC INFECTION ON NUTRIENT AVAILABILITY AND UTILIZATION

Infections in children induce alterations in the metabolism of carbohydrates, proteins, lipids, and micronutrients. In normal conditions, metabolic pathways are largely regulated by circulating hormones, neurotransmitters, changes in organ blood flow and body composition, and by physical activity.[46] During acute or chronic infectious illness, the presence of inflammatory mediators alters hormone secretion and action. The presence of stress augments the sympathetic tone; increases circulating cortisol, glucagon, and the catecholamines; and decreases secretion of insulin-like growth factor-1 and promotes resistance to the combined effects of insulin and growth hormone[60] and growth hormone alone.[61–63] Such humoral and neural changes induce antagonism of the normal growth drive of pediatric subjects, including a decrease in anabolism and increased catabolism of body protein by several mechanisms, including anorexia and starvation, decreased immobility, and catabolism of endogenous nutrient reserves by stress and inflammation.[39,62,64] Those changes include decreased nutrient intake, diminished response to nutrients, increased metabolic requirements, depletion and constant utilization of endogenous metabolic stores, and chronic macronutrient and micronutrient deficits.

EFFECTS ON APPETITE, ABSORPTION, AND REQUIREMENTS

Infection has been shown to induce anorexia and decreased activity.[39] This is a direct effect on the central nervous system through the neuroendocrine axis by inflammatory mediators and stress and metabolic hormones, such as cytokines, interleukins, leptin, and cortisol. Leptin regulates satiety and connects nutrition and immunity through the hypothalamic–pituitary–adrenal axis. Reduced circulating leptin levels have been described in patients with PEM and have been associated with impaired macrophage functions, increases in serum levels of stress hormones, and possibly with increased susceptibility to infection by *Mycobacterium tuberculosis*.[4]

Infection and malnutrition, alone and in combination, have been shown to induce changes in the intestinal microbiota and metabolites, impairing normal metabolism of nutrients and leading to loss of the integrity of the intestinal barrier and to a deficient surface antibody response. This may lead to malabsorptive syndromes and further macronutrient and micronutrient losses and increased susceptibility to infections. Intestinal infection and reinfections maintain a perennial state of inflammation, aggravating the presence of malnutrition.

Requirements of several macronutrients and micronutrients increase during an acute illness, and chronic disease induces deficiency states that increase the susceptibility to infections. Pediatric patients have increased macronutrient and micronutrient requirements to sustain growth during developmental stages that have rapid growth velocity. The presence of infections and growth in such individuals, together with depleted stores in the presence of malnutrition, and the need of additional substrate for catch-up growth in the presence of stunting, may suggest overall increased requirements to establish well-being, when infection and malnutrition coincide in the pediatric patient.

ACQUIRED NUTRITIONAL DEFICIENCIES

Increased requirements in pediatric patients with malnutrition–infection may lead to acquired nutritional deficiencies that may or may not respond to supplementation.[20]

Major macronutrient deficits occur during illness due to those increased requirements, and those deficits accumulate over time.[19] The sustained imbalance of increased protein requirements during infection eventually leads to loss of lean body mass and is associated with growth failure in children.[12,46]

Protein, lipids, and glucose need to be supplied during acute infection to avoid catabolism and macronutrient body depletion. Inflammation induces protein breakdown from endogenous protein stores, and the skeletal muscle releases AAs and nitrogen to the systemic circulation to supply AAs for whole body protein metabolism.[46,62,65,66] Circulating plasma AAs are cleared from the circulation for oxidation and energy production, gluconeogenesis, fuel and substrate for immune cells and enterocytes, and to supply the hepatic needs for nitrogen to synthesize acute-phase reactants. If enough energy is not provided, AAs are oxidized for energy production.[66] Therefore, circulating plasma AA concentrations are lower in patients with infectious and critical illness.[67,68] Lower circulating plasma AA concentrations have been reported in acute measles and dengue.[15,56] Other AAs, such as arginine and methionine, seem to become conditionally deficient in acute infective states.[4,68] During infection, whole body protein synthesis is increased, due to high protein synthesis in the liver and immune cells. If dietary protein is not provided, the splanchnic bed does not receive AAs from absorbed protein, and the synthesis of visceral protein, such as albumin, and prealbumin decreases and intestinal epithelial breakdown occurs.[69,70] Kwashiorkor malnutrition has selective deficiencies in AAs, and it is associated with opportunistic diseases such as pertussis and tuberculosis. In children, the immune response that the body mounts against infection compounds an imbalance in the AA pool essential for protein synthesis and growth.[5,71]

Malnutrition and several other infections may cause specific nutrient deficiencies. A mutual requirement for iron in the bacteria and the host leads to iron deficiency and anemia.[5] Vitamin A deficiency increases the risk of diarrhea, *Plasmodium falciparum* malaria, measles, and overall child mortality from pneumonia and diarrhea. Recently, the United Nations Children's Fund and the World Health Organization published recommendations for the prevention and treatment of diarrhea; breastfeeding, zinc, and vitamin A were included as beneficial interventions for the reduction of child mortality from diarrhea.[72] A study by Mda et al. of 118 children <2 years of age in South Africa concluded that daily supplementation with multivitamins containing vitamins A, B complex, C, D, and E; folic acid; copper; iron; and zinc caused a significant reduction in the duration of hospitalization in children admitted with diarrhea or pneumonia.[73] A recent meta-analysis by Imdad et al. found that vitamin A supplementation in preschool children showed substantial reductions in diarrhea morbidity and mortality; however, there was no difference in children with pneumonia.[74] Measles in a child is more likely to exacerbate any existing nutritional deficiency, but vitamin A deficiency and child death for measles are closely associated.[1,3] Studies on the effect of vitamin A supplementation on growth have yielded various results. In a randomized controlled study by Hadi et al., a single dose of vitamin A or placebo was given every 4 months to 1405 children in Indonesia aged 6–48 months; the authors concluded that vitamin A supplementation improves the linear growth of children who have a low intake of vitamin A, but the impact is muted with increasing levels of respiratory infections.[75] Another randomized controlled trial by Villamor et al.

of 687 Tanzanian children aged 6–60 months admitted to the hospital with pneumonia found that supplementation with vitamin A improved linear and ponderal growth in infants who are infected with HIV and malaria, and decreased the risk of stunting associated with persistent diarrhea.[76]

Low blood zinc concentrations occur in patients with tuberculosis, Crohn's disease, diarrheal disease, and pneumonia.[3] Zinc deficiency affects B-cell lymphopoiesis and induce potent atrophy of the thymus and a decline in the number of peripheral T lymphocytes.[10] The majority of these nutritional deficiencies will have an impact in the immune response perpetuating the interaction between malnutrition and infection. Effects of infection on metabolic substrate such as lipids (e.g., fatty acids, cholesterol, or fat-soluble vitamins), glucose, or oligo elements (e.g., zinc, copper, and iron) will cause secondary immunodeficiencies. Several studies have reported results of zinc supplementation in children with diarrhea,[77–79] while other authors have reported the use of a combination of zinc and other micronutrients in infants and children with diarrhea.[80,81] Two randomized controlled trials in Indian children aged 3–36 months by Bhandari et al. and Bhatnagar et al. found a beneficial effect of zinc supplementation in the incidence and severity of prolonged diarrhea.[77,78] Most recently, Malik et al. in a randomized, double-blind, placebo-controlled trial reported the use of a short-course prophylactic zinc supplementation in Indian children aged 6–11 months with diarrhea; the authors found that zinc supplementation for 2 weeks may reduce diarrhea morbidity in infants for up to 5 months, in populations with a high prevalence of wasting and stunting.[77–79] A randomized controlled trial by Chhagan et al. reported results of the use of zinc alone or zinc plus multiple micronutrients, to vitamin A in the incidence of diarrhea in stunted or HIV-infected children in rural South Africa; the authors concluded that compared with vitamin A alone, supplementation with zinc, and with zinc and multiple micronutrients, had reduced diarrhea morbidity in this population.[80]

Vitamin E (α-tocopherol) and the trace element selenium (Se) function synergistically in tissues to reduce damage to lipid membranes by the formation of reactive oxygen species (ROS) during infections.[82] Vitamin E is a lipid-soluble antioxidant, and deficiency results in increased free radical–induced membrane damage to red blood cells.[83] Supplementation with vitamin E to those believed to have marginal status increased skin test response, enhanced mitogen-induced lymphocyte proliferation and IL-2 production, and improved the antibody responses to vaccines, while decreasing the synthesis of the immunosuppressive eicosanoid PGE_2.[84,85]

Selenium plays a role in balancing the redox state of the cell and removing ROS, which likely contributes to its anti-inflammatory effects.[86] Alterations in immune function are associated with selenium deficiency and may explain the pathogenesis of some chronic inflammatory and viral diseases.[87] Substantial evidence has accumulated to explain a beneficial effect of supplementing selenium during HIV-1 infection, where it has been demonstrated to reduce oxidative stress, modulate cytokine synthesis, improve T-cell proliferation and differentiation, and reduce cytokine-induced HIV-1 replication.[88] In a recent randomized controlled trial of 847 HIV-infected children in Uganda, 426 children were supplemented with 14 micronutrients, including selenium, compared with 421 children that received six multivitamins; the results indicated no difference in mortality, growth, or CD4 counts between the two groups.[89]

Several systematic reviews of the use of micronutrient supplementation including selenium, in patients with cystic fibrosis, HIV, and kwashiorkor, have shown no clear benefit of the effectiveness of supplementary micronutrients.[90–92]

Several inflammatory conditions in humans, such as clinical sepsis, have been associated with significantly decreased selenium status.[93,94] Also, low blood selenium concentrations in preterm infants have been suggested as a potential risk factor for sepsis, chronic neonatal lung disease, and retinopathy of prematurity.[95] Intervention with selenium supplementation has been proposed as an inexpensive means to mitigate the effects of critical illness stress-induced immune suppression (CRISIS) and other conditions involving sepsis.[20,96] A systematic review of three randomized controlled trials in preterm neonates[97] and a randomized double-blind controlled trial in critically ill children (CRISIS prevention trial)[20] concluded that supplementation with selenium had a beneficial effect in reducing sepsis without improved survival.

NUTRIENT UTILIZATION

In the presence of infection, even when AAs are provided, insulin resistance; the effects of stress, cortisol, and cytokines; and alterations in growth hormone may limit an adequate response to protein provision.[46,61] Injury, sepsis, and inflammation diminish the anabolic response to hormones and nutrients that stimulate protein deposition in the major protein reservoir, skeletal muscle.[62,63]

Although certain AAs may modulate a specific cellular or physiologic effect, AA imbalances may also be detrimental for metabolic homeostasis. All 20 protein AAs and their metabolites are required for normal cell physiology and function.[45] Infants and infected children have a high protein turnover owing to increased whole body protein synthesis and breakdown.[98] In contrast to the net increase in whole body protein synthesis during inflammation, in skeletal muscle, protein synthesis decreases and protein degradation increases to decrease utilization and release and shuttle AAs and nitrogen to visceral tissues and immune cells.[62,99] Partitioning in protein metabolism also occurs, as different organ systems may have specific AA requirements or certain AAs may exert particular functions.[62,70,98]

Micronutrients such as zinc; copper; vitamins A, D, and E; and iron will be preferentially used for respiratory and intestinal epithelial repair and sustenance of the cellular immune response.

NUTRIENT DISTRIBUTION AND REPRIORITIZATION

Inflammation induces protein breakdown from endogenous protein stores, and the skeletal muscle releases AAs and nitrogen to the systemic circulation to supply AAs for whole body protein metabolism.[46,62,65,66] Circulating plasma AAs are cleared from the circulation for oxidation and energy production, gluconeogenesis, fuel and substrate for immune cells and enterocytes, and to supply the hepatic needs for nitrogen to synthesize acute-phase reactants. If enough energy is not provided, AAs can be oxidized for energy production.[66]

During infections, macronutrients and micronutrients are shifted toward the immune response, and less energy and protein are utilized for growth purposes;

survival becomes essential and growth faltering during times of acute inflammation becomes an adaptive mechanism.[100] However, chronic infections and repeated episodes of infection will put the child in a state of growth suppression and failure to thrive.

Nutritional interventions in childhood decrease the burden of the synergy between infection and malnutrition. The current consensus is that improved nutrition can ameliorate or eliminate the negative consequences of infection on growth. The mechanisms by which adequate nutrition reduce the effect of infection include (i) support of the immune system; (ii) compensating for malabsorption, reallocation, or losses of key nutrients; (iii) catch-up growth after infection; (iv) augmenting appetite; and (v) supporting the growth of beneficial gut microorganisms.[100]

Supplementation of high-caloric-density macronutrients in combination with multiple micronutrients to malnourished mothers antenatally and to malnourished children has been shown to reduce LBW and improve adolescent growth.[31,32]

CONCLUSIONS

Childhood infectious disease is the most common cause of morbidity and mortality in developing countries.[36] Protein–calorie malnutrition is the main reason for increased susceptibility to infections and is directly related to the socioeconomic factors of a society rooted in poverty.[59] The risk factors for childhood malnutrition are maternal malnutrition, a lack of exclusive breast-feeding, inappropriate complementary feeding practices, and high burden of infectious diseases.[31] The high incidence and severity of infections in malnourished children is mainly due to the worsening of the immune system; limited production and diminished function of the cellular immune system is a common feature in malnutrition.[36]

Globally, the high burden of diarrheal disease, respiratory infections, and HIV are major contributors for the prevalence of growth stunting in children. However, limited access to adequate nutrition to cover growth requirements impose deficits that lead to stunting.[100] Moreover, providing adequate nutritional supplementation with interventions aimed to prevent and control infections will be the most effective approach for optimizing child growth and development. Social and ecologic systems that promote poverty, food insecurity, and an environment with poor sanitation perpetuate the prevalence of malnutrition and infection in children, and efforts to provide a thriving environment for children should accompany nutritional and anti-infective interventions.[59]

Macronutrients and micronutrients are essential for maintaining the function of immune cells, and it is plausible to think that variations in nutrient intake contribute to the differences in immune responses between individuals.[25] As our understanding of the function of specific nutrients in host resistance to infectious diseases improves, specific recommendations will be formulated to attain the immune response required to prevent and treat specific infectious diseases in the population, particularly in the most vulnerable, the malnourished children.

More research is needed on the efficacy and effectiveness of interventions that combine nutritional therapies with strategies aimed at the prevention and control of infections, including better hygiene; education; improvement in sanitary conditions and water quality; and actions directed to the prevention and treatment of gastrointestinal diseases, respiratory illnesses, measles, malaria, and HIV infection.[100]

REFERENCES

1. Scrimshaw, N.S. Historical concepts of interactions, synergism and antagonism between nutrition and infection. *J Nutr* **133**, 316S–321S (2003).
2. Hammond, R.A. & Dube, L. A systems science perspective and transdisciplinary models for food and nutrition security. *Proc Natl Acad Sci U S A* **109**, 12356–12363 (2012).
3. Katona, P. & Katona-Apte, J. The interaction between nutrition and infection. *Clin Infect Dis* **46**, 1582–1588 (2008).
4. Schaible, U.E. & Kaufmann, S.H. Malnutrition and infection: Complex mechanisms and global impacts. *PLoS Med* **4**, e115 (2007).
5. Blackburn, G.L. Pasteur's Quadrant and malnutrition. *Nature* **409**, 397–401 (2001).
6. Gordon, J.I., Dewey, K.G., Mills, D.A. & Medzhitov, R.M. The human gut microbiota and undernutrition. *Sci Transl Med* **4**, 137ps112 (2012).
7. Zeisel, S.H. Epigenetic mechanisms for nutrition determinants of later health outcomes. *Am J Clin Nutr* **89**, 1488S–1493S (2009).
8. Lillycrop, K.A. & Burdge, G.C. Epigenetic mechanisms linking early nutrition to long term health. *Best Pract Res Clin Endocrinol Metab* **26**, 667–676 (2012).
9. Sim, K. et al. The neonatal gastrointestinal microbiota: The foundation of future health? *Arch Dis Child Fetal Neonatal Ed* **98**, F362–F364 (2012).
10. Wolowczuk, I. et al. Feeding our immune system: Impact on metabolism. *Clin Dev Immunol* **2008**, 639803 (2008).
11. Kelly, P. Nutrition, intestinal defence and the microbiome. *Proc Nutr Soc* **69**, 261–268 (2010).
12. Evans, W.J. et al. Cachexia: A new definition. *Clin Nutr* **27**, 793–799 (2008).
13. Jahoor, F., Badaloo, A., Reid, M. & Forrester, T. Protein metabolism in severe childhood malnutrition. *Ann Trop Paediatr* **28**, 87–101 (2008).
14. Mizock, B.A. Metabolic derangements in sepsis and septic shock. *Crit Care Clin* **16**, 319–336, vii (2000).
15. Klassen, P., Furst, P., Schulz, C., Mazariegos, M. & Solomons, N.W. Plasma free amino acid concentrations in healthy Guatemalan adults and in patients with classic dengue. *Am J Clin Nutr* **73**, 647–652 (2001).
16. Levy, O. Innate immunity of the newborn: Basic mechanisms and clinical correlates. *Nat Rev Immunol* **7**, 379–390 (2007).
17. Caulfield, L.E., de Onis, M., Blossner, M. & Black, R.E. Undernutrition as an underlying cause of child deaths associated with diarrhea, pneumonia, malaria, and measles. *Am J Clin Nutr* **80**, 193–198 (2004).
18. Smith, M.I. et al. Gut microbiomes of Malawian twin pairs discordant for kwashiorkor. *Science* **339**, 548–554 (2013).
19. Mehta, N.M. et al. Nutritional practices and their relationship to clinical outcomes in critically ill children—An international multicenter cohort study*. *Crit Care Med* **40**, 2204–2211 (2012).
20. Carcillo, J.A. et al. The randomized comparative pediatric critical illness stress-induced immune suppression (CRISIS) prevention trial. *Pediatr Crit Care Med* **13**, 165–173 (2012).
21. Hall, M.W. et al. Immunoparalysis and nosocomial infection in children with multiple organ dysfunction syndrome. *Intensive Care Med* **37**, 525–532 (2010).
22. Typpo, K.V., Petersen, N.J., Petersen, L.A. & Mariscalco, M.M. Children with chronic illness return to their baseline functional status after organ dysfunction on the first day of admission in the pediatric intensive care unit. *J Pediatr* **157**, 108–113.e101 (2010).
23. Kyle, U.G., Jaimon, N. & Coss-Bu, J.A. Nutrition support in critically ill children: Underdelivery of energy and protein compared with current recommendations. *J Acad Nutr Diet* **112**, 1987–1992 (2012).

24. Hulst, J. et al. Malnutrition in critically ill children: From admission to 6 months after discharge. *Clin Nutr* **23**, 223–232 (2004).
25. Field, C.J., Johnson, I.R. & Schley, P.D. Nutrients and their role in host resistance to infection. *J Leukoc Biol* **71**, 16–32 (2002).
26. Davis, T.A. & Fiorotto, M.L. Regulation of muscle growth in neonates. *Curr Opin Clin Nutr Metab Care* **12**, 78–85 (2009).
27. Orellana, R.A. et al. Development aggravates the severity of skeletal muscle catabolism induced by endotoxemia in neonatal pigs. *Am J Physiol Regul Integr Comp Physiol* **302**, R682–R690 (2012).
28. El-Kadi, S.W. et al. Anabolic signaling and protein deposition are enhanced by intermittent compared with continuous feeding in skeletal muscle of neonates. *Am J Physiol Endocrinol Metab* **302**, E674–E686 (2012).
29. Prentice, A.M. et al. Critical windows for nutritional interventions against stunting. *Am J Clin Nutr* **97**, 911–918 (2013).
30. Gahagan, S. Failure to thrive: A consequence of undernutrition. *Pediatr Rev* **27**, e1–e11 (2006).
31. Imdad, A., Sadiq, K. & Bhutta, Z.A. Evidence-based prevention of childhood malnutrition. *Curr Opin Clin Nutr Metab Care* **14**, 276–285 (2011).
32. Palmer, A.C. Nutritionally mediated programming of the developing immune system. *Adv Nutr* **2**, 377–395 (2011).
33. Ghazal, P., Dickinson, P. & Smith, C.L. Early life response to infection. *Curr Opin Infect Dis* **26**, 213–218 (2013).
34. Zeller, W.P., Goto, M., Witek-Janusek, L. & Hurley, R.M. Mortality, temporal substrate and insulin responses to endotoxic shock in zero, ten and twenty-eight day old rats. *Surg Gynecol Obstet* **173**, 375–383 (1991).
35. Victora, C.G. et al. Potential interventions for the prevention of childhood pneumonia in developing countries: Improving nutrition. *Am J Clin Nutr* **70**, 309–320 (1999).
36. Rodriguez, L., Cervantes, E. & Ortiz, R. Malnutrition and gastrointestinal and respiratory infections in children: A public health problem. *Int J Environ Res Public Health* **8**, 1174–1205 (2011).
37. Muscaritoli, M. et al. Consensus definition of sarcopenia, cachexia and pre-cachexia: Joint document elaborated by Special Interest Groups (SIG) "cachexia–anorexia in chronic wasting diseases" and "nutrition in geriatrics." *Clin Nutr* **29**, 154–159 (2010).
38. Schefold, J.C., Bierbrauer, J. & Weber-Carstens, S. Intensive care unit–acquired weakness (ICUAW) and muscle wasting in critically ill patients with severe sepsis and septic shock. *J Cachexia Sarcopenia Muscle* **1**, 147–157 (2010).
39. Laviano, A. et al. Neural control of the anorexia–cachexia syndrome. *Am J Physiol Endocrinol Metab* **295**, E1000–E1008 (2008).
40. Martorell, R. & Young, M.F. Patterns of stunting and wasting: Potential explanatory factors. *Adv Nutr* **3**, 227–233 (2012).
41. Olofin, I. et al. Associations of suboptimal growth with all-cause and cause-specific mortality in children under five years: A pooled analysis of ten prospective studies. *PLoS One* **8**, e64636 (2013).
42. Waterlow, J.C. Classification and definition of protein–calorie malnutrition. *Br Med J* **3**, 566–569 (1972).
43. Fujita, Y. et al. Studies of nitrogen balance in male highlanders in Papua New Guinea. *J Nutr* **116**, 536–544 (1986).
44. Liu, B. & Qian, S.B. Translational regulation in nutrigenomics. *Adv Nutr* **2**, 511–519 (2011).
45. Wu, G. Amino acids: Metabolism, functions, and nutrition. *Amino Acids* **37**, 1–17 (2009).
46. Wolfe, R.R. Regulation of skeletal muscle protein metabolism in catabolic states. *Curr Opin Clin Nutr Metab Care* **8**, 61–65 (2005).

47. Medzhitov, R., Schneider, D.S. & Soares, M.P. Disease tolerance as a defense strategy. *Science* **335**, 936–941 (2012).

48. Stearns, S.C. Evolutionary medicine: Its scope, interest and potential. *Proc Biol Sci* **279**, 4305–4321 (2012).

49. Schneider, D.S. & Ayres, J.S. Two ways to survive infection: What resistance and tolerance can teach us about treating infectious diseases. *Nat Rev Immunol* **8**, 889–895 (2008).

50. Chambers, M.C. & Schneider, D.S. Balancing resistance and infection tolerance through metabolic means. *Proc Natl Acad Sci U S A* **109**, 13886–13887 (2012).

51. Ko, D.C. et al. Functional genetic screen of human diversity reveals that a methionine salvage enzyme regulates inflammatory cell death. *Proc Natl Acad Sci U S A* **109**, E2343–E2352 (2012).

52. Holmes, E. et al. Therapeutic modulation of microbiota–host metabolic interactions. *Sci Transl Med* **4**, 137rv136 (2012).

53. Hooper, L.V., Littman, D.R. & Macpherson, A.J. Interactions between the microbiota and the immune system. *Science* **336**, 1268–1273 (2012).

54. Nicholson, J.K. et al. Host–gut microbiota metabolic interactions. *Science* **336**, 1262–1267 (2012).

55. Relman, D.A. Microbiology. Undernutrition—Looking within for answers. *Science* **339**, 530–532 (2013).

56. Phillips, R.S., Enwonwu, C.O., Okolo, S. & Hassan, A. Metabolic effects of acute measles in chronically malnourished Nigerian children. *J Nutr Biochem* **15**, 281–288 (2004).

57. Trehan, I. et al. Antibiotics as part of the management of severe acute malnutrition. *N Engl J Med* **368**, 425–435 (2013).

58. Tilg, H. & Moschen, A.R. Malnutrition and microbiota—A new relationship? *Nat Rev Gastroenterol Hepatol* **10**, 261–262 (2013).

59. WHO. Integrating poverty and gender into health programmes: A sourcebook for health professionals (module on noncommunicable diseases). http://www.wpro.who.int/publications/PUB_978+929061+245+2.htm (2010).

60. Shangraw, R.E. et al. Differentiation between septic and postburn insulin resistance. *Metabolism* **38**, 983–989 (1989).

61. Jenkins, R.C. & Ross, R.J. Acquired growth hormone resistance in adults. *Baillieres Clin Endocrinol Metab* **12**, 315–329 (1998).

62. Lang, C.H., Frost, R.A. & Vary, T.C. Regulation of muscle protein synthesis during sepsis and inflammation. *Am J Physiol Endocrinol Metab* **293**, E453–E459 (2007).

63. Teng Chung, T. & Hinds, C.J. Treatment with GH and IGF-1 in critical illness. *Crit Care Clin* **22**, 29–40, vi (2006).

64. Rogers, E.J., Gilbertson, H.R., Heine, R.G. & Henning, R. Barriers to adequate nutrition in critically ill children. *Nutrition* **19**, 865–868 (2003).

65. Hasselgren, P.O. & Fischer, J.E. Sepsis: Stimulation of energy-dependent protein breakdown resulting in protein loss in skeletal muscle. *World J Surg* **22**, 203–208 (1998).

66. Hoffer, L.J. & Bistrian, B.R. Appropriate protein provision in critical illness: A systematic and narrative review. *Am J Clin Nutr* **96**, 591–600 (2012).

67. Druml, W., Heinzel, G. & Kleinberger, G. Amino acid kinetics in patients with sepsis. *Am J Clin Nutr* **73**, 908–913 (2001).

68. Argaman, Z. et al. Arginine and nitric oxide metabolism in critically ill septic pediatric patients. *Crit Care Med* **31**, 591–597 (2003).

69. Schreiber, G. et al. The acute phase response of plasma protein synthesis during experimental inflammation. *J Biol Chem* **257**, 10271–10277 (1982).

70. Verbruggen, S.C. et al. Albumin synthesis rates in post-surgical infants and septic adolescents; influence of amino acids, energy, and insulin. *Clin Nutr* **30**, 469–477 (2011).

71. Orellana, R.A. et al. Amino acids augment muscle protein synthesis in neonatal pigs during acute endotoxemia by stimulating mTOR-dependent translation initiation. *Am J Physiol Endocrinol Metab* **293**, E1416–E1425 (2007).

72. WHO/UNICEF. Diarrhoea: Why children are still dying and what can be done. http://www.unicef.org/media/files/Final_Diarrhoea_Report_October_2009_final.pdf (2009).

73. Mda, S., van Raaij, J.M., de Villiers, F.P., MacIntyre, U.E. & Kok, F.J. Short-term micronutrient supplementation reduces the duration of pneumonia and diarrheal episodes in HIV-infected children. *J Nutr* **140**, 969–974 (2010).

74. Imdad, A., Herzer, K., Mayo-Wilson, E., Yakoob, M.Y. & Bhutta, Z.A. Vitamin A supplementation for preventing morbidity and mortality in children from 6 months to 5 years of age. *Cochrane Database Syst Rev*, CD008524 (2010).

75. Hadi, H., Stoltzfus, R.J., Moulton, L.H., Dibley, M.J. & West, K.P., Jr. Respiratory infections reduce the growth response to vitamin A supplementation in a randomized controlled trial. *Int J Epidemiol* **28**, 874–881 (1999).

76. Villamor, E. et al. Vitamin A supplements ameliorate the adverse effect of HIV-1, malaria, and diarrheal infections on child growth. *Pediatrics* **109**, E6 (2002).

77. Bhandari, N. et al. Substantial reduction in severe diarrheal morbidity by daily zinc supplementation in young north Indian children. *Pediatrics* **109**, e86 (2002).

78. Bhatnagar, S. et al. Zinc with oral rehydration therapy reduces stool output and duration of diarrhea in hospitalized children: A randomized controlled trial. *J Pediatr Gastroenterol Nutr* **38**, 34–40 (2004).

79. Malik, A., Taneja, D.K., Devasenapathy, N. & Rajeshwari, K. Short-course prophylactic zinc supplementation for diarrhea morbidity in infants of 6 to 11 months. *Pediatrics* **132**, e46–e52 (2013).

80. Chhagan, M.K. et al. Effect of micronutrient supplementation on diarrhoeal disease among stunted children in rural South Africa. *Eur J Clin Nutr* **63**, 850–857 (2009).

81. Luabeya, K.K. et al. Zinc or multiple micronutrient supplementation to reduce diarrhea and respiratory disease in South African children: A randomized controlled trial. *PLoS One* **2**, e541 (2007).

82. Reddanna, P. et al. The role of vitamin E and selenium on arachidonic acid oxidation by way of the 5-lipoxygenase pathway. *Ann N Y Acad Sci* **570**, 136–145 (1989).

83. Beharka, A., Redican, S., Leka, L. & Meydani, S.N. Vitamin E status and immune function. *Methods Enzymol* **282**, 247–263 (1997).

84. Meydani, S.N. et al. Vitamin E supplementation enhances cell-mediated immunity in healthy elderly subjects. *Am J Clin Nutr* **52**, 557–563 (1990).

85. Meydani, S.N. et al. Vitamin E supplementation and *in vivo* immune response in healthy elderly subjects. A randomized controlled trial. *JAMA* **277**, 1380–1386 (1997).

86. Parnham, M.J. & Graf, E. Seleno-organic compounds and the therapy of hydroperoxide-linked pathological conditions. *Biochem Pharmacol* **36**, 3095–3102 (1987).

87. McKenzie, R.C., Rafferty, T.S. & Beckett, G.J. Selenium: An essential element for immune function. *Immunol Today* **19**, 342–345 (1998).

88. Baum, M.K., Miguez-Burbano, M.J., Campa, A. & Shor-Posner, G. Selenium and interleukins in persons infected with human immunodeficiency virus type 1. *J Infect Dis* **182 Suppl 1**, S69–S73 (2000).

89. Ndeezi, G., Tylleskar, T., Ndugwa, C.M. & Tumwine, J.K. Effect of multiple micronutrient supplementation on survival of HIV-infected children in Uganda: A randomized, controlled trial. *J Int AIDS Soc* **13**, 18 (2010).

90. Irlam, J.H., Visser, M.M., Rollins, N.N. & Siegfried, N. Micronutrient supplementation in children and adults with HIV infection. *Cochrane Database Syst Rev*, CD003650 (2010).

91. Odigwe, C.C., Smedslund, G., Ejemot-Nwadiaro, R.I., Anyanechi, C.C. & Krawinkel, M.B. Supplementary vitamin E, selenium, cysteine and riboflavin for preventing kwashiorkor in preschool children in developing countries. *Cochrane Database Syst Rev*, CD008147 (2010).

92. Shamseer, L., Adams, D., Brown, N., Johnson, J.A. & Vohra, S. Antioxidant micronutrients for lung disease in cystic fibrosis. *Cochrane Database Syst Rev*, CD007020 (2010).

93. Maehira, F. et al. Alterations of serum selenium concentrations in the acute phase of pathological conditions. *Clin Chim Acta* **316**, 137–146 (2002).

94. Hollenbach, B. et al. New assay for the measurement of selenoprotein P as a sepsis biomarker from serum. *J Trace Elem Med Biol* **22**, 24–32 (2008).

95. Tarnow-Mordi, W., Isaacs, D. & Dutta, S. Adjunctive immunologic interventions in neonatal sepsis. *Clin Perinatol* **37**, 481–499 (2010).

96. Huang, Z., Rose, A.H. & Hoffmann, P.R. The role of selenium in inflammation and immunity: From molecular mechanisms to therapeutic opportunities. *Antioxid Redox Signal* **16**, 705–743 (2012).

97. Darlow, B.A. & Austin, N.C. Selenium supplementation to prevent short-term morbidity in preterm neonates. *Cochrane Database Syst Rev*, CD003312 (2003).

98. van Waardenburg, D.A. et al. Assessment of whole body protein metabolism in critically ill children: Can we use the [15N]glycine single oral dose method? *Clin Nutr* **23**, 153–160 (2004).

99. Verbruggen, S.C. et al. Current recommended parenteral protein intakes do not support protein synthesis in critically ill septic, insulin-resistant adolescents with tight glucose control. *Crit Care Med* **39**, 2518–2525 (2011).

100. Dewey, K.G. & Mayers, D.R. Early child growth: How do nutrition and infection interact? *Matern Child Nutr* **7 Suppl 3**, 129–142 (2011).

15 Aging and Effects of Nutrient–Infection Interactions

Sung Nim Han

CONTENTS

Introduction 357
Infectious Diseases in the Elderly 358
Immunological Changes in the Elderly 358
    Aging and Innate Immunity 358
    T cells and Aging 359
Changes in Nutritional Status in the Elderly 360
Influence of Infection on the Nutritional Status 361
Influence of Nutritional Status on Host Defense against Infection 361
    Vitamin D and Infection 361
    Vitamin E and Infection 362
    Selenium and Infection 363
    Zinc and Infection 363
Nutrient Supplementation and Infectious Disease in the Elderly 364
    Vitamin D Supplementation and Infectious Diseases 364
    Vitamin E Supplementation and Infectious Diseases 364
    Selenium Supplementation and Infectious Diseases 369
    Zinc Supplementation and Infectious Diseases 370
    Multivitamin and Multimineral Supplementation and Infectious Diseases 371
Conclusions 371
References 372

INTRODUCTION

During the 20th century, infectious disease mortality has declined gradually, yet large periodic spikes in the infectious disease curve suggest that factors that influence the emergence and reemergence of infectious diseases are dynamic.[1] Human life expectancy has increased significantly, and as a result, the number of persons aged over 65 years has been increasing rapidly in most countries. In the United States, >12% of the population were 65 years or older in 2011.[2] Between 2000 and 2010, the population aged 65 and older grew by 15.1%.[3] Increase in the population aged 65 or older emphasizes the importance of better understanding the infectious diseases in the elderly. Despite a general decrease in infectious disease mortality during the 20th century, increases in the infectious disease mortality among persons aged >65 years have been reported during the 1980s and 1990s due to increases in pneumonia and influenza deaths.[1] Therefore, infectious disease is a continuing threat to the older population. Multiple factors, including decline of immune function, comorbidities, changes in nutritional status due to alterations in intake and metabolism of nutrients, contribute to the increased susceptibility to infection in the elderly. In this chapter, we discuss the changes in immunity and nutritional status that accompany aging and the interaction between nutrient and infection. We review how nutritional status influences susceptibility to infectious diseases and the impact of nutritional supplementation on infectious diseases in the elderly.

INFECTIOUS DISEASES IN THE ELDERLY

The elderly population is more susceptible to infectious diseases. Improvement in medical care, vaccination, living condition, and sanitation, contributed to the overall decline in infectious diseases mortality during the last century. Among the infectious diseases, influenza and pneumonia contributed the most to the infectious disease mortality, averaging 44.4% of all infectious diseases deaths from 1900 to 1996. Pronounced year-to-year fluctuation in infectious disease mortality among the old age group suggested large contributions of pneumonia and influenza to mortality in this group.[1] Deaths among persons aged >65 years accounted for 87.9% of the overall estimated average annual influenza-associated deaths with underlying pneumonia and influenza causes during 1976–2007.[4] Hospitalization rate due to infectious disease increased during 1998–2006 from 152.5 to 162.2.[5] Approximately $865 billion in hospital charges were associated with primary infectious disease hospitalizations during this period. Infectious disease hospitalization rate was highest among those aged >80 years, followed by those <1 year, >70 years, and then >60 years. These mortality and hospitalization rates clearly show that infectious disease is a major health issue in the elderly. In addition to pneumonia and influenza, certain infections, including urinary tract infection, diverticulitis, endocarditis, and bacteremia, are more prevalent in the elderly compared with younger adults.[6] The proportion of older human immunodeficiency virus (HIV)-infected patients has increased, and thus understanding the interaction between aging and HIV progression is important.[7]

IMMUNOLOGICAL CHANGES IN THE ELDERLY

One of the hallmarks of physiological changes with aging is decline of immune function. Many components of the immune system are affected by aging. Impaired adaptive immunity with aging has been well described; however, how aging affects innate immunity has been less clear.

AGING AND INNATE IMMUNITY

Innate immunity serves as the first line of defense against infection. Neutrophils, macrophages, natural killer (NK) cells, and dendritic cells are important cellular components of the innate immune system, and aging has been reported to affect several aspects of these cells.[8,9] The total number of circulating neutrophils does not seem to be affected by aging. Age-related changes in effector functions such as decreased chemotaxis, phagocytosis of microbes, and generation of reactive oxygen species in response to stimulation have been reported in human neutrophils. However, excessive inflammatory response due to increased infiltration of neutrophils and excessive chemokine production after infection have been observed in aged animals.

Macrophages play a key role in innate immunity by phagocytosing intracellular pathogens and in inflammatory responses through the release of a variety of inflammatory mediators, including prostaglandins and proinflammatory cytokines. An age-associated decrease in macrophage function especially through Toll-like receptor (TLR) 4 activation, evidenced by decreased inflammatory cytokine production upon lipopolysaccharide (LPS) stimulation, has been reported.[8,9] However, enhanced bactericidal activity after *Salmonella* uptake by macrophages, and increased production of nitric oxide production after LPS stimulation have also been observed in macrophages from the aged animals.[10] Macrophages from old mice produced significantly higher levels of prostaglandin E_2 (PGE_2) compared with young mice, which was due to increased cyclooxygenase (Cox)-2 activity. Increased Cox-2 activity was due to higher Cox-2 protein and mRNA levels.[11] PGE_2 suppresses T-cell proliferation by inhibiting the early stages of T-cell activation,[12,13] and can modulate Th1/Th2 cytokine secretion.[14]

Proper NK activity is important for the early control of viral infections. Increased number of NK cells, however, decreased NK cytolytic activity and decreased cytokine and chemokine production after activation has been reported in elderly humans.[8,9] Dendritic cells play an important role in bridging innate immunity and adaptive immunity by functioning as antigen-presenting cells and by producing cytokines to regulate T-cell response. Among dendritic cells, plasmacytoid dendritic cells (pDCs) are the most potent producer of type I interferon (IFN) and key cellular responders of viral infection. A compromised function of pDCs with aging, including impaired IFN-α generation, has been reported.[7,8]

T CELLS AND AGING

Aging significantly affects T-cell function. Age-associated changes in T cells occur at multiple levels, including changes in population, functionality, signal transduction, and gene transcription. The effects of aging on T cells have been extensively reviewed.[15–17] Aging causes a shift toward greater proportions of antigen-experienced memory T cells with fewer T cells of naive phenotype. T cells from old mice go through lower activation-induced cell division, have fewer IL-2+ cells, and produce less IL-2 per cell. These age-associated changes in T cells were only observed within naive T-cell subpopulations.[18] Several changes in T-cell gene expression with aging have been identified.[16,19] Lower expression of CD28 and TCR-related genes, higher expression of apoptotic *Gadd45*, and lower expression of antiapoptotic *Bcl2*, decreased expression of genes of TCR signaling including *AKT*, *PDK2*, *ITK*, *Erk*, *Dlgh1*, *p38*, and *PI3K*, and higher expression of cytokines of the tumor necrosis factor (TNF) and transforming growth factor-β families have been observed. Aged T cells cannot effectively form immunologic synapses or recruit signaling molecules.[20] Age-related impairment of activation and expansion of CD4 T cells can extend to reduced B-cell response by hindering the T cells' help to B cells. The decreased ability of CD8 T cells to proliferate and to produce IFN-γ upon viral challenge contributes to impaired antiviral response in the aged.[21,22]

CHANGES IN NUTRITIONAL STATUS IN THE ELDERLY

Elderly persons are at a greater risk for poor nutritional status because of insufficient dietary intake and altered nutrient metabolism. Physiological changes that occur with aging or associated with comorbidities contribute to the alteration in nutrient metabolism. Various factors, such as inability to purchase enough foods, poor appetite, and decreased capability to absorb nutrients, can contribute to insufficient dietary intake. Lower status of several nutrients is a particular problem among the older population. Protein–energy malnutrition and lower plasma levels of zinc, vitamin D, and vitamin B_{12} have been reported to be more common in the elderly.[23,24]

When serum zinc levels of 578 nursing home residents with an average age of 84.6 years were measured, about 30% of the subjects had low (<70 µg/dL) zinc levels.[25] These elderly nursing home residents with lower zinc status had higher all-cause mortality. Dietary intake analysis using National Health and Nutrition Examination Survey between 1988 and 1994 revealed that population >71 years old were at a greater risk of inadequate zinc intake.[26] Dietary zinc intakes based on analysis of 24-h dietary recall of 29,103 persons (among them, 2623 were >71 years old) showed that the mean zinc intake from the food was 9.2 mg/d for those >71 years old. The proportion of population with adequate zinc intake was 42.5% for persons >71 years old, while 60.7% of adults (19–50 years old) had adequate zinc intake. Bogden et al.[27] investigated the zinc concentrations in plasma, erythrocytes, mononuclear cells, polymorphonuclear cells, and platelets from 100 subjects with a mean age of 72.1 years. In these subjects, the average plasma zinc concentration was 84.8 µg/dL and the percentage of those who had plasma zinc levels < 70 µg/dL was 14.7%. Lower nutritional status in the elderly has been reported in different countries. Among the elderly (n = 352, mean age 74.4 years old) living in the Quito area in Ecuador, a significant proportion of the subjects had lower than the reference range of circulating vitamin C (59.8% in men and 32.8% in women), vitamin B_6 (27% in men and 16.1% in women), vitamin B_{12} (20.5% in men and 19.6% in women), folate (37% in men and 27.4% in women), vitamin D (18.8% in men and 9.4% in women), and zinc (41.3% in men and 45.4% in women) concentrations.[28]

Bates et al.[29] measured plasma selenium concentrations from 1134 British elderly during 1994–1995, and the overall mean concentration was 0.90 µmol/L. This level is lower than the mean concentration of 1.09 µmol/L in British adults (19–64 years old, n = 1216).[30] However, the significance of the difference could not be determined and direct comparison would be impossible, as the measurements in adults were done during 2000–2001. Nevertheless, decline in plasma selenium concentration with age was evident in the elderly population. A significant inverse correlation between plasma selenium and age was observed in both free-living and institutionalized elderly.[29] Selenium status in the elderly seemed to be associated with mortality.

When 632 women between 70 and 79 years old were followed for mortality during 60 months, higher baseline selenium levels were associated with a significantly lower risk of mortality (hazard ratio [HR] 0.71, 95% CI 0.56–0.90).[31]

Older adults are at higher risk of having lower than optimal levels of vitamin D because of the decreased ability to produce vitamin D as well as decreased exposure to sunlight due to reduced mobility. Of homebound elderly in Baltimore, 54% of community dwellers and 38% of nursing home residents had the serum 25-hydroxyvitamin D levels < 25 nmol/L (10 ng/mL).[32]

INFLUENCE OF INFECTION ON THE NUTRITIONAL STATUS

Infection leads to decreased nutritional status. Prospective studies that investigated nutritional changes after infection in humans, especially in the elderly, are limited. Cross-sectional studies that compared infectious disease patients with the healthy controls reported lower plasma nutrient concentrations in the patients. Lower plasma vitamin E levels in patients with viral hepatitis were observed.[33] Serum selenium concentration was significantly lower in adults with hepatitis B and C virus infection compared with healthy controls.[34] In animals infected with influenza virus, decreases in concentrations of glutathione, vitamin C, and vitamin E from the lung were observed especially in the early stages of the infection, which was attributed to the increased production of oxidants.[35] Serum zinc concentrations of the hospitalized elderly patients were lower than those of healthy community-dwelling controls with similar age.[36] Six hundred sixty-eight elderly patients with a mean age of 80.9 years were compared with 104 healthy elderly with a mean age of 80.4 years. While 20.2% of the patients had a serum zinc concentration < 70 µg/dL, none of the healthy controls had lower zinc concentration. Among hospitalized patients, those with respiratory disease had the highest percentage of patients with <70 µg/dL zinc concentrations. Among patients with infectious diseases, 21.2% had serum zinc levels < 70 µg/dL. Significant decreases in carotenoids and β-carotene levels were observed in HIV-seropositive patients, and a decrease in vitamin and trace element level was related to the severity of disease.[37]

INFLUENCE OF NUTRITIONAL STATUS ON HOST DEFENSE AGAINST INFECTION

Malnutrition or nutritional deficiency can delay the recovery from infectious diseases.[38–40] In some cases, nutrient deficiency has a beneficial role in controlling infection by depriving nutrients required for the survival of pathogens or potentiating the mechanisms, such as oxidative stress, for the control of pathogens.[41,42]

VITAMIN D AND INFECTION

The impact of vitamin D on infectious disease could vary depending on the pathogens involved since the influence of vitamin D on different arms of the immune system could be either inhibitory or activating.[43] Generally, vitamin D has an inhibitory influence on adaptive immunity but an activating role on innate immune response.

According to a systematic review of clinical studies in which the association between vitamin D deficiency and susceptibility to acute respiratory infection in humans was investigated, observational studies predominantly reported statistically significant associations between low vitamin D status and increased risk of both upper and lower respiratory tract infections.[44] In a retrospective cohort study on 23,603 patients (mean age 61.2 years old), the association between preadmission serum 25-hydroxyvitamin D (measured between 7 and 365 days before hospital admission) and 30-day all-cause mortality after hospital admission was determined.[45] Prehospital vitamin D level was a strong predictor of mortality after adjustment for age, sex, and race. Those who had <15 ng/mL (37.4 nmol/L) vitamin D had increased odds of 30-day mortality (adjusted odds ratio [OR] 1.45, 95% CI 1.21–1.74) and increased odds of community-acquired bloodstream infection (adjusted OR 1.29, 95% CI 1.06–1.57) compared with those who had a vitamin D level of > 30 ng/mL (74.9 nmol/L). Remmelts et al.[38] investigated the impact of vitamin D status on community-acquired pneumonia outcome in a prospective cohort study, which involved 272 hospitalized patients with a mean age of 63.5 years. More than half of the patients (53%) were vitamin D deficient (<50 nmol/L). Vitamin D deficiency was associated with an increased risk of intensive care unit admission and 30-day mortality. The pneumonia severity index (PSI) calculated on admission was higher in patients with low vitamin D status, and the combination of PSI score and vitamin D status provided a superior prediction of 30-day mortality in community-acquired pneumonia. Leow et al.[46] also investigated the associations between mortality and serum vitamin D status in a prospective cohort study with 112 patients admitted with community-acquired pneumonia. The mean age of the subjects was 76 years (range 16–97 years). Vitamin D levels were determined from the blood samples taken within 24 h of admission. Overall, 44% of patients had vitamin D levels < 50 nmol/L, and 15% of the patients were severely vitamin D deficient (<30 nmol/L). Patients with severe vitamin D deficiency had significantly higher 30-day mortality compared with patients with mildly deficient (30–49 nmol/L) or sufficient vitamin D (≥50 nmol/L) levels. The unadjusted 30-day mortality was 5 of 17 among severely vitamin D–deficient patients, while it was 2 of 32 among mildly vitamin D–deficient and 2 of 63 among vitamin D–sufficient patients.

Vitamin E and Infection

In animal models, vitamin E deficiency has been shown to increase the pathogenicity of several pathogens such as *Citrobacter rodentium*,[47] *Trypanosoma cruzi* (Y strain),[48] and coxsackievirus B3 (CVB3/20) (associated with myocarditis).[49] On the other hand, vitamin E deficiency may protect against malarial infection by increasing oxygen radical production causing oxidative damage to the parasite.[41,42] Higher vitamin E levels seemed to have an undesirable effect on HIV-1-infected Kenyan women.[50] Among 67 Kenyan women, those with higher preinfection vitamin E status at 16–59 days before HIV-1 infection had a higher mortality risk (adjusted HR 1.58, 95% CI 1.15–2.16) when followed for 45–85 months. Reduced RANTES (regulated on activation, normal T cell expressed and secreted; also known as CCL5, chemokine [C–C motif] ligand 5) production, which would reduce the

RANTES-mediated internalization of CCR5 (C–C chemokine receptor 5), one of the main coreceptors for HIV-1,[51] was suggested as a possible mechanism to explain the findings in Kenyan women.

SELENIUM AND INFECTION

Selenium deficiency has been linked to the occurrence, virulence, and pathogenesis of certain viral infections, including coxsackievirus, influenza virus, and HIV.[52–55] Keshan disease is a cardiomyopathy observed in selenium-deficient areas in China.[56] Selenium supplementation in the form of sodium selenite tablet prevented the disease. Keshan disease seemed to be caused by multiple factors, and infections may be one of the etiologies. Coxsackievirus has been isolated from the blood and tissues of persons with Keshan disease.[57] In mice, Beck et al.[52] showed that the avirulent coxsackievirus (CVB3/0) mutates to the virulent cardiotoxic form when it is passaged through an Se-deficient host and exerts similar effects to that of the virulent type, CVB3/20. The observation that Keshan disease occurs in Se-deficient areas of China suggested that nutrient (Se)–viral interaction is involved in the development of the disease. Selenium deficiency had no effect on viral titer or antibody response in influenza-infected mice, but increased the lung pathology.[53] Selenium has been indicated in susceptibility to and pathogenesis of HIV. Among HIV-1-seropositive drug users, selenium deficiency was significantly associated with mortality even after all the factors that could affect survival were considered together.[55]

ZINC AND INFECTION

The zinc status of the elderly can influence the incidence of infectious diseases. Plasma zinc concentration was significantly different between the elderly responders and nonresponders to individual skin test antigens.[27] These results clearly suggested that zinc status can influence the *in vivo* immune response. Among elderly nursing home residents, those with lower zinc status (<70 μg/dL) had higher risk of pneumonia, a longer duration of pneumonia episodes, and a greater number of new antibiotic prescriptions during a 1-year period while they received daily micronutrient supplementation containing 50% of the recommended dietary allowance.[25] Several mechanisms by which zinc may play a role in the maintenance of host resistance to infection have been proposed. These mechanisms include the interaction of zinc with metallothioneins, inducible nitric oxide synthase, and poly(ADP)-ribose polymerase.[58]

Zinc status can modulate the response to bacterial infection and sepsis. Liu et al.[59] showed that animals fed the zinc-deficient diet developed excessive inflammation to polymicrobial sepsis. Significant increase in serum IL-6, keratinocyte-derived chemokine, TNF-α, and monocyte chemotactic protein-1 was observed in zinc-deficient animals compared with the control animals after LPS injection or cecal ligation and puncture treatment. Transcript levels of NF-κB target genes also increased in zinc-deficient animals. This overactivation was mainly due to inappropriate control of IκB kinase activity. There was a significant increase in phosphorylated IκBα, IκBα degradation, and ERK phosphorylation with zinc deficiency.

NUTRIENT SUPPLEMENTATION AND INFECTIOUS DISEASE IN THE ELDERLY

The impact of intervention with single- or multinutrient supplements on the incidence of infectious diseases in the elderly has been investigated in several studies. However, the number of studies is limited, and the results have not been consistent. A list of studies that investigated the impact of nutrient supplementation on infectious diseases or antibody response to vaccination is shown in Table 15.1.

VITAMIN D SUPPLEMENTATION AND INFECTIOUS DISEASES

Recently, the association between vitamin D and the risk of acute respiratory infections, and the results from a clinical trial of vitamin D supplementation for the prevention of acute respiratory infections have been reviewed.[44] Many of the prospective clinical trials were conducted in children or included a wide age range of subjects. A few of the studies conducted in the older population are summarized in Table 15.1.

In a randomized, placebo-controlled, prospective study conducted by Li-Ng et al.,[60] 162 adults received either placebo or 50 µg vitamin D for 12 weeks. The age range of subjects was from 18 to 80, and the mean age of the vitamin D–supplemented group was 59.3 years and that of the placebo group was 58.1 years. A biweekly questionnaire was used to assess the incidence, severity, and duration of the upper respiratory infections. There was no effect of vitamin D supplementation on the incidence, duration, or severity of upper respiratory infections in this study. Baseline vitamin D status was high, with mean vitamin D levels > 60 nmol/L in both the supplemented and placebo groups. Higher baseline vitamin D status and high influenza vaccination rate (56.4% in vitamin D group and 64.3% in placebo group) might have contributed to a diminished difference between the supplemented and placebo groups. In observational studies, an increased risk of infectious diseases was observed when vitamin D status was low. Therefore, supplementation of vitamin D might not have conferred any added benefits of upper respiratory infection prevention to the population with already sufficient vitamin D status. In another study with a 2 × 2 factorial design, the effect of 2000 IU vitamin D supplementation combined with standard or extended physiotherapy for 12 months among old patients with hip fracture on rate of falls and hospital readmissions were compared with a 800 IU vitamin D–supplemented group.[61] The baseline mean vitamin D levels were 30.2 nmol/L in the 800 IU–supplemented group and 32.7 nmol/L in the 2000 IU–supplemented group. The overall hospital readmission rate was significantly lower in the high dose group, which was due to fewer readmissions associated with fall-related injury and due to fewer infections. While 18 fall-related injuries and 10 infections occurred among 87 patients in 800 IU group, 7 fall-related injuries and 1 infection were observed among 2000 IU–supplemented patients (n = 86).

VITAMIN E SUPPLEMENTATION AND INFECTIOUS DISEASES

Among the nutrients, vitamin E is one of the most studied for its clinical effect on infectious diseases. Vitamin E deficiency is rarely observed in humans, and the elderly do not have lower vitamin E status than the young. However, vitamin E has

TABLE 5.1

Impact of Nutrient Supplementation on Infections and Response to Vaccination in the Elderly

Nutrient	Subjects and Age	Amount and Duration of Supplementation	Effects	Reference
Vitamin E	Elderly (n = 88), ≥65 years old	Placebo, 60, 200, or 800 mg/d for 235 days	⇑ DTH and antibody titer to hepatitis B with 200 and 800 mg	Meydani et al.[62]
	Nursing home residents (n = 617), ≥65 years old	Placebo or 200 IU/d for 1 year	⇓ Numbers of subjects with all and upper respiratory infections ⇓ Incidence of common cold ⇔ Lower respiratory infection	Meydani et al.[63]
	Hepatitis C virus patients (n = 23), mean age of 55	Placebo or 800 IU/d for 12 weeks per phase (cross-over design)	⇓ ALT level (24% decrease) ⇓ AST level (19% decrease)	von Herbay et al.[64]
	Hepatitis C virus patients (n = 17), mean age of 62	500 mg/d for 3 months (no placebo)	⇓ ALT level in patients with ALT >70 IU/L at baseline ⇔ ALT level in patients with ALT <70 IU/L at baseline	Mahmood et al.[65]
Vitamin D	Healthy subjects (n = 162), aged 18–80, mean age of 59.3 for the treatment group and 58.1 for the placebo group	Placebo or 50 μg/d vitamin D3 for 12 weeks	⇔ Incidence of upper respiratory infection ⇔ Duration or severity of upper respiratory infection symptoms	Li-Ng et al.[60]
	Patients with acute hip fracture (n = 173), >65 years old, mean age of 84	2000 IU vs. 800 IU/d vitamin D, extended physiotherapy vs. standard physiotherapy (2 × 2 factorial design) for 12 months	⇓ Hospital readmissions due to fall-related injury and infections	Bischoff-Ferrari et al.[61]
Zinc	Healthy subjects (n = 50), aged 55–87	Placebo or 45 mg Zn/d for 12 months	⇓ Total incidence of infection	Prasad et al.[66]

(continued)

TABLE 5.1 (Continued)
Impact of Nutrient Supplementation on Infections and Response to Vaccination in the Elderly

Nutrient	Subjects and Age	Amount and Duration of Supplementation	Effects	Reference
Selenium	Critically ill patients (n = 35), mean age of 58 for the treatment group and 54 for the placebo group	2000 μg bolus at enrollment and 1600 μg/d for 10 days	⇓ Sequential organ failure score ⇓ Number of episodes of ventilator-associated pneumonia	Manzanares et al.[67]
	Critically ill patients (n = 150), mean age of 60	1000 μg at day 1 and 500 μg/d on days 2–14	⇓ C-reactive protein ⇔ Mortality	Valenta et al.[68]
Multinutrient	Noninstitutionalized individuals (n = 652), >60 years old	200 mg/d vitamin E, multivitamin–mineral supplement[a] for a median of 441 days (2 × 2 factorial design, placebo controlled)	⇔ Incidence and severity of acute respiratory infections	Graat et al.[69]
	Male smokers (n = 21,796, ATBC study cohort), 50–69 years old	50 mg/d vitamin E, 20 mg/d β-carotene for 4-year follow-up (2 × 2 factorial design, placebo controlled)	⇔ Overall self-reported common cold incidence ⇓ Incidence of common cold among older city dwellers who smoked <15 cigarettes per day	Hemila et al.[70]
	Male smokers (n = 29,133, ATBC study cohort) (898 hospital-treated pneumonia cases), 50–69 years old	50 mg/d vitamin E, 20 mg/d β-carotene for median of 6.1 years (2 × 2 factorial design, placebo controlled)	Vitamin E: ⇔ Overall incidence of pneumonia ⇓ Risk of pneumonia among the subjects who had initiated smoking at a later age (>21) β-Carotene: ⇔ Overall incidence of pneumonia ⇑ Risk of pneumonia among the subjects who had initiated smoking at a later age (>21)	Hemila et al.[71]
	Elderly (n = 5292, 3444 participants responded to the questionnaire), mean age of 77	800 IU/d vitamin D$_3$, 1000 mg/d calcium for a median of 18 months follow-up (2 × 2 factorial design, placebo controlled)	⇔ Self-reported infection and antibiotic use	Avenell et al.[72]

Study population	Intervention	Outcome	Reference
Institutionalized elderly (n = 725), >65 years old	Trace element (20 mg zinc + 100 μg selenium), vitamin (120 mg ascorbic acid + 6 mg β-carotene + 15 mg α-tocopherol) for 2 years (2 × 2 factorial design, placebo controlled)	⇑ Resistance to respiratory infections with trace element supplementation	Girodon et al.[73]
Elderly (n = 910), >65 years old	Placebo or one multivitamin and multimineral supplement[b] tablet per day for 1 year	⇔ Contacts with primary care; ⇔ Self-reported days of infection	Avenell et al.[74]
Nursing home residents (n = 763), >65 years old	Placebo or one multivitamin and multimineral supplement[c] tablet per day for 18 months	⇔ Incidence of infection; ⇓ Number of antibiotic courses and antibiotic days	Liu et al.[75]
Community-living elderly (n = 217), 65–85 years old	Placebo, dietary intervention, or micronutrient supplement[d] for 3 months intervention with a 3-month follow-up	⇓ Number of general practitioner and hospital visits in the dietary intervention and micronutrient supplement groups; ⇓ Number of weeks with symptoms of infection in the dietary intervention group only	Forster et al.[76]

a   Retinol 600 μg, β-carotene 1.2 mg, ascorbic acid 60 mg, vitamin E 10 mg, cholecalciferol 5 μg, vitamin K 30 μg, thiamin mononitrate 1.4 mg, riboflavin 1.6 mg, niacin 18 mg, pantothenic acid 6 mg, pyridoxine 2 mg, biotin 150 μg, folic acid 200 μg, cyanocobalamin 1 folate 400 μg, zinc 10 mg, selenium 25 μg, iron 4 mg, magnesium 30 mg, copper 1 mg, iodine 100 μg, calcium 74 mg, phosphor 49 mg, manganese 1 mg, chromium 25 μg, molybdenum 25 μg, silicium 2 μg.

b   Vitamin A 800 μg, vitamin C 60 mg, vitamin D_3 5 μg, vitamin E (D,L-α-tocopheryl acetate) 10 mg, thiamin (mononitrate) 1.4 mg, riboflavin 1.6 mg, niacin (nicotinamide) 18 mg, pantothenic acid (calcium D-pantothenate) 6 mg, pyridoxine (hydrochloride) 2 mg, vitamin B_{12} 1 μg, folic acid 200 μg, iron (fumarate) 14 mg, iodine (potassium iodide) 150 μg, copper (gluconate) 0.75 mg, zinc (oxide) 15 mg, manganese (sulfate) 1 mg.

c   Vitamin A 400 retinol equivalent, β-carotene 16 mg, vitamin D 4 μg (160 IU), vitamin E 44 mg (741 IU), vitamin C 80 mg, thiamin 2.2 mg, riboflavin 1.5 mg, niacin 16 mg, vitamin B_6 3 mg, vitamin B_{12} 4 μg, folate 400 μg, calcium (elemental) 200 mg, magnesium 100 mg, iron (elemental) 16 mg, iodine 200 μg, copper 1.4 mg, zinc 14 mg, selenium 20 μg.

d   β-Carotene 1500 μg, vitamin E 2 mg, vitamin C 80 mg, zinc (sulfate) 2 mg, selenium (selenomethionine) 25 μg.

been reported to enhance the immune function in the aged. Therefore, the clinical implication of vitamin E supplementation has been investigated in several studies looking at its impact on the incidence of infectious diseases; however, results in the elderly have demonstrated mixed outcomes.

In a randomized, double-blind study, 617 persons aged >65 residing at nursing homes received either a placebo or 200 IU of vitamin E (DL-α-tocopherol) daily for 1 year.[63] All participants received a capsule containing half the recommended daily allowance of essential vitamins and minerals. The main outcomes of the study were incidence of respiratory tract infections, number of persons and number of days with respiratory infections (upper and lower), and number of new antibiotic prescriptions for respiratory infections. The presence and type of respiratory infections, or absence, was documented by infectious disease specialists based on a review of data gathered by trained research nurses during weekly subject interviews, review of medical records, and physical examination focused on respiratory infections using standardized case definition. Vitamin E supplementation had no significant effect on the incidence or number of days with infection for all, upper, or lower respiratory tract infections. However, significantly fewer vitamin E–supplemented subjects acquired one or more respiratory tract infections (65% vs. 74%; RR 0.88, 95% CI 0.75–0.99, p = .04), or upper respiratory tract infections (50% vs. 62%; RR 0.81, 95% CI 0.66–0.96, p = .01). The vitamin E–supplemented group had a lower incidence of common cold (0.66 vs. 0.83 per person-year; RR 0.80, 95% CI 0.64–0.98, p = .04), and fewer subjects in the vitamin E group acquired one or more colds (46% vs. 57%; RR 0.80, 95% CI 0.64–0.96, p = .02). The results of this clinical trial showed that vitamin E supplementation had a protective effect on upper respiratory infections in the elderly. Because of the high rate and more severe morbidity associated with common colds in this age group, these findings have important implications for the well-being of the elderly as well as for the economic burden associated with their care.

A retrospective study showed that subjects with plasma vitamin E levels > 16.7 mg/L had a significantly lower mean number of infections compared with those with plasma vitamin E levels < 12.2 mg/L (1.0 vs. 2.3, 95% CI 0.12–2.48).[77] Hemila et al.[70] evaluated the effect of long-term vitamin E and β-carotene supplementation on the incidence of common cold episodes among a cohort of 21,796 male smokers from the Alpha-Tocopherol Beta-Carotene (ATBC) Cancer Prevention Study. Common cold episodes were queried three times per year during a 4-year follow-up period. Neither 50 mg of vitamin E (DL-α-tocopheryl acetate) nor 20 mg of β-carotene supplementations had an overall effect on the incidence of common cold. However, vitamin E supplementation alone resulted in a lower incidence of cold among older subjects who smoked fewer than 15 cigarettes per day and living in a city (RR 0.72, 95% CI 0.62–0.83). In a subsequent study, Hemila et al.[71] evaluated whether vitamin E or β-carotene supplementation had an impact on the risk of pneumonia among 29,133 men aged 50–69 years. During the 6.1 years of the intervention period (median), 898 cases of hospital-treated pneumonia were retrieved. Overall, neither vitamin E nor β-carotene supplementations had an effect on the incidence of pneumonia. However, vitamin E supplementation alone decreased the risk of pneumonia among subjects who had initiated smoking after age 21 years (n = 7469, 196 pneumonia cases) by 35% (RR 0.65, 95% CI 0.49–0.86). Contrary to vitamin E's effect, β-carotene supplementation increased the risk by 42% in the same subjects. Compared with other studies in which the effect of vitamin E was investigated, the vitamin E supplementation level was not high, but the duration of intervention was longer in the above two studies by Hemila et al.[70,71] The effects of vitamin E on infectious diseases were seen in subgroups with less amount of smoking or with later initiation of smoking, which suggested that the effect of 50 mg vitamin E supplementation was observed in those with less oxidative stress.

In a randomized, double-blind, placebo-controlled, 2×2 factorial trial in the elderly (>60 years old) living in the community, neither daily multivitamin–mineral supplementation nor 200 mg of vitamin E (DL-α-tocopheryl acetate) showed a beneficial effect on the incidence and severity of acute respiratory infections.[69] In this study, subjects self-reported their infections by telephone, and then the infections were confirmed by nurse visits. Absence of infection in those not reporting was not confirmed, and types of infections were not differentiated. Generally, the study population in the study by Graat et al.[69] seemed to be a healthier population since only 2% of the subjects were institutionalized and the percentages of subjects with suboptimal concentrations of vitamin C or vitamin E were very low. Plasma levels of zinc were not reported.

Vitamin E supplementation has been reported to improve the clinical outcomes of viral hepatitis in older adults. In a randomized, double-blind, placebo-controlled, cross-over design study by von Herbay et al.,[64] treatment of hepatitis C virus (HCV) patients (mean age 55 years) with 800 IU vitamin E (RRR-α-tocopherol) per day for 12 weeks improved clinical parameters indicative of liver damage. In average, alanine aminotransferase (ALT) levels were lowered by 24% and aspartate aminotransferase (AST) levels were lowered by 19% after 12 weeks of vitamin E treatment. Of 23 patients, 11 were responders with 46% decrease in ALT and 35% decrease in AST. Nonresponders did not show significant decreases. Cessation of vitamin E resulted in the increase of enzyme levels, and retreatment led to reproducible decrease in levels, which suggested that the decrease was a vitamin E–specific effect. In another study, 17 HCV patients (mean age 62 years) receiving anti-inflammatory therapy for at least 6 months were supplemented with daily 500 mg vitamin E (D-α-tocopherol) for 3 months.[65] All patients were supplemented with vitamin E, and there was no placebo control. When patients were divided into two groups based on the baseline ALT levels (low-ALT group with levels < 70 IU/L and high-ALT group with >70 IU/L), the ALT level decreased with vitamin E treatment in the high-ALT group but the effect of vitamin E was not observed in the low-ALT group.

Results from the vitamin E intervention studies on the incidence or clinical outcomes of respiratory infections or hepatitis virus infections imply that vitamin E's effects are dependent on the subjects' baseline characteristics, such as nutritional and health status. Subgroup analysis from the ATBC study presented evidence that heterogeneity in vitamin E's effect on pneumonia was strong among different subgroups.[78]

SELENIUM SUPPLEMENTATION AND INFECTIOUS DISEASES

Recently, results from a meta-analysis to assess the efficacy of parenteral selenium supplementation administered to critically ill septic patients on mortality were published.[79] Nine trials with 965 subjects in total were analyzed. Parenteral selenium supplementation significantly reduced the all-cause mortality in critically ill patients with sepsis (RR 0.83, 95% CI 0.70–0.99). Most of the selenium intervention studies conducted in critically ill patients included patients older than 18 years and were not specifically intended for the elderly. In the study by Valenta et al.,[68] the mean age of the critically ill subjects was 60 years. Seventy-five septic patients received additional selenium for 14 days (1000 μg on day 1 and 500 μg on days 2–14) in the form of Na-selenite pentahydrate in addition to the Na-selenite added in the parenteral nutrition, which was <75 μg per day. The placebo group received only the selenium added in the parenteral nutrition. A more pronounced decrease in C-reactive protein was observed in the selenium-supplemented group. However, mortality was not reduced by selenium supplementation. In a study by Manzanares et al.,[67] selenium supplementation significantly reduced the Sequential Organ Failure Assessment score and the number of episodes of ventilator-associated pneumonia in systemic inflammatory response syndrome patients admitted to the intensive care unit. Patients received 2000 μg selenium (as selenite) on day 1 as bolus and 1600 μg/d as continuous infusion for 10 days, and the mean ages of the patients were 58 years for the selenium group and 54 years for the placebo group.

In a randomized, double-blind, placebo-controlled study, effective increase in serum selenium after selenium supplementation suppressed the progression of HIV-1 viral burden.[80] Two hundred sixty-two HIV-1-seropositive subjects received either 200 μg/d selenium or placebo for 9 months. The mean ages of the subjects were 40.5 years in the selenium group (n = 141) and 40.6 years in the placebo group (n = 121). Among subjects in the selenium-supplemented group, those with an increase in serum selenium <26.1 μg/L were defined as nonresponders and those with an increase >26.1 μg/L were defined as responders. While the placebo group and non-responders had viral load elevation and decreased CD4 count, responders had no change in viral load and increase in CD4 count.

ZINC SUPPLEMENTATION AND INFECTIOUS DISEASES

Many studies that investigated the effect of zinc supplementation on infectious diseases have been mostly conducted in children. Improved antibody response during acute shigellosis,[81] reduced pneumonia incidence,[82] and no overall effect on duration of hospitalization or of clinical signs associated with pneumonia[83] have been reported with zinc supplementation in children.

In the elderly, 45 mg elemental zinc supplementation in the form of zinc gluconate for 12 months resulted in a lower total incidence of infection.[66] Elderly subjects aged between 55 and 87 were included in the study, and the mean ages of the subjects were 65 years for the supplemented group and 67 years for the placebo group. Subjects that appeared to have infections were evaluated by nurse practitioners. During the 12-month study period, the mean incidence of infections per subject was 0.29 in the supplemented group, while it was 1.4 in the placebo group. Among different types of infections, the incidence of common cold tended to be lower in the zinc-supplemented group. The number of subjects who had no evidence of any infections were different between the supplemented (17 of 24) and placebo (3 of 25) groups.

The mean plasma zinc levels at baseline were 92.9 µg/dL in the supplemented group and 95.7 µg/dL in the placebo group, and about 35% of the subjects in the study were zinc deficient.

Large doses of zinc supplementation could have adverse effects. Among institutionalized patients being treated for pressure ulcer, 26 received 440 mg/d oral zinc sulfate (equivalent to 100 mg elemental zinc) as part of the pressure ulcer treatment protocol and 44 patients received similar care for pressure ulcer without zinc supplementation.[84] The odds of an infection requiring antibiotic treatment were 7.8 times greater in patients receiving the zinc supplement.

MULTIVITAMIN AND MULTIMINERAL SUPPLEMENTATION AND INFECTIOUS DISEASES

In a 1-year multivitamin and multimineral supplement intervention study conducted among the elderly in Scotland, 456 subjects received a vitamin and mineral supplement that provided 50%–210% of UK reference nutrient intakes and the 454 subjects received a sorbitol placebo. The supplemented group did not show significant differences in the contact with the primary care team for the infections and the self-reported days of infection compared with the placebo group.[74] In a study conducted by Liu et al.,[75] 763 institutionalized elderly (mean ages were 85.4 years for the supplemented group and 84.7 years for the placebo group) received either a multivitamin and mineral supplement or a placebo for 18 months. The supplement contained 16%–200% of the dietary reference intake of nutrients (the composition of the nutrients is described in the footnotes to Table 15.1). Episodes of infections were recorded using retrospective chart reviews. There was no significant difference in the rate of infections between the supplemented and placebo groups. However, the number of antibiotic courses and antibiotic days were significantly lower in the supplemented group. Foster et al.[76] conducted a study to determine the effect of a dietary intervention and a micronutrient supplementation on infections in the elderly. Two hundred seventeen elderly between 65 and 85 years old participated, and their mean age was 72.6 years. Subjects received a placebo, dietary intervention (provided with a selection of foods and nutritional advice to increase the intake of zinc, selenium, carotenoids, and vitamins C and E), or a micronutrient supplement (containing β-carotene, vitamin E, vitamin C, zinc, and selenium) for 3 months and followed for 3 months. Measures of infections were self-reported. Weeks in which illness affected life and the number of hospitals and general practitioner visits were significantly lower in the dietary intervention and micronutrient supplement group compared with the placebo group. The number of weeks in which symptoms of an infection were described was significantly lower in the dietary intervention group compared with the micronutrient supplement and placebo groups.

CONCLUSIONS

The elderly population has higher susceptibility to and higher mortality from infectious diseases. The major factors contributing to increased risk are decline in immune functions and changes in nutritional status. Changes in innate immunity and decline of T-cell functions are responsible for impaired viral clearance and severity of infections. Observational studies clearly suggest that deficiencies of several nutrients in the elderly correlate with a higher incidence of and mortality from infectious diseases. On the other hand, infection can lead to decreased nutritional status. Therefore, infection in the elderly can further exacerbate the course of the disease, as they have less reserve of nutrients to maintain proper immune functions. However, results from the studies that investigated the impact of nutrient supplementation on the incidence or clinical outcomes of infectious diseases in the older population have not been always consistent. Baseline nutritional status, changes in blood or tissue levels of nutrients, supplement dose, health status of the subjects, methods to assess and confirm incidence, and clinical outcomes can affect the results. Better understanding of the interaction between nutrient and infection in the elderly will provide an improved targeted approach for intervention with nutrients for protection against infections.

REFERENCES

1. Armstrong GL, Conn LA, Pinner RW. Trends in infectious disease mortality in the United States during the 20th century. *JAMA* 1999;281:61–6.
2. U.S. Census Bureau. Population by Age and Sex: From 2011 US Census Bureau; 2011.
3. U.S. Census Bureau. Age and Sex Composition: 2010; 2011.
4. MMWR. Estimates of deaths associated with seasonal influenza—United States, 1976–2007; 2010.
5. Christensen KL, Holman RC, Steiner CA, Sejvar JJ, Stoll BJ, Schonberger LB. Infectious disease hospitalizations in the United States. *Clin Infect Dis* 2009;49:1025–35.
6. Gavazzi G, Krause KH. Ageing and infection. *Lancet Infect Dis* 2002;2:659–66.
7. Leng J, Goldstein DR. Impact of aging on viral infections. *Microbes Infect* 2010; 12:1120–4.
8. Mahbub S, Brubaker AL, Kovacs EJ. Aging of the innate immune system: An update. *Curr Immunol Rev* 2011;7:104–15.
9. Shaw AC, Joshi S, Greenwood H, Panda A, Lord JM. Aging of the innate immune system. *Curr Opin Immunol* 2010;22:507–13.
10. Smallwood HS, Lopez-Ferrer D, Squier TC. Aging enhances the production of reactive oxygen species and bactericidal activity in peritoneal macrophages by upregulating classical activation pathways. *Biochemistry* 2011;50:9911–22.
11. Hayek MG, Mura C, Wu D et al. Enhanced expression of inducible cyclooxygenase with age in murine macrophages. *J Immunol* 1997;159:2445–51.
12. Choudhry MA, Ahmed Z, Sayeed MM. PGE(2)-mediated inhibition of T cell p59(fyn) is independent of cAMP. *Am J Physiol* 1999;277:C302–9.
13. Choudhry MA, Hockberger PE, Sayeed MM. PGE2 suppresses mitogen-induced Ca^{2+} mobilization in T cells. *Am J Physiol* 1999;277:R1741–8.
14. Betz M, Fox BS. Prostaglandin E2 inhibits production of Th1 lymphokines but not of Th2 lymphokines. *J Immunol* 1991;146:108–13.
15. Herndler-Brandstetter D, Ishigame H, Flavell RA. How to define biomarkers of human T cell aging and immunocompetence? *Front Immunol* 2013;4:136.
16. Chen G, Lustig A, Weng NP. T cell aging: A review of the transcriptional changes determined from genome-wide analysis. *Front Immunol* 2013;4:121.
17. Moro-Garcia MA, Alonso-Arias R, Lopez-Larrea C. When aging reaches CD4+ T-cells: Phenotypic and functional changes. *Front Immunol* 2013;4:107.
18. Adolfsson O, Huber BT, Meydani SN. Vitamin E-enhanced IL-2 production in old mice: Naive but not memory T cells show increased cell division cycling and IL-2-producing capacity. *J Immunol* 2001;167:3809–17.

19. Han SN, Adolfsson O, Lee CK, Prolla TA, Ordovas J, Meydani SN. Age and vitamin E-induced changes in gene expression profiles of T cells. *J Immunol* 2006;177:6052–61.

20. Maue AC, Yager EJ, Swain SL, Woodland DL, Blackman MA, Haynes L. T-cell immunosenescence: Lessons learned from mouse models of aging. *Trends Immunol* 2009;30:301–5.

21. Jiang J, Fisher EM, Murasko DM. Intrinsic defects in CD8 T cells with aging contribute to impaired primary antiviral responses. *Exp Gerontol* 2013;48:579–86.

22. Han SN, Wu D, Ha WK et al. Vitamin E supplementation increases T helper 1 cytokine production in old mice infected with influenza virus. *Immunology* 2000;100:487–93.

23. Labossiere R, Bernard MA. Nutritional considerations in institutionalized elders. *Curr Opin Clin Nutr Metab Care* 2008;11:1–6.

24. High KP. Nutritional strategies to boost immunity and prevent infection in elderly individuals. *Clin Infect Dis* 2001;33:1892–900.

25. Meydani SN, Barnett JB, Dallal GE et al. Serum zinc and pneumonia in nursing home elderly. *Am J Clin Nutr* 2007;86:1167–73.

26. Briefel RR, Bialostosky K, Kennedy-Stephenson J, McDowell MA, Ervin RB, Wright JD. Zinc intake of the U.S. population: Findings from the third National Health and Nutrition Examination Survey, 1988–94. *J Nutr* 2000;130:1367S–73S.

27. Bogden JD, Oleske JM, Munves EM et al. Zinc and immunocompetence in the elderly: Baseline data on zinc nutriture and immunity in unsupplemented subjects. *Am J Clin Nutr* 1987;46:101–9.

28. Hamer DH, Sempertegui F, Estrella B et al. Micronutrient deficiencies are associated with impaired immune response and higher burden of respiratory infections in elderly Ecuadorians. *J Nutr* 2009;139:113–9.

29. Bates CJ, Thane CW, Prentice A, Delves HT. Selenium status and its correlates in a British national diet and nutrition survey: People aged 65 years and over. *J Trace Elem Med Biol* 2002;16:1–8.

30. Bates CJ, Prentice A, Birch MC, Delves HT, Sinclair KA. Blood indices of selenium and mercury, and their correlations with fish intake, in young people living in Britain. *Br J Nutr* 2006;96:523–31.

31. Ray AL, Semba RD, Walston J et al. Low serum selenium and total carotenoids predict mortality among older women living in the community: The women's health and aging studies. *J Nutr* 2006;136:172–6.

32. Gloth FM, 3rd, Gundberg CM, Hollis BW, Haddad JG, Jr., Tobin JD. Vitamin D deficiency in homebound elderly persons. *JAMA* 1995;274:1683–6.

33. von Herbay A, Stahl W, Niederau C, von Laar J, Strohmeyer G, Sies H. Diminished plasma levels of vitamin E in patients with severe viral hepatitis. *Free Radic Res* 1996;25:461–6.

34. Khan MS, Dilawar S, Ali I, Rauf N. The possible role of selenium concentration in hepatitis B and C patients. *Saudi J Gastroenterol* 2012;18:106–10.

35. Hennet T, Peterhans E, Stocker R. Alterations in antioxidant defences in lung and liver of mice infected with influenza A virus. *J Gen Virol* 1992;73 (Pt 1):39–46.

36. Belbraouet S, Biaudet H, Tebi A, Chau N, Gray-Donald K, Debry G. Serum zinc and copper status in hospitalized vs. healthy elderly subjects. *J Am Coll Nutr* 2007;26:650–4.

37. Sappey C, Leclercq P, Coudray C, Faure P, Micoud M, Favier A. Vitamin, trace element and peroxide status in HIV seropositive patients: Asymptomatic patients present a severe beta-carotene deficiency. *Clin Chim Acta* 1994;230:35–42.

38. Remmelts HH, van de Garde EM, Meijvis SC et al. Addition of vitamin D status to prognostic scores improves the prediction of outcome in community-acquired pneumonia. *Clin Infect Dis* 2012;55:1488–94.

39. Woo J, Ho SC, Mak YT, Law LK, Cheung A. Nutritional status of elderly patients during recovery from chest infection and the role of nutritional supplementation assessed by a prospective randomized single-blind trial. *Age Ageing* 1994;23:40–8.

40. Correia MI, Waitzberg DL. The impact of malnutrition on morbidity, mortality, length of hospital stay and costs evaluated through a multivariate model analysis. *Clin Nutr* 2003;22:235–9.
41. Herbas MS, Ueta YY, Ichikawa C et al. Alpha-tocopherol transfer protein disruption confers resistance to malarial infection in mice. *Malar J* 2010;9:101.
42. Shankar AH. Nutritional modulation of malaria morbidity and mortality. *J Infect Dis* 2000;182 Suppl 1:S37–53.
43. Mora JR, Iwata M, von Andrian UH. Vitamin effects on the immune system: Vitamins A and D take centre stage. *Nat Rev Immunol* 2008;8:685–98.
44. Jolliffe DA, Griffiths CJ, Martineau AR. Vitamin D in the prevention of acute respiratory infection: Systematic review of clinical studies. *J Steroid Biochem Mol Biol* 2013;136:321–9.
45. Lange N, Litonjua AA, Gibbons FK, Giovannucci E, Christopher KB. Pre-hospital vitamin D concentration, mortality, and bloodstream infection in a hospitalized patient population. *Am J Med* 2013;126:640.e19–27.
46. Leow L, Simpson T, Cursons R, Karalus N, Hancox RJ. Vitamin D, innate immunity and outcomes in community acquired pneumonia. *Respirology* 2011;16:611–6.
47. Smith AD, Botero S, Shea-Donohue T, Urban JF, Jr. The pathogenicity of an enteric *Citrobacter rodentium* infection is enhanced by deficiencies in the antioxidants selenium and vitamin E. *Infect Immun* 2011;79:1471–8.
48. Carvalho LS, Camargos ER, Almeida CT et al. Vitamin E deficiency enhances pathology in acute *Trypanosoma cruzi*–infected rats. *Trans R Soc Trop Med Hyg* 2006;100: 1025–31.
49. Beck MA, Kolbeck PC, Rohr LH, Shi Q, Morris VC, Levander OA. Vitamin E deficiency intensifies the myocardial injury of coxsackievirus B3 infection of mice. *J Nutr* 1994;124:345–58.
50. Graham SM, Baeten JM, Richardson BA et al. Higher pre-infection vitamin E levels are associated with higher mortality in HIV-1-infected Kenyan women: A prospective study. *BMC Infect Dis* 2007;7:63.
51. Portales P, Guerrier T, Clot J et al. Vitamin E supplementation increases the expression of the CCR5 coreceptor in HIV-1 infected subjects. *Clin Nutr* 2004;23:1244–5.
52. Beck MA, Shi Q, Morris VC, Levander OA. Rapid genomic evolution of a non-virulent coxsackievirus B3 in selenium-deficient mice results in selection of identical virulent isolates. *Nat Med* 1995;1:433–6.
53. Beck MA, Nelson HK, Shi Q et al. Selenium deficiency increases the pathology of an influenza virus infection. *Faseb J* 2001;15:1481–3.
54. Nelson HK, Shi Q, Van Dael P et al. Host nutritional selenium status as a driving force for influenza virus mutations. *Faseb J* 2001;15:1846–8.
55. Baum MK, Shor-Posner G, Lai S et al. High risk of HIV-related mortality is associated with selenium deficiency. *J Acquir Immune Defic Syndr Hum Retrovirol* 1997;15: 370–4.
56. Ge K, Yang G. The epidemiology of selenium deficiency in the etiological study of endemic diseases in China. *Am J Clin Nutr* 1993;57:259S–63S.
57. Beck MA, Levander OA, Handy J. Selenium deficiency and viral infection. *J Nutr* 2003;133:1463S–7S.
58. Mocchegiani E, Muzzioli M, Giacconi R. Zinc and immunoresistance to infection in aging: New biological tools. *Trends Pharmacol Sci* 2000;21:205–8.
59. Liu MJ, Bao S, Galvez-Peralta M et al. ZIP8 regulates host defense through zinc-mediated inhibition of NF-kappaB. *Cell Rep* 2013;3:386–400.
60. Li-Ng M, Aloia JF, Pollack S et al. A randomized controlled trial of vitamin D3 supplementation for the prevention of symptomatic upper respiratory tract infections. *Epidemiol Infect* 2009;137:1396–404.

61. Bischoff-Ferrari HA, Dawson-Hughes B, Platz A et al. Effect of high-dosage cholecalciferol and extended physiotherapy on complications after hip fracture: A randomized controlled trial. *Arch Intern Med* 2010;170:813–20.

62. Meydani SN, Meydani M, Blumberg JB et al. Vitamin E supplementation and *in vivo* immune response in healthy elderly subjects. A randomized controlled trial. *JAMA* 1997;277:1380–6.

63. Meydani SN, Leka LS, Fine BC et al. Vitamin E and respiratory tract infections in elderly nursing home residents: A randomized controlled trial. *JAMA* 2004;292:828–36.

64. von Herbay A, Stahl W, Niederau C, Sies H. Vitamin E improves the aminotransferase status of patients suffering from viral hepatitis C: A randomized, double-blind, placebo-controlled study. *Free Radic Res* 1997;27:599–605.

65. Mahmood S, Yamada G, Niiyama G et al. Effect of vitamin E on serum aminotransferase and thioredoxin levels in patients with viral hepatitis C. *Free Radic Res* 2003;37:781–5.

66. Prasad AS, Beck FW, Bao B et al. Zinc supplementation decreases incidence of infections in the elderly: Effect of zinc on generation of cytokines and oxidative stress. *Am J Clin Nutr* 2007;85:837–44.

67. Manzanares W, Biestro A, Torre MH, Galusso F, Facchin G, Hardy G. High-dose selenium reduces ventilator-associated pneumonia and illness severity in critically ill patients with systemic inflammation. *Intensive Care Med* 2011;37:1120–7.

68. Valenta J, Brodska H, Drabek T, Hendl J, Kazda A. High-dose selenium substitution in sepsis: A prospective randomized clinical trial. *Intensive Care Med* 2011;37:808–15.

69. Graat JM, Schouten EG, Kok FJ. Effect of daily vitamin E and multivitamin–mineral supplementation on acute respiratory tract infections in elderly persons: A randomized controlled trial. *JAMA* 2002;288:715–21.

70. Hemila H, Kaprio J, Albanes D, Heinonen OP, Virtamo J. Vitamin C, vitamin E, and beta-carotene in relation to common cold incidence in male smokers. *Epidemiology* 2002;13:32–7.

71. Hemila H, Virtamo J, Albanes D, Kaprio J. Vitamin E and beta-carotene supplementation and hospital-treated pneumonia incidence in male smokers. *Chest* 2004;125:557–65.

72. Avenell A, Cook JA, Maclennan GS, Macpherson GC. Vitamin D supplementation to prevent infections: A sub-study of a randomised placebo-controlled trial in older people (RECORD trial, ISRCTN 51647438). *Age Ageing* 2007;36:574–7.

73. Girodon F, Galan P, Monget AL et al. Impact of trace elements and vitamin supplementation on immunity and infections in institutionalized elderly patients: A randomized controlled trial. MIN. VIT. AOX. geriatric network. *Arch Intern Med* 1999;159:748–54.

74. Avenell A, Campbell MK, Cook JA et al. Effect of multivitamin and multimineral supplements on morbidity from infections in older people (MAVIS trial): Pragmatic, randomised, double blind, placebo controlled trial. *BMJ* 2005;331:324–9.

75. Liu BA, McGeer A, McArthur MA et al. Effect of multivitamin and mineral supplementation on episodes of infection in nursing home residents: A randomized, placebo-controlled study. *J Am Geriatr Soc* 2007;55:35–42.

76. Forster SE, Powers HJ, Foulds GA et al. Improvement in nutritional status reduces the clinical impact of infections in older adults. *J Am Geriatr Soc* 2012;60:1645–54.

77. Chavance M, Herbeth B, Fournier C, Janot C, Vernhes G. Vitamin status, immunity and infections in an elderly population. *Eur J Clin Nutr* 1989;43:827–35.

78. Hemila H, Kaprio J. Subgroup analysis of large trials can guide further research: A case study of vitamin E and pneumonia. *Clin Epidemiol* 2011;3:51–9.

79. Huang TS, Shyu YC, Chen HY et al. Effect of parenteral selenium supplementation in critically ill patients: A systematic review and meta-analysis. *PLoS One* 2013;8:e54431.

80. Hurwitz BE, Klaus JR, Llabre MM et al. Suppression of human immunodeficiency virus type 1 viral load with selenium supplementation: A randomized controlled trial. *Arch Intern Med* 2007;167:148–54.

81. Rahman MJ, Sarker P, Roy SK et al. Effects of zinc supplementation as adjunct therapy on the systemic immune responses in shigellosis. *Am J Clin Nutr* 2005;81:495–502.

82. Bhutta ZA, Black RE, Brown KH et al. Prevention of diarrhea and pneumonia by zinc supplementation in children in developing countries: Pooled analysis of randomized controlled trials. Zinc Investigators' Collaborative Group. *J Pediatr* 1999;135:689–97.

83. Bose A, Coles CL, Gunavathi et al. Efficacy of zinc in the treatment of severe pneumonia in hospitalized children <2 y old. *Am J Clin Nutr* 2006;83:1089–96; quiz 207.

84. Houston S, Haggard J, Williford J Jr, Meserve L, Shewokis P. Adverse effects of large-dose zinc supplementation in an institutionalized older population with pressure ulcers. *J Am Geriatr Soc* 2001;49:1130–2.

16 Future Strategies and Research Directions in Nutrition–Infection Interactions That Will Enhance Human Health

Mohan Pammi, Jesus G. Vallejo, and Steven A. Abrams

CONTENTS

Systems Biology and Nutrition 377
Nutrigenomics 379
Nutritional Immunology 379
Epigenetics in Human Nutrition 381
Dysbiosis, Genetic Variations in Immunity, and Inflammatory Bowel Disease 381
Personalized Nutrition and Nutrigenetics 382
Conclusions 383
References 384

The study of nutrition has progressed from being essentially a study of epidemiology and physiology to discerning the molecular mechanisms for nutrient effects and responses. Macronutrients and micronutrients previously considered as fuel for energy or cofactors, respectively, are now considered potent signals that influence the expression of genes, proteins, and metabolites of the cells, tissues, and ultimately the whole organism. This study of the molecular effects of nutrients has been facilitated significantly by the availability of high-throughput technologies such as transcriptomics (microarrays, whole-exome sequencing, and RNAseq), proteomics, and metabolomics. This concept is depicted in Figure 16.1.

SYSTEMS BIOLOGY AND NUTRITION

Systems biology is a holistic approach where all the cellular responses that can be determined by proteomics, metabolomics, transcriptomics, or other methods are integrated to understand the broad picture of homeostasis in the whole organism [1–4].

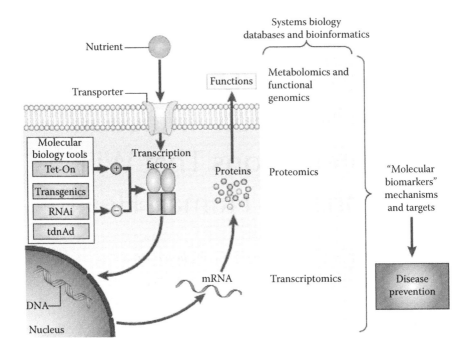

FIGURE 16.1 **(See color insert.)** Nutrigenomics and systems biology in nutrition: "the smart" combination of molecular nutrition and nutrigenomics. Molecular biology tools related to transcriptomics, proteomics, metabolomics, and functional genomics will determine the effects of nutrients, "nutrient signatures." These signatures will enhance the discovery of nutritional biomarkers that relate to personalized or general strategies for disease prevention and assessment of disease risk. These biomarkers may allow early dietary intervention to reverse the onset of diet-related diseases and to regain homeostasis. (Reprinted by permission from McMillan Publishers Ltd., *Nat Rev Genet*, Muller, M. and S. Kersten, Nutrigenomics: Goals and strategies, 4, 4, 315–22, copyright 2003.)

Systems biology emphasizes the interactions of the complex biological networks in the organism, which is diametrically opposite to the reductionist approach where the study is reduced to one individual protein or metabolite. A complex team of experts in cellular biology, bioinformatics, proteomics, statistics, and mathematics try to put together pieces of information that applies to the whole organism. The systems biology approach to nutrition will help us understand the complex interactions of diet–gene–epigenetic influences in the homeostasis of the whole human organism. The availability of high-throughput "omics" technology has facilitated the systems biology approach to a great extent. By identifying biomarkers, we may eventually understand the nutritional process and develop new interventional strategies that target the whole organism. This will lead to a better understanding of how infection and inflammation affect the dietary responses in the organism and vice versa. Another facet of this holistic approach is the possibility of mathematical modeling *in silico* to predict the nutrient–infection interactions with better analysis and integration of data to predict success of interventional strategies [5].

NUTRIGENOMICS

Nutrigenomics describes the impact of nutrition on health status, at the level of gene transcription, protein expression, and metabolism, or understanding the mechanism of action of nutrients, their receptors, and signaling pathways [6–8]. In essence, nutrigenomics is an embodiment and component of the systems biology approach. Nutrients can be viewed as dietary signals to which the cells respond variably in health and disease that results in patterns of cellular gene, protein, and metabolic responses, which can be termed "dietary signatures." The study of these responses at the cellular level is now possible with the use of laser microdissection techniques, where individual cells can be dissected and studied [9,10]. In this context, it will be interesting to understand how infection or inflammation triggered by infection affects these dietary signatures. The complex triad of nutrient, gene, and infection/inflammation is an emerging area of research that needs to be explored more in the future (Figure 16.2). A significant area of interest is how ongoing or persisting inflammation and its mediators predispose to cardiovascular morbidity, diabetes, obesity, and cancer [11]. The ultimate goal would be to alter these dietary or infectious signals to achieve optimum cellular homeostasis and clinical benefit.

NUTRITIONAL IMMUNOLOGY

Immunology and nutrition are two major complex biological systems that often interact, especially in the context of human infections [2]. Immune cells require macronutrients and micronutrients for their sustenance and survival and when deprived during malnutrition states, cause immune dysfunction and predisposition to chronic infections [12,13]. In malnutrition, immune deficiencies include decreased expression of integrins and chemokines and subsequent neutrophil migration [14–17].

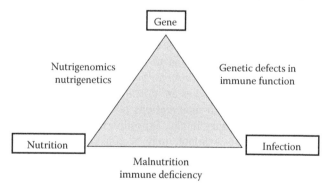

FIGURE 16.2 Gene, nutrition, and infection interactions: Interplay of gene, diet, and infection that influences human health. Nutrigenetics such as SNPs or epigenetic mechanisms may determine an individual's variations in the metabolic response to nutrition. Similarly genetic mechanisms that lead to defects in immune function may predispose to infection. Malnutrition, both undernutrition and excess nutrition, may predispose to immune deficiencies that lead to infection. Infection that leads to poor intake or absorption of nutrients leads to malnutrition completing this triad.

Replenishment of the nutrient deficiency can restore immune function [18–20]. Deprivation of glucose and glutamine to macrophages or neutrophils decreases cytokine production and phagocytosis [21,22].

One example of nutrition affecting the immune response is the role of polyunsaturated fatty acids (PUFAs) in inflammation [23–27]. Ω-6 PUFAs mediate proinflammatory functions such as chemotaxis and neutrophil migration, and production of reactive oxygen species and proinflammatory cytokines [28]. On the contrary, Ω-3 PUFAs are anti-inflammatory and promote wound healing and resolution of inflammation. Competitive inhibition of Ω-6 PUFAs by Ω-3 PUFAs, and hence a decrease in inflammation, has also been noted [29]. In contrast to undernutrition, nutrient excess can activate stress responses and activate inflammation such as those that occur in obesity. High glucose levels and excess extracellular and intracellular free fatty acids may induce cytokine production, including interleukin (IL)-6, IL-18, and tumor necrosis factor-α production by monocytes [30–34].

Immunonutrients that enhance immunity may foster novel preventive strategies against infections, especially those nutrients whose deficiency states are associated with increased infection risk. Deficiency of micronutrients, including minerals and vitamins, may increase susceptibility to infection by causing deficits in immune function [35]. For example, deficiency of the mineral zinc causes deficits in macrophage phagocytosis and intracellular killing [36–38]. Vitamin D (1,25(OH)D3) is another micronutrient involved in immune responses, which also may influence autophagy [39]. Vitamin D deficiency decreases appropriate antimycobacterial host responses [40–42]. Hence, vitamin D supplementation is being explored as an adjunct in the treatment of tuberculosis [43]. Glutamine improves improved neutrophil migration and phagocytosis after parenteral nutrition and glycogen-induced peritonitis in mice and contributes to cellular superoxide production [44,45]. Glutamine may also be beneficial in individuals in a proinflammatory state, such as after sepsis or after surgery [46,47]. The role of immunonutrients, namely glutamine, arginine, and nucleotides, in the perinatal period has been reviewed elsewhere [48].

Another important area of research is the discovery of biomarkers to identify both nutrient deficiency and excess and to predict infection risk resulting from an immunodeficient state. A biomarker can be defined as a molecule that can be measured objectively and evaluated as an indicator of normal biological or pathological processes or responses to interventions [49–53]. Important biomarkers in nutrition research relate to dietary intake, exposure, nutrient deficiencies, and bioactivity. Biomarkers currently available may be considered as recovery biomarkers when they are recovered from urine or feces (e.g., radiolabeled isotopes) or concentration biomarkers when they are estimated in body fluids such as plasma, serum, or blood (e.g., retinol in the serum). However, to evaluate disease risk and its association with future clinical outcomes, a complex set of biomarkers is likely to be necessary. Existing nutritional biomarkers include serum retinol, homocysteine levels, and vitamin D but more are needed to understand the complex role of nutrition in human health. Changes in nutritional biomarkers in infectious and/or inflammatory states also need to be explored. Metabolic profiling using state-of-the-art metabolomics has the potential to expedite biomarker discovery in human diseases [54].

EPIGENETICS IN HUMAN NUTRITION

Epigenetics refers to the study of a group of biological processes (DNA methylation, chromatin remodeling, and regulation of gene expression by noncoding RNA) that induce changes in gene expression without altering the DNA sequence and that can be inherited both mitotically and meotically [55–57]. Epigenetic changes are reversible by endogenous and exogenous stimuli and referred to as meta-stable, unlike genetic mutations that are nonreversible. Epigenetic mechanisms may be responsible for diseases associated with cancer, cardiovascular diseases, and other diseases associated with the aging process. Nutrients involved in one-carbon metabolism (e.g., folate, vitamin B12, vitamin B6, riboflavin, methionine, choline, and betaine) are involved in DNA methylation by regulating the levels of the universal methyl donor *S*-adenosyl-methionine and methyltransferase inhibitor *S*-adenosyl-homocysteine [55]. Retinoic acid, resveratrol, curcumin, sulforaphane, and tea polyphenols may alter the levels of *S*-adenosylmethionine and *S*-adenosylhomocysteine or direct the enzymes that catalyze DNA methylation and histone modifications [58]. One example may be the response to caloric restriction and longevity and recent evidence pointing to DNA methylation in specific loci related to delayed aging and longevity [59]. Epigenetic alterations in the perinatal period (the period of maximum plasticity) may contribute to developmental programming that lasts throughout life, e.g., low-birth-weight babies are at risk for later development of hypertension in adulthood [54,56,57]. In adulthood, obesity, predisposition, weight loss, and clinical outcomes have been repeatedly shown to be associated with changes in epigenetic patterns [56,60]. However, explorations of epigenetic processes in many areas of human nutrition are lacking and remain a prime priority for future research.

DYSBIOSIS, GENETIC VARIATIONS IN IMMUNITY, AND INFLAMMATORY BOWEL DISEASE

The gut microbiota plays a significant role in intestinal mucosal immunity and secondarily on systemic immunity, to prevent colonization with pathogenic bacteria and promote health. Gut dysbiosis occurs when the microbiome is disturbed by antibiotics or other stressors and may lead to human disease. The concept of enterotypes, patterns of microbiota, in humans has been suggested by Arumugam et al. based on a study from a European cohort [61]. Humans can be clustered into two or three distinct types based on their gut microbial communities. If subjects can be classified into simple enterotypes, then clinical studies can proceed to group each enterotype to explore scientific questions. Similar enterotypes were suggested by the Human Microbiome Project at the genus level; however, variation at the subgenus level can potentially confound enterotypes and the appropriate level of taxonomic resolution for metagenome association studies remains an open question [62,63].

A classic example for the interplay of nutrition, inflammation, and intestinal dysbiosis is inflammatory bowel disease (IBD), which is characterized by chronic inflammation of the gastrointestinal tract (Crohn's disease and ulcerative colitis) [64–66]. Genome-wide association studies (GWAS) have identified 99 different variants associated with IBD. Many variants involved the innate immunity pattern recognition receptor NOD2, autophagy genes (*ATG16L1* and *IRGM*), and IL23/IL17 signaling. IBD is treated with anti-inflammatory agents (mesalazine and steroids) or by dietary modifications. Fecal microbiota transplant, which favors the reestablishment of beneficial microbiota from healthy donors, has been efficacious in ameliorating disease, suggesting a role for dysbiosis in the pathogenesis of IBD [67–69].

PERSONALIZED NUTRITION AND NUTRIGENETICS

Nutrigenetics is the study of the effect of genetic variations on nutrient–gene interactions [70–72]. Nutritional requirements and responses vary from individual to individual due to genetic variability, and the most commonly studied variation is the single nucleotide polymorphisms (SNPs). SNPs are essentially single point mutations that occur at a frequency of ≥1% in the human population [73]. More than 16 million SNPs have been identified in humans thus far (http://www.ncbi.nlm.nih.gov/SNP/index.html). Every person has about 50,000 SNPs in the genome that may contribute to the interindividual variations in metabolic responses. Methods to understand this interindividual variation include DNA microarrays, which are readily available and less expensive than before. GWAS use genetic variations such as SNPs and the human genomic data, using dense gene arrays to identify allele frequency differences between groups (http://www.genome.gov/gwastudies). The goal is to understand human biological variability resulting from genetic and epigenetic variations that influence nutritional and immunological health and predispose to infections (Figure 16.3). A typical example of this GWAS approach is the study of adiponectin, which is decreased in obesity, type 2 diabetes, metabolic syndrome, and other diseases [74–79]. An approach that combines GWAS with metabolomics and stratification of individuals into genetically determined metabolotypes has also been explored [4,80,81]. Similarly, dietary requirements of choline vary; men and postmenopausal women develop liver and muscle dysfunction when deficient in dietary choline [82,83]. Premenopausal women have estrogen that induces the pathway for endogenous synthesis of choline (phosphatidyl-ethanolamine-*N*-methyltransferase [PEMT]) and do not seem to develop choline deficiency except when they have SNPs in PEMT [82–84].

Several genetic polymorphisms may have an effect on the nutritional and metabolic status of the individual, e.g., folate metabolism, iron homeostasis, bone, lipid metabolism, and immune function [85–88]. Although genotypes may influence nutrient–gene interactions, in most situations, little evidence exists for nutritional interventions that can modify nutrient–gene interactions for health benefits. The current evidence and ethics of this approach has recently been summarized by Gorman et al. [89].

The most widely studied genetic polymorphism and metabolic variability is the *MTHFR* (methyl-tetrahydrofolate reductase) gene C677T polymorphism and its effect on folate metabolism and homocysteine levels [90,91]. The MTHFR enzyme in 677T individuals has only 35% of enzymatic activity, and low dietary folate leads to high homocysteine levels. Adequate folate (400–600 μg/day) supplementation is associated with lower homocysteine levels. Although a high homocysteine level has been recognized as a cardiovascular risk factor, a causal relation between decrease

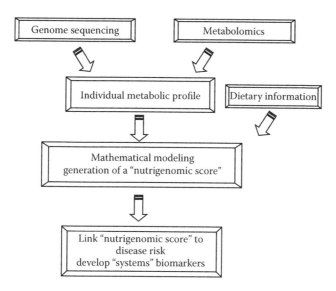

FIGURE 16.3 Nutrigenomic biomarker selection. The scheme illustrates an approach in which various nutrigenomic methods could be used to incorporate genetic, metabolic, and dietary information for an individual so as to assess health status or disease risk. Integrating these different data could produce a "systems" biomarker that is based on multiple interrelated measurements. (Reprinted by permission from McMillan Publishers Ltd., *Eur J Clin Nutr*, Hesketh, J., Personalised nutrition: How far has nutrigenomics progressed? 67, 430–5, copyright 2013.)

in homocysteine levels by folate supplementation and improvement in cardiovascular morbidity is yet to be proven [91–93]. In addition, secondary prevention using folate supplementation in elderly individuals did not show any benefit [94].

Another example is the well-studied gene–diet interaction in the prevention of lung cancer by intake of cruciferous vegetables and the genes *GSTT1* and *GSTM1*, which are involved in elimination of isothiocyanates [95]. Cruciferous vegetables were protective in *GSTT1*- and *GSTM1*-null individuals, but not in individuals who have working copies of both these genes [95]. Other authors have demonstrated gene–diet–interactions that decrease DNA damage and decrease prostate cancer risk [96–99].

CONCLUSIONS

Personalized nutrition requires an understanding of many facets of an individual and includes nutrigenetics, ethnicity, sex, health status, and age. A scheme to develop personalized dietary requirements based on genetic susceptibility to disease is proposed by Hesketh et al. (Figure 16.4) [100]. There is evidence that genotype-based personalized dietary advice may promote better compliance than standard recommendations [89]. Dietary recommendations for micronutrients and macronutrients are based on observational epidemiological data that do not consider the individual GDP–genetic metabolotype. As our understanding of nutrigenomics increases,

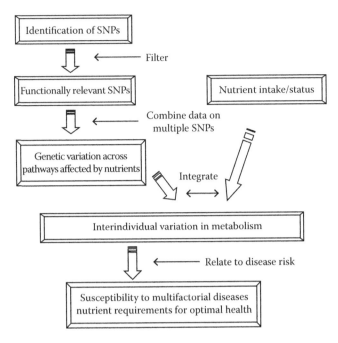

FIGURE 16.4 Scheme illustrating the need to (i) focus on SNPs with known functional effects, (ii) consider multiple variants within relevant biochemical pathways, (iii) integrate both genetic and dietary information, and (iv) then relate both genetic and dietary factors to disease risk. (Reprinted by permission from McMillan Publishers Ltd., *Eur J Clin Nutr*, Hesketh, J., Personalised nutrition: How far has nutrigenomics progressed? 67, 430–5, copyright 2013.)

it may be possible to eventually make specific dietary recommendations for specific populations based on a given GDP [80]. More research and evidence will be needed before personalized nutrition based on nutrigenetics can be recommended or adopted as a public health policy. Given our current understanding of nutrigenomics, it is almost certain that our learning curve will be extremely steep for the foreseeable future.

REFERENCES

1. Kang, J.X., Nutrigenomics and systems biology. *J Nutrigenet Nutrigenom*, 2012. **5**(6): I–II.
2. Afacan, N.J., C.D. Fjell, and R.E. Hancock, A systems biology approach to nutritional immunology—Focus on innate immunity. *Mol Aspects Med*, 2012. **33**(1): 14–25.
3. From systems biology and functional genomics to personalized health. 5th Biologie Prospective Santorini Conference, Island of Santorini, Greece, September 30–October 2, 2010. *Drug Metabol Drug Interact*, 2011. **26**(1): 41–2.
4. Nicholson, J.K. and J.C. Lindon, Systems biology: Metabonomics. *Nature*, 2008. **455**(7216): 1054–6.
5. Yan, Q., Bioinformatics for transporter pharmacogenomics and systems biology: Data integration and modeling with UML. *Methods Mol Biol*, 2010. **637**: 23–45.

6. Bouchard, C. and J.M. Ordovas, Fundamentals of nutrigenetics and nutrigenomics. *Prog Mol Biol Transl Sci*, 2012. **108**: 1–15.

7. Fenech, M. et al., Nutrigenetics and nutrigenomics: Viewpoints on the current status and applications in nutrition research and practice. *J Nutrigenet Nutrigenomics*, 2011. **4**(2): 69–89.

8. Muller, M. and S. Kersten, Nutrigenomics: Goals and strategies. *Nat Rev Genet*, 2003. **4**(4): 315–22.

9. Coop, R.L. and I. Kyriazakis, Nutrition–parasite interaction. *Vet Parasitol*, 1999. **84**(3–4): 187–204.

10. Else, K.J., Have gastrointestinal nematodes outwitted the immune system? *Parasite Immunol*, 2005. **27**(10–11): 407–15.

11. Jackson, J.A. et al., Gastrointestinal nematode infection is associated with variation in innate immune responsiveness. *Microbes Infect*, 2006. **8**(2): 487–92.

12. Cunningham-Rundles, S., D.F. McNeeley, and A. Moon, Mechanisms of nutrient modulation of the immune response. *J Allergy Clin Immunol*, 2005. **115**(6): 1119–28; quiz 1129.

13. Russell, B.J. et al., Evaluation of hospitalisation for indigenous children with malnutrition living in central Australia. *Aust J Rural Health*, 2004. **12**(5): 187–91.

14. Bhaskaram, P., Micronutrient malnutrition, infection, and immunity: An overview. *Nutr Rev*, 2002. **60**(5 Pt 2): S40–5.

15. Buys, H. et al., The role of nutrition and micronutrients in paediatric HIV infection. *SADJ*, 2002. **57**(11): 454–6.

16. Duggal, S., T.D. Chugh, and A.K. Duggal, HIV and malnutrition: Effects on immune system. *Clin Dev Immunol*, 2012. **2012**: 784740.

17. Goto, R., C.G. Mascie-Taylor, and P.G. Lunn, Impact of intestinal permeability, inflammation status and parasitic infections on infant growth faltering in rural Bangladesh. *Br J Nutr*, 2009. **101**(10): 1509–16.

18. High, K.P., Nutritional strategies to boost immunity and prevent infection in elderly individuals. *Clin Infect Dis*, 2001. **33**(11): 1892–900.

19. Katona, P. and J. Katona-Apte, The interaction between nutrition and infection. *Clin Infect Dis*, 2008. **46**(10): 1582–8.

20. Thomas, A.M. and S.C. Mkandawire, The impact of nutrition on physiologic changes in persons who have HIV. *Nurs Clin North Am*, 2006. **41**(3): 455–68, viii.

21. Kafwembe, E.M. et al., The vitamin A status of Zambian children in a community of vitamin A supplementation and sugar fortification strategies as measured by the modified relative dose response (MRDR) test. *Int J Vitam Nutr Res*, 2009. **79**(1): 40–7.

22. Hughes, S. and P. Kelly, Interactions of malnutrition and immune impairment, with specific reference to immunity against parasites. *Parasite Immunol*, 2006. **28**(11): 577–88.

23. Malafaia, G., Protein–energy malnutrition as a risk factor for visceral leishmaniasis: A review. *Parasite Immunol*, 2009. **31**(10): 587–96.

24. Calder, P.C. et al., Lipid emulsions in parenteral nutrition of intensive care patients: Current thinking and future directions. *Intensive Care Med*, 2010. **36**(5): 735–49.

25. Botero-Garces, J.H. et al., Giardia intestinalis and nutritional status in children participating in the complementary nutrition program, Antioquia, Colombia, May to October 2006. *Rev Inst Med Trop Sao Paulo*, 2009. **51**(3): 155–62.

26. Stephenson, L.S., M.C. Latham, and E.A. Ottesen, Malnutrition and parasitic helminth infections. *Parasitology*, 2000. **121 Suppl**: S23–38.

27. Amare, B. et al., Micronutrient levels and nutritional status of school children living in Northwest Ethiopia. *Nutr J*, 2012. **11**: 108.

28. Calder, P.C., Polyunsaturated fatty acids and inflammatory processes: New twists in an old tale. *Biochimie*, 2009. **91**(6): 791–5.

29. Hesham, M.S., A.B. Edariah, and M. Norhayati, Intestinal parasitic infections and micronutrient deficiency: A review. *Med J Malaysia*, 2004. **59**(2): 284–93.
30. Esposito, K. et al., Inflammatory cytokine concentrations are acutely increased by hyperglycemia in humans: Role of oxidative stress. *Circulation*, 2002. **106**(16): 2067–72.
31. Morohoshi, M. et al., Glucose-dependent interleukin 6 and tumor necrosis factor production by human peripheral blood monocytes *in vitro*. *Diabetes*, 1996. **45**(7): 954–9.
32. Ozcan, U. et al., Chemical chaperones reduce ER stress and restore glucose homeostasis in a mouse model of type 2 diabetes. *Science*, 2006. **313**(5790): 1137–40.
33. Schaeffler, A. et al., Fatty acid-induced induction of Toll-like receptor-4/nuclear factor-kappaB pathway in adipocytes links nutritional signalling with innate immunity. *Immunology*, 2009. **126**(2): 233–45.
34. Shi, H. et al., TLR4 links innate immunity and fatty acid-induced insulin resistance. *J Clin Invest*, 2006. **116**(11): 3015–25.
35. Shankar, A.H. and A.S. Prasad, Zinc and immune function: The biological basis of altered resistance to infection. *Am J Clin Nutr*, 1998. **68**(2 Suppl): 447S–63S.
36. Caulfield, L.E., S.A. Richard, and R.E. Black, Undernutrition as an underlying cause of malaria morbidity and mortality in children less than five years old. *Am J Trop Med Hyg*, 2004. **71**(2 Suppl): 55–63.
37. Grommes, J. et al., Balancing zinc deficiency leads to an improved healing of colon anastomosis in rats. *Int J Colorectal Dis*, 2011. **26**(3): 295–301.
38. Sharir, H. et al., Zinc released from injured cells is acting via the Zn^{2+}-sensing receptor, ZnR, to trigger signaling leading to epithelial repair. *J Biol Chem*, 2010. **285**(34): 26097–106.
39. Hewison, M., Antibacterial effects of vitamin D. *Nat Rev Endocrinol*, 2011. **7**(6): 337–45.
40. Liu, P.T. et al., Cutting edge: Vitamin D-mediated human antimicrobial activity against *Mycobacterium tuberculosis* is dependent on the induction of cathelicidin. *J Immunol*, 2007. **179**(4): 2060–3.
41. Yang, C.S. et al., NADPH oxidase 2 interaction with TLR2 is required for efficient innate immune responses to mycobacteria via cathelicidin expression. *J Immunol*, 2009. **182**(6): 3696–705.
42. Yu, J. et al., Host defense peptide LL-37, in synergy with inflammatory mediator IL-1beta, augments immune responses by multiple pathways. *J Immunol*, 2007. **179**(11): 7684–91.
43. Nursyam, E.W., Z. Amin, and C.M. Rumende, The effect of vitamin D as supplementary treatment in patients with moderately advanced pulmonary tuberculous lesion. *Acta Med Indones*, 2006. **38**(1): 3–5.
44. Ikeda, S. et al., Glutamine improves impaired cellular exudation and polymorphonuclear neutrophil phagocytosis induced by total parenteral nutrition after glycogen-induced murine peritonitis. *Shock*, 2003. **19**(1): 50–4.
45. Pithon-Curi, T.C. et al., Glutamine plays a role in superoxide production and the expression of p47phox, p22phox and gp91phox in rat neutrophils. *Clin Sci (Lond)*, 2002. **103**(4): 403–8.
46. Hu, Y.M. et al., Glutamine administration ameliorates sepsis-induced kidney injury by downregulating the high-mobility group box protein-1-mediated pathway in mice. *Am J Physiol Renal Physiol*, 2012. **302**(1): F150–8.
47. Calder, P.C., Immunonutrition in surgical and critically ill patients. *Br J Nutr*, 2007. **98 Suppl 1**: S133–9.
48. Huang, Y., X.M. Shao, and J. Neu, Immunonutrients and neonates. *Eur J Pediatr*, 2003. **162**(3): 122–8.
49. Ganesh, V. and N.S. Hettiarachchy, Nutriproteomics: A promising tool to link diet and diseases in nutritional research. *Biochim Biophys Acta*, 2012. **1824**(10): 1107–17.

50. Rubio-Aliaga, I., S. Kochhar, and I. Silva-Zolezzi, Biomarkers of nutrient bioactivity and efficacy: A route toward personalized nutrition. *J Clin Gastroenterol*, 2012. **46**(7): 545–54.

51. Kussmann, M., A. Panchaud, and M. Affolter, Proteomics in nutrition: Status quo and outlook for biomarkers and bioactives. *J Proteome Res*, 2010. **9**(10): 4876–87.

52. Kussmann, M. and S. Blum, OMICS-derived targets for inflammatory gut disorders: Opportunities for the development of nutrition related biomarkers. *Endocr Metab Immune Disord Drug Targets*, 2007. **7**(4): 271–87.

53. Biomarkers and surrogate endpoints: Preferred definitions and conceptual framework. *Clin Pharmacol Ther*, 2001. **69**(3): 89–95.

54. Zeisel, S.H. et al., Highlights of the 2012 Research Workshop: Using nutrigenomics and metabolomics in clinical nutrition research. *JPEN J Parenter Enteral Nutr*, 2013. **37**(2): 190–200.

55. Park, L.K., S. Friso, and S.W. Choi, Nutritional influences on epigenetics and age-related disease. *Proc Nutr Soc*, 2012. **71**(1): 75–83.

56. Milagro, F.I. et al., Dietary factors, epigenetic modifications and obesity outcomes: Progresses and perspectives. *Mol Aspects Med*, 2012. **34**: 782–812.

57. Gomes, M.V. and R.A. Waterland, Individual epigenetic variation: When, why, and so what? *Nestle Nutr Workshop Ser Pediatr Program*, 2008. **62**: 141–50; discussion 151–5.

58. Afman, L.A. and M. Muller, Human nutrigenomics of gene regulation by dietary fatty acids. *Prog Lipid Res*, 2012. **51**(1): 63–70.

59. Li, Y., M. Daniel, and T.O. Tollefsbol, Epigenetic regulation of caloric restriction in aging. *BMC Med*, 2011. **9**: 98.

60. Niculescu, M.D. and D.S. Lupu, Nutritional influence on epigenetics and effects on longevity. *Curr Opin Clin Nutr Metab Care*, 2011. **14**(1): 35–40.

61. Arumugam, M. et al., Enterotypes of the human gut microbiome. *Nature*, 2011. **473**(7346): 174–80.

62. Stower, H., Microbiology: The human microbiome project. *Nat Rev Genet*, 2012. **13**(8): 518.

63. Human Microbiome Project Consortium. Structure, function and diversity of the healthy human microbiome. *Nature*, 2012. **486**(7402): 207–14.

64. Gruber, L. et al., Nutrigenomics and nutrigenetics in inflammatory bowel diseases. *J Clin Gastroenterol*, 2012. **46**(9): 735–47.

65. Neuman, M.G. and R.M. Nanau, Inflammatory bowel disease: Role of diet, microbiota, life style. *Transl Res*, 2012. **160**(1): 29–44.

66. Ferguson, L.R., Nutrigenomics and inflammatory bowel diseases. *Expert Rev Clin Immunol*, 2010. **6**(4): 573–83.

67. Brandt, L.J., *American Journal of Gastroenterology* Lecture: Intestinal microbiota and the role of fecal microbiota transplant (FMT) in treatment of *C. difficile* infection. *Am J Gastroenterol*, 2013. **108**(2): 177–85.

68. Weissman, J.S. and W. Coyle, Stool transplants: Ready for prime time? *Curr Gastroenterol Rep*, 2012. **14**(4): 313–6.

69. Gough, E., H. Shaikh, and A.R. Manges, Systematic review of intestinal microbiota transplantation (fecal bacteriotherapy) for recurrent *Clostridium difficile* infection. *Clin Infect Dis*, 2011. **53**(10): 994–1002.

70. Phillips, C.M., Nutrigenetics and metabolic disease: Current status and implications for personalised nutrition. *Nutrients*, 2013. **5**(1): 32–57.

71. Farhud, D. and M. Zarif Yeganeh, Nutrigenomics and nutrigenetics. *Iran J Public Health*, 2010. **39**(4): 1–14.

72. Rimbach, G. and A.M. Minihane, Nutrigenetics and personalised nutrition: How far have we progressed and are we likely to get there? *Proc Nutr Soc*, 2009. **68**(2): 162–72.

73. Frazer, K.A. et al., Human genetic variation and its contribution to complex traits. *Nat Rev Genet*, 2009. **10**(4): 241–51.

74. Chung, C.M. et al., A genome-wide association study reveals a quantitative trait locus of adiponectin on CDH13 that predicts cardiometabolic outcomes. *Diabetes*, 2011. **60**(9): 2417–23.

75. Jee, S.H. et al., Adiponectin concentrations: A genome-wide association study. *Am J Hum Genet*, 2010. **87**(4): 545–52.

76. Wu, Y. et al., Genome-wide association study for adiponectin levels in Filipino women identifies CDH13 and a novel uncommon haplotype at KNG1-ADIPOQ. *Hum Mol Genet*, 2010. **19**(24): 4955–64.

77. Heid, I.M. et al., Clear detection of ADIPOQ locus as the major gene for plasma adiponectin: Results of genome-wide association analyses including 4659 European individuals. *Atherosclerosis*, 2010. **208**(2): 412–20.

78. Richards, J.B. et al., A genome-wide association study reveals variants in ARL15 that influence adiponectin levels. *PLoS Genet*, 2009. **5**(12): e1000768.

79. Ling, H. et al., Genome-wide linkage and association analyses to identify genes influencing adiponectin levels: The GEMS Study. *Obesity (Silver Spring)*, 2009. **17**(4): 737–44.

80. Collino, S. et al., Nutritional metabonomics: An approach to promote personalized health and wellness. *Chimia (Aarau)*, 2011. **65**(6): 396–9.

81. Rezzi, S. et al., Nutritional metabonomics: Applications and perspectives. *J Proteome Res*, 2007. **6**(2): 513–25.

82. Zeisel, S.H., Nutritional genomics: Defining the dietary requirement and effects of choline. *J Nutr*, 2011. **141**(3): 531–4.

83. Zeisel, S.H., Nutrigenomics and metabolomics will change clinical nutrition and public health practice: Insights from studies on dietary requirements for choline. *Am J Clin Nutr*, 2007. **86**(3): 542–8.

84. Corbin, K.D. and S.H. Zeisel, The nutrigenetics and nutrigenomics of the dietary requirement for choline. *Prog Mol Biol Transl Sci*, 2012. **108**: 159–77.

85. Lattka, E. et al., Genetic variations in polyunsaturated fatty acid metabolism—Implications for child health? *Ann Nutr Metab*, 2012. **60 Suppl 3**: 8–17.

86. Vanden Heuvel, J.P., Nutrigenomics and nutrigenetics of omega3 polyunsaturated fatty acids. *Prog Mol Biol Transl Sci*, 2012. **108**: 75–112.

87. Garcia-Rios, A. et al., Nutrigenetics of the lipoprotein metabolism. *Mol Nutr Food Res*, 2012. **56**(1): 171–83.

88. Davis, C.D. and J.A. Milner, Nutrigenomics, vitamin D, and cancer prevention. *J Nutrigenet Nutrigenomics*, 2011. **4**(1): 1–11.

89. Gorman, U. et al., Do we know enough? A scientific and ethical analysis of the basis for genetic-based personalized nutrition. *Genes Nutr*, 2013. **8**: 373–81.

90. Williams, K.T. and K.L. Schalinske, Homocysteine metabolism and its relation to health and disease. *Biofactors*, 2010. **36**(1): 19–24.

91. Collaboration, H.-L.T., Dose-dependent effects of folic acid on blood concentrations of homocysteine: A meta-analysis of the randomized trials. *Am J Clin Nutr*, 2005. **82**(4): 806–12.

92. Wald, D.S. et al., Folic acid, homocysteine, and cardiovascular disease: Judging causality in the face of inconclusive trial evidence. *BMJ*, 2006. **333**(7578): 1114–7.

93. Wald, D.S. et al., Randomized trial of folic acid supplementation and serum homocysteine levels. *Arch Intern Med*, 2001. **161**(5): 695–700.

94. Wald, D.S., A. Kasturiratne, and M. Simmonds, Serum homocysteine and dementia: Meta-analysis of eight cohort studies including 8669 participants. *Alzheimers Dement*, 2011. **7**(4): 412–7.

95. Brennan, P. et al., Effect of cruciferous vegetables on lung cancer in patients strati-fied by genetic status: A Mendelian randomisation approach. *Lancet*, 2005. **366**(9496): 1558–60.
96. Fenech, M., Nutrition and genome health. *Forum Nutr*, 2007. **60**: 49–65.
97. Steinbrecher, A. et al., Dietary glucosinolate intake, polymorphisms in selected bio-transformation enzymes, and risk of prostate cancer. *Cancer Epidemiol Biomarkers Prev*, 2010. **19**(1): 135–43.
98. Steinbrecher, A. et al., Effects of selenium status and polymorphisms in selenoprotein genes on prostate cancer risk in a prospective study of European men. *Cancer Epidemiol Biomarkers Prev*, 2010. **19**(11): 2958–68.
99. Lampe, J.W. et al., Modulation of human glutathione *S*-transferases by botanically defined vegetable diets. *Cancer Epidemiol Biomarkers Prev*, 2000. **9**(8): 787–93.
100. Hesketh, J., Personalised nutrition: How far has nutrigenomics progressed? *Eur J Clin Nutr*, 2013. **67**: 430–5.

Index

Page numbers followed by f and t indicate figures and tables, respectively.

A

Abacavir, 129t, 143t, 149t
Absorption
    of drugs, 113t, 117, 120
    of nutrients, 259
Acetate, 253
Acidic beverages, 138
Acquired immune system, 82
Acquired immunodeficiency syndrome (AIDS),
        65, 188
Acquired nutritional deficiencies, 348–351
Acrodermatitis enteropathica (AE) and zinc
        deficiency, 276–277
Acyclovir, 132t
Adaptive immune system, 342
Adenosine triphosphate binding cassette (ABC),
        114
Adipocytes, 18
Adiponectin, 21
Adipose tissue in obesity, 19
Adiposity and overweight/obesity. *See also*
        Infection-nutrition interaction
    and immune function, 71–72
    increased, 73
Adolescence and puberty, nutrition in, 8–9. *See
        also* Nutrition in human health and
        disease
Adolescents, 340
Adrenergic receptors, 25
Age on immune system. *See also* Diet and
        immunity
    immune response
        changes with aging, 24
        in neonates, 23–24
        stress, 24–25
Aging and nutrient-infection interactions
    immunological changes in elderly
        aging and innate immunity, 360–361
        T cells and aging, 361–362
    infection on nutritional status, 363
    infectious diseases in elderly, 360
    nutrient supplementation/infectious diseases
        in elderly
        multivitamin/multimineral supplement, 373
        selenium supplementation, 371–372
        vitamin D supplementation, 366

vitamin E supplementation, 366, 370–371
zinc supplementation, 372–373
    nutritional status in elderly, 362–363
    nutritional status on host defense against
        infection
        selenium, 365
        vitamin D, 363–364
        vitamin E, 364–365
        zinc, 365
    overview, 359–360
AIDS-related deaths, 155
    children, 158
Alanine aminotransferase (ALT), 371
Albendazole, 126t
α-lipoic acid, 21
Allogenic hematopoietic stem cell
        transplantation, 269
Alpha-Tocopherol Beta-Carotene (ATBC) Cancer
        Prevention Study, 370
Amantadine, 132t
Amino acid (AA), 341, 349, 351
Aminoglycosides, 120, 122t, 139
Amniotic fluid, 290
Amoebiasis, 236
Amoxicillin/clavulanic acid, 122t
Amphotericin B, 125t
Amprenavir, 127t
Anabolic block, 191
Anemia, 5, 7, 8, 42, 200, 261
    hemoglobin and, 165–166
Angular cheilitis, 276
Animal studies, undernutrition, 183
Anorexia nervosa, 9
Antenatal supplementation, 339
Anthelmintics, 126t
Anthropometric indices, 66
Anthropometry, 163–165
Antibiotics, 116, 122t, 136, 253. *See also* Gut
        microbiome in nutrition
    use of, 6–7
Antifungals, 125t
Antigen presentation, efficient, 26–27. *See also*
        Diet and immunity
Antigen-presenting cell (APC), 23, 26
Anti-infectives
    agents, 44, 133t
    examples, 113t

Anti-inflammatory hormone, 21
Antimalarials, 126t
Antimycobacterial therapy, 211
Antioxidant micronutrients and trace elements,
        323–324
Antioxidants, 28
    dietary. *See* Dietary antioxidants
    endogenous and exogenous, 85t
    and immune functions, 88t
    natural, in foods, 97–99
    protective role of, 84–87, 85t, 86f. *See also*
            Oxidative stress and inflammation
    vitamins, 317
Antiprotozoals, 127t
Antiretroviral therapy (ART), 144, 145, 153, 154
    heterogeneous or unspecified, 159, 162, 164
Anti-*Toxoplasma* compound, 98
Antitubercular agents, 131
Antivirals, 132t
Appetite, 348
    alterations in, 142–144, 143t
Arginine, 316t, 318–319
Artemether and lumefantrine, 126t
Arterial oxygenation, 321
Artificial nutrition. *See* Immunonutrients
Ascariasis, 235–236
Ascorbic acid, 89, 111t, 210
Aspartate aminotransferase (AST), 371
Atazanavir, 127t
Atovaquone, 127t
Autoimmune enteropathy (AIE). *See also* Enteric
            syndromes
    and immune dysregulation,
            polyendocrinopathy, enteropathy
            X-linked (IPEX) syndrome, 265–267
    treatment, 268–269
    type 2, 267, 268f
    type 3 (without or with extraintestinal
            manifestations), 268
Autoimmunity, 20
Azithromycin, 113

B

Baby Friendly Hospital Initiative, 4
Bacille Calmette–Guerin (BCG) vaccination,
        183
Bacillus subtilis, 295
Bacterial overgrowth, 138
Bacteroidaceae, 250
Bacteroides enterotype, 251
Bacteroides fragilis, 292
Bacteroides thetaiotaomicron, 296
Bacteroidetes, 292
B-cell homeostasis, 52
Beverages on drug bioavailability, 137–138
Bifidobacterium lactis, 299

Bile acid biotransformation, 291
Bile acids, 291
Binding proteins, 117
Biomarker, 31
    defined, 382
Birth outcomes, 165
Birth weight, 339
B-lymphocyte development and function, 48
Body mass index (BMI), 3, 11, 71, 182, 186
Bone deficits, 272
Bone health, 50
Bone marrow transplantation, 269
Borage oil, 322
Bovine colostrum, 30
Brain-derived neurotrophic factor (BDNF), 294
Branched-chain amino acids, 316t
Breast cancer therapy, 31
Breast-feeding, 4, 339
Butyrate, 253

C

Cachexia, 342–344
Calcitriol, 206
Calcium, 3
    homeostasis, 50
    supplementation, 139
Caloric restriction (CR), 28
Campylobacteraceae, 250
Campylobacterales, 252
Cancer cell proliferation, 22f
Carbohydrates, 111t, 134
β-Carotene, 88t, 90t, 92, 166
Case-control studies, undernutrition, 184–185
Case series, undernutrition, 184
Caspofungin, 125t
Catechins, 98, 99
Catecholamine, 25
Cathelicidin, 51
Catheter-related blood stream infection (CRBSI),
        275
Celiac disease (CD), 259–263, 260t, 261f, 261t.
            See also Enteric syndromes
        diseases and syndromes, 260t
        extraintestinal manifestation of, 261
Cell-mediated immunity, 40, 41
Cell membranes, 84
Cells and processes in nutrition, 18–19, 19t
Cell-surface chemokine receptor (CCR9), 45
Cellular immunity
        vitamin A and, 45–46
        vitamin D and, 51–52
Cellular iron, 96
Central venous catheters (CVC), 274
Cephalosporins, 122t, 139
Chemosensory nerves, 142
Chemotherapy, 191

Chest x-ray (CXR), 184
Children
    and adolescents, growth and development, 340
    HIV transmission, 163
Chloramphenicol, 122t
Chloroquine phosphate, 126t
Chromium supplementation, 169
Chronic diseases and long-term health outcomes,
    169–170
Cidofovir, 132t
Ciprofloxacin, 135
Clindamycin, 122t
Clinical morbidities and assessments. *See
    also* HIV and micronutrient
    supplementation
    chronic diseases and long-term health
        outcomes, 169–170
    clinical indicators, signs, symptoms, 170
    diarrhea, 167–169
Clofazimine, 122t, 133t
Clostridium difficile, 274
Clostridium difficile infections (CDI), 254
Cochrane database review, 239
Cochrane Pregnancy and Childbirth Group's
    Trials Register, 9
Cochrane systematic review, 7, 10
Cocoa flavonoids, 99
Cohort studies, undernutrition, 184
Colonic lesions, 267
Colostrum, 29
Colostrum-supplemented diets, 30
Comfort feedings for patient, 12
Commensal bacteria, 293
Commensal organisms, 292
Communication, 293
Compensatory anti-inflammatory response
    syndrome (CARS), 312
Complete nutrition, 27
Concomitant iron deficiency, 262
Confidence interval (CI), 7
Consumption, for tuberculosis, 65
Copper, 88t, 94t, 97, 237t
Copper deficiency, 97, 262
Cotrimoxazole prophylaxis, 274
Coxsackievirus, 93, 365
Coxsackievirus infection, 68
Critical illness stress-induced immune
    suppression (CRISIS), 351
Cruciferous vegetables, 385
Cutaneous lesions, 266
Cycloserine, 131

D

Daily food supplement, 167
Dairy products, 137
Dapsone, 122t

Deaths in elderly, 360
Debility, 12
Delavirdine, 130t
Delayed-type hypersensitivity (DTH), 188
Dendritic cell (DC), 23, 51, 295
Dermatitis, 266
Diabetes mellitus (DM), 21, 23, 181, 186–188
Diarrhea, 49, 167–169, 168
    oral zinc supplementation, 67
Diarrheal diseases, 238
Didanosine, 129t
Diet and immunity
    age on immune system
        immune response changes with aging,
            24
        immune response in neonates, 23–24
        stress, 24–25
    antigen presentation, efficient, 26–27
    gut, largest immune organ, 25
    gut-associated lymphoid tissue (GALT), 26
    immune health, benefits of, 20–21
    immune health impacts
        diabetes mellitus, 21, 23
        malnutrition/overnutrition, 21, 22f, 22t
    at multiple levels
        active modulation of immune system,
            28–30
        complete nutrition, 27
        macronutrients and micronutrients,
            optimizing, 27–28, 29f
        personalized nutrition, 30–31
Dietary antioxidants, 87–97. *See also* Oxidative
    stress and inflammation
    and immune functions, 88t
    trace elements and host resistance to
        infection, 92–97, 94t–95t
    vitamins and host resistance to infection,
        89–92, 90t–91t
Dietary fat, 135–136
Dietary manipulation on pharmacokinetics,
    121–134
Dietary restrictions, 137
Dietary signatures, 381
Dietary zinc intakes, 362
1,25-dihydroxyvitamin D3, 50
Disease tolerance, 344–346
DNA methylation, 383
Docosahexaenoic acid, 30
Double-edged sword, 194
Drosophila melanogaster, 18
Drug absorption, 113t, 117
Drug and grapefruit juice interactions,
    136–137
Drug and nutrient transport systems, 113–114.
    See also Nutrient-drug interactions
Drug biotransformation, 112
Drug distribution, 120

Drug interactions, probiotics, 298
Drug-metabolizing enzymes, 110
Drug therapy
    in marasmus, 119–120
    nutritional factors and, 108f
Dual-energy x-ray absorptiometry (DEXA), 191,
        272
d-xylose absorption, 264
Dysbiosis, 290, 383
Dyslipidemia, 141t, 169

E

Eating, poor, 61
Ecological studies, undernutrition, 183–184
Efavirenz, 130t
Electrolyte disturbances, medication-associated
        fluid and, 139
Emtricitabine, 129t
Endocrine tissue, 118
Endomysial antibodies (EMA), 260
End-stage renal disease (ESRD), 11
Enfurvitide, 131t
Enteral feedings and medications, 114–115. *See
        also* Nutrient-drug interactions
Enteral formulas, 324–326
Enteral glutamine, 314
Enteral nutrition, 312
    omega-3 fatty acids, 321–323
Enteric syndromes
    acrodermatitis enteropathica (AE) and zinc
        deficiency, 276–277
    autoimmune enteropathy (AIE)
        and immune dysregulation,
            polyendocrinopathy, enteropathy
            X-linked (IPEX) syndrome, 265–267
        treatment, 268–269
        type 2, 267, 268f
        type 3, 268
    celiac disease (CD), 259–263, 260t, 261f,
        261t
    inflammatory bowel disease (IBD), 271–274,
        271f
    intestinal failure (IF), 274–276
    intestinal lymphangiectasia, 269–271
    overview, 259
    tropical sprue (TS), 264–265
Enterobacteriaceae, 99
Enterochromaffin cells, 293
Enterotypes, 251
Environmental enteropathy, 346
Environmental hostility/undernutrition and
        infection, 346–347, 347f
Epidemiological transition, 63
Epigallocatechin-3-gallate (EGCG), 98
Epigenetics in human nutrition, 383
Epstein–Barr virus, 99

Erythropoiesis, 200
Escherichia coli, 116
Estrogen, 384
Ethambutol, 131t
Ethionamide, 131t
Etravirine, 130t
Evolution, nature of, 60
Exclusive enteral nutrition (EEN) therapy, 273
Extended-release niacin (ERN), 169
Exudative enteropathy, 270
Ex vivo bioinactivations, 112, 114

F

Famciclovir, 132t
Fast foods, 8
Fat, 111t, 140–142, 141t. *See also* Medications on
        nutrient status
    composition, 191
Fatty meals, 136
Febrile illnesses, 65
Fecal bacteriotherapy, 300
Fecal microbiome transplantation (FMT), 254,
        255
Ferric iron, 273
Ferritin, 42
Ferroportin, 42
Fetal gastrointestinal tract, 290
Fetal health, nutrition and, 3. *See also* Nutrition
        in human health and disease
Fetal period, growth and development, 338–339
Firmicutes, 292
First-pass effect (presystemic clearance), 109, 134
Fish oil, 320
Fluconazole, 125t
Flucytosine, 125t
Folate, 264, 265
Folic acid, 9, 10, 262
Food
    deserts, 8
    on drug absorption, 121
    insecurity, 61
Forkhead transcription factor (FOXO), 18
Fosamprenavir, 127t
Fractures, 12
Free radicals, 85, 87
Fuazolidine, 133t

G

γ-aminobutyric acid (GABA), 139
Ganciclovir, 132t
Gastric emptying and intestinal transit
        time, 109. *See also* Nutrient-drug
        interactions
Gastrointestinal complications, 142–144, 143t
Gastrointestinal hormones, 275

Gastrointestinal infections, 65
Gastrointestinal motility, 293
Gastrointestinal tract, 290
Genetic variations in immunity, 383
Genome-wide association studies (GWAS), 383
Gentamicin, 115
Geriatrics, nutrition in, 11–13. *See also* Nutrition
    in human health and disease
Germ-free animals, 26
Ghrelin, 192, 193t, 194
Giardia intestinalis, 65
Giardiasis, 236
Gliadin antibodies (DGP), 260
Glucocorticoid (GC) hormones, 25
Glucose, 140, 140t. *See also* Medications on
    nutrient status
  levels, 382
  metabolism, 140t
Glutamine, 27, 314, 316t, 318, 382
Glutathione peroxidase, 92, 93, 211
Gomez classification, malnutrition, 2t, 3
G-protein-coupled receptor, 291
Granuloma, 271
Grapefruit juice interactions, drug and, 136–137
GRAS (Generally Recognized as Safe), 297
Green, harry, 44
Green tea, 98, 99
Griseofulvin, 125t
Growth and development, infection on,
    337–347. *See also* Infection-nutrient
    interactions in infants/children/
    adolescents
  cachexia/chronic diseases/immune
    compromise, 342–344
  disease tolerance/alterations in microbiota,
    344–346
  environmental hostility/undernutrition/
    infection, 346–347, 347f
  ontogeny of circle of malnutrition/infection,
    338–342
Guanosine pentaphosphate (ppGpp), 116
Gut, largest immune organ, 25. *See also* Diet and
    immunity
Gut-associated lymphoid tissue (GALT), 26,
    296
Gut dysbiosis, 383
Gut microbes, 291
Gut microbiome in nutrition
  antibiotics, 253
  malnourished children altering microbiomes,
    250–251
  malnutrition and altered microbiome,
    251–253, 251t
  microbiomes, changing, 254–255
  overview, 249–250
Gut microbiota, 60, 293, 294, 298, 345
Gut microorganisms, 249

H

Hazard ratio (HR), 7
Helicobacteraceae, 250
Helicobacter pylori, 21, 71, 89
Hematological indicators. *See also* HIV and
    micronutrient supplementation
  hemoglobin and anemia, 165–166
  micronutrient concentrations, 166–167
Hemoglobin, 9
  and anemia, 165–166
Hepatic drug clearance, 118
Hepatic metabolism, 110, 111t. *See also* Nutrient-
    drug interactions
Hepatic transporters, 114
Hepatitis C virus (HCV), 68, 371
Hepatocarcinoma, 96
Hepcidin, 41, 42
Hidden hunger, 8, 62. *See also* Nutrition in
    human health and disease
High-density lipoproteincholesterol (HDL-C),
    169
Hippocrates, 20
HIV, 65, 74, 144–145, 186
  infection, 89, 92
  infection in elderly, 360
HIV and micronutrient supplementation
  discussion, 171–172
  methods, 154
  overview, 153–154
  results, 154–170, 155f
    birth outcomes, 165
    clinical morbidities and assessments,
      167–170
    hematological indicators, 165–167
    HIV progression, 155–163, 160t–161t
    mortality, 155, 156t–157t
    transmission, 163–165
HIV progression
  AIDS-related deaths, 155
  disease stage changes, 158
  HIV viral load, infected cells, DNA, RNA,
    158–159
  T-lymphocyte subsets, 159–163, 160t–161t
HIV transmission
  anthropometry, 163–165
  children, 163
Homocysteine, 384
Hookworm infections, 235
Hormones, 25
Host resistance to infection. *See also* Dietary
    antioxidants
  trace elements and, 92–97, 94t–95t
  vitamin effect, 90t–91t
  vitamins and, 89–92, 90t–91t
Hot meals, 134
Human immunodeficiency virus. *See* HIV

Human leukocyte antigens (HLA), 312
Human Microbiome Project, 250, 300
Human milk oligosaccharides (HMO), 299
Human studies, undernutrition, 183
Humoral immunity, 267
    vitamin A and, 46
    vitamin D and, 52
HuT-78 cells, 48
Hydroxychloroquine, 126t
Hydroxytyrosol (3,4-dihydroxyphenyl ethanol), 98
25-hydroxyvitamin D, 10, 12, 68
Hyperferritinemia, 42
Hyperglycemia, 139
Hyperhomocysteinemia, 262
Hyperinflammation, 312
Hypoalbuminemia, 118
Hypocalcemia, 3, 139
Hypochromic anemia, 166
Hypoferremia, 42
Hypomagnesemia, 139
Hypothalamic–pituitary–adrenal (HPA), 294
Hypovitaminosis, 272

I

IFN-γ. *See* Interferon-γ
Immunaid®, 325
Immune brinksmanship, 69
Immune compromise, 342–344
Immune deficiency, 20
Immune dysregulation, polyendocrinopathy,
        enteropathy X-linked (IPEX)
        syndrome, 265–267
Immune-enhancing enteral formulas, 324
Immune functions, dietary antioxidants and, 88t
Immune health
    benefits of, 20–21
    impact
        diabetes mellitus, 21, 23
        malnutrition/overnutrition, 21, 22f, 22t
Immune impairment
    in macronutrient deficiency, 237t
    in micronutrient deficiency, 237t
Immune-modulating effects, 50
Immune reconstitution inflammatory syndrome,
        145
Immune response
    changes with aging, 24
    in neonates, 23–24
Immune response modifiers (IRM), 26
Immune system, 18–19, 19t, 84
    active modulation of, 28–30
Immune weakness, 341–342
Immunity
    iron deficiency and, 40–41
    iron homeostasis in, 41–43
Immunization, 6, 263

Immunodeficiency, 25
Immunological changes in elderly. *See also*
        Aging and nutrient-infection
        interactions
    aging and innate immunity, 360–361
    T cells and aging, 361–362
Immunology and nutrition, 381
Immunomodulation, 295–296
Immunomodulators, 273
Immunonutrients, 382
    immune-modulating artificial nutrition,
        313–326
        antioxidant micronutrients and trace
            elements, 323–324
        arginine, 318–319
        enteral formulas, 324–326
        glutamine, 314, 318
        N-acetyl cysteine, 319
        Omega-3 fatty acids from fish oil, 319–323
    immunonutrition, 312–313, 313f
    overview, 311–312
Immunonutrition, 28, 312–313, 313f. *See also*
        Immunonutrients
Immunopathology, 344
Immunosenescence, 24, 28
Immunosuppressive therapy, 268, 269
Impaired immune defense mechanisms, 340
Indinavir, 128t
Infancy, early, 4. *See also* Nutrition in human
        health and disease
Infants, 339
Infection-nutrient interactions in infants/children/
        adolescents
    on growth and development, 337–347
        cachexia/chronic diseases/immune
            compromise, 342–344
        disease tolerance/alterations in
            microbiota, 344–346
        environmental hostility/undernutrition/
            infection, 346–347, 347f
        ontogeny of circle of malnutrition/
            infection, 338–342
    on nutrient availability and utilization,
        347–352
        acquired nutritional deficiencies, 348–351
        appetite/absorption/requirements, effects
            on, 348
        nutrient distribution and reprioritization,
            351–352
        nutrient utilization, 351
    overview, 335–336, 336f
Infection-nutrition interactions
    coadaptation in evolution, nature of, 60–61
    malnutrition
        and infection interaction, classic narrative
            of, 62
        and infectious disease, 62–63

nutrition transition, 63
overnutrition paradigms
    adiposity and overweight/obesity, immune
        function and, 71–72
    adiposity and overweight/obesity,
        increased, 73
    enhanced risk of, 70
    iron supplementation and increased
        reserves, 73–74
    social power and physical well-being, 61
undernutrition paradigms
    and aggravation of infectious
        consequences, 66–68
    and diminished infectious consequences,
        68–70
    enhanced risk of, infection and, 64–66
Infectious consequences
    aggravation of, 66–68
    diminished, 68–70
Infectious diseases, 3
    in elderly, 360. *See also* Aging and nutrient-
        infection interactions
    severe malnutrition and, 6–7
    zinc and, 49
Inflammation, 30
Inflammatory bowel disease (IBD), 262,
    271–274, 271f, 383–384. *See also*
    Enteric syndromes
Infliximab, 273
Influenza, 72
Innate and acquired immune response, 83f
Innate immune system, 82, 340, 341, 346
Innate immunity, aging and, 360–361
Integrase Inhibitor Raltegravir, 131t
Interferon (IFN), 43, 83, 361
Interferon-γ (IFN-γ), 193t, 194–195, 236
Interferon-γ (IFN-γ) release assays (IGRA), 185,
    189–190
Interleukin (IL)-6, 194
Interleukin (IL), 41
Interleukin (IL)-2 expression in HuT-78 cells, 48
Interspecies, 60
Intestinal environment, 290. *See also* Probiotics
    diseases and microbial perturbation, 294t
    functions of, 290–295, 291f
Intestinal failure (IF), 274–276. *See also* Enteric
    syndromes
Intestinal infection, 348
Intestinal lymphangiectasia, 269–271. *See also*
    Enteric syndromes
Intestinal microbiota, 28
    functions of, 291f
    metabolic role of, 290
Intestinal motility, 293
Intestinal transit time, gastric emptying and,
    109
Intestine, adult, 60

Intrauterine growth restriction (IUGR), 338
Intrauterine growth retardation (IUGR), 1
Iodine deficiency, 6
Iodine deficiency disorders (IDD), 227
Iron, 88t, 95t, 96, 111t, 200, 237t. *See also*
    Micronutrient deficiency
    iron deficiency and immunity, 40–41
    iron homeostasis in immunity, 41–43
Iron deficiency, 96, 272
    and immunity, 40–41
    during pregnancy, 3
Iron deficiency anemia (IDA), 227, 261, 262
Iron dosing, 273
Iron–folic acid (IFA) supplementation, 239
Iron loading of macrophages, 42
Iron supplementation, 73–74
    malaria and, 7
    pregnancy, 9
Isoniazid, 138
Isoniazid preventive therapy (IPT), 185
Isothiocyanates, 114
Itraconazole, 125t
Ivermectin, 126t

K

Keratinization, 44
Keshan disease, 93, 365
Ketoconazole, 125t
Kidney, 118
Kwashiorkor, 6
    on pharmacokinetics, 119
Kwashiorkor malnutrition, 349

L

Lactobacillus reuteri, 292
Lactobacillus rhamnosus, 298
Lactoferrin, 42
Lamivudine, 129t
Latent TB infection (LTBI), 182, 185
Leishmania chagasi, 236
Leishmaniasis, 236
Leptin, 21, 192, 193t, 348
Leukocytosis, 266
Linezolid, 123t
Lipids, 135
    emulsions, 320
    peroxidation, 85
Lipocalin-2, 42
Lipophilicity of drug, 120
Lipopolysaccharide (LPS), 18, 361
Lipoprotein receptor (LPR), 142
Listeria monocytogenes, 93
Long-chain polyunsaturated fatty acids
    (LC-PUFA), 299
Lopinavir and ritonavir, 128t

Lorazepam, 110
Low birth weight (LBW), 5, 338
Low-fat diets, 135
Lymphocytic infiltration, 265

M

Macrocytic anemia, 166
Macrolides, 123t
Macrominerals
    iron, 200
Macronutrients, 27–28, 29f, 145
    effects of TB on
        nutritional supplementation for wasting
            treatment, 195, 196t–199t
        potential mediators of wasting, 192–195,
            193t
        protein-energy malnutrition and wasting
            mechanisms, 190–192
    in pulmonary tuberculosis, 196t–199t
Macrophage function, 45, 50–51, 187
Macrophages, 361
Magnesium deficiency, 139
Malabsorption, 270
Malaria, 73, 74
    and iron supplementation, 7
Malaria and parasitic infections
    macronutrient/micronutrient deficiencies
        micronutrients, 238–239
        protein-energy malnutrition, 238
    malaria/nutrition and immunity, 232–233,
        232f
    malaria on PEM, impact of, 231–232
    and malnutrition
        areas of high incidence of malaria, 228f
        malaria, case definitions, 229
        nutrition, 227, 229
    malnutrition, burden of, 226–227
        iodine deficiency disorders (IDD), 227
        iron deficiency anemia (IDA), 227
        protein-energy malnutrition (PEM), 227
        vitamin A deficiency (VAD), 227
    malnutrition, parasitic infections, and
        immunity, 237–238, 237t
    micronutrients and malaria, 233, 233t, 234t
    nutritional interventional programs and
        parasitic infections, 239–240
    parasitic infections, 234–236
        amoebiasis, 236
        giardiasis, 236
        leishmaniasis, 236
        nematodes, 235–236
    parasitic infections, burden of, 224–226,
        224f, 225t–226t
    PEM on malaria, 229–231
        animal studies, 230
        human studies, 230–231

Malnourishment of children, 249
    altering microbiomes, 250–251. *See also* Gut
        microbiome in nutrition
    treatment for, 255
Malnutrition, 20, 21, 22f, 22t, 25, 340, 381f. *See
    also* Diet and immunity; Nutrient-
        drug interactions
    and altered microbiome, 251–253, 251t. *See
        also* Gut microbiome in nutrition
    burden of, 226–227
        iodine deficiency disorders (IDD), 227
        iron deficiency anemia (IDA), 227
        protein-energy malnutrition (PEM), 227
        vitamin A deficiency (VAD), 227
    in children, 259
    definitions, 2–3, 2t
    in elderly, 11
    and infection, 62
    and infection interaction
        classic narrative of, 62
        infectious diseases, 62–63, 336
    malaria and
        areas of high incidence of malaria, 228f
        malaria, case definitions, 229
        nutrition, 227, 229
    parasitic infections and immunity, 237–238,
        237t
    on pharmacokinetic parameters, 115–117
    and risk for TB, 182–188. *See also*
        Tuberculosis (TB) and human
        nutrition
    obesity/diabetes mellitus and, 186–188
    undernutrition, 183–186
    social and economic impacts, 11
    in women, 1
Malnutrition and TB testing
    IFN-γ release assays, 189–190
    TST, effects on, 188–189
Malnutrition–TB–malnutrition interaction, 182f
Mammalian target of rapamycin (mTOR), 18
Marasmus, 6
    drug therapy in, 119–120
Maraviroc, 131t
Marinol, 9
Maternal malnutrition, 342
Maternal nutritional deficits, 338
Maternal undernutrition, 4, 5, 338
Meal timing and drug absorption, 112–113, 113t.
    See also Nutrient-drug interactions
Mean upper arm circumference (MUAC), 3
Measles, 349
Mebendazole, 126t
Medications
    altering glucose metabolism/response, 140t
    associated with dyslipidemia, 141t
    decreasing appetite, 143t
    enteral feedings and, 114–115

Medications on nutrient status. *See also* Nutrient-
  drug interactions
  fat, 140–142, 141t
  glucose, 140, 140t
  medication-associated fluid and electrolyte
    disturbances, 139
  nutrient absorption, 138
  nutrient metabolism, 138–139
  nutrient transport, 138
Medium-chain triglycerides (MCT), 265, 319
Mellanby, Edward, 44
Menkel, J. F., 20
Mental Development Index, 170
Metabolic activities, probiotics, 298
Metabolic syndrome, 11
Metabolism, 118
Metalloproteins, 92
Metallothionein, 48, 69
Methenamine, 133t
Methyl-tetrahydrofolate reductase (MTHFR),
    384
Metronidazole, 119, 123t
Micafungin, 125t
Mice fed milk bioactives, 29
Microbes, 60
Microbial ecosystem therapeutics (MET), 300
Microbial organisms, 289
Microbiomes, changing, 254–255. *See also* Gut
    microbiome in nutrition
Microbiota, 292, 344
  alterations in, 344–346
Microbiota composition, nutrition-associated
    modifications of, 251t
Microbiota–host immune relation, 345
Micronutrient concentrations, 166–167
Micronutrient deficiency, 8
  defined, 39
  iron
    iron deficiency and immunity, 40–41
    iron homeostasis in immunity, 41–43
  overview, 39–40
  vitamin A, 43–47
    and cellular immunity, 45–46
    and humoral immunity, 46
    mucosal immunity, 44–45
    vitamin A deficiency, 43–44
    vitamin A function, 44
  vitamin D
    and cellular immunity, 51–52
    and dendritic cells, 51
    and humoral immunity, 52
    and macrophage function, 50–51
  zinc, 47–50
    and B-lymphocyte development and
      function, 48
    IL-2 expression in HuT-78 cells, 48
    and infectious disease, 49

  and sickle cell disease (SCD), 49
  zinc deficiency, in vivo and in vitro
    models of, 47–48
Micronutrients, 27–28, 29f, 185–186, 351. *See
    also* Malaria and parasitic infections
  and malaria, 233, 233t, 234t
  selenium deficiency and parasitic infections,
    239
  supplement, 162
  VAD and parasitic infections, 239
  zinc deficiency and parasitic infections,
    238–239
Microorganisms, 252
Mid-upper arm circumference (MUAC), 164
Mild malnutrition, 3
Milk bioactives, 29
Millennium Development Goals, 1
Minerals, 27, 136
Mini Nutritional Assessment, 12
Moderate malnutrition, 3
Molecular biology tools, 380f
Monoamine oxidase inhibitor (MAO-I), 135
Monocyte chemoattractant protein (MCP), 322
Monosodium glutamate (MSG), 66
Monotherapy, 269
Morbidity, 347
Mortality, 155, 156t–157t. *See also* HIV and
    micronutrient supplementation
  in children, 347
Mother-to-child transmission (MTCT), 163
Motility disorders, 274
Mucosal immunity, vitamin A and, 44–45
Multinutrient, 368t
Multiple-micronutrient supplementation, 10
Multivitamin/multimineral supplement and
    infectious diseases, 373
Multivitamins, 158, 162, 164, 165
Mycobacteria, 43
Mycobacterium bovis, 189
Mycobacterium marinum, 345
Mycobacterium tuberculosis (MTb), 74, 181, 348
Myeloperoxidase, 41

N

N-acetyl cysteine, 316t, 319
Nalidixic acid, 133t
National Health and Epidemiologic Follow-up
    Study (NHEFS), 184
National Health and Nutrition Examination
    Survey (NHANES), 8, 184
National Institutes of Health, 297
Natural antioxidants in foods, 97–99
Natural killer (NK), 83f
  cell activity, 23
  cell lytic activity, 48
N-demethylation of diazepam, 110

Necrotizing enterocolitis (NEC), 296
Nelfinavir, 128t
Nematodes
  ascariasis, 235–236
  hookworm infections, 235
  trichuriasis, 236
Neomycin, 123t
Neonatal deficiency, 23
Neonatal immune responses, 23
Neurotransmitter, 138
Neutrophil function, 187
Neutrophils, 291
Nevirapine, 131t
Newborn and infant, 339
N-3 fatty acids, 9
Niacin, 169
Nitazoxanide, 127t
Nitric oxide (NO), 41, 85
Nontuberculous mycobacteria (NTM), 189
NO synthase (NOS), 87
Nramp1, 42
Nuclear factor-κB (NF-κB), 296, 312
Nucleotide-binding oligomerization domain
      receptors (NOD-like receptors), 83
Nucleotides, 316t
Nutrient absorption, 138
Nutrient availability and utilization, infection on
  acquired nutritional deficiencies, 348–351
  appetite/absorption/requirements, effects on,
      348
  nutrient distribution and reprioritization,
      351–352
  nutrient utilization, 351
Nutrient distribution and reprioritization, 351–352
Nutrient-drug interactions
  affecting drug pharmacokinetics
    gastric emptying and intestinal transit
        time, 109
    hepatic metabolism, 110, 111t
    presystemic clearance, 109–110
  dietary manipulation on pharmacokinetics,
      121–134
  drug and nutrient transport systems, 113–114
  enteral feedings and medications, 114–115
  examples, 122t–133t
  gastrointestinal complications
    alterations in appetite, 142–144, 143t
  human immunodeficiency virus (HIV), 144–145
  malnutrition on pharmacokinetic parameters,
      115–117
  meal timing and drug absorption, 112–113, 113t
  medications on nutrient status
    fat, 140–142, 141t
    glucose, 140, 140t
    medication-associated fluid and
        electrolyte disturbances, 139
    nutrient absorption, 138

nutrient metabolism, 138–139
nutrient transport, 138
nutrients on pharmacokinetics
  beverages on drug bioavailability, 137–138
  carbohydrates, 134
  dietary fat, 135–136
  dietary restrictions, 137
  drug and grapefruit juice interactions,
      136–137
  minerals, 136
  parenteral nutrition, 138
  protein, 134–135
  vegetables, 136
nutritional factors and drug therapy, relation,
      108f
nutritional status on pharmacokinetic properties
  absorption, 117
  clearance of medications, 118–119
  distribution, 117–118
  drug therapy in marasmus, 119–120
  kwashiorkor on pharmacokinetics, 119
  metabolism, 118
  obesity, 120–121
  principles of, 112
  tuberculosis, 144
Nutrient malabsorption, 264
Nutrient metabolism, 18, 138–139
Nutrients in immune-modulating artificial
      nutrition, 316t–317t
Nutrients on pharmacokinetics
  beverages on drug bioavailability, 137–138
  carbohydrates, 134
  dietary fat, 135–136
  dietary restrictions, 137
  drug and grapefruit juice interactions, 136–137
  minerals, 136
  parenteral nutrition, 138
  protein, 134–135
  vegetables, 136
Nutrient stress, 116
Nutrient supplementation/infectious diseases in
      elderly. See also Aging and nutrient-
      infection interactions
  multivitamin/multimineral, 373
  selenium, 371–372
  vitamin D, 366
  vitamin E, 366, 370–371
  zinc, 372–373
Nutrient transport, 138
Nutrient utilization, 351
Nutrigenetics, 381f
  personalized nutrition and, 384–385, 385f
Nutrigenomic biomarker selection, 385f
Nutrigenomics, 380f, 381, 381f
Nutrition. See also Diet and immunity
  complete, 27
  malaria and, 227, 229

personalized, 30–31
  systems biology and, 379–380, 380f
Nutritional deficiency, 64, 66, 84, 363
Nutritional immunity, 41, 69
Nutritional immunology, 381–382
Nutritional interventional programs and parasitic
    infections, 239–240
Nutritional status, 84. *See also* Aging and
    nutrient-infection interactions
  in elderly, 362–363
  on host defense against infection
    selenium and infection, 365
    vitamin D and infection, 363–364
    vitamin E and infection, 364–365
    zinc and infection, 365
  infection on, 363
Nutritional status on pharmacokinetic properties.
    See also Nutrient-drug interactions
  absorption, 117
  clearance of medications, 118–119
  distribution, 117–118
  drug therapy in marasmus, 119–120
  kwashiorkor on pharmacokinetics, 119
  metabolism, 118
  obesity, 120–121
Nutritional supplementation for wasting
    treatment, 195, 196t–199t
Nutrition and immunity. *See also* Diet and
    immunity
  cells and processes, 18–19, 19t
  diet and immunity, 20–31
    active modulation of immune system, 28–30
    age on immune system, 23–25
    complete nutrition, 27
    gut, largest immune organ, 25
    gut-associated lymphoid tissue (GALT),
      26–27
    immune health, benefits of, 20–21
    immune health impacts, 21–23, 22f, 22t
    macronutrients and micronutrients,
      optimizing, 27–28, 29f
    personalized nutrition, 30–31
  malaria and, 232–233, 232f
  overview, 17–18
Nutrition and immunocompetence, 73
Nutrition and infection, 336f
Nutrition-infection interactions, research and
    strategy in
  dysbiosis, 383
  epigenetics in human nutrition, 383
  genetic variations in immunity, 383
  inflammatory bowel disease (IBD), 383–384
  nutrigenomics, 381, 381f
  nutritional immunology, 381–382
  personalized nutrition and nutrigenetics,
    384–385, 385f
  systems biology and nutrition, 379–380, 380f

Nutrition in human health and disease
  adolescence and puberty, 8–9
  adults, 11
  in ages 1-5 (critical years), 4–7
    antibiotics, use of, 6–7
    malaria and iron supplementation, 7
    severe malnutrition and infectious
      diseases, 6–7
  fetal health, 3
  geriatrics, 11–13
  infancy, early, 4
  malnutrition, definitions, 2–3, 2t
  overview, 1–2
  pregnancy, 9–10
  school-age children, 7–8
    hidden hunger, 8
Nutrition therapy, 273
Nutrition transition, 63

O

Obesity, 11, 21, 61
  adipose tissue in, 19
  alterations in immune system in, 22t
  defined, 73
  on drug pharmacokinetics, 115
  energy storage overnutrition, 70
  and immune disequilibrium, 337
  lung mechanics, 71
  malnutrition and risk for TB, 186–188
  nutritional status on pharmacokinetic
    properties, 120–121
  and overnutrition, 343t
  periodontitis, 71
Oleuropein, 98
Oligosaccharides, 299
Olive oil, dietary antioxidant in, 98
Omega-3 fatty acids, 30
Omega-3 fatty acids from fish oil, 317t, 319–323.
    See also Immunonutrients
  in enteral nutrition, 321–323
  in parenteral nutrition, 319–321
Ontogeny of circle of malnutrition/infection,
    338–342
  children and adolescents, 340
  failure to thrive and hindered development,
    340–341
  fetal period, 338–339
  immune weakness and recurrence of
    infections, 341–342
  newborn and infant, 339
Oral arginine supplementation, 318
Oral iron supplementation, 73, 74
Oral zinc supplements, 167
Organic aniontransporting polypeptides (OATP),
    137
Oseltamivir, 132t

Osmolality of stomach secretions, 115
Overnutrition, 21, 22f, 22t, 237t. *See also* Diet
    and immunity; Infection-nutrition
    interaction
    adiposity and overweight/obesity
        immune function and, 71–72
        increased, 73
    causing cancer, 22f
    enhanced risk of, 70
    iron supplementation and increased reserves,
        73–74
Overweight
    burden of, 63
    hepatitis C virus (HCV) liver disease, 71
Overweight/obesity, adiposity and. *See* Adiposity
    and overweight/obesity
Oxidant/antioxidant balance, 86
Oxidative stress, 24, 27, 211
Oxidative stress and inflammation
    acquired immune system, 82
    antioxidants, protective role of, 84–87, 85t, 86f
    defined, 84
    dietary antioxidants, 87–97, 88t, 90t–91t,
        94t–95t
        and immune functions, 88t
        trace elements and host resistance to
            infection, 92–97, 94t–95t
        vitamins and host resistance to infection,
            89–92, 90t–91t
    immune system, 84
    innate and acquired immune response, 83f
    innate immune system, 82
    natural antioxidants in foods, 97–99
    nutritional status, 84
Oxygenase metabolism, 111t
Oxygen radicals, 85

P

Parasitic infections, 234–236. *See also* Malaria
    and parasitic infections
    amoebiasis, 236
    burden of, 224–226, 224f, 225t–226t
    giardiasis, 236
    leishmaniasis, 236
    malaria, and immunity, 237–238, 237t
    nematodes, 235–236
    nutritional interventional programs and,
        239–240
    selenium deficiency and, 239
    VAD and, 239
    zinc deficiency and, 238–239
Parathyroid hormone (PTH), 139
Parenteral antioxidants, 324
Parenteral glutamine, 314
Parenteral nutrition (PN), 138, 266
    omega-3 fatty acids in, 319–321

Pathogen-associated molecular patterns (PAMP),
    25, 82, 341
Pathogen sensing, 18
Pathogen tolerance, 344–345
Pattern recognition receptors (PRR), 82
Pediatric patients, 337, 348
PEM. *See* Protein-energy malnutrition (PEM)
Penicillins, 124t
Pentamidine, 133t
Peptide YY, 193
Peptidoglycans, 292
Peripheral blood mononuclear cell (PBMC), 210
Peroxynitrite (ONOO⁻), 85
Persistent diarrhea, 259
Personalized medicine, 31
Personalized nutrition, 30–31
    and nutrigenetics, 384–385, 385f
P-glycoprotein (P-gp), 110
Phagocytosis, 211
Pharmacodynamics
    defined, 109
Pharmacokinetics
    defined, 109
    dietary manipulation on, 121–134
    kwashiorkor on, 119
    malnutrition on, 115–117
    nutrients on. *See* Nutrients on
        pharmacokinetics
Phenolic components, 98
Phorbol myristate acetate, 48
Phosphatidyl-ethanolamine-*N*-methyltransferase
    (PEMT), 384
Phosphoric acid, 137
Physical well-being, social power and, 61
Phytohemagglutinin, 48
Pill esophagitis, 142
Plasmacytoid dendritic cells (pDC), 361
Plasma zinc concentration, 365
Plasmodiun infections, 69, 74
Pneumocystis jiroveci, 274, 344
Pneumocystis jiroveci pneumonia, 269
Pneumonia, 49
Pneumonia severity index (PSI), 364
Polymorphisms, 185
Polyphenols, 97, 98, 99
Polyunsaturated fatty acids (PUFA), 87, 135, 382
Porphyromonadaceae, 250
Posaconazole, 125t
Poverty, 337, 346
Preadipocytes, 18
Prebiotics, 28, 29f, 254
    risks and benefits, 297f
Pregnancy and nutrition, 9–10. *See also*
    Nutrition in human health and
    disease
Premenopausal women, 384
Prenatal regulation of gene expression, 338

Presystemic clearance, 109–110. *See also*
    Nutrient-drug interactions
Presystemic metabolism, 118
Preterm infants, 290
Prevotella enterotype, 251
Primaquine phosphate, 126t
Primary lymphangiectasia (PIL), 269
Probiotics, 254, 295–299. *See also* Intestinal
    environment
    drug interactions, 298
    immunomodulation, 295–296
    metabolic activities, 298
    risks and benefits, 297f
    safety of, 296–297, 297f
    and synbiotics, 299–300
Procyanidins, 99
Proinflammatory cytokines, 192
Prophylactic antimicrobial therapy, 270
Propionate, 253
Protease inhibitors, 142, 145
Protein, 111t, 134–135
    breakdown, 190, 349
    deprivation, 118
Protein-energy malnutrition (PEM), 6, 62, 65,
    115, 227, 238, 340, 362. *See also*
    Malaria and parasitic infections
    acute/chronic, 343t
    immune impairment, 237t
    on malaria, 229–231
        animal studies, 230
        human studies, 230–231
    and wasting mechanisms, 190–192
Protein-energy undernutrition, 19
    examples, 19t
Protein YY (PYY), 194
Pruritis, 266
Pseudomonas aeruginosa, 116, 117, 314
Psychomotor Development Index, 170
Psychoneuroimmunology, 24
Public health indicators, 340
Pulmonary tuberculosis
    macronutrient in, 196t–199t
    randomized controlled trials (RCT)
        and micronutrients supplementation,
        201t–203t, 204t–205t
        and vitamin D supplementation,
        208t–209t
Purified protein derivate (PPD), 189
Putative mechanism, 22f
Pyridoxine, 111t
Pyrimethamine, 126t

Q

Quantiferon (QFT) tests, 189
Quinine, 119
Quinolones, 124t

R

Randomized clinical trials (RCT), 211
Randomized control trials (RCT), 154, 169
Reactive nitrogen species (RNS), 84–85
Reactive oxygen species (ROS), 84, 85, 86,
    350
Ready-to-use therapeutic food (RUTF), 6, 252,
    254, 346
Recommended daily allowance (RDA), 155
Refeeding, 119
Renal disease, 266
Renal elimination, 118
Renal wasting of magnesium, 139
Reprioritization, nutrient distribution and,
    351–352
Respiratory infections, 65
Resveratrol, 99
Retinoic acid, 45, 46
Retinoic acid–inducible gene-like helicases
    (RIG-like helicases), 83
Retinoic acid receptors (RAR), 44
Retinoic acid response elements (RARE), 44
Retinoid X receptors (RXR), 44
Riboflavin, 111t
Ribonucleotide reductase, 40
Rickets, 3, 260
Rifabutin, 132
Rifampin, 132t
Rilpivirine, 131t
Ritonavir, 128t
Rouxen-Y gastric bypass (RYGB), 120
Ruminococcus-dominated enterotype, 251

S

Safety of probiotics, 296–297, 297f
SAMP8 mouse, 21
Saquinavir, 128t
Schistosoma haematobium, 65
Schistosoma mansoni, 65
School-age children, nutrition in, 7–8
Scrimshaw, Nevin, 62
Scrimshaw–Taylor–Gordon thesis, 62
Selenium, 88t, 93, 94t, 211, 237t, 350, 368t
    and infection, 365
    supplementation and infectious diseases,
        371–372
    supplements, 172
Selenium deficiency, 68, 93
    and parasitic infections, 239
Selenoenzyme glutathione peroxidase, 93
Sepsis, 87
Sequential Organ Failure Assessment score,
    372
Serum zinc concentrations, 363
Severe acute malnutrition (SAM), 119

Severe malnutrition, 3
  and infectious diseases, 6–7
Short-bowel syndrome, 274
Short-chain fatty acids (SCFA), 252, 290, 293, 296
Sickle cell disease (SCD), 49
SIGNET trial, 318
Single nucleotide polymorphisms (SNP), 384
Skin lesions, 276
Skin prick tests, 267
Social ecosystems, 346, 347f
Social power and physical well-being, 61
Soft drinks, 137
Solubilization of drug, 121
Soybean oil, 319
Splenic atrophy, 263
Splenomegaly, 266
Staphylococcus aureus, 71
Starvation, 116
  chronic, 118
Stavudine, 129t
Stress, 24–25. *See also* Diet and immunity
Stresson®, 325
Stunting, 2t, 3, 5, 273, 340
Sulfadoxine and pyrimethamine, 127t
Sulfonamides, 124t
Synbiotics, 297
    probiotics and, 299–300
Systemic inflammatory response syndrome
    (SIRS), 311
Systems biology and nutrition, 379–380, 380f

T

Tanzania, studies on, 163–164, 168
Target of rapamycin (TOR), 18
Taurine, 317t
TB. *See* Tuberculosis (TB)
T-cell-dependent antibody, 48
T-cell immunocompetence, 239
T-cell proliferation assays, 267
T cells and aging, 361–362
Tenofovir disoproxil fumarate, 129t
Tetracyclines, 124t
T-helper type 1 (Th1), 23
Thiamine, 111t
Thrombin-activatable fibrinolysis inhibitor
    (TAFI), 262
Thymulin, 47, 49
Thymus, 24
Tipranavir, 129t
Tissue transglutaminase (tTG), 260
T lymphocytes, 82
T-lymphocyte subsets, 159–163, 160t–161t
TNF-α, 193t, 194
Tolerogenic phenotype, 51
Toll-like receptor (TLR), 83, 292, 361
Toll-like receptor 4 (TLR4), 42

Trace elements, 88t, 317t. *See also* Dietary
    antioxidants
  antioxidant micronutrients and, 323–324
  and host resistance to infection, 92–97, 94t–95t
    copper, 97
    iron, 96
    selenium, 93
    zinc, 96–97
  selenium, 211
  zinc, 210–211
Transforming growth factor (TGF), 23
Transforming growth factor-β (TGF-β), 183
Trastuzumab, 31
T-regulatory (Treg) cells, 52, 265
Trichuriasis, 236
Trichuris dysentery syndrome, 236
Trimethoprim, 124t, 139
Tropical sprue (TS), 264–265. *See also* Enteric
    syndromes
Trypanosoma cruzi, 238
T-Spot.TB (T-Spot TB), 189
TST. *See* Tuberculin skin testing (TST)
Tube feeding, 312
Tuberculin skin testing (TST), 185, 188–189
Tuberculosis (TB), 62, 74, 144, 164
Tuberculosis (TB) and human nutrition
  macronutrients, effects on
    nutritional supplementation for wasting
        treatment, 195, 196t–199t
    potential mediators of wasting, 192–195, 193t
    protein-energy malnutrition and wasting
        mechanisms, 190–192
  malnutrition and risk for TB, 182–188
    obesity/diabetes mellitus and, 186–188
    undernutrition, 183–186
  malnutrition and TB testing
    IFN-γ release assays, 189–190
    TST, effects on, 188–189
  micronutrients and TB, 200–211, 201t–203t,
      204t–205t
    macrominerals, 200
    trace elements, 210–211
    vitamins, 200, 206–207, 210
  overview, 181–182, 182f
Tumor necrosis factor (TNF-α), 311, 312
Type 1 diabetes mellitus (T1DM), 265
Tyramine, 135

U

UDP-glucuronosyltransfersae (UGT), 110
Ulcerative colitis (UC), 271
Undernutrition, 4, 9
    and aggravation of infectious consequences,
        66–68
    and diminished infectious consequences,
        68–70

on drug pharmacokinetics, 115
enhanced risk of, infection and, 64–66
environmental hostility, and infection,
    346–347, 347f
and risk for TB. *See also* Tuberculosis (TB)
    and human nutrition
    animal studies, 183
    case-control and cohort studies, 184–185
    case series, 184
    ecological studies, 183–184
    human studies, 183
    micronutrients, 185–186
Underweight, 3
Urinary tract infections (UTI), 72

V

Vaccine responses, 24
VAD. *See* Vitamin A deficiency (VAD)
Valacyclovir, 132t
Valganciclovir, 133t
Vegetables, 136
Venous thrombosis, 262
Video capsule endoscopy, 270
Viral load, 159
Vitamin(s), 27, 88t, 200
    and host resistance to infection, 89–92,
        90t–91t. *See also* Dietary antioxidants
    β-Carotene, 92
    vitamin C, 89
    vitamin E, 89, 92
Vitamin A, 43–47, 90t, 162, 169, 171, 200, 206.
    See also Micronutrient deficiency
    and cellular immunity, 45–46
    and humoral immunity, 46
    immune impairment, 237t
    mucosal immunity, 44–45
    vitamin A deficiency, 43–44
    vitamin A function, 44
Vitamin A deficiency (VAD), 5, 43–44, 227,
    349
    and parasitic infections, 239
Vitamin B12, 262
    deficiency, 273
Vitamin C, 88t, 89, 90t, 210
    immune impairment, 237t
Vitamin D, 3, 8, 10, 162, 166, 185, 206–207,
    272, 367t. *See also* Micronutrient
    deficiency
    and cellular immunity, 51–52
    deficiency, 382
    and dendritic cells, 51
    and humoral immunity, 52
    and infection, 363–364
    and macrophage function, 50–51
    tuberculosis control, 68
Vitamin D receptor (VDR), 50, 51, 52, 185

Vitamin D supplementation and infectious
    diseases, 366
Vitamin E, 88t, 89, 91t, 92, 111t, 210, 350, 367t
    immune impairment, 237t
    and infection, 364–365
    supplementation and infectious diseases, 366,
        370–371
Vitamin K, 272
Voriconazole, 125t

W

Wasting, 2t, 3
Wasting, potential mediators of, 192–195, 193t.
    See also Tuberculosis (TB) and human
    nutrition
    factor in pathogenesis of wasting, 193t
    Ghrelin, 192, 194
    IFN-γ, 194–195
    interleukin (IL)-6, 194
    Leptin, 192
    Protein YY (PYY), 194
    TNF-α, 194
Wasting mechanisms, protein-energy
    malnutrition and, 190–192
Wasting syndrome, 268
Wasting treatment, nutritional supplementation
    for, 195, 196t–199t
Waterlow classification, malnutrition, 2t, 3
WHO classification, malnutrition, 2t, 3

Z

Zalcitabine, 129t
Zidovudine, 130t, 145
Zinc, 47–50, 88t, 95t, 96–97, 210–211, 237t,
    367t. *See also* Micronutrient
    deficiency
    ameliorative effect of, 50
    and B-lymphocyte development and function,
        48
    IL-2 expression in HuT-78 cells, 48
    and infection, 365
    and infectious disease, 49
    and sickle cell disease (SCD), 49
    sufficiency, 47
    zinc deficiency, in vivo and in vitro models
        of, 47–48
Zinc deficiency, 21, 23, 96, 210, 350
    acrodermatitis enteropathica (AE), 276–277
    and parasitic infections, 238–239
    in vivo and in vitro models of, 47–48
Zinc replacement therapy, 276
Zinc supplementation, 49, 158, 162, 189
    and infectious diseases, 372–373
    oral, 67
Z-Scores (standard deviation), 2t, 3

Printed and bound by CPI Group (UK) Ltd, Croydon, CR0 4YY

18/10/2024

01776257-0015